Glaucoma In Infants And Children

MARVIN L. KWITKO, B.A., M.D., F.A.A.O., F.A.C.S., F.I.C.S., F.R.C.S. (C)

Consultant in Ocular Pathology
St. Mary's Hospital;
Project Director (Ophthalmology)
Lady David Institute
for Medical Research;
Montreal, Canada

Foreword by

Harold G. Scheie, M.D.
Professor and Chairman
Department of Ophthalmology
University of Pennsylvania
Philadelphia, Pennsylvania

Glaucoma In Infants And Children

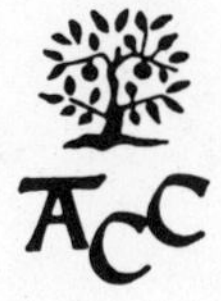

APPLETON-CENTURY-CROFTS
Educational Division
MEREDITH CORPORATION
New York

73 74 75 76/10 9 8 7 6 5 4 3 2 1

Library of Congress Catalog Card Number: 74-171664

PRINTED IN THE UNITED STATES OF AMERICA
390-53034-4

Dedicated to

JACQUELINE BETH KWITKO

GEOFFREY MALCOM KWITKO

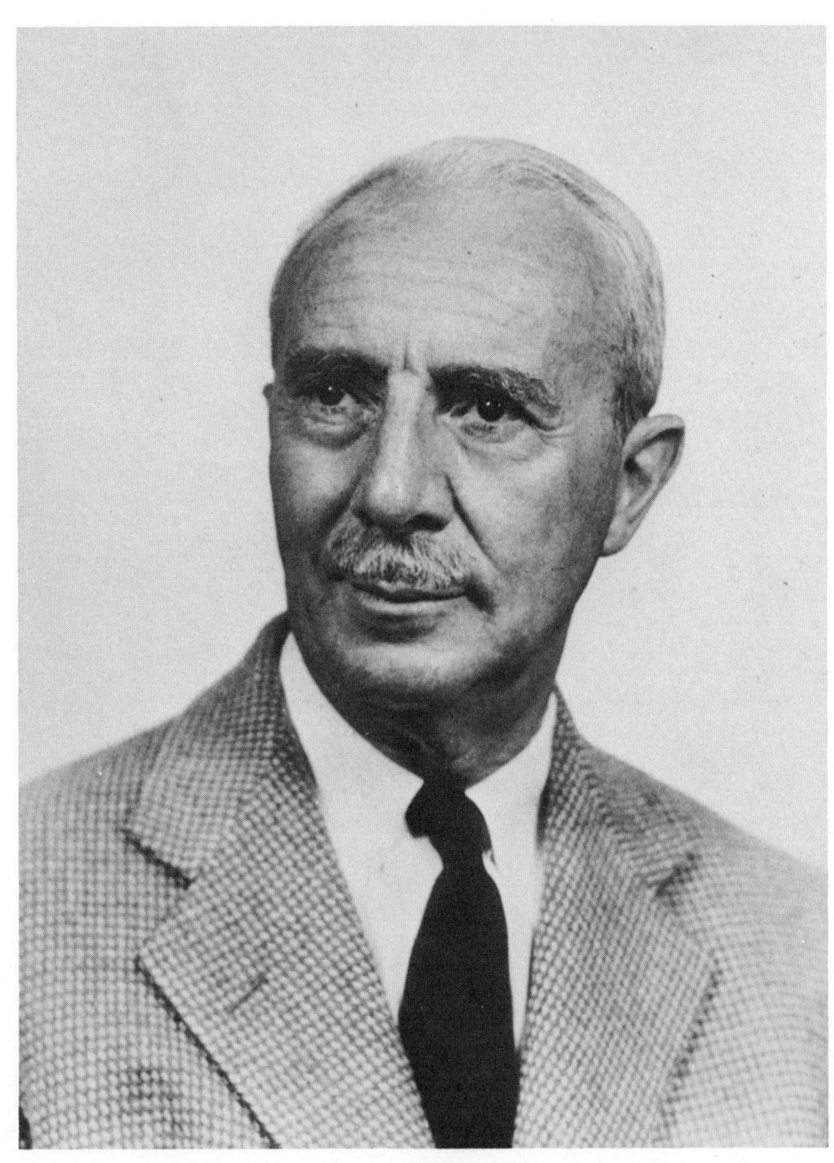

Dr. Otto Barkan

PREFACE

"Oeil de boeuf est une maladie d'oeil quand il est gros et eminent sortant hors la teste comme on voit les boeufs les avoir."
Ambroise Paré (1517-1590).

Although the enlarged eye was observed and described by many of the early medical historians including Hippocrates, Celsus and Galen, it was not until 1744 that Berger observed an increased ocular tension which distinguished this condition from other entities such as megalocornea, anterior staphyloma, etc. However, credit goes to von Muralt, who in 1869 classified congenital glaucoma as part of the variety of conditions that give rise to raised intraocular pressure.

Congenital glaucoma in the past resulted in a high percentage of blindness due to lack of an adequate operation. In 1939 J. Ringland Anderson wrote a clear detailed monograph on the subject. He stated: "There is no division of opinion regarding the severity of the visual loss and its progressive nature in spite of treatment. Seefelder found that 81 per cent of his series of 60 eyes were quite or almost blind. Ten of the 46 patients were in blind asylums. In only 15 was the corrected vision as good as 6/60." He offered the following prognosis. "Little hope of preserving sufficient sight to permit the earning of a livelihood can be held out to them."

About the time of the appearance of this book, Otto Barkan adopted the de Vincentiis procedure and introduced the goniotomy operation for the treatment of congenital glaucoma which completely changed the outlook for this condition. But even today the practicing ophthalmologist sees only an occasional patient with congenital glaucoma, and the ophthalmic resident comes into contact with so few cases during his period of training that he obtains little more than a passing acquaintance with the subject. Under these conditions it is difficult to attain proficiency in the diagnosis and treatment of this disease, so that too often the congenital glaucoma specialist is confronted with a mis-handled case that requires re-operation, when an adequate reference source might have prevented such a complication.

Over the past several years I have given an instruction course on the diagnosis and treatment of glaucoma in infants and children at the Annual Meeting of the American Academy of Ophthalmology and Otolaryngology. The frequent queries from ophthalmic residents and colleagues has been the prime motivating force for producing this book. The effort has been made to provide a comprehensive discussion to which the inquiring ophthalmologist can be referred.

The other facet of this subject is that, as the title suggests, this is not just an ocular problem but frequently involves a study of the young patient as a whole. The problems of diagnosis and treatment are diverse and cover many disciplines. The approach to the clinical description and understanding is therefore to discuss the pediatric aspects as well as the ocular. This interdisciplinary approach is of special value in this situation since the ophthalmologist is usually not the first one to see the patient. The nurse in the newborn nursery, the public health nurse, the pediatrician, optometrist or general practitioner may be in a better position to make the diagnosis than the ophthalmologist. This was made evident to me during my own period of training as a resident in pediatrics. Once the patient has been referred for treatment and hospitalized, the pediatric cardiologist, endocrinologist, geneticist and anesthesiologist must all be called upon to assess the case since glaucoma at this early age may be associated with other anomalies such as congenital heart disease, homocystinuria, Lowe's syndrome, and so forth. In addition there are numerous pediatric conditions where the eye simulates congenital glaucoma, such as familial dysautonomia (Riley-Day Syndrome), Block Sulzberger's syndrome and so forth, so that an awareness of the differential diagnosis is essential.

In this book I have tried to bring together a discussion and summary of present day thinking on glaucoma and allied conditions in infants and children. This has been done from an interdisciplinary point of view involving the pediatrician and pediatric subspecialist as well as the ophthalmologist, in practice or still in training. The purpose is to eliminate the pitfalls in making the diagnosis so that treatment can be initiated quickly and safely under ideal conditions. This is essential since as Barkan pointed out, "ultimate visual acuity depends largely upon how soon after onset the raised (intraocular) pressure and cloudiness (of the cornea) are relieved."

The author wishes to indicate his great appreciation to the following persons for their very earnest support in the preparation of this book: Dr. Alan Finley of the Montreal Children's Hospital and Dr. Harry Thompson of the Toronto Sick Children's Hospital during the early years, Dr. Frank D. Costenbader and Dr. Marshall M. Parks during the later years at the Children's Hospital of the District of Columbia, Dr. Benjamin Rones, at the Washington Hospital Center, Dr. Lorenz E. Zimmerman, at the Armed Forces Institute of Pathology, Dr. Mark I. H. Kaufman, Dr. Gaston Duclos, Dr. Kurt E. Schirmer and Dr. H. L. Tannenbaum of Montreal. The author is also grateful to Jose A. Ruiz, who prepared the illustrations, and to Nathan Fifer and Harold E. Coletta for their photography.

CONTENTS

FOREWORD

I am pleased to write a foreword to this book because it covers the kind of information and precise instruction which the ophthalmologist and pediatrician need to know, but which often is hard to find in one volume.

The subject of glaucoma in infants and children is usually dealt with in books on the comprehensive field of glaucoma and in pediatric textbooks. At best these books can give but limited coverage.

I quite agree with Dr. Kwitko that special training, special techniques, special vigilance and an everlasting attention to all details which affect the patient's welfare are required.

Concentrated in one volume are the various aspects of glaucoma in young children. From firsthand knowledge, available research data, and an exhaustive review of the literature, the author presents the clinical and practical aspects of the disease. Citing specific and concrete examples, he discusses the more common syndromes as well as the rare diseases.

The advent of new instruments and techniques such as the high power operating microscopes and the scanning electron microscope have given us a better understanding of the basic science of this condition. This new information has been reviewed.

A child born today should anticipate not only a long life—70 years or more—but also a full and productive one, not restricted by preventable or curable physical handicaps. The detection of visual dysfunction, however, cannot be left with the medical profession alone. The solution lies in a coordinated effort and the promotion of understanding among all persons in the child-oriented professions—ophthalmologists, pediatricians, family physicians, optometrists, hospital nurses, school health officials, social workers, public health nurses and other paramedical personnel. Dr. Kwitko wisely emphasizes the advantage of consultations with other medical specialists in order to solve the complex problems which may arise. Satisfactory teamwork must be developed. Accordingly, the author has set himself the difficult task of writing an account for a wide spectrum of disciplines, yet one that will be interesting to each. I feel that he has been successful in his aim to make available the basic practical information necessary to enable those concerned to manage their young patients satisfactorily.

He deserves a debt of gratitude from those who will benefit most, the children about whom he has written.

Harold G. Scheie, M.D.

Glaucoma In Infants And Children

Legends for colorplates

Chap. 1

FIG. 3.A. Glaucoma in an albino New Zealand rabbit.*

Chap. 9

FIG. 7. Unilateral microphthalmos and microcornea. This eye was operated on for a congenital cataract. (Courtesy of M. A. Galin.)*

FIG. 20. Bilateral aniridia.*

FIG. 27. Coloboma of the retina in the typical location. (Courtesy of D. Boyanner.)*

FIG. 54. Sturge-Weber's Syndrome. Gross section illustrating choroidal hemangioma with intraocular hemorrhage. (Courtesy of R. Cordero-Morino.)‡

FIG. 55. Sturge-Weber's syndrome. Filtration apparatus filled with blood. (Courtesy of R. Cordero-Morino.)‡ X 50.

FIG. 63. Homocystinuria. The body is notably longer below the waist than above. A malar flush is evident. (Courtesy of G. E. Gaull.)*

FIG. 64. Homocystinuria with buphthalmia. (Courtesy of G. E. Gaull.)*

*From Kwitko. **Can. J. Ophthalmol.** 2:91, 1967.
‡From Kwitko. **Can. J. Ophthalmol.** 4:231, 1969.

Chap. 10

FIG. 3. Congenital nonluetic interstitial keratitis.†

FIG. 23. Congenital corneal dystrophy. (Courtesy of J. S. Speakman.)†

FIG. 25. Congenital idiopathic corneal edema. (Courtesy of J. S. Speakman.)†

FIG. 32. Child with one large myopic eye and an opposite normal eye. (Courtesy of A. J. McKenna.)†

FIG. 33. Megalocornea, profile.†

FIG. 37. Keratoconus.†

Chap. 11

FIG. 1. Tear gas burn of the eye. Note the sclerosed conjunctiva. (Courtesy of R. Cordero-Morino.)‡

FIG. 2. Contusion injury to pupil margin with rupture of sphincter muscle.‡

FIG. 4. Gonioscopic photograph of postcontusion angle deformity; facility of outflow has been altered. (Courtesy of M. G. Alper.)‡

FIG. 5. Total anterior chamber hemorrhage with raised intraocular pressure. (Courtesy of H. M. Byron.)‡

FIG. 10. Retinoblastoma.‡

FIG. 12. Neuroblastoma. (Courtesy of C. M. Alexander.)‡

FIG. 13. Retinopathy of prematurity.‡

†From Kwitko. **Can. J. Ophthalmol.** 3:120, 1968.
‡From Kwitko. **Can. J. Ophthalmol.** 4:231, 1969.

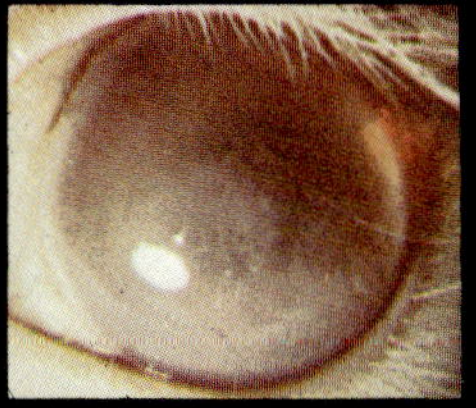

Chap. 1, Fig. 3.A

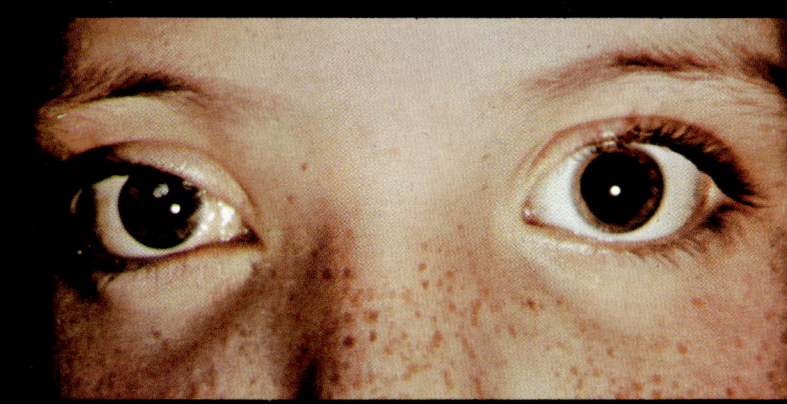

Chap. 9, Fig. 7

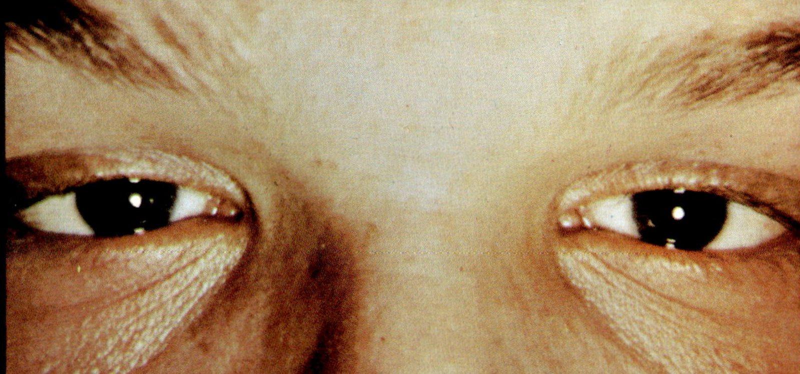

Chap. 9, Fig. 20

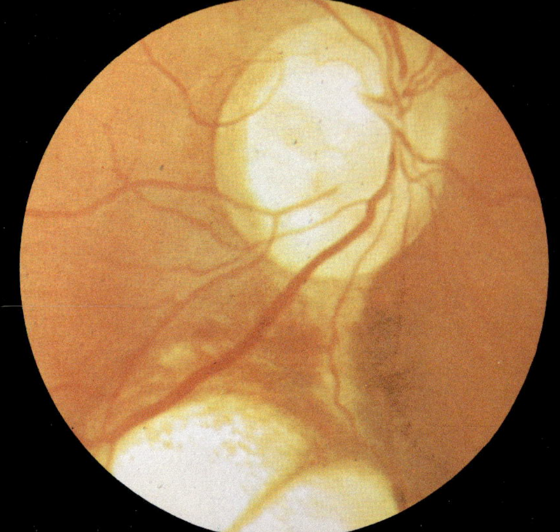

Chap. 9, Fig. 27

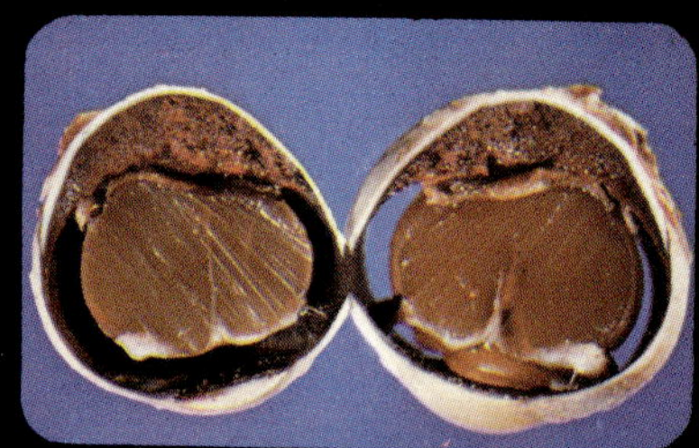

Chap. 9, Fig. 54

Chap. 9, Fig. 55

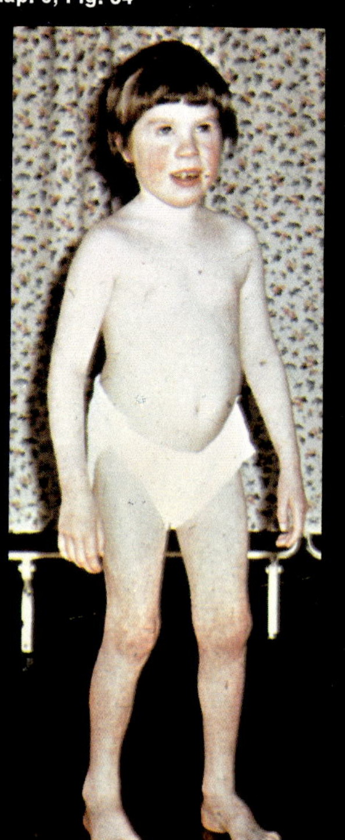

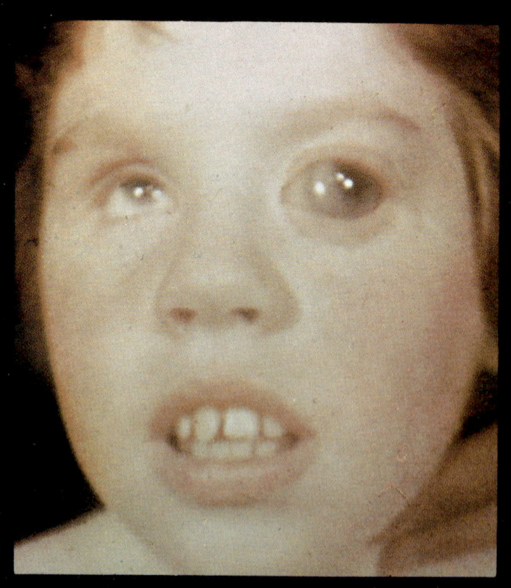

Chap. 9, Fig. 64

Chap. 9, Fig. 63

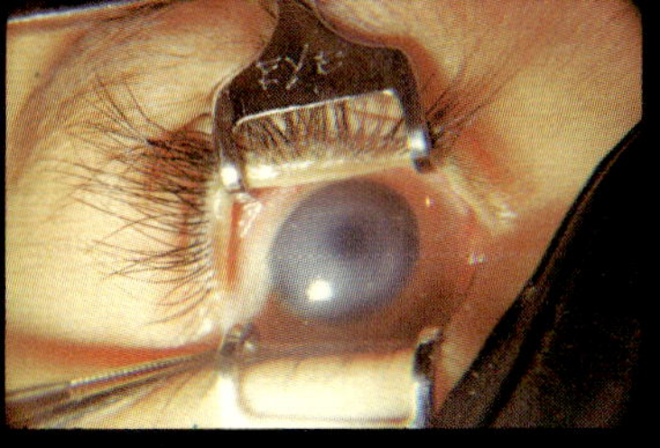

Chap. 10, Fig. 3

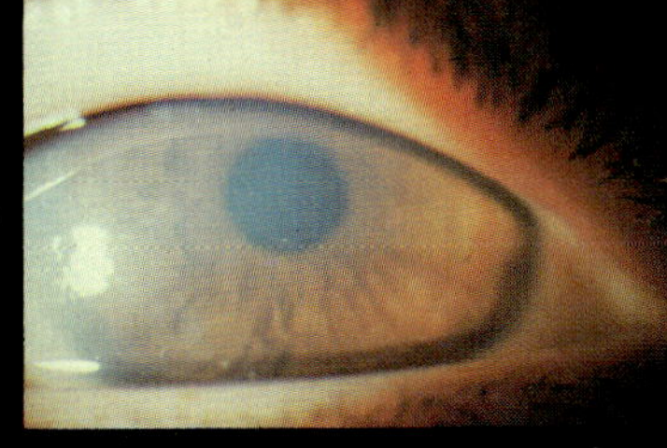

Chap. 10, Fig. 23

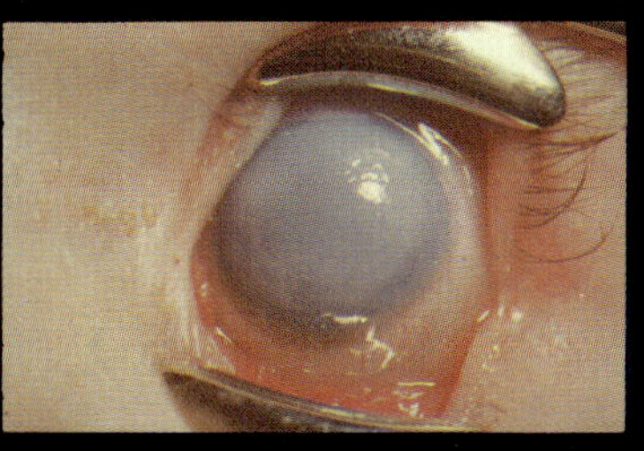

Chap. 10, Fig. 25

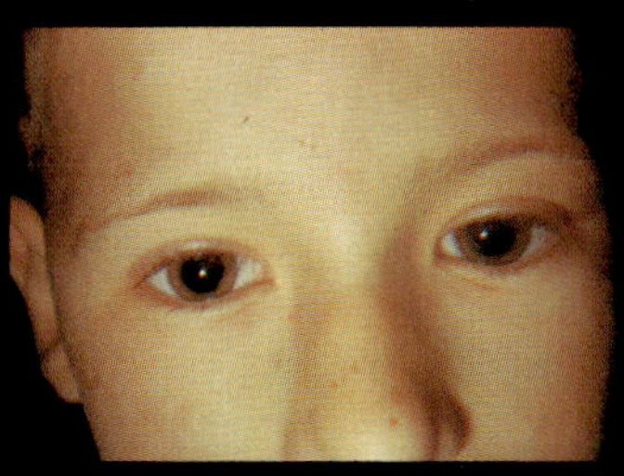

Chap. 10, Fig. 32

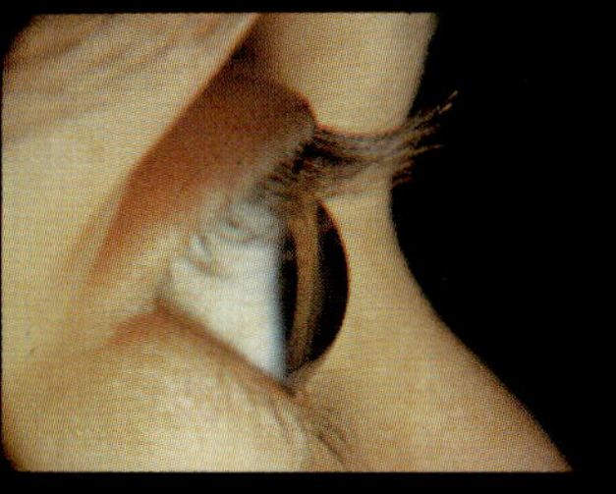

Chap. 10, Fig. 33

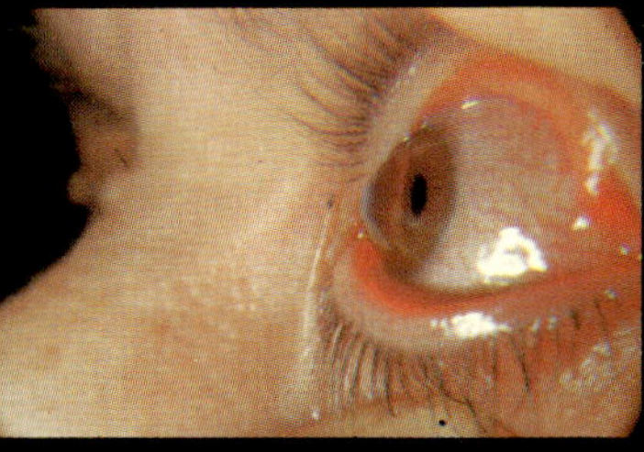

Chap. 10, Fig. 37

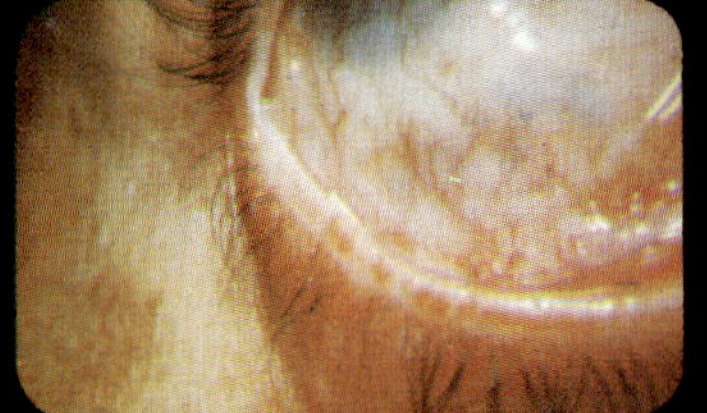

Chap. 11, Fig. 1

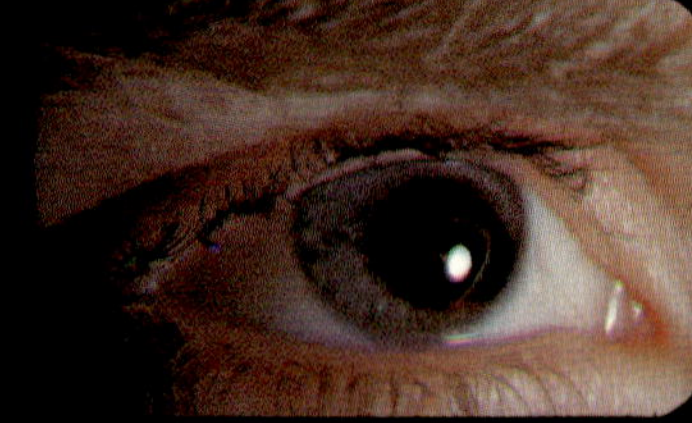

Chap. 11, Fig. 2

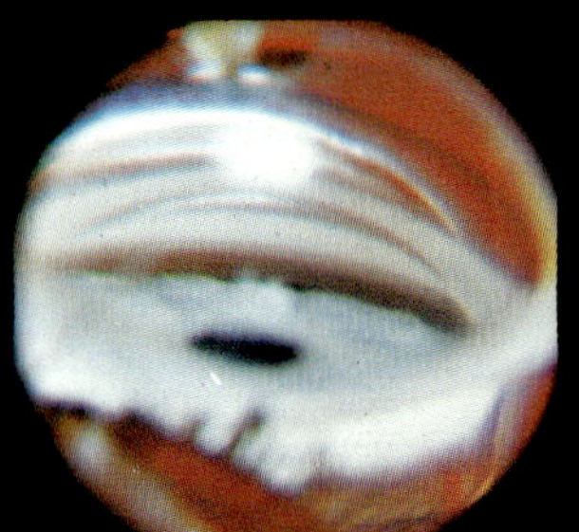

Chap. 11, Fig. 4

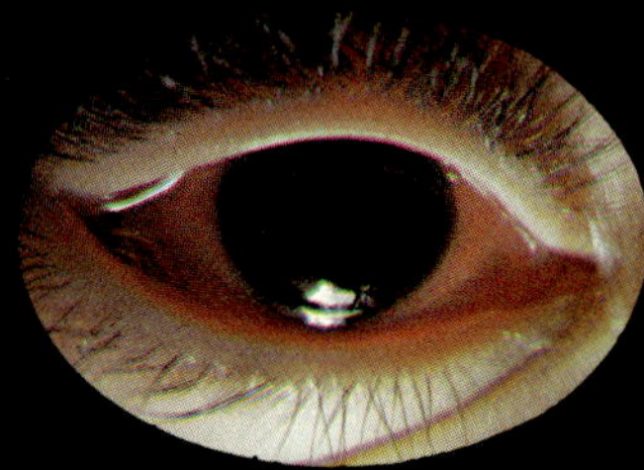

Chap. 11, Fig. 5

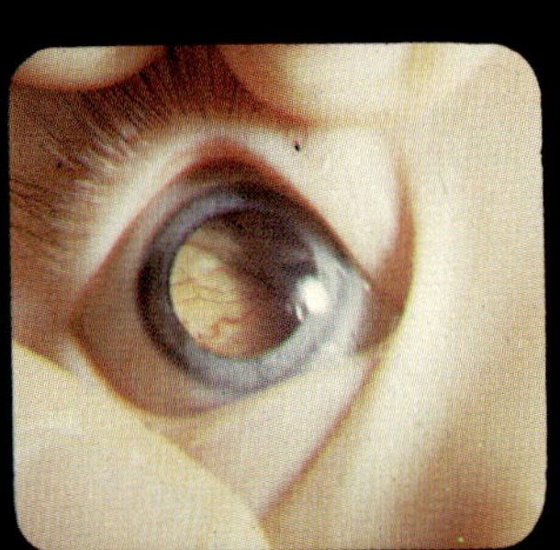

Chap. 11, Fig. 10

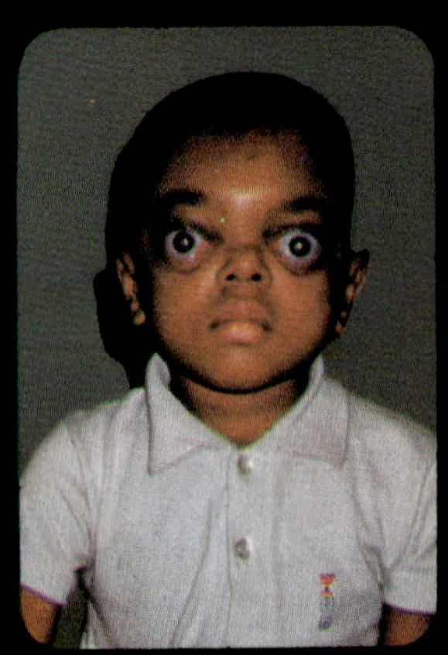

Chap. 11, Fig. 12

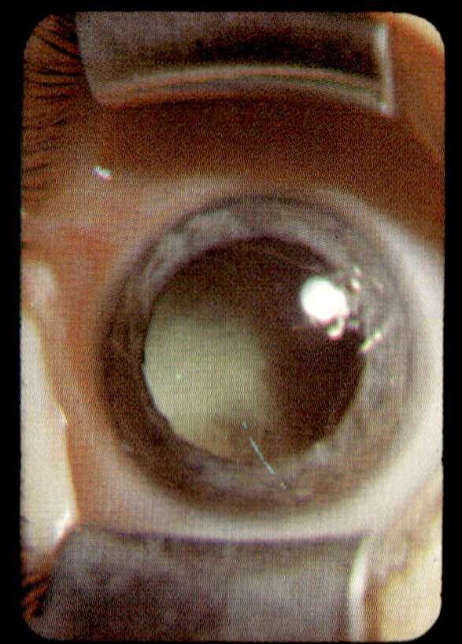

Chap. 11, Fig. 13

1

Causes of Congenital Abnormalities

The surge of knowledge about the influence of the various teratogenic agents has had fruitful consequences for clinical medicine. These consequences are all the more significant because there has been a striking reduction in the importance of pathogenic organisms as causes of disease. For one population, that of Northern Ireland, it has been estimated that one-quarter of all chronic hospital beds are now used by people with genetic diseases.

Birth defects in the United States constitute a leading cause of hospitalization of children and are the leading cause of deaths in the first year of life. Of all live-born infants, an estimated 7 percent have defects which are recognized at birth, during childhood, or in adult life. Fewer than half of these defects are evident at birth. While the great majority of birth defects are caused by a combination of heredity and environment, one of

TABLE 1.

EXPOSURE TO SELECTED POTENTIAL TERATOGENS IN 240 PREGNANCIES

Potential Teratogen	Exposure: First Trimester		Exposure: Entire Pregnancy	
	No.	%	No.	%
Radiation	29	12	72	30
Appetite suppressants	31	13	65	27
Antiemetics	36	15	38	16
Tranquilizers	22	9.2	51	21
Analgesics	28	12	155	65
Antibiotics	29	12	101	42
Antihistamines	41	17	62	26
Insecticides	50	21	125	52
Acute illness	28	12	129	54
Vitamins*	156	65	214	89

*Not scored as teratogen when taken in normal quantities.

five birth defects is caused by heredity alone. "Environment" includes not only the mother's environment but that of the fetus as well. Maternal infections and the taking of certain medications during pregnancy are among the factors that can adversely affect fetal development. Table 1 illustrates a series of 240 mothers observed by Nora et al. which reveals a high frequency of exposure to potential teratogens.

Of the total American population approximately 15,000,000 people have one or more congenital defects which affect their daily lives. This includes 500,000 people who were born blind or with serious loss of vision.

Genetic counseling can perhaps limit the number of the afflicted, but it cannot do more than reduce future generations of genetic defectives. What can be done for those already born with defects? In some instances, successful control of the disease has been achieved by medical intervention. In phenylpyruvic oligophrenia, for instance, dietary control instituted within one to three months of birth can prevent the irreparable and secondary damage that is caused by the genetic inability to carry out parahydroxylation. In other genetic diseases, particularly in clotting defects such as hemophilia and afibrinogenemia, we can help the afflicted by supplying the molecule which he lacks. However, in general, the treatment of genetic disease is still in its infancy and much remains to be learned about the exact molecular nature, the evolutionary significance, and the control of these diseases. We can at this stage recognize in the common features of these diseases the general phenomenon of polymorphism.

The individuality of man's mind finds a counterpart in biochemical individuality, which has been among the biologic discoveries of the 20th century. In the last two decades molecular polymorphism has been found not only in macromolecules of membranes but also in an ever-growing list of soluble proteins and enzymes. Thus DNA enshrines—in its universal code—the common evolutionary heritage of all living beings, but it also contains the differences that result in the biochemical fingerprints by which members of the same species differ from one another.

As a rule, individuals who have different forms of a given molecule are indistinguishable in terms of their biochemical effectiveness. At the fringe of polymorphism, however, lies a narrow zone in which changed molecular structure results in a functionally inefficient molecular structure. This type of polymorphism leads to dysfunction and thus to a group of diseases which we call inborn errors of metabolism.

The borderline between functional effectiveness and ineffectiveness (i.e., between the "normal" and the "abnormal") is not well defined and is, in fact, relative to the demands made on the individual. Sometimes the borderline is extended by environmental conditions, sometimes by pharmacologic challenge.

Not only nature but also man's technology can create conditions which impinge on the expression of polymorphism. The effect of pharmacologic challenge is illustrated in the case of the polymorphism of pseudocholinesterase. There is a relatively rare (a gene frequency of 0.019) form of this enzyme which seems to function quite adequately until certain drugs are administered. The enzyme is unable to convert these drugs and the affected individual is unable to cope adequately with the environmental challenge of pharmacologic intervention. Thus polymorphic forms which are ordinarily adequate can become a source of danger if the internal molecular environment is altered by pharmacologic interference.

In general, polymorphic forms of molecules function equally well, but in some instances one molecular form may function much better or much worse than another in the face of exceptional environmental changes. As a consequence, certain types of polymorphism are naturally maintained owing to their survival value.

Genetic disease has been found in several of the biologic systems. Examples are provided by various clotting deficiencies such as congenital afibrinogenemia, hemophilia, Christmas disease, absence of Factors V, VII, VIII, and X, and by such metabolic deficiencies as total albinism (tyrosinase), Von Gierke's disease (glucose-6-phosphatase), familial goitrous cretinism (iodotyrosine deshalogenase), phenylketonuria (phenylalanine hydroxylase), Crigler-Najjar syndrome (glucuronyltransferase), and acatalasemia. It is clear from this list and from the association with defined molecular defects that we can regard most inborn errors of metabolism as instances of polymorphism in which a polymorphic form of a biologically active molecule is ineffective and thus breaks an interlocking chain of reactive molecules. One might therefore hope that in many cases we could control genetic disease by administering the molecule which is lacking. Although this has been a very effective way of managing most diabetics, it has been relatively ineffective in the treatment of other types of inborn errors, often because "resistance" to the molecule has developed—even against molecules of human origin.

The extent of this resistance has differed in the different individuals who suffer from the "same" genetic disease. Indeed, this difference in responsiveness suggests a degree of heterogeneity within the disease entity itself. At any rate, it would be useful to be able to apply criteria by which one could predict resistance to supportive measures.

GENERAL CONSIDERATIONS

Etiologic Factors

In general only a relatively few reactions in the developing embryo are responsible for the diversity of embryonic disorders. Each type of disorder has a critical phase during which hereditary as well as environmental factors exert their influence. The pattern of damage depends on the degree of differentiation of the structure at the moment the insult takes place. At an early stage the organ rudiments are highly sensitive and minimum doses of a teratogenic agent can produce severe damage. As the organ develops, damage can be produced only by a corresponding increase in dosage. There is, in addition, a specificity of action of various teratogenic agents with certain substances acting on a selective basis on organs that show hypersensitivity to that agent. Many of these factors have a widespread influence that includes effects on the heart and the central nervous system. Therefore, a large undetected percentage of malformed embryos die in utero and are prematurely expelled while others are carried to term but not as viable organisms.

A study of 233 congenitally blind children by Robinson et al. over a 21-year period showed that genetic, prenatal, and perinatal causes account for over 60 percent of the cases. The three major lesions associated with congenital blindness are: retinopathy of prematurity (35.6 percent), congenital cataracts (21.0 percent), and optic nerve atrophy (10.3 percent). The first two lesions have varied in relative importance over the 21-year period so that congenital cataracts are presently the commonest lesion. Although of less importance than 10 to 15 years ago, retinopathy of prematurity appears to be increasing again. Optic atrophy occupies second place, having maintained its position throughout the period of study. The etiology of congenital blindness was unknown in almost 40 percent of cases. Of children suffering from retinopathy of maturity, 43 percent had no useful vision, which accounts for this condition's causing the most severe visual loss. More than 50 percent of the children had a second handicap such as deafness, developmental retardation, cerebral palsy, epilepsy, or congenital heart disease; 16 percent had two such handicaps. The rubella syndrome is responsible for the majority of multihandicapped children; a common association of hearing impairment and heart disease was noted with congenital cataracts. Retinopathy of maturity and optic nerve atrophy were associated with cerebral palsy and epilepsy. Developmental retardation—that is, the inability of the child to perform on a par with his peers—was the most important additional handicap, which affected 35.2 percent of the children. Fraser and Friedman studied a group of 776 blind children in Great Britain. They found that a single gene defect accounted for 38 percent of the cases, prenatal defects accounted for 5 percent, perinatal defects accounted for 33 percent, and 11 percent were due to postnatal acquired causes. The commonest eye lesions were retinopathy of prematurity (23 percent), chorioretinal degeneration (15 percent), congenital and infantile cataracts (14 percent), and optic atrophy (7 percent).

Since anomalies in man are not usually studied in utero but after they are fully developed, it is not always possible to deduce the cause from the final state of the condition. The factors are primarily hereditary and environmental. Neel showed in his series of more than 16,000 children that 20 percent of malformations were due to hereditary causes, 10 percent to chromosomal aberrations, and 10 percent to the effect of viruses. The cause could not be determined in the remaining 60 percent. Hereditary factors are easily identified in the case of a dominant inherited anomaly while recessive factors are often difficult to detect. Environmental factors include x-rays, substances such as aminopterin and thalidomide, viruses such as the rubella virus, parasites such as *Toxoplasma gondii*, syphilis, anoxia, hyperoxia, social conditions and religious factors, and maternal disease. Table 2 illustrates the incidence of a variety of congenital malformations as they appear in several regions of the world. It is clear that the varying incidence of specific types of anomalies reflects not only geographic location but racial differences as well.

TABLE 2.

THE INCIDENCE PER 1,000 BIRTHS OF FIVE RELATIVELY COMMON CONGENITAL MALFORMATIONS IN VARIOUS REGIONS OF THE WORLD

Author	Place	Spina bifida	Hydro-cephalus	Anen-cephaly	Cleft lip	Mongol-ism
McIntosh (1954)	New York	1.57	0.87	1.40	0.87	1.92
Coffey & Jessop (1959)	Dublin	4.20	3.50	5.10	0.88	0.64
Pleydell (1957)	Northamptonshire	1.86	0.45	0.87	1.57	1.63
Edwards (1958)	Scotland	1.70	1.90	2.80	—	—
Pitt (1961)	Melbourne	1.08	0.54	0.58	1.25	0.98
Neel (1958)	Japan	0.20	0.19	0.63	1.68	—
Wong (1964)	Singapore	0.17	0.12	0.21	1.36	0.88

Another important factor is the so-called "biological clock mechanism." The most familiar rhythmic phenomenon is the menstrual cycle, which follows an approximate lunar rhythm of twenty-nine days. Body temperature is normally lowest in the early hours of the morning and rises to a peak around 9:00 PM. Both mind and body are more sluggish when the temperature is low and become more alert with temperature rise. Not everyone shows this temperature rise at precisely the same time so that there will be a difference in response among different individuals to certain drugs, hormones, and x-rays at different times of the day or night. Hague described the retino-hypothalamo-hypophyseal mechanism involving the effect of day length upon animal behavior. Various animal activities such as reproduction, growth, and development are related to the weather or light cycle. When the day reaches a certain length, certain natural rhythms take place. Intraocular pressure measurements in humans, for example, follow definite patterns from day to day and at different times of the same day in both normal and glaucomatous individuals. Animals are able to sense and respond to very small increments of day or night length, as shown by the fact that while the day length may increase by only minutes, marked changes take place in the animal's behavior. A number of photosensitive parameters in birds and mammals including the reproductive system, pituitary gland, hypothalamus, adrenal cortex, and pineal body as well as behavior are known to be profoundly affected by the photoperiod.

Incidence

The incidence of major anomalies is dependent upon the length of the postnatal period chosen. Stillborn infants and infants who die during the postnatal period have an incidence of detectable malformations of 1.0 to 1.5 percent. Neel examined more than 16,000 children at the age of 9 months and found major anomalies in 3 percent, while McIntosh et al. gave an incidence of 7.5 percent in 5,964 infants. In infants born after the twenty-eighth week of gestation and observed for a period of one year after birth, 4.0 to 5.0 percent showed malformations. Taking into account those anomalies which do not become manifest until late infancy, adolescence, or in adult life, Lamy and Frezal found the incidence to be 5.0 to 6.0 percent. LeVann noted an increase for neonatal congenital physical abnormalities from 7.9 per 1,000 births in 1959 to 13.8 per 1,000 births in 1961. In analyzing the 1961 results he found that in geographic areas where precipitation was highest, 15.5 per 1,000 births showed physical defects. In areas where precipitation was lowest, 11.9 per 1,000 infants were born with physical defects. Increases of radioactive dust containing cesium–137, cerium–144, and strontium–90 were associated with above-ground Soviet thermonuclear Arctic explosions. Le Vann presented the hypothesis that higher levels of rainfall contaminated by radioactive dust caused more babies to be subjected to man-made radioactive elements in utero.

Animal Experiments

The evidence for linking various agents with the production of congenital malformations is often strongly suggestive. In addition to the use of careful statistical evaluation, animal experiments are required to determine more reliably what reports are more likely the result of chance association between unrelated events and what reports are conclusive. Analysis of the literature reveals that about 60 different methods have been successfully employed to produce malformations in laboratory animals. The most varied factors—physical, chemical, nutritional, infectious as well as metabolic disorders and disorders of the endocrine glands—can affect the development of the eye. In the occurrence of these malformations, as in that of all other anomalies, the sensitivity of the primordium, which varies in the course of development and the specific toxicity of each teratogenic agent must be considered of particular importance. To these essential factors must be added the animal's genotype, which influences more or less appreciably the reaction to the teratogenic agent and can therefore result in considerable variations in degree and type of malformations.

Causative Factors

X-Irradiation

The action of x-rays gives a very clear demonstration of the great sensitivity of the optic primordium. As little as 25 R are sufficient to disturb ocular development, whereas the teratogenic insult for other organs requires 100 R or more. Malformations caused by x-rays depend upon the state of development at the moment of irradiation. Pregnant mice were subjected to a single irradiation of 200 R at intervals of 24 hrs by Russell and Russell, the treatment beginning half a day after fertilization. In the preimplantation phase the majority of embryos were killed and only a small number were born as normal animals. With the beginning of embryogenesis the number of prenatal deaths decreased while the malformations rose sharply, reaching a peak when irradiation was carried out on the ninth day. At birth, all these animals suffered from severe malformations which were frequently multiple and lethal. When irradiation took place on the tenth day, more than 60 percent of the animals died at birth. Embryos that were subjected to irradiation after the thirteenth day were born with only slight disorders

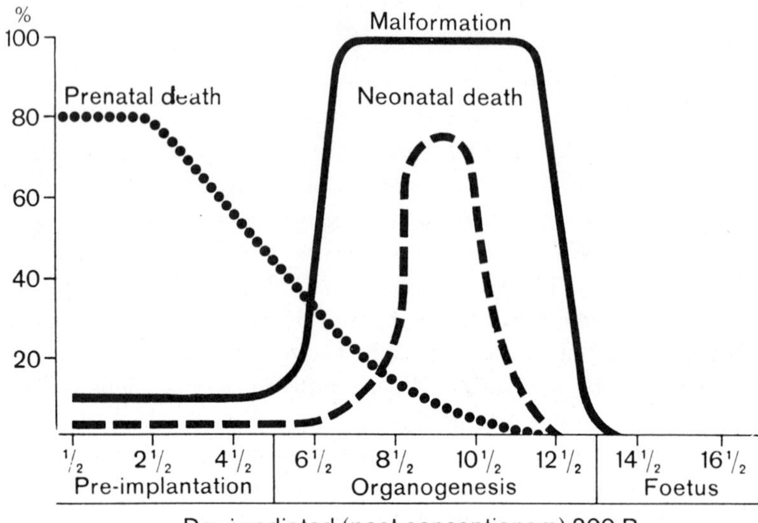

FIG. 1. Behavior of mouse embryos subjected to x-irradiation. Time intervals: 12, 36, 84 hrs etc. (Adapted from Tondury. **Triangle** 7:90, 1965. After Russell and Russell. **J. Cell. Comp. Physiol.** 43, Suppl 1:103, 1954.)

(Fig. 1). The malformation curve may be applied to the developing human embryo (Fig. 2).

Ocular experiments with x-irradiation early in pregnancy results in total absence of development of the optic primordium, primary anophthalmia, microphthalmia, and a variety of other anomalies–among them the persistence of the choroidal fissure.

A single dosage of 100 R in rats on the tenth day of pregnancy results in fetal anophthalmia. More or less complex damage to the retina results after irradiation on the eleventh and twelfth days. When mice are irradiated with 300 R on the thirteenth day of gestation, massive destruction of the future retinal cells is observed 4 hrs after treatment. After 24 hrs the cellular degeneration continues and active phagocytosis appears. However, after 72 hrs most fetal eyes begin to repair the damage so that the retina appears almost normal. The eyes remain small, but in general, morphologic proportions are maintained.

Certain agents such as cysteamine diminish and others such as cortisone augment the sensitivity to x-rays.

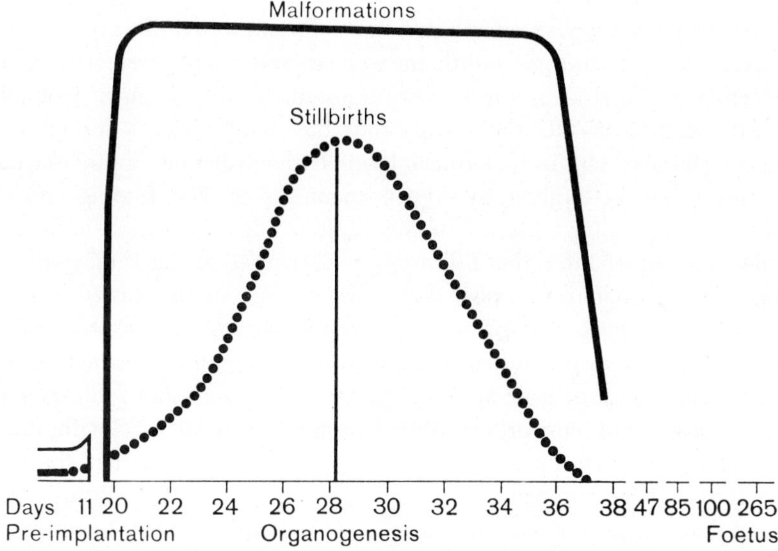

FIG. 2. Malformation curve of Fig. 1 applied to the development of human beings. (Adapted from Tondury. **Triangle** 7:90, 1965.)

Exogenous and Endogenous Substances

ESTRADIOL. In animal experiments it has been shown that estradiol attacks the cells of the matrix of the neural tube and the blastema of the extremities during differentiation. The surviving embryos are microcephalic, with small eyes and crippled limbs.

d-LYSERGIC ACID DIETHYLAMIDE (LSD-25). Numerous experiments on animals with d-lysergic acid diethylamide (LSD-25) have shown the agent to have a profound effect at relatively low doses. Auerbach and Rugowski injected mice intraperitoneally with LSD-25 on the seventh day of pregnancy. Four days later embryos of the injected mice had a deformity rate of 57 percent as compared to a rate of 10 percent in the control embryos. The stage of pregnancy found sensitive to embryonic malformations by LSD-25 corresponds to human pregnancy of 16 to 22 days, a period of embryonic development when pregnancy is frequently unsuspected.

TRYPAN BLUE. Microphthalmia, exophthalmia, and anophthalmia are known to occur in mice and rats involved in trypan blue experiments.

VITAMINS. Rat embryos subjected to hypervitaminosis A from the fifth to the eighth day show anophthalmia. From the eighth to the eleventh day, anophthalmia and microphthalmia occur, and from the eleventh to the fourteenth day aplasia of the eyelids is noted. If the treatment is applied from the eighteenth to the twenty-first day only cataract formation is observed. Similar but not identical lesions to retrolental fibroplasia have been produced in rabbits by hypervitaminosis A. The findings include intraocular hemorrhage, fibrosis of the vitreous body, alteration in the lens, and detachment of the retina followed by degeneration. Lack of vitamin A causes microphthalmia in pigs and a variety of malformations in rats including colobomas, fibrosis of the vitreous body, and puckering of the retina. Deficiency in pantothenic acid results in anophthalmia and microphthalmia. Deficiency of folic acid may result in eversions and folding of the retina. Nelson and co-workers observed colobomas in rats with retinal cysts after x-methylfolic acid administration. It was noted that the most vulnerable stage of the ocular primordia was on the eighth and ninth days. Microphthalmia in the cat has been observed after similar experiments. Vitamin B_2 deficiency obtained by the use of the antivitamin galactoflavin also produces ocular malformations.

HORMONAL FACTORS. Unbalanced thyroid activity (hypoactivity or hyperactivity) has been shown to have a definite influence on the development of the eye. Cataracts have resulted after the administration of thyroxine. Hypothyroidism obtained by thyroidectomy has produced retinal folds in the rat.

The effects of other hormones including corticosteroids, sexual hormones, pituitary-stimulating substances, and insulin still remain a matter of controversy.

HYPOGLYCEMIC SULFONAMIDES. Carbutamide BZ 55 causes anomalies in the rat, of which 95 percent involve the eye. Other hypoglycemic sulfonamides including tolbutamide cause ocular damage but to a lesser degree.

ACTINOMYCIN D. The highest percentage of malformations may be obtained in experimental animals by intraperitoneal injection of 20 μg of actinomycin D on the eighth and ninth days of gestation. Ocular malformations include: anophthalmia, coloboma, abnormal orientation of the primordia, wrinkling of the retina, and cataract formation.

OTHER SUBSTANCES. Other substances known to produce anomalies in animal experiments include: adrenalin, busulphan, chlorambucil, and cyclophosphamide streptomycin. Various antimitotics have proved to be harmful to the eye including 1-methyl-4-aminopyrazolo (3.4d)-pyrimidin and triethylenmelamin.

Infections

TOXOPLASMA GONDII. Microphthalmia, persistence of the pupillary membrane, chororetinitis, and cataracts have been observed in experimental animals following toxoplasmosis infection.

VIRUSES. Viruses may cause malformations when the organ rudiments reach the phase of maximum sensitivity. Chicken embryo experiments have shown several viruses to be teratogenic, namely: (1) influenza A virus; animals exhibit pronounced microcephalia and a more or less crooked body axis; (2) mumps virus; vacuolation of lens cortex has been noted with the presence of eosinophilic inclusion bodies in lenticular fibers undergoing differentiation; and (3) the chicken pest virus; malformations in the neural tube, lens, and otocysts have been noted. The critical phase lies between the thirty-sixth and forty-eighth hour, with older embryos showing no malformations. Viruses which induce formation of tumors in avian and mammalian hosts include Rous sarcoma of fowl, avian erythromyeloblastosis, and murine leukemia. These viruses contain ribonucleic acid (RNA). Those tumor-forming viruses containing desoxyribonucleic acid (DNA) include polyoma, papilloma, and the adenoviruses. Growth retardation and nonchromosomally inherited physiologic defects have been reported in animal embryos following viral infections.

Glaucoma in Rabbits

Malformation of the anterior segment of the eye of rabbits was recorded as early as 1886. In breeding experiments, Kolker et al. noted that none of the offspring from the mating of buphthalmic and normal rabbits showed any evidence of glaucoma, as determined by corneal diameter, intraocular pressure, and outflow facility. When these hybrid rabbits were bred back to their buphthalmic parent, both normal and buphthalmic offspring were produced. This would indicate an autosomal recessive inheritance. The gene for transmission of this disease is reported to be semilethal, and affected offspring are frequently less healthy and grow and breed more poorly than their normal litter mates. Possible confirmation of this observation was the 25 percent mortality rate in the offspring obtained in this series. Kolker et al. later bred normally pigmented rabbits to albino buphthalmic rabbits. All the offspring of such matings were normal, although several were pigmented. On breeding the pigmented rabbits back to buphthalmic rabbits one buphthalmic male rabbit was obtained. Clinically, glaucoma in the rabbit is characterized by an elevation in the intraocular pressure, decreased aqueous outflow facility, enlargement of the intraocular pressure, decreased aqueous outflow facility, enlargement of the globe, deep anterior chamber, and excavation of the optic disc, so that the disorder resembles glaucoma in the human. Kolker et al. showed that the glaucomatous condition could not be detected clinically at birth and was usually not obvious until three or four months of age. At that time, with the intraocular pressure at a normal level, a marked impairment in the facility of outflow could be noted. The intraocular pressure did not reach high levels until about five to six months of age (Fig. 3A).

The gonioscopic appearance of the chamber angle and microscopic sections of two normal and three buphthalmic rabbit eyes were studied by Lee. In the normal eyes the anterior chamber was open (Fig. 3B). As the rabbits approached the adult age of one year, the uveal tract began to differentiate anatomically. Fine fibers of uveal tissue, iris processes, and pectinate ligaments were seen extending forward from the periphery of the iris to the surface of the trabecular meshwork. On maturity the uveal meshwork lost much of its early homogeneous sheetlike appearance to become coarser and more open in structure, adhering more closely to the ciliary body band and trabecular meshwork.

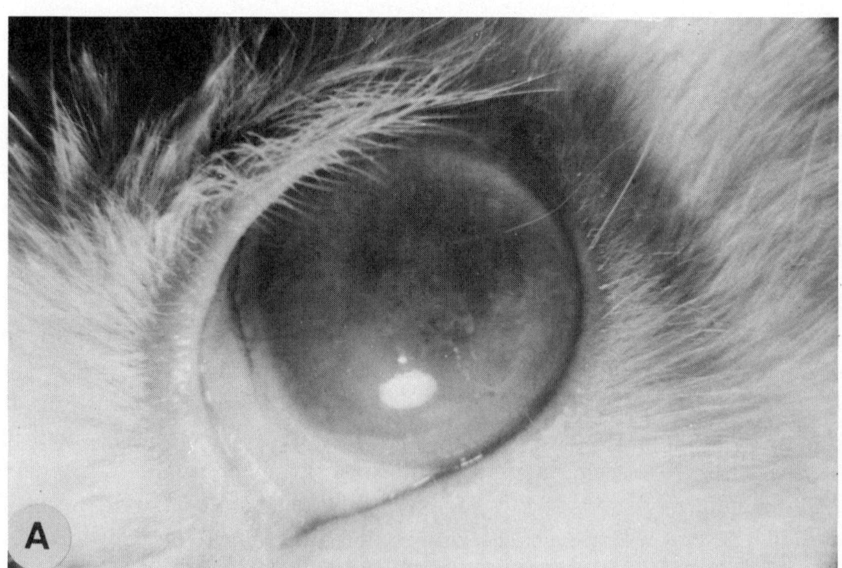

FIG. 3.A. Glaucoma in an albino New Zealand rabbit.

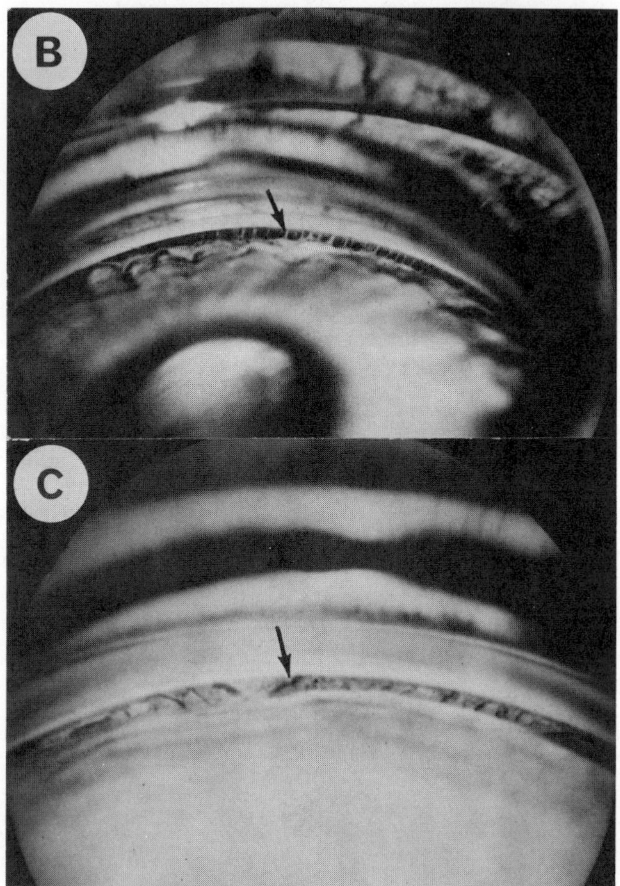

FIG. 3. (Cont.) B. Filtration angle in eye of normal rabbit. Goniophotograph shows open filtration angle. Pectinate ligaments (*arrow*) are clearly visible. There are no abnormal vessels. **C.** Filtration angle in eye of buphthalmic rabbit. Goniophotograph shows filtration angle packed with undifferentiated uveal tissue which contains many capillaries (*arrow*). (From Lee. **Arch. Ophthalmol.** 79:775, 1968.)

In buphthalmic eyes, the iris tissue and capillaries were attached to the trabecular meshwork, forming an abnormal anterior insertion of uveal tissue on or anterior to the trabecular meshwork (Fig. 3C). The uveal tissue in the filtration angle was more prominent, richer in blood vessels, and usually extended forward in the plane from the periphery of the iris to the surface of the trabecular meshwork. As the buphthalmic rabbit approached the age of one to two years, the undifferentiated vascularized uveal tissue lost its glistening sheetlike surface and appeared as a gray, cobweblike vascularized

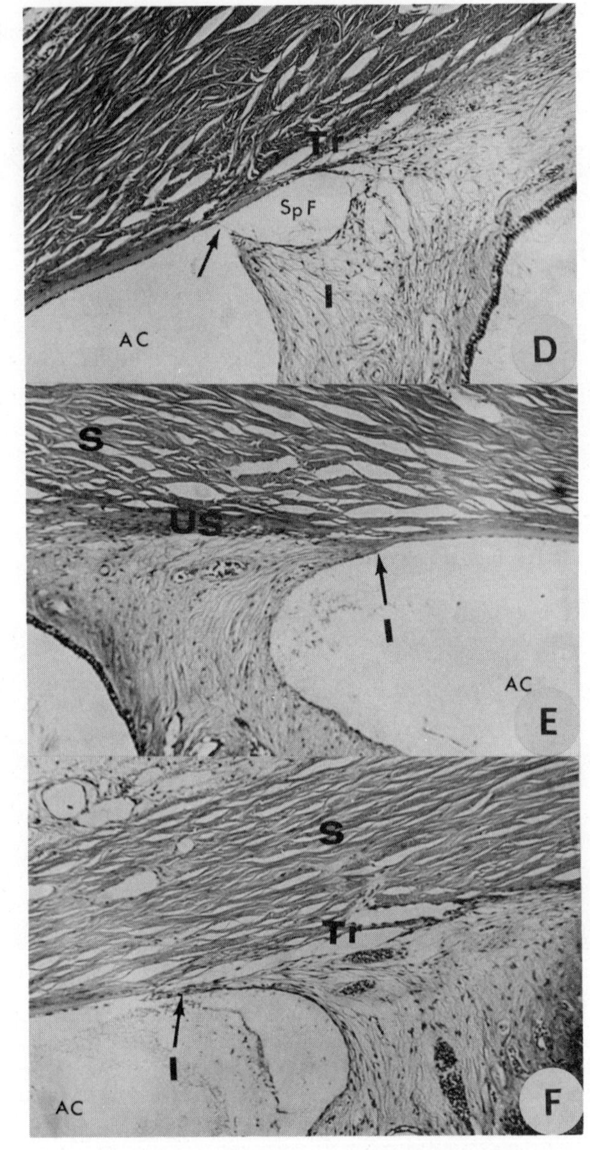

FIG. 3. (Cont.) D. Histologic section of filtration angle of same (Fig. 3B) normal rabbit. Space of Fontana (SpF), pectinate ligaments (*arrow*), drainage channel (Tr), and normal insertion of iris (I) are clearly visible. Anterior chamber (AC) and sclera (S) are seen. **E.** Histologic section of filtration angle of same (Fig. 3C) buphthalmic rabbit. Space of Fontana is absent; abnormal anterior insertion (I) of uveal tissue, rich in capillaries. Undifferentiated uveal tissue closely attached to sclera and filtration angle (US). Drainage channel cannot be identified in this section. Anterior chamber (AC) and sclera (S) are shown. **F.** Histologic section of filtration angle of same (Fig. 3C) buphthalmic rabbit. Space of Fontana is absent; abnormal anterior insertion (I) of uveal tissue, rich in capillaries. Drainage channel (Tr) is clearly visible in this section. Anterior chamber (AC) and sclera (S) are shown. (From Lee. **Arch. Ophthalmol.** 79:775, 1968.) H & E, X70.

fibrotic membrane overlying the ciliary body band and trabecular meshwork. The abnormal vessels in the peripheral iris typically had one end at the base or just beyond the root of the iris and the other end in the embryonic uveal tissue on the trabecular meshwork. The looped vessels had both ends in the iris. They did not bridge the filtration angle and did not extend beyond the angle wall.

On histologic examination the normal eyes showed well-developed spaces of Fontana and trabecular channels (Fig. 3D). Uveal fibers extending from the iris root were loosely applied to the ciliary body and filtration angle. The peripheral iris and filtration angle showed no abnormal vessels or residual uveal tissue.

Buphthalmic eyes exhibited the following features: absence of the spaces of Fontana, abnormal anterior insertion of uveal tissues, and poorly developed trabecular channels (Figs. 3E and F). Undifferentiated uveal tissue was closely attached to the filtration angle and sclera. The peripheral iris was richly vascularized in a manner not unlike that of hemorrhagic glaucoma in humans. The ciliary body was smaller than normal.

Studies by Rochon-Duvegneaud and McMaster have implicated dense tissue and fibrosis as a cause of glaucoma in rabbits. According to Lee, it is conceivable that this finding is actually undifferentiated uveal tissue. Lee's studies show that glaucoma in the rabbit is associated with incomplete cleavage of the anterior chamber angle and an abnormal insertion of uveal tissue anteriorly with malformation of the outflow channels.

Glaucoma in Other Animals

AVIAN GLAUCOMA. Jensen and Matson showed in 1957 that chicks reared in continuous light develop a glaucomalike condition characterized by buphthalmos, increased eye weight, flattening of the cornea with shallow anterior chamber, a narrow iridocorneal angle, and decreased aqueous outflow facility. When domestic fowl are reared under continuous light for prolonged periods of time, histological evidence of pathology is found in the retina, ciliary body, and optic nerve. Manifestations include retinal detachment, fibrous metaplasia of intraocular structures, and intraocular bone formation. Lauber et al. kept a group of chicks in continuous light and treated them with various miotics and oral acetazolamide. Glaucoma was not prevented by the miotics but the use of acetazolamide prevented the development of an enlarged eye. In addition, light-induced buphthalmia developed in spite of covering the eyes with an occluder from hatching to six weeks of age. Smith et al. reported that the administration of oral acetazolamide prevented a rise in intraocular pressure but did not prevent the shallow chamber from developing. Frankelson and his co-workers performed iridectomies on young chicks subsequently reared under either diurnal or continuous lighting conditions. The experiments showed that the iridectomy did not prevent the development of glaucoma nor did it alter its course. These authors concluded that the shallow anterior chamber and narrow iridocorneal angle did not seem to be the primary mechanism involved in the development of buphthalmia in domestic fowl. According to Frankelson et al., the influence of light on aqueous fluid dynamics might be mediated by a photosensitive endocrine or neural mechanism which could alter the aqueous humor secretion rate. The pathway for such a response is open to speculation but a number of observations have been made. Biochemical alterations occur in the rat pineal gland when adult rats are kept in continuous light. These effects of light exposure are abolished by bilateral enucleation. However, in newborn rats the alterations in the pineal gland still occur in blinded rats but are abolished when cloth hoods are placed over the rat's head. This would suggest that an extraretinal pathway involving the head influences the pineal gland in the newborn rat, according to Cohen et al. and Zweig et al.

GLAUCOMA IN MONKEYS. The chamber angle of the higher monkeys is structurally similar to that of man and differs considerably from that of lower monkeys and other mammals, according to Rohen. Glaucoma was first described in the monkey by Smythe. Barany and Rohen described two cases of secondary glaucoma and one case considered to be "simple glaucoma" in a series of monkeys (*Cercopithecus aethiops*). This latter case showed large pressure increases in both eyes on infusion. The one eye reached a plateau after 10 min and the other eye not until 16 min had elapsed. The pressure increase in this eye was 23 mm Hg. Histologic characteristics of the anterior segment of this monkey did not differ markedly from those of the normal eye.

GLAUCOMA IN THE PIG. Koby described hydrophthalmia in one eye of a pig. The other eye was microphthalmic. The glaucomatous condition was associated with an extensive pupillary membrane. The filtration angle was blocked by a broad adherence of the iris to the peripheral cornea. The ciliary processes and ciliary body showed extremely poor development. Only the lens capsule was present as a remnant of the lens. Schlemm's canal could not be identified.

Hypothermia

Smith lowered the body temperature of hamsters below 0°C for 45 min between Day 1½ and Day 8½ of pregnancy. Ocular malformations were noted in the animals, among which were unilateral or bilateral anophthalmia.

Hypoxia

Werthemann and Reiniger subjected rats to low atmospheric pressures (460 to 350 mm Hg) between the first and eighth days of pregnancy. Ocular malformations were observed including puckering of the retina and degeneration of the lens. Ingals and co-workers subjected mice to low atmospheric pressures of 280 to 260 mm Hg for 5 hrs on the eighth day of gestation. The fetuses showed lesions in the lens and retina.

Material Nutritional Deficiencies

Abnormalities of the cornea and crystalline lens have been noted in experimental animals placed on a diet deficient in tryptophan. Sugars such as galactose produce cataracts in rats which also show a defect in the migration of the optic nerve fibers toward the diencephalon.

CLINICAL MANIFESTATIONS

Reactions in the animal are of great importance for investigative purposes, but at the present time it is not possible to compare these reactions in man. A mouse can complete a generation within two months, a fruit fly within two weeks, and a microorganism within 20 min, but man has a generation time of at least 20 years. In lower forms it is possible to make test matings to acquire desired information or to test hypotheses, but in humans nature makes the experiment and the investigator can only record the outcome. A mouse can produce scores of offspring in its lifetime, a fruit fly hundreds, and a microorganism millions. Human families average about 3 children each. Human intrauterine development takes 40 weeks, while in the mouse it requires only 21 days. Embryogenesis lasts only four days in the mouse and the sensitive phase during which the organism reacts lasts only a few hours. In man this period stretches from the fifteenth to the forty-second day. Reactions resulting in the appearance of major malformations generally reach a peak on the twenty-first day and remain at this level until the thirty-eighth day (Fig. 2).

CAUSATIVE FACTORS

Viral Infections

Viral diseases in pregnancy range from unapparent maternal infections to severe and sometimes fatal acute illnesses. Fetal infections may occur as a result of transplacental invasion of the fetus subsequent to maternal viraemia or by transmission of the virus to the infant during delivery. Fetal injury or death in the absence of overt fetal infection may result from an unfavorable environment caused by the systemic toxicity associated with severe maternal viral infections. Abnormality in maternal acid-base, electrolyte, and fluid balances, as well as severe febrile response and maternal anoxia contribute to fetal loss and injury. The effects induced by viral disease are determined in part by the gestational age at the time of infection and in part by the virulence of the infecting organism. There appears to be a definite time specificity for the occurrence of the teratogenic effects. The earlier the infection, the greater the risk of damage to the fetus.

CYTOMEGALIC INCLUSION DISEASE. Cytomegalic inclusion disease is a common, mild, usually unapparent infection. About 30 to 60 percent of women of child-bearing age have serologic evidence of previous infection and another approximately 6 percent show serologic evidence of infection during pregnancy. Fetal infection apparently occurs during the viraemic phase of the primary infection, as it does not occur in subsequent pregnancies. Ophthalmic manifestations following this disease include the ocular complications associated with microcephaly and chorioretinitis. Other manifestations include cerebral palsy, mental retardation, jaundice, hepatitis, hepatosplenomegaly, thrombocytopoenic purpura, and cerebral calcification. The infection is chronic and cytomegaloviruria is persistent. Cytomegalovirus antibody has been demonstrated in the sera of microcephalic infants and children who have not shown typical symptoms of generalized congenital cytomegalic inclusion disease, indicating that the in-utero infection may selectively damage the central nervous system without producing systemic disease.

MUMPS. Tondury found damage to the crystalline lens in embryos of mothers who had contracted mumps during the early stages of pregnancy.

HERPES ZOSTER. Herpes zoster infection in the first trimester is thought to be associated with an increased incidence of congenital cataracts.

RUBELLA VIRUS. Gregg first described the congenital rubella syndrome in a study of mothers who had contracted German measles during the early months of pregnancy. He found small, malnourished infants with congenital cataracts, sluggish pupillary response to light, nystagmus, microphthalmos, heart disease (particularly patent ductus arteriosus), and an intolerance to atropine. Swan extended these studies and showed that the syndrome also included deaf mutism, microcephaly, mental retardation, primary congenital aphakia, chorioretinal scarring with vitreous haze, strabismus, shallow anterior chambers, corneal opacities, corneal haze associated with elevation of the intraocular pressure, corneal haze without intraocular pressure elevation, optic atrophy, anterior uveitis with posterior synechiae, and coloboma of the iris and retina.

The rubella virus has been identified and methods have been developed to propogate the organism in tissue culture. Seltzer reported the isolation of the rubella virus from an aborted human fetus. Although many cells in the preparation were in a state of degeneration, the virus could still be detected three to four weeks after the infection. Sever et al. were able to isolate the virus from an embryo at three weeks, and Heggie and Weir 57 days after onset of the disease. Neva et al. isolated the virus from 24 fetuses or placentas, which they had obtained within 49 days after infection of the mothers. In four cases the virus was isolated postnatally from the oropharynx and urine.

Montif et al. reported a successful postmortem isolation of the rubella virus in various organs of three damaged infants aged 22, 27, and 59 days. The rubella virus has also been recovered from the cataractous lens by Bellanti and co-workers. Rudolph et al. were able to isolate the virus as long as nine months after birth. These cases were definitely infectious to susceptible individuals.

Histopathologic observations made on eyes obtained from proven cases of rubella have provided an anatomic basis for many of the clinically observed changes. Boniuk and Zimmerman noted that microphthalmos, iris hypoplasia, and incomplete development of the chamber angle—that is, generalized retardation of ocular development—appeared similar to the generalized growth retardation that is typical of the congenital rubella syndrome. Arrested development of the chamber angle with incomplete cleavage was a common feature in their cases and was found to be associated with atrophy of the inner retinal layers, posterior bowing of the lamina cribrosa, atrophy of the corneal endothelium with breaks in Descemet's membrane and hydrops, and moderate atrophy of the midzonal and pupillary portions of the iris.

Because none of the cases of congenital glaucoma had associated cataracts, it is possible that these cases were associated with a rubella infection in the latter part of the first trimester. The development of the lens capsule during the fifth week of embryonic life could protect the lens from invasion of the rubella virus. It was also noted that many of these children with glaucoma did not have the full-blown clinical picture of the rubella syndrome.

In 1946 Guerry reported a case in which bilateral congenital glaucoma occurred in association with congenital cataracts. In this instance the mother had contacted rubella between the first and second month of pregnancy. Examination of each eye revealed extreme glaucomatous optic atrophy, fairly dense cataractous changes confined to the nuclear region, and an intraocular pressure of over 40 mm Hg in each eye. However, the cornea, although cloudy, was only 10 mm in diameter and the anterior chamber was shallow. The cornea cleared immediately after the eye was opened during surgery and responded well to a filtering operation. In their series of cases, Boniuk and Zimmerman noted that the lenticular changes include persistence of pyknotic and karyorrhetic nuclei in the cells of the lens nucleus together with an absence of posterior migration of lens epithelium, and though there was widespread cortical degeneration. This was thought to be due to persistence of the virus in the lenticular cells. The cataractous lens often appears swollen in the anteroposterior diameter. This spherophakia could result in pupil block and secondary glaucoma.

Changes in the ciliary body include focal necrosis of the pigment epithelium with infiltrates of lymphocytes and plasma cells in the iris ciliary body. Secondary changes due to inflammation in the iris include vacuolization and necrosis of the iris pigment epithelium as well as stromal atrophy. The iris also shows signs of hypoplasia, characterized by shortening of the iris leaves and an absence of pigment in the peripheral portion of the posterior layer of the pigment epithelium.

Wolter et al. also noted the lenses to be smaller than normal with a distinct extension of the ciliary processes. They described one case of widespread rubella involvement in only one of two nonidentical twins nursed by one placenta.

Cooper and co-workers noted that 271 out of 344 children whose mothers had suffered from a rubella infection during the first trimester had at least one significant abnormality. Hearing loss, congenital heart disease, cataract, glaucoma, psychomotor retardation, and neonatal thrombocytopenic purpura were the more significant conditions found. The incidence of cataract formation was 10 times more frequent than glaucoma, the conditions appearing to be mutually exclusive. The group found that 84 percent of the children were still excreting rubella virus in throat secretions during the first month. This incidence dropped to 11 percent by one year and to zero after two years. In lens tissue, however, the virus could be found up to 30 months, long after it was undetectable anywhere else in the body. The overall mortality rate in this group was 13 percent. Scheie reported that intraocular cultures have yielded virus in almost 50 percent of congenital rubella patients more than one year old.

Roy et al. described three eyes in which the anterior limiting membrane of the iris was hypoplastic, with complete absence in one case. The iris stroma in all three eyes was diminished in blood vessels, cellular structure, and loose connected tissue. The iris sphincter muscle was very thin in one eye and markedly diminished in size in another. The iris dilator muscle was almost absent in all three eyes. There was diminution of ciliary processes and the ciliary body in one eye was markedly hypoplastic.

Alfano described four patients who were operated upon for congenital glaucoma following rubella infection. One of the eyes was examined histologically. The anterior chamber was deep and the trabeculum was partially obstructed by thin fibrous bands stretching from the anterior iris surface. Schlemm's canal was present and the meridional muscle of the ciliary body appeared to insert normally into the scleral spur.

Continued development of the chamber angle after birth could account for the transient nature of glaucoma that has been noted clinically. Roy and co-workers described a case of congenital glaucoma with a cloudy cornea where the initial pressure was 35 mm Hg with the patient under general anaesthesia. At a later date a pressure of 18 mm Hg was recorded and the cornea had cleared spontaneously.

Geltzer et al. pointed out that the high incidence of associated multiple defects in the rubella syndrome should be considered in determining the timing of possible surgical intervention. It was noted that there was a very high correlation of eye and heart involvement in this series.

Genetics

In 1865 Mendel reported the results of his experiments with plant hybrids, providing the basis of the entire field of modern genetics. Advances in the past 10 years in the visualization of human chromosomes has made it possible to associate recognizable chromosomal abnormalities with a variety of developmental errors, so that chromosome analysis is now a commonly used guide for the diagnosis of certain abnormal conditions.

Of the 23 pairs of chromosomes in man, 22 pairs are autosomes and the remaining pair are sex chromosomes. Genes in the same positions on a pair of chromosomes contain similar genetic information. They are homozygous if their information is identical, and heterozygous if it is different. When a disorder results from genetic heterozygosity the gene is dominant. Homologous genes must be present for recessive inheritance of a disease to occur. Because genetic information does not always break through, a dominant gene can be present without manifesting itself in an individual, who may then pass it on to his children. A pathogenic gene may also cause severe disease in one individual and mild symptoms in another. Von Recklinghausen's neurofibromatosis is an example of such a condition.

There are three main patterns of disease inheritance. Autosomal dominant inheritance has the following characteristics. The gene which is in the heterozygous state is on one of the autosomes. The disease occurs in successive generations and males and females are both involved. Fifty percent of children of an affected parent are themselves affected. Autosomal dominant disorders include: achondrophasia, familial polyposis of the colon, hereditary hemorrhagic telangiectasia, hereditary spherocytosis, Huntington's chorea, Marfan's syndrome, congenital lymphedema (Milroy's disease), myotonic muscular dystrophy, osteogenesis imperfecta, and von Recklinghausen's neurofibromatosis. Autosomal recessive inheritance has the following characteristics. The gene which is in the homozygous state is on one of the autosomes. The disease tends to appear in one sibship of one generation only. Parents of an affected individual are both heterozygous carriers. Heterozygote carriers produce children of whom 25 percent are affected, 50 percent are carriers, and 25 percent are normal (average rates). Males and females are both affected. Autosomal recessive disorders include: albinism, alkaptonuria, cystic fibrosis, cystinuria, galactosemia, phenylketonuria, pseudoxanthoma elasticum, Tay-Sach's disease (amaurotic family idiocy, infantile type), and Wilson's disease (hepatolenticular degeneration). Sex-linked (X-linked) inheritance has the following characteristics. The gene is on the X chromosome. Females usually carry the gene without developing the disease. Generations may be skipped and affected males may have unaffected carrier daughters who pass the gene to half their sons. The disease is never passed from father to son but affected males may have affected male relatives on the maternal side of the family. Sex-linked disorders include: agammaglobulinemia (Bruton type), glucose-6-phosphate dehydrogenase deficiency (favism; primaquin sensitivity), hemophilia A (classical), hemophilia B (Christmas disease), ocular albinism and pseudohypertrophic muscular dystrophy. With few exceptions such as vitamin D-resistant rickets and Alport's disease, sex-linked diseases are recessive.

A new era in medical genetics opened in 1959, when Lejeune and co-workers demonstrated that mongols had 47 chromosomes instead of the normal 46. At the present time it is possible to identify individuals with an increased genetic risk in reproduction. These factors, often multiple, are listed below.

A. The past occurrence of a genetic disease in the family.
B. A poor reproductive history of chronic infertility, recurrent abortions, or fetal demise.
C. Mutagenic exposure either during gametogenesis or early fetal development.
D. Epidemiological problems of parental age, season, and geographic location.

Since the chromosomes are considered to be bearers and transmitters of hereditary instructions, any chromosomal deviation from normal may result in abnormal patterns recognizable clinically in certain human diseases. Best known are the chromosomal aberrations which subsequently present the clinician with such conditions as Down's, Klinefelter's, Turner's syndrome, and trisomy 13-15 syndrome.

GENETIC METHODS OF INVESTIGATION

The principal methods of investigation are twin studies employed for elucidating the degree of hereditary determination, family studies used for uncovering the mode of inheritance, and chromosomal analysis.

TWIN STUDIES. Superficially, twin studies would appear to be a very easy form of investigation, since only two people need be examined and not some 50 or so people as in family studies. Nevertheless, the difficulties involved in conducting a systematic study of a large group of twins with a view to obtaining results which are statistically significant should not be underestimated. It is frequently assumed that only studies on identical twins are of importance. However, for determining the role played by heredity, comparison between identical and fraternal twins is, in fact, highly informative. For this purpose the so-called "concordance quotient" is calculated. As applied to twin studies there is concordance when only one twin is affected. Only a comparison of concordantly affected identical twins with concordantly affected fraternal twins yields the concordance quotient, usually expressed as a percentage, which affords an indication of the degree to which heredity is responsible.

FAMILY STUDY. As the term "family study" suggests, it is quite inadequate to proceed from anamnestic data elicited perhaps from only one person. It is important that all members of the family are investigated, including those allegedly free from any signs of the disease.

CHROMOSOMAL ANALYSIS. METHODS OF CHROMOSOMAL STUDY. Buccal smears, peripheral blood, and in some instances bone marrow, skin, and testis tissue are used to study chromosomes. Barr and co-workers discovered in their work with chromatin (a chromosomal derivative) that the XX pair in the female and the XY pair in the male cause different imprints on the nuclear chromatin. Microscopic examination of buccal smears show that normal females have a dark-staining area at the periphery of some cell nuclei, while normal males do not have this dark area, called the "Barr body" or sex chromatin body. It was found that the number of "Barr bodies" is equal to the number of X chromosomes minus one. Thus abnormal females with only one X chromosome have no sex chromatin body, and abnormal males with two X chromosomes and one Y chromosome have one "Barr body." Abnormal buccal smears are usually an indication that more detailed chromosome studies are required.

This information can be obtained by analysis of the chromosomes from cell cultures. Cells for chromosomal analysis, usually peripheral white blood cells, are cultured and incubated for three days. Colchicine is then added to arrest cells in metaphase when the chromosomes are best analyzed. After further incubation for 3 to 5 hrs, the cells are placed in a hypotonic solution which causes them to swell and the chromosomes to disperse within the cell. Following fixation and staining, microscopic analysis is performed. To show clearly the karyotype of an individual, the chromosomes are cut from enlarged photomicrographs and arranged in pairs, and then rephotographed.

TRISOMY AND MONOSOMY. The most common clinical condition caused by a chromosomal defect is Down's syndrome, also known as mongolism and trisomy 21. Typically in Down's syndrome there are three chromosomes instead of two of the number 21 autosomes. The most common cause of trisomy is failure of a pair of chromosomes to separate during reduction division (meiosis) in the formation of egg or sperm cells. As a result of this failure, called "meiotic nondisjunction," one germ cell contains both of a pair of chromosomes and the other is missing this chromosome. If the cell with an extra chromosome unites with a normal germ cell, the fetus will have 47 chromosomes. The incidence of trisomy 21 is about once in 600 live births, and the chance of having a mongoloid child increases with the advancing age of the mother.

Trisomy of most of the autosomes is not compatible with survival of the human embryo, but two other trisomies are found in the newborn, one in the 17-18 autosome group and the other in the 13-15 group. Infants with these conditions usually die within the first year of life because of severe malformations.

If a germ cell lacking a chromosome unites with a normal germ cell, the new individual will have only 45 chromosomes. This condition is termed "monosomy." Loss of a sex chromosome resulting in a YO error is fatal. The XO error is the most common abnormality found in spontaneous abortuses, but only 1 in 40 embryos survives. The XO error, or monosomy X, is identified clinically with Turner's syndrome.

Opposite to the XO error is trisomy X. These women may appear normal and neither fertility nor growth is affected, but there is a higher than normal incidence of mental retardation.

SEX CHROMOSOMAL ABNORMALITIES IN THE MALE. When the sex chromosomes fail to separate during production of sperm, four types of chromosomally abnormal sperm can occur: XY, XX, YY, and O. Fertilization of a normal X-bearing ovum by an XY-carrying sperm produces a male with XXY sex chromosomes which clinically is identified as Klinefelter's syndrome. These patients appear normal until puberty, but the testes fail to develop and sterility is the rule. Other chromosomal complexes have been found in patients with Klinefelter's syndrome, but the XXY error is the most common.

OTHER CHROMOSOMAL DEFECTS. Chromosomal defects can occur at times other than during the formation of the ovum or sperm. If there is a failure of two chromosomes to separate in the first cell division after conception, a condition known as mosaicism occurs, that is, half the individual's cells are trisomic and half are monosomic for that particular chromosome. Mosaicism may also result from loss of a chromosome. This can result in an XX/XO mosaicism in the female. These patients appear to have Turner's syndrome, but their buccal smear is chromatin positive.

Two other types of chromosomal abnormalities are called "deletion" and "translocation." In deletion, a section of a chromosome is lost, and in translocation, an exchange of fragments occurs between two broken chromosomes. The clinical syndrome known as cri du chat, characterized by the typical "cat cry" of the child, results from loss of a segment of the short arm of a chromosome in the 4-5 group. These physically and mentally retarded children usually die in childhood.

GENETICS IN GLAUCOMA

According to Sorsby, most cases of buphthalmos are sporadic. A substantial difficulty in assessing the significance of heredity arises from the fact that there are probably different pathological entities grouped in the same pedigree under one clinical designation. This is suggested by the

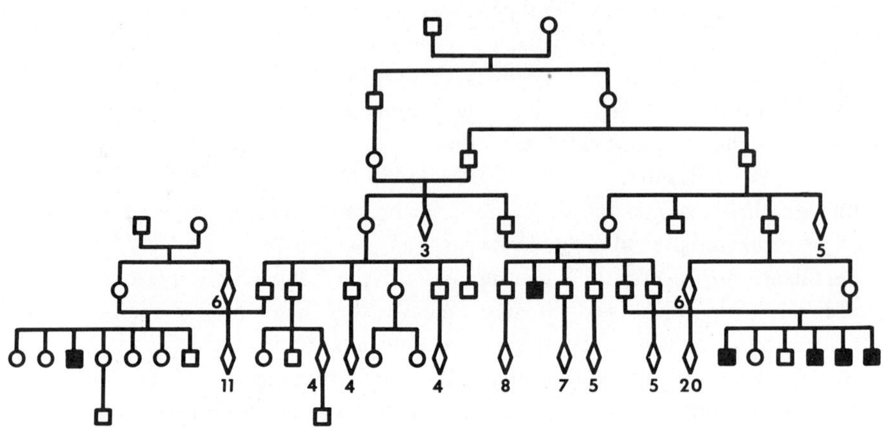

FIG. 4. Buphthalmos. Pedigree heavily intermarried, illustrates recessive inheritance in three collateral branches of family. Affected person indicated by black square or circle. (From Sorsby. **Ophthalmic Genetics**, 2nd ed. 1970. Courtesy of Appleton-Century-Crofts.)

following factors: (1) The developmental anomaly in the angle of the anterior chamber which gives rise to buphthalmos may lead to a distended globe that is already present at birth or to distention that becomes manifest in infancy. There is a gradual transition to juvenile glaucoma in which there is no distention. (2) There is the classical distinction between primary and secondary buphthalmos. (3) The distinction between buphthalmos and megalocornea is not always readily made. (4) It is recognized that buphthalmos may be an aspect of widespread ocular or even systemic disorders. Twin material, though slight in extent, records concordance in monozygotic twins. The evidence for the existence of a recessive variety (Figs. 4 and 5) is considerable. Aside from the many records of familial cases of the classical primary type of buphthalmos, there is an incidence of parental consanguinity of the order of 10 percent in the more substantial series on record.

In a recessive disorder, transmission is not to be expected (except in the unusual situation shown in the pedigree recorded in Fig. 6). What little information there is on this aspect supports this expectation (Fig. 7) but observations suggest that the affection has been transmitted (without necessarily being fully expressed). It is possible that some of the cases of direct transmission are examples of "pseudodominance".

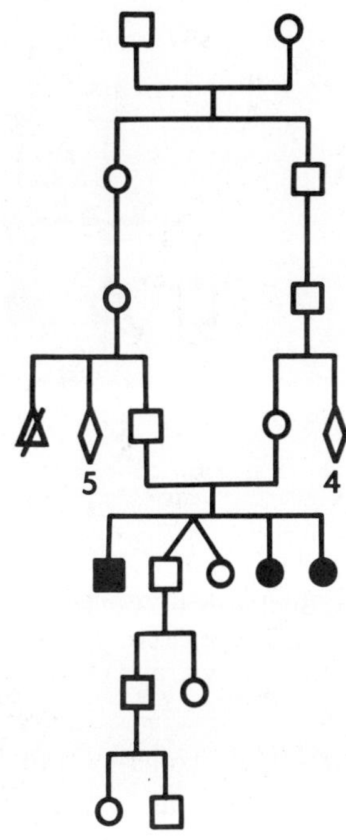

FIG. 5. Buphthalmos. Pedigree illustrates recessive inheritance in offspring of parents who were second cousins. Affected person indicated by black square or circle. (From Sorsby. **Ophthalmic Genetics**, 2nd ed. 1970. Courtesy of Appleton-Century-Crofts.)

In a study of juvenile glaucoma, Keerl found heredity to be a factor in 18 percent of his patients. Abnormality of the anterior segment of the eye in a large pedigree has resulted from a dominant inheritance, according to Falls. Franceschetti has also attributed such anomalies to a genetic basis. Audet and co-workers studied 1,261 descendents of one family in Quebec, and noted 54 persons suffering from glaucoma and 22 who were blind. Stokes concluded from his study of a pedigree of five generations that hereditary primary glaucoma results from a simple dominant gene that is not sex linked. The age at which the rise of intraocular pressure appears varies so that the onset occurs in early youth, adolescence, and adult life. Allen and Ackerman reported a pedigree of three generations in which the average age of onset was 11.6 years. Löhlein reported a family of four sisters, the youngest having marked hydrophthalmos. Glaucoma developed in the other three girls at ages 10, 15, and 17. Derby reported a glaucomatous father with a family of 11 children, three blind with glaucoma and one with hydrophthalmos. Berg reported a pedigree of six generations with 21 affected members of whom two had hydrophthalmos. Scheerer reported hydrophthalmos in a father, daughter, and cousin, as well as juvenile glaucoma that appeared in another cousin at the age of 18. Korte reported on a family in which the father and

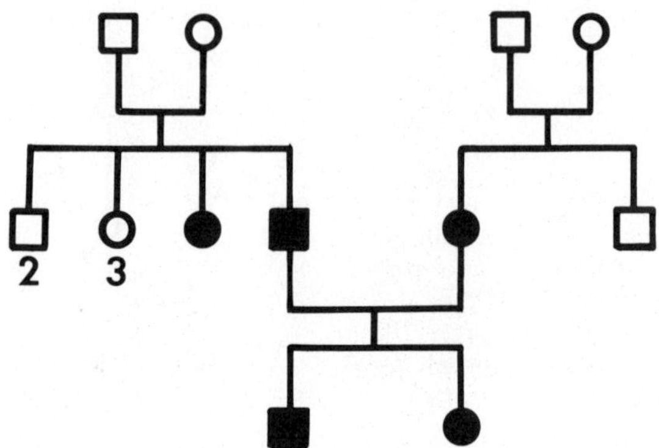

FIG. 6. Buphthalmos. Pedigree illustrates recessive inheritance. Affected person indicated by black square or circle. (From Sorsby. **Ophthalmic Genetics**, 2nd ed. 1970. Courtesy of Appleton-Century-Crofts.)

daughter had glaucoma and buphthalmos developed in two grandchildren, one male and the other female. Posner and Schlossman reviewed 474 glaucoma cases and found 50 patients who showed hereditary tendencies to

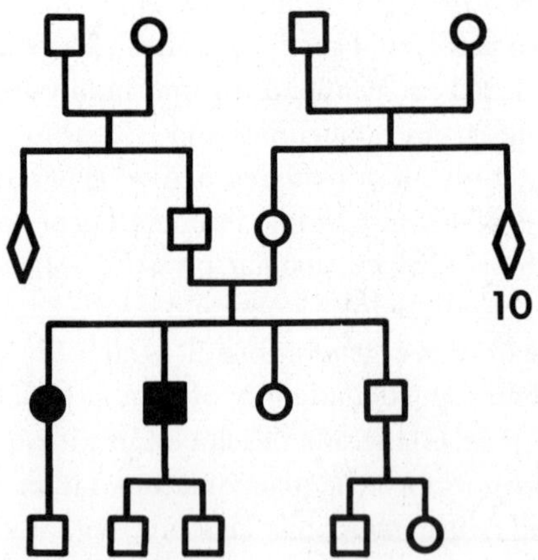

FIG. 7. Buphthalmos. Pedigree shows normal offspring of affected woman and also of her affected brother. (From Sorsby. **Ophthalmic Genetics**, 2nd ed. 1970. Courtesy of Appleton-Century-Crofts.)

the disorder. The pedigrees studied exhibited dominant inheritance. In 23 patients the age of onset was under 35 years.

Exogenous Substances and X-Irradiation

Reed and co-workers observed a case of congenital glaucoma (as well as deafness, mental deficiency, and cardiac anomaly) following an attempted abortion with quinine.

Cases of microphthalmia have been reported in children born to women who have undergone therapeutic x-irradiation during the first weeks of pregnancy. The fetal eye is particularly vulnerable to the effect of x-irradiation around the twenty-eighth day of pregnancy.

References

Albaugh, G. H. Congenital anomalies following maternal rubella in early weeks of pregnancy: with special emphasis on congenital cataract. J. A. M. A., 129:719, 1945.

Alfano, J. E. Ocular aspects of the maternal rubella syndrome. Trans. Am. Acad. Ophthalmol. Otolaryngol., 70:235, 1966.

Alford, C. A., Neva, F. A., and Weller, T. H. Virologic and serologic studies on human products of conception after maternal rubella. N. Engl. J. Med., 271:1275, 1964.

Allen, L., Burian, H. M., and Braley, A. E. A new concept of the development of the anterior chamber angle. Arch. Ophthalmol. 53:783, 1955.

and Burian, H. M., and Braley, A. E. The anterior border ring of Schwalbe and pectinate ligament. Arch. Ophthalmol., 53:799, 1955.

Allen, T. D., and Ackerman, W. G. Hereditary glaucoma in a pedigree of three generations. Arch. Ophthalmol., 27:139, 1942.

Audet, J., Dugré, J., and Coté, G. Une étude sur le glaucome familial. Annual Meeting of the Canadian Ophthalmological Society, Quebec, Canada, June 27, 1967.

Auerbach, R., and Rugowski, J. A. Lysergic acid diethylamide: effect on embryo. Science, 157:1325, 1967.

Axelrod, J., Wurtman, R. J., and Snyder, S. Control of hydroxyindole-o-methyl transferase activity in the rat pineal gland by environmental lighting. J. Biol. Chem., 240:949, 1965.

Bakker, A. Eine methode die Linsen erwachsener kaninchen Auberhalb des Korpers am Leben zu erholten. Graefes Arch. Ophthal., 135:581, 1936.

Die Regeneration der verwundeten Linsenkapsel von kaninchenlinsen in der Durchstromungskultur. Graefes Arch. Ophthal., 136:333, 1936.

Bamatter, F. La chorioretinite toxoplasmique. Ophthalmologica, 114:340, 1947.

Bannon, S. L., Higginbottom, R. M., McConnel, J. A., and Kaan, H. W. Development of galactose cataract in the albino rat embryo. Arch Ophthalmol., 33:224, 1945.

Barany, E. H., and Rohen, J. W. Glaucoma in monkeys (Cercopithecus aethiops). Arch. Ophthalmol., 69:630, 1963.

Becker, B., and Constant, M. A. Experimental tonography. Arch. Ophthalmol., 54:321, 1955. and Shaffer, R. N. Diagnosis and Therapy of the Glaucomas, 2nd ed. Mosby, St. Louis, 1965, p. 111.

Bell, J. The Treasury of Human Inheritance. Ed. by K. Pearson, Vol. 11, Pt. V. Cambridge Univers., London, 1933.
Bellanti, J. A., Artenstein, M. S., Olsen, L. C., Buescher, E. L., Luhrs, C. E., and Milstead, K. L. Congenital rubella. Am. J. Dis. Child., 110:464, 1965.
Benoit, J. The role of the eye and of the hypothalamus in the photostimulation of gonads in the duck. Ann. New York Acad. Sci., 117:204, 1964.
Berg, F. Ehbliches jugendlichen Glaukom. Acta. Ophthal., 10:568, 1932.
Biggs, R., and MacFarlane, R. G. Human Blood Coagulation and its Disorders, 3rd ed. Blackwell Scientific, Oxford, 1962.
Boniuk, M. Cited by Zimmerman, L. E., and Font, R. L. Congenital malformations of the eye: some recent advances in knowledge of the pathogenesis and histopathological characteristics. J. A. M. A., 196:684, 1966.
and Zimmerman, L. E. Ocular pathology in the rubella syndrome. Arch. Ophthalmol., 77:455, 1967.
Brons, H. Uber die Vererbung des Hydrophthalmus Congenitus. Thesis, Tubingen, 1937.
Browman, L. G., and Ramsey, F. Embryology of microphthalmos in rattus nowegicus. Arch Ophthalmol., 30:338, 1943.
Cinader, B. Specificity and inheritance of antibody response: a possible steering mechanism. Nature (London), 188:619, 1960.
Dependence of antibody responses on structure and polymorphism of autologous macromolecules. Br. Med. Bull., 19:219, 1963.
Dubinski, S., and Wardlaw, A. C. Allotypy and eniotypy. Nature (London), 210:1291, 1966.
Cohen, R. A. Wurtman, R. J., Axelrod, J., and Snyder, S. H. Some clinical, biochemical and physiological actions of the pineal gland. Ann. Intern. Med., 61:1144, 1964.
Cohlan, S. Q. Excessive intake of vitamin A as a cause of congenital anomalies in the rat. Science, 117:535, 1953.
Cooper, L. Z., Green, R. H., and Krugman, S. Neonatal thrombosytopenic purpura and other manifestations of rubella contracted in utero. Am. J. Dis. Child., 110:416, 1965.
and Krugman, S. Diagnosis and management: congenital rubella. Pediatrics, 37:335, 1966.
Courtney, R. H., and Hill, E. Hereditary juvenile glaucoma simplex. J. A. M. A., 97:1602, 1931.
Custodis, E. Die einseitige Hydrophthalmus heritarius und seine Erbpflege. Klin. Monatsbl. Augenheilk 102:242, 1939.
de Meyer, R. Action tératogène du galactose administré a la rate gravide. An. Endocrinol., 20:203, 1959.
Derby. H. C. Three cases of hydrophthalmos treated with iridectomy. Arch. Ophthalmol. 11:37, 1882.
Derer, J. Familiarny glaucom juvenilny. Bratislav. Lekarske Listy, 10:600, 1930.
Drance, S. M. The significance of the diurnal tension variations in normal and glaucomatous eyes. Arch. Ophthalmol., 64:494, 1960.
Editorial. Genetic disease. Canad. Med. Assoc. J., 98:414, 1969.
Eichenwald, H. F. The placental barrier and infections of the fetus. Birth Defects Original Artical Series, 1:74, 1965.
Engelking, E. Augenarztlich wichtige Rontgenschadigungen der Frucht nach bestrahlung schwangerer. Klin. Monatsbl. Augenheilk., 94:151, 1935.
Ericson, L. A. Twenty four hours variations of the aqueous flow. Acta Ophthal. Supp., 50, 1958.
Erickson, C. A. Rubella early in pregnancy causing congenital malformations of the eyes and heart. J. Pediat., 25:281, 1944.
Falls, H. F. A gene producing various defects of the anterior segment of the eye. Am. J.

Ophthalmol., 32:41, 1949.
Farner, D. A. The photoperiodic control of reproductive cycles in birds. Amer. Sci., 52:137, 1964.
Felden, E., and Halmai, O. Association of unilateral simple glaucoma with scleroderma on the same side. Szemeszet, 104:313, 1967.
Ferraro, A., and Roizin, L. Ocular involvement in rats on diets deficient in amino acids: 1. tryptophan. Arch. Ophthalmol., 38:331, 1947.
Follmann, P., and Vadasz, Z. Spontanes Glaucom beim Kaninchen, Klin. Monatsbl. Augenheilk., 146:355, 1965.
Franceschetti, A. Kurzes Handbuch der Ophthalmologie. Springer, Berlin, 1930. p. 712.
Frankelson, E. N., Lauber, J. K., and Boyd, T. A. S. The role of angle closure in light induced avian glaucoma. Can. J. Ophthalmol., 4:59, 1969.
Fraser, G. R., and Friedman, A. I. The Causes of Blindness in Childhood: A Study of 776 Children With Severe Visual Handicaps. Johns Hopkins Press, Baltimore, 1967.
Garrod, A. E., and Harris, H. Garrod's Inborn Errors of Metabolism. Oxford Univers., London, 1963.
Geltzer, A. I., Guber, D., and Sears, M. L. Ocular manifestations of the 1964-1965 rubella epidemic. Am. J. Ophthalmol., 63:221, 1967.
Geri, G. Considerazioni e recerche bull eredita dell idroftalmia nel coniglio. Ricerca Scientifica, 24:2299, 1954.
Gilbert, C., and Gillman, J. The morphogeneses of trypan blue induced defects of the eye. S. Afr. J. Med. Sci., 19:147, 1954.
Giroud, A., and de Rothschild, B. Repercussions de la thyroxine sur l'oeil du foetus. Co. R. Soc. Biol., 145:525, 1951.
and Martinet, M. Alterations de l'epithelium et des fibres du crystallin après thyroxine. Arch. d'Oph., 14:247, 1954.
and Martinet, M. Tératogénèse par hautes doses de Vitamin A en fonction de stades du developpement. Arch. Anat. Micr. Morph. Exp., 45:77, 1956.
and Martinet, M. Malformations oculaires avec fibrose du vitré chez des embryons de lapin soumis à l'hypervitaminose A. Bull. Soc. Opht. (Paris), 3:191, 1959.
Gregg, N. M. Congenital cataract following German measles in the mother. Trans. Ophthalmol. Soc. Aus., 3:35, 1941.
Further observations on congenital defects in infants following maternal rubella. Trans. Ophthalmol. Soc. Aus., 4:119, 1944.
Guerry, D. Congenital glaucoma following maternal rubella: a report of two cases. Am. J. Ophthalmol., 29:190, 1946.
Gyllensten, L. J., and Hellstrom, B. E. Experimental approach to the pathogenesis of retrolental fibroplasia: IV. the effects of gradual and of rapid transfer from concentrated oxygen to normal air on the oxygen-induced changes in the eyes of young mice. Am. J. Ophthalmol., 41:619, 1956.
Hague, E. B. The retino-hypothalamo-hypophyseal mechanism: new concepts. Kresge Eye Inst. Bull., 10:3, 1966.
Hale, F. The relation of Vitamin A to anophthalmos in pigs. Am. J. Ophthalmol., 18:1087, 1935.
Hamburg, M. The embryology of trypan blue induced abnormalities in mice. Anat. Record., 119:409, 1954.
Hanna, B. L., Sawin, P. B., and Sheppard, B. Recessive buphthalmos in the rabbit. Genetics, 47:519, 1962.
Hanshaw, J. B. Cytomegalovirus complement–fixing antibody in microcephaly. N. Engl. J. Med., 275:476, 1966.
Hardy, J. B. Viral infections in pregnancy: a review. Am. J. Obstet. Gynecol., 93:1052, 1965.
Haskin, D. Some effects of nitrogen mustard on the development of external body form

in the fetal rat. Anat. Record., 102:493, 1948.

Heggie, A. D., and Weir, W. C. Isolation of rubella virus from a mother and fetus. Pediat., 34:278, 1964.

Hicks, S. P. Developmental malformations produced by radiation: a timetable of their development. Am. J. Roentgen., 69:272, 1953.

The effects of ionizing radiation, certain hormones and radiomimetic drugs on the developing nervous system. J. Cell. Comp. Physiol., 43:151, 1954.

Holm-Pedersen, E. Glaucoma juvenile, glaucoma adultum, glaucoma juvenile i tre generationer. Nordisk Med., 39:1615, 1948.

Hsia, D. Y. Inborn Errors of Metabolism, 2nd ed. Year Book, Chicago, 1966.

Ingalls, T. H., Curley, F. J., and Prindle, R. A. Experimental production of congenital abnormalities, timing and degree of anoxia as factors causing fetal deaths and congenital abnormalities in the mouse. N. Engl. J. Med., 247:758, 1952.

Jacobsen, L. Diagnostic radiology as a potential teratogen. Exerpta Med. Internat. Cong. Ser. No. 89, 1965. p. 6.

Jensen, L. S. and Matson, W. E. Enlargement of the avian eye by subjecting chicks to continuous incandescent illumination. Science, 125:741, 1957.

Kalow, W. Pharmacogenetics; Heredity and the Response to Drugs. Saunders, Philadelphia, 1962.

Kalter, H., and Warkany, J. Congenital malformations in inbred strains of mice induced by riboflavin-deficient galactoflavin-containing diets. J. Expt. Zool., 136:531, 1957.

Kalter, H. Drugs and congenital malformations. Abbottempo, 3:8, 1967.

Keerl, M. Das glaukom der jugendlichem. Inaug. Dissert. Leipzig. Emil Lehrmann, 1920.

Koby, F. E. Hydrophthalmia chez un porc, coincident avec une microphtalmie de l'autre coté. An. Oculist, 166:200, 1929.

Kolker, A. E., Moses, R. A., Constant, M. A., and Becker B. The development of glaucoma in rabbits. Invest. Ophthalmol., 2:316, 1963.

Korte, W. Beitrage zur erblichkeit des glaukoms. Klin. Monatsbl. Angenheilk., 102:664, 1939.

Kwitko, M. L. Anterior segment anomalies, a clinical pathologic report of conditions simulating congenital glaucoma. Can. J. Ophthalmol., 3:120, 1967.

Kwitko, M. L. Genetic aspects of the anterior chamber cleavage syndrome. Exerpta Medica No. 154. Amsterdam. Exerpta Medica Found., 1967, p. 80.

Lamy, M., and Frezal, J. The frequency of congenital malformations. First International Conference on Congenital Malformations, London, 1960. (Lippincott, Philadelphia, 1961.)

Langman, J. and van Faassen, F. Congenital defects in the rat embryo after partial thyroidectomy of the mother animal: a preliminary report on the eye defects. Am. J. Ophthalmol., 40:65, 1955.

Lauber, J. K., Schutze, J. V., and McGinnis, J. Effects of exposure to continuous light on the eye of the growing chick. Proc. Soc. Exp. Biol. Med., 106:871, 1961.

and McGinnis, J. Eye lesions in domestic fowl reared under continuous light. Vision Res., 6:619, 1966.

McGinnis, J., and Boyd, J. E. Influence of miotics, diamox and vision occluders on light-induced buphthalmos in domestic fowl. Proc. Soc. Exp. Biol. Med., 120:572, 1965.

Laurent, C., Royer, J., and Noel. G. Syndrome de Turner et glaucome congenitale. Bull. Soc. d'Ophtalmol de France, 5:367, 1961 (No. 5-6).

Lee, P. Gonioscopic study of hereditary buphthalmia in rabbits. Arch. Ophthalmol., 79:775, 1968.

Lefebvres, J. Role tératogène de la déficience en acide pantothenique chez le rat. An. Méd., 52:225, 1951.

Lehmann, H., and Huntsman, R. G. Man's Haemoglobins: Including the Haemoglobinopathies and Their Investigation. Lippincott, Philadelphia, 1966.
Lejeune, J., Gauthier, M., and Turpin, R. Les chromosomes humains en culture de tissues. Co. R. Acad. Sci., 248:602, 1959.
Le Vann, L. J. Congenital abnormalities in children born in Alberta during 1961: a survey and hypothesis. Can. Med. Assoc. J., 89:120, 1963.
Lohlein, W. Das Glaukom der Jugendlichen. Graefe's Arch. Ophthal., 85:393, 1913.
On juvenile glaucoma. Bericht. 39, Versanmlung der Ophthalmologischen Gesellschaft, Heidelberg, 1913, p. 96-113.
Lowe, C. U., Terrey, M., and MacLachlan, E. A. Organic-aciduria, decreased renal ammonia production, hydrophthalmos and mental retardation. Am. J. Dis. Child., 83:164, 1952.
MacMahon, B. Prenatal x-ray exposure and childhood cancer. J. Nat. Cancer Inst., 28:1173, 1962.
McIntosh, R., Merritt, K. K., Richards, M. R., Samuels, M. H., and Bellows, M. T. The incidence of congenital malformations: a study of 5,964 pregnancies. Pediatrics, 14:505, 1954.
McMaster, P. R. B. Decreased aqueous outflow in rabbits with hereditary buphthalmia. Arch. Ophthalmol., 64:388, 1960.
and Macri, F. J. The rate of aqueous humor formation in buphthalmic rabbit eyes. Invest. Ophthalmol., 6:84, 1967.
Medearis, D. N. Observations concerning human cytomegalovirus infection and disease. Bull. Johns Hopkins Hosp., 114:181, 1964.
Viral infections during pregnancy and abnormal human development. Am. J. Obstet. Gynecol., 90:1140, 1964.
Menaker, M. Extraretinal light perception in the sparrow: I. entrainment of the biological clock. Proc. Nat. Acad. Sci. U.S.A., 59:414, 1968.
Mendel, G. Versuche uber Pflanzen-hybriden. Verh. natur-forsch. ver., Brunn, 4:3, 1866 (Meeting of February 8th and March 8th, 1865).
Miller, M., Robbins, J., Fishman, R., Medenis, R., and Rosenthal, I. A chromosomal anomaly with multiple ocular defects. Am. J. Ophthalmol., 55:901, 1963.
Montif, G. R. C., Avery, G. B., Korones, S. B., and Sever, J. L. Postmortem isolation of rubella virus from three children with rubella syndrome defects. Lancet, 1:723, 1965.
Murphy, M. L., and Karnofsky, D. A. Effect of azaserine and other growth inhibiting agents on fetal development of the rat. Cancer, 9:955, 1956.
A comparison of the teratogenic effects of five polyfunctional alkylating agents on the rat fetus. Pediatrics, 23:231, 1959.
Neel, I. V. A study of major congenital defects in Japanese infants. Amer. J. Hum. Genet., 10:398, 1958.
Nelson, M. M., Wright, H. V., Asling, C. W., and Evans, H. M. Multiple congenital abnormalities resulting from transitory deficiency of pteroylglutamic acid during gestation in the rat. J. Nutr. 56:349, 1955.
Baird, C. D. C., Wright, H. V., and Evans, H. M. Multiple congenital abnormalities in the rat resulting from riboflavin deficiency induced by the antimetabolite galactoflavin. J. Nutr. 58:125, 1956.
Neva, F. A., Alford, C. A., and Weller, F. H. Emerging perspective of rubella. Bacteriol. Rev., 28:444, 1964.
Nora, J. J., Nora, A. H., Sommerville, R. S., Hill, R. M., and McNamara, D. G. Maternal exposure to potential teratogens. J. A. M. A., 202:1065, 1967.
Oksche, A., Laws, D. F., Kamemoto, F. I., and Farner, D. S. The hypothalamohypophyseal neurosecretory system of the white-crowned sparrow, zontrichia, Leucophyrs Gambelli. Z. Zellforsch., 51:1, 1959.

Parkman, P. D., Beuscher, E. L., and Artenstein, M. S. Recovery of rubella virus from army recruits. Proc. Soc. Exper. Biol. Med., 111:225, 1962.

Pike, R. L. Congenital cataract in albino rats fed different amounts of tryptophan and niacin. J. Nutr., 44:191, 1951.

Posner, A., and Schlossmann, A. The clinical course of glaucoma: a review of 474 cases from private practice. Am. J. Ophthalmol., 31:915, 1948.

Reed, H., Briggs, J. N., and Martin, J. K. Congenital glaucoma, deafness, mental deficiency and cardiac anomaly following attempted abortion. J. Pediat., 46:182, 1955.

Reese, A. B. Congenital cataract and other anomalies following German measles in the mother. Am. J. Ophthalmol., 27:483, 1944.

and Ellsworth, R. M. The anterior chamber cleavage syndrome. Arch. Ophthalmol., 75:307, 1966.

Roberts, A. L. Viruses and pregnancy. Therapeutic Notes, 74c:59, 1967.

Robinson, G. C., Watt, J. A., and Scott, E. A study of congenital blindness in British Columbia: methodology and medical findings. Can. Med. Assoc. J. 99:831, 1968.

Rochon-Duvigneaud, A. Un cas de buphthalmie chez le lapin: étude anatomique et physiologique. An. Oculist, 158:401, 1921.

Rochen, J. W. Kammerwinkelstudien. Graefe Arch. Ophthal., 158:310, 1957.

Rohen, J. W. Das Sehorgan der Primaten, in Primatologia: Handbuch der Primatenkunde, Vol. 2, part 6. Karger, Basel, 1962.

Rones, B. The relationship of German measles during pregnancy to congenital ocular defects. Med. An. D. C., 13:285, 1944.

Roy, F. H., Hiatti, R. L., Korones, S. B., and Roane, J. Ocular manifestations of congenital rubella syndrome. Arch. Ophthalmol. 75:601, 1966.

Fuste, F., Hiatti, R. L., Deutsch, A. R., and Korones, S. B. The congenital rubella syndrome with virus recovery: ocular pathology and literature review. Am. J. Ophthalmol., 62:222, 1966.

Ruch, R., and Wolff, J. Reparation of the fetal eye following radiation insult. Arch. Ophthalmol., 54:351, 1955.

X-irradiation effects of the human fetus. J. Pediat., 52:531, 1958.

Rudolph, A. J., Yow, M. D., Phillips, A., Desmond, M. M., Blattner, R. J., and Melnick, J. L. Transplacental rubella infection in newly born infants. J. A. M. A., 191:843, 1965.

Russell, L. B., and Russell, W. L. An analysis of the changing radiation response of the developing mouse embryo. J. Cell. Comp. Physiol., 43, Suppl. 1:103, 1954.

Saba, G. C., Saba, P., Carnicelli, A., and Marescotti, V. Diurnal rhythm in the adrenal cortical secretion and in the rate of metabolism of corticosterone in the rat: I: in normal animals. Acta. Endocr., 44:413, 1963.

Scheerer, A. Demonstration klinischer falle. Klin. Monatsbl. Augenheilk, 89:829, 1932.

Scheie, H. G. Address to Meeting of the Research for Prevention of Blindness, New York, 1968.

Schloesser, C. Acutes secundar-glaucom Beimkaninchen. Z. Vergl. Augenheilk., 4:79, 1886.

Schwalbe, E. Allgemeine Mibbildungslehre (Teratologie) ein Einfuhrung in das Studium der abnormen Entwicklung. Fisher, Jena, 1906.

Sedan, J., and Sedan-Baury, S. Depistage d'une glaucomatose latente chez deux jeune gens ayant une heredite de trois et quatre generations pour cette affection. Bull. Soc. Ophthal. France, 29, 1949.

Selzer, G. Virus isolation, inclusion bodies, and chromosomes in rubella infected human embryo. Lancet, 2:336, 1963.

Sever, J. L., Schiff, G. M., and Traub, R. G.: Rubella virus. J. A. M. A., 182:663, 1962.

Schiff, G. M., Bell, J. A., and Huebner, R. J. Rubella: frequency of antibody among children and adults and isolation of the virus from fetal tissue. J. Pediat., 65:1027, 1964.

Sheppard, B. L. The anatomy and histology of the normal rabbit eye with special reference to the ciliary zone (part 2). Arch. Ophthalmol., 67:87, 1962.
Siegel, M., Fuerst, H. T., and Peress, N. D. Comparative fetal mortality in maternal virus disease. N. Engl. J. Med., 274:768, 1966.
and Fuerst, H. T. Low birth weight and maternal virus diseases, a prospective study of rubella, measles, mumps, and hepatitis. J. A. M. A., 197:680, 1966.
Smith, A. U. The effect on foetal development of freezing pregnant hamsters (Mesocricetus Auratus). J. Embryol. Expt. Morphol., 5:311, 1957.
Smith, J. H. The blood aqueous barrier in hydrophthalmic rabbits.Ophthalmol.,108:293, 1944.
Smith, J. L., Cavanaugh, J. J. A., and Stone, F. C. Ocular manifestations of the Pierre Robin syndrome. Arch. Ophthalmol., 63:884, 1960.
Smith, M. E., Becker, B., and Podos, S. M.: Light-induced angle closure glaucoma in domestic fowl. Invest. Ophthalmol., 7:121, 1968.
Smythe, R. H. Veterinary Ophthalmology. Ballière, London, 1956, p. 215.
Sorsby, A. Opthalmic Genetics, 2nd ed. Appleton-Century-Crofts, New York, 1970, p. 31.
Stokes, W. H., Hereditary primary glaucoma: a pedigree with five generations. Arch. Ophthalmol., 24:885, 1940.
Swan, C., Tostevin, A. L., Moore, B., Mayo, H., and Barham Black, C. H. Congenital defects in infants following infectious diseases during pregnancy. Med. J. Aus., 2:201, 1943.
Congenital malformations in infants following maternal rubella during pregnancy. Trans. Ophthalmol. Soc. Aus., 4:132, 1944.
Study of three infants dying from congenital defects following maternal rubella in early stages of pregnancy. J. Path. Bact., 56:289, 1944.
Thiersch, J. B. Effect of certain 2, 4 diaminopyrimidine antagonists of folic acid on pregnancy and rat fetus. Proc. Soc. Expt. Biol. Med., 87:571, 1954.
Thompson, J. S., and Thompson, M. W. Genetics in Medicine. Saunders, Philadelphia, 1966, p. 2.
Tondury, G. Embryopathien über die Wirkungsweise (Infektionsweg und Pathogenese) von Viren auf den menschlicken Keimling. Springer, Berlin, 1962.
Aetiological factors in human malformations. Triangle, 7:90, 1965.
Tuchmann-Duplessis, H., and Mercier-Parot, L. Influence de trois sulfamides hypoglycémiants sur la ratte gestante. Co. R. Acad. Sci., 247:1134, 1958.
and Mercier-Parot, L. Production of congenital eye malformations, particularly in rat fetuses, in The Structure the Eye, G. K. Smelser, ed. Academic, New York, 1961, p. 507-520.
Unger, H. H., and Jankovsky, F. Capillary aneurysms in glaucoma. Arch. Klin. Exp. Ophthalmol., 173:323, 1967.
Van Duyse, M. L'heredite en ophtalmologie. Traite Ophthal., 1:896, 905, 984, 1939.
Waardenberg, P. J. Beobachtungen uber Vererburg im Grenzgebiete zwischen jugendlichem und altersglaukom, sowie zwischen kindliehem und jugendlichen Glaucom. Graefe Arch. Ophthal., 140:662, 1939.
Franceschetti, A., and Klein, D. Genetics and Ophthalmology. Thomas, Springfield, 1961, p. 565.
Warkany, J. and Schraffenberger, E. Congenital malformations induced in rats by maternal vitamin A deficiency: 1. defects in the eye. Arch. Ophthalmol., 35:150, 1946.
Weiss, D. I., Cooper, L. Z., and Green, R. H. Infantile glaucoma: a manifestation of congenital rubella. J. A. M. A., 195:725, 1966.
Weller, T. H., and Neva, F. A. Propagation in tissue culture of cytopathic agents from patients with rubella-like illness. Proc. Soc. Exper. Biol. Med., 111:215, 1962.
and Hanshaw, J. B. Virologic and clinical observations on cytomegalic inclusion disease. N. Engl. J. Med., 266:1233, 1962.

Werthemann, A., and Reiniger, M. Uber Augenentwicklungsstorungen bei Rattenembryonen durch Sauerstoffmangel in der Fruhschwangerschaft. Acta Anat., 11:329, 1950.
Westerlund, E. Etude clinique et genetique du glaucome primitif. Arch Ophthalmol, 9:495, 1959.
Wilson, J. G. Teratogenic activity of several azo dyes chemically related to trypan blue. Anat. Record., 123:313, 1955.
Experimental studies on congenital malformations. J. Chronic Dis., 10:111, 1959.
Wolter, J. R., Insel, P. A., Willey, E. N., and Brittain, H. P. Eye pathology following maternal rubella: a study of four children J. Ped. Ophthalmol., 3:29, 1966.
Wood, J. W., Keehn, R. N., Kawamoto, S., and Johnson, K. G. The growth and development of children exposed in utero to the atomic bombs. A.M.P.H. 57:1374, 1966.
Woolam, D. H. M., Millen, J. W., and Fozzard, J. A. F. The influence of cortisone on the teratogenic activity of x-radiation. Br. J. Radiol., 32:47, 1959.
Zweig, M., Snyder, S. H., and Azelrod, J. Evidence of a non-retinal pathway of light to the pineal gland of newborn rats. Proc. Nat. Acad. Sci., 56:575, 1966.

Embryology as Applied to Anterior Segment Abnormalities

CENTRAL NERVOUS SYSTEM DEVELOPMENT

After closure of the neural tube, brain tissue and spinal cord display a particular capacity for increasing their surface area by vigorous growth. In these two main components of the embryonic central nervous system, such growth progresses in a distinct manner depending on the locations of the various parts of the neural tube relative to each other and to their environment. Organogenesis therefore takes place under a variety of influences, one of the most important of which is called induction, the process by which groups of cells affect the growth and differentiation of surrounding cells. For example, ectoderm in the midline is inhibited from forming ocular rudiments by the surrounding notocord and mesoderm.

During the first month of life the brain anlage is embedded in a highly vascularized mesenchyma. At this time the neural tube is the most voracious consumer of nutriment in the entire cephalic region. This results in a rapid development noted especially in the area of the head, which grows much faster than its mesenchymal bed through which nutrient is obtained. The basal arteries and veins thus remain short while the neural tube and especially the brain anlage increase in length to a considerable degree.

For this reason, by the time the embryo has grown to 6 mm, (Fig. 1A) the brain, which is "bridled" by vascular trunks, appears bent. As a result of this flexed position the forehead hangs in front of the stomoschisis as far as the umbilical cord.

This pattern of development of the large blood vessels leads to the bellows type folds and bulges seen in the brain of a 10-mm embryo (Fig. 1B). Ectoderm does not participate in this folding, so that its basement membrane is stretched stiffly–resulting in an extreme lateral bulge. This is the beginning of the small and large hemispheres. Between the ectoderm and the inward folds of the upper neural tube the mesenchyme is swollen and

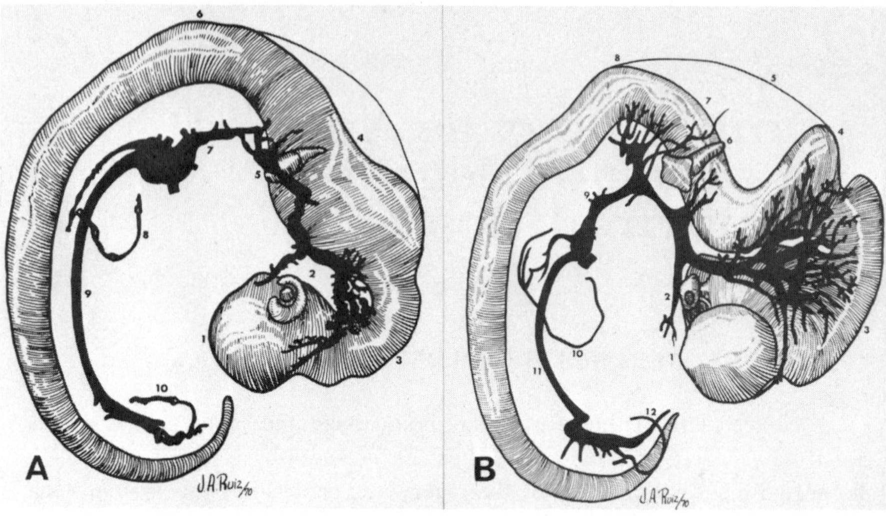

FIG. 1.A. In 6.3-mm embryo neural tube has lengthened faster than vascular system (black). (1) Cerebral hemisphere; (2) eye; (3) mesencephalon; (4) IVth ventricle; (5) ear vesicle; (6) cervical flexure; (7) supracardinal vein; (8) peripheral vein of arm anlage; (9) subcardinal vein; (10) peripheral vein of leg anlage. **B.** In the 10-mm embryo anchorage by the aortic arch takes place over ocular rudiment and superior to ear by the Vth cranial nerve. Brain anlage is thus flexed and forms forebrain, midbrain, hindbrain (prosencephalon, mesencephalon, opisthencephalon). Hindbrain, already appearing as rhombencephalon, results in marked lateral encroachment on pontine region, as do cerebral hemispheres. (1) Cerebral hemispheres; (2) eye; (3) mesencephalon; (4) cerebellum; (5) roof of IVth ventricle; (6) ear vesicle; (7) medulla oblongata; (8) cervical flexure; (9) supracardinal vein; (10) peripheral vein of arm anlage; (11) subcardinal vein; (12) peripheral vein of leg anlage.

only here is there sufficient room for the vascular system to proliferate. The vessels form fanlike plexuses which are connected with neighboring fans of vessels by archlike formations of mesenchymal funiculi in the convexity of the head. The connections are made through the peripheral processes of the fanlike structures.

The growth of the surface area of the neural tube takes place against three principal forms of resistance: that offered by the enveloping tissues, that arising in the wall of the brain interior, and the pressure exerted by the cerebrospinal fluid. The neural tube cells developed by mitoses in the vicinity of the ventricle form plasmic processes which can be visualized with the electronmicroscope. These cells push upward to the nutritive surface of the pia mater. They quickly ramify to form an extensive marginal velum (the

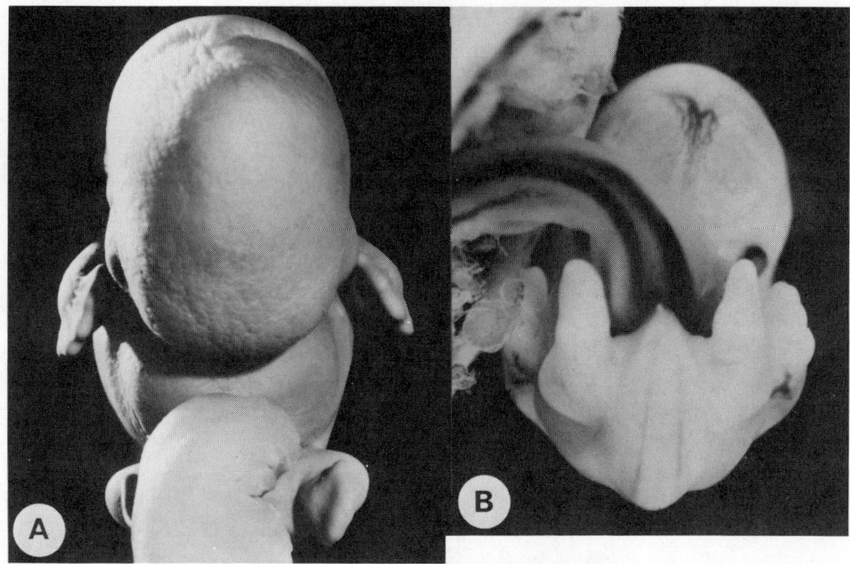

FIG. 2.A. Human embryo of 16.2 mm. Most of the head, which is bent forward almost down to navel, consists of brain; frontal region has already begun to assume form of twin cerebral hemispheres. **B.** Human embryo of 16.8 mm. Size of head is still large compared with trunk. (Courtesy of E. Blechschmidt.)

epicortical white) where the capsule of the brain yields laterally to the pressure of the pulsating blood vessels in the pia mater. The cell bodies become less crowded together underneath this marginal velum so that those pushing up from below have the opportunity as well as the inducement for emigrating provided by their need for nutrition. Thus the cortex begins to form. At the middle of the second month of pregnancy the human embryo of 16.2 mm has a spinal cord which comprises a narrow black inner zone near the central canal, a wide gray middle zone, and a white outer zone. The head at this stage is bent forward almost down to the navel (Fig. 2A). The frontal region of the brain has already begun to assume the form of twin cerebral hemispheres. As the embryo enlarges to 16.8 mm (Fig. 2B) the size of the head is still large compared with the trunk, and has a length only slightly larger than its width and breadth. At 27.2 mm (Fig. 3) the brain is large in size compared with the thin paries. The heavily capillarized pia mater fits closely along the entire brain and spinal cord. In the temporal region the brain has become laterally concave while near the falx cerebri, expansion is slight.

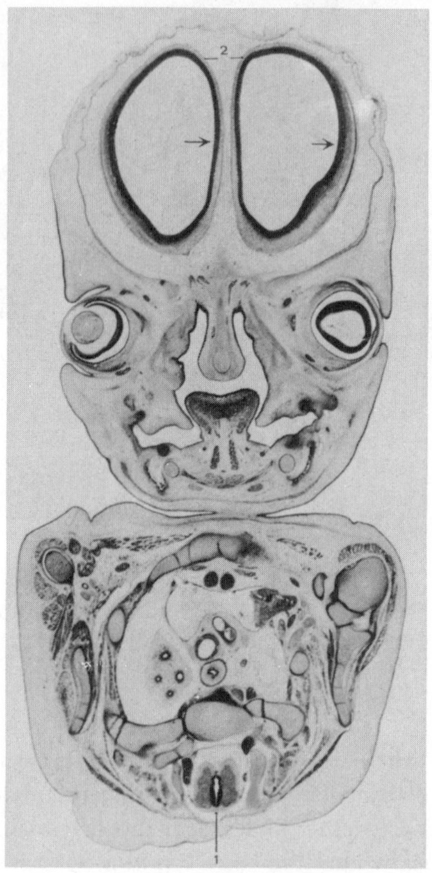

FIG. 3. Human embryo of 27.2 mm. Section cuts through strongly inclined brain and spinal cord at right angles. Note large size of brain compared with thin paries, and very small section of spinal cord (1) which is in turn very narrow compared with lining of trunk. Heavily capillarized pia mater (2) fits closely along entire brain and spinal cord. As in the following photographs, arrows indicate layer of mitoses taking place near ventricles. Cells thus multiply in order to send out processes toward surface of the pia mater. (Courtesy of E. Blechschmidt.) X 11.2.

In the medial section of each hemisphere the transition from the black zone to a white zone is direct (Fig. 4), while in the lateral region an intermediate gray zone is also present. The nuclei of the medial section as well as the thin processes of the cell bodies are almost all perpendicular to the pial surface of the brain. The black zone stains intensively due to the large number of cell nuclei.

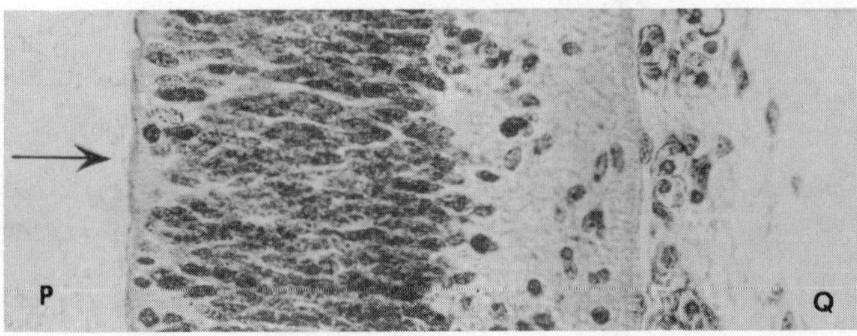

FIG. 4. Medial cerebral wall of 16-mm embryo. Position corresponds to left-hand arrow in Fig. 3. Between (P) lateral ventricles and (Q) pia mater is intensively stained inner zone on left which is rich in nuclei and therefore appears almost black; pale-staining white outer zone on right. Nuclei as well as thin processes of cell bodies (which are just barely visible under light microscope) are almost all perpendicular to pial surface of brain (Courtesy of E. Blechschmidt.) X 450.

The developmental potential of the pia mater of the lateral cerebral wall is greater than in the medial wall. Growth of the surface area is therefore more intensive laterally than medially. In addition, the surrounding body wall yields slightly to the pressure of growth exerted by the pulsating upper surface of the brain. Owing to the ingrowth of cells from the deep layer, the area near the pia mater appears to be much larger than in the area proximal to the ventricles. In the gray zone, the cell bodies no longer appear to be all perpendicular to the surface but usually assume a spherical form (Fig. 5). Both the spinal cord and the brain are separated

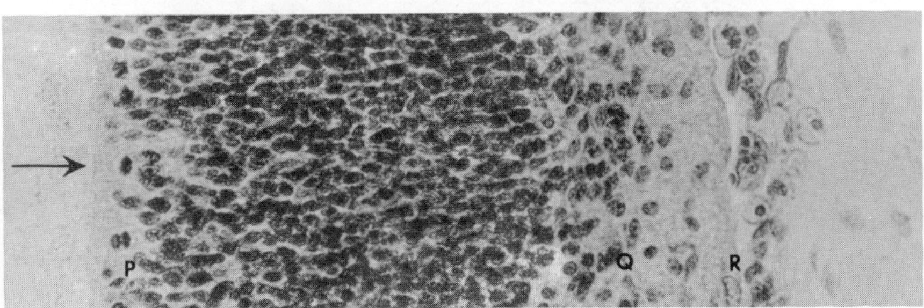

Fig. 5. Lateral cerebral wall of 16-mm embryo. Owing to ingrowth of cells from deep layer, layer near pia mater appears to be much larger than in proximity of ventricles. In gray zone all cell bodies no longer appear to be perpendicular to the surface, but usually assume spherical form, as the cell bodies have obtained more space. (P) black layer; (Q) gray layer; (R) white layer. (Courtesy of E. Blechschmidt.) X 450.

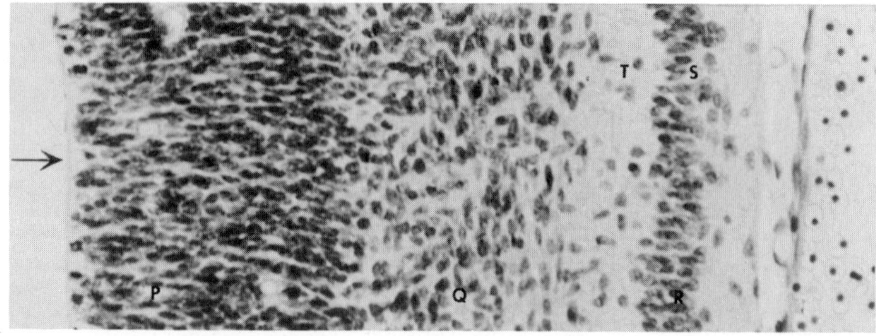

FIG. 6. Lateral cerebral wall of 27.2-mm embryo. Wide cell bodies with correspondingly large nuclei are now at (S) in white zone (T). Cortex has attached itself to pia mater in form of what might be called a marginal velum and separated itself from middle gray zone (Q) with growth of surface area of the pia mater, similar to the process illustrated in Fig. 7. (Courtesy of E. Blechschmidt.)

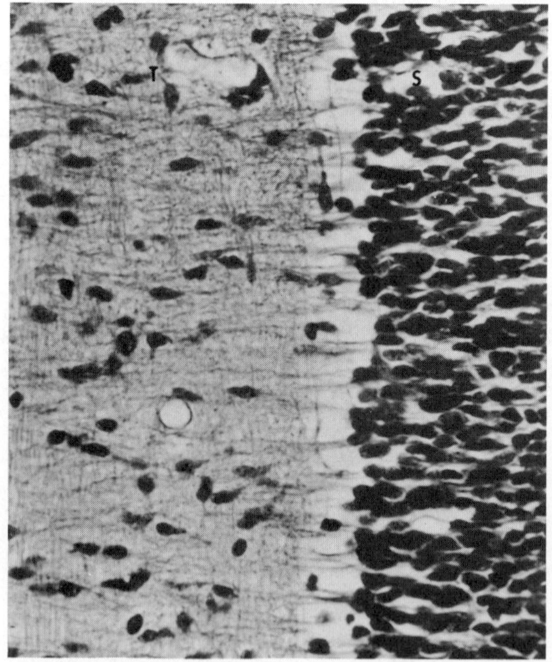

FIG. 7. Cortical zone of outer layer of 50-mm embryo and neighboring subcortical layer, corresponding to (T) and (S) in Fig. 6. Zone of cleavage corresponds to kinetic field (T) in Fig. 6 and is rich in intercellular substance. (Courtesy of E. Blechschmidt.) X 701.

from their environment at this stage by the pia mater, which is provided with a rich network of capillaries.

The gray zone in the brain as well as the spinal cord is a mixed area of thick cell bodies containing nuclei and narrow processes. When the embryo has reached the 27-mm stage (Fig. 6), the wide cell bodies with their correspondingly large nuclei have migrated to the white zone.

By the 50-mm stage growth is rapid and with reasonable precision takes the path of least resistance offered dorsally, while laterally it is inhibited at the sclerotomes. The formation of processes from the cell bodies is determined by the particular method by which the neural tube is embedded locally and is thus directly dependent upon the development of the pia mater. As the brain grows and its area increases, the cell bodies on the border between the subcortical and cortical layers separate parallel to the surface (Fig. 7). With the increase in circumference of the pia mater the cortex parts from its subcortical structures to which it is indirectly attached by the dendrites of the marginal velum. The cells in the mitotic layer near the ventricles which extend their processes in the direction of the upper surface of the pia mater are the first glia cells. From these arise the first ganglioblasts as anlagen of embryonal neurons.

OCULAR DEVELOPMENT

The eye is derived from three sources. The parts forming the outer coats and accessory structures come from mesoderm, while the parts concerned directly with visual function come from the neural tube and surface ectoderm.

Once the optic primordium is formed, the ocular rudiments develop by a budding-out process of the primitive forebrain as two hollow diverticula projecting from the lateral aspects of the forebrain during the third week before the anterior end of the neural tube closes. After closure, these structures are known as optic vesicles and project from the sides of the head. The distal portion expands while the proximal part, called the optic stock, remains narrow—forming a tract along which fibers of the optic nerve grow (Fig. 8).

The cornea, ciliary body, pupillary membrane, and iridocorneal recess do not exist in the first month of embryonic life. About the end of the fourth week, a small area of ectoderm overlying the optic vesicle begins to thicken. It is the proximity of this portion of surface ectoderm to the optic vesicle that stimulates the lens placode. A depression appears in the center of this thickening which deepens and invaginates so that its edges come together and fuse, enclosing a hollow sphere called the lens vesicle, which

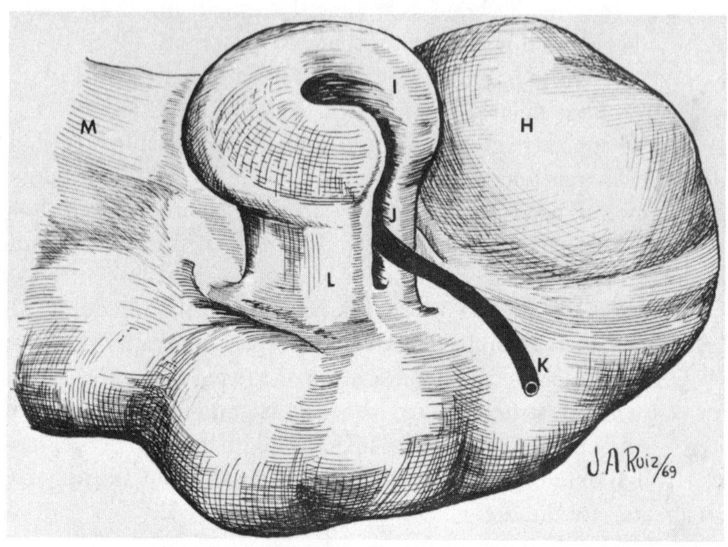

FIG. 8. Optic cup and choroidal fissure of human embryo about five weeks old, ventral aspect. (H) Telencephalon; (I) edge of optic cup; (J) choroidal fissure; (K) hyaloid vessel; (L) optic stalk; (M) thalamencephalon.

soon looses its connection with the surface ectoderm. When the surface ectoderm fails to react, true or primary aphakia results. This is quite rare and when present is associated with malformation of other parts of the anterior segment. Teratogenic agents acting during fetal life may result in a reabsorption of the lens subsequent to its development (secondary aphakia). Here the lens is represented by a wrinkled capsule which may be partially invaded and destroyed by vascular mesoderm.

The outer wall of the optic vesicle thickens and undergoes invagination forming a gobletlike structure called the optic cup, which consists of two strata of cells that are continuous with each other at the cup margin. The margins of the optic cup extend in front of the lens, reaching as far forward as the future aperture of the pupil. The invagination is not limited to the outer wall of the vesicle but also involves the caudal surface; it extends in the form of a groove for some distance along the optic stock, thus forming a wide gap called the choroidal fissure. Anophthalmos occurs during the period of organogenesis, that is, between the second and sixth week. Primary anophthalmos results from a failure of the optic vesicle to invaginate; only neuroectodermal elements and those surface ectodermal structures stimu-

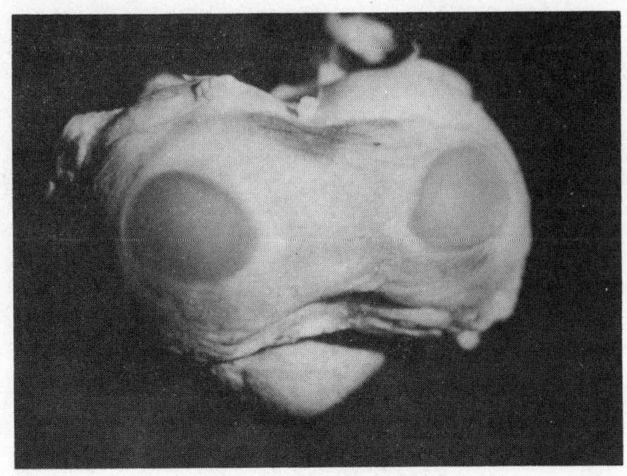

FIG. 9. Synophthalmus. (Courtesy of I. Michaelson.)

lated by the optic vesicle e.g., the lens is missing. Other mesodermal structures such as the corneal stroma, sclera, and extraocular muscles are present. Secondary anophthalmos is associated with a complete suppression of the entire forebrain. It is environmental in origin and generally not compatible with life. Malformation of the primitive forebrain is a rare occurrence that may result in a fusing of the optic vesicles to a varying degree. Cyclopia refers to those cases where there is complete fusion of the ocular rudiments to form what appears to be a single eye in the middle of the forehead. When there is incomplete fusion of elements of the two eyes the condition is referred to as synophthalmus, an example of which is shown in Fig. 9. Fig. 10 illustrates the variety of cyclopic defects that may be found. Another anomaly associated with failure of the optic cup to invaginate is congenital cystic eye. In this case, the lens is excluded from the optic cup or only partially invaginated. When a primary failure in lid formation takes place, mesoderm in front of the embryonal lens becomes transformed into skin, resulting in cryptophthalmia.

Mesenchyme extends into the optic stock and optic cup through the choroidal fissure, carrying with it the hyaloid artery (Fig. 8). As growth and development proceeds, the edges of the fissure become approximated and close during the seventh week. The artery is included in the distal portion of the stock. A highly critical period exists between the fifth and ninth week of intrauterine life. Should the fetus be affected between the sixth and seventh week, before the choroidal fissure closes, ocular structure in the region of the fissure remain undeveloped, giving rise to a congenital coloboma

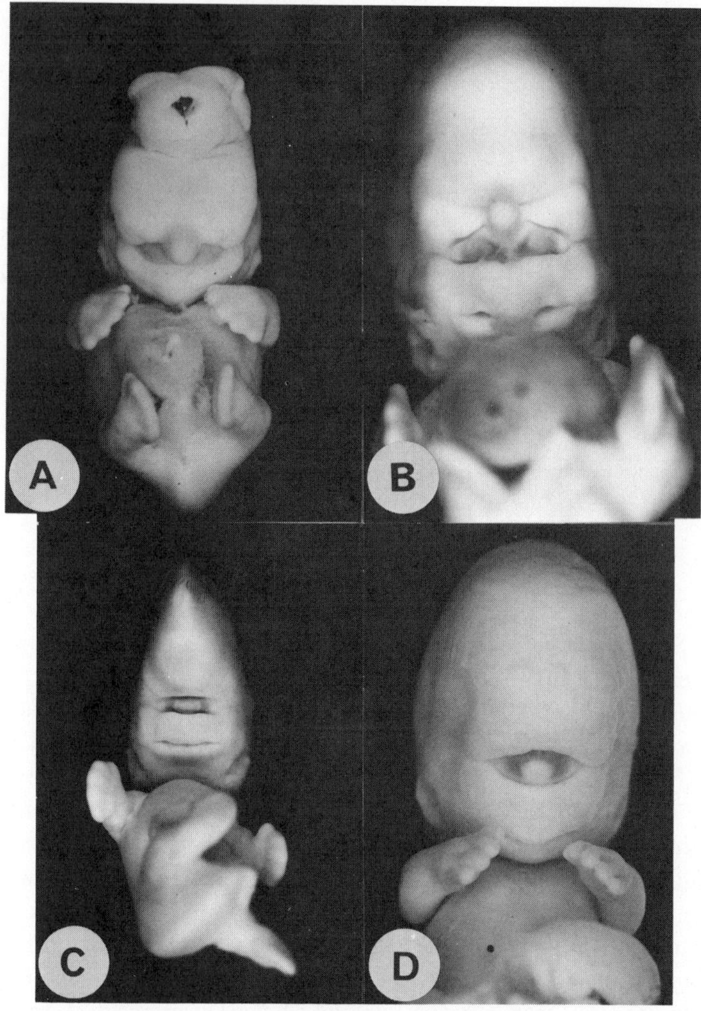

FIG. 10.A. Embryo; CR length 13 mm. X 4.5. **B.** Embryo; CR length 11 mm. X 7.5. **C.** Embryo; CR length 14 mm. X 3.8. **D.** Embryo; CR length 18 mm. X 4.5 (Courtesy of H. Nishimura.)

involving several structures, e.g., retina, choroid, lens and iris. After the seventh week, a coloboma of the iris alone occurs. With defective closure of the anterior portion of the choroidal fissure, the ciliary body is affected so that a portion is absent. Associated with this defect is a loss of zonular fibers which leads to an unequal pull on the lens capsule and a notch on the

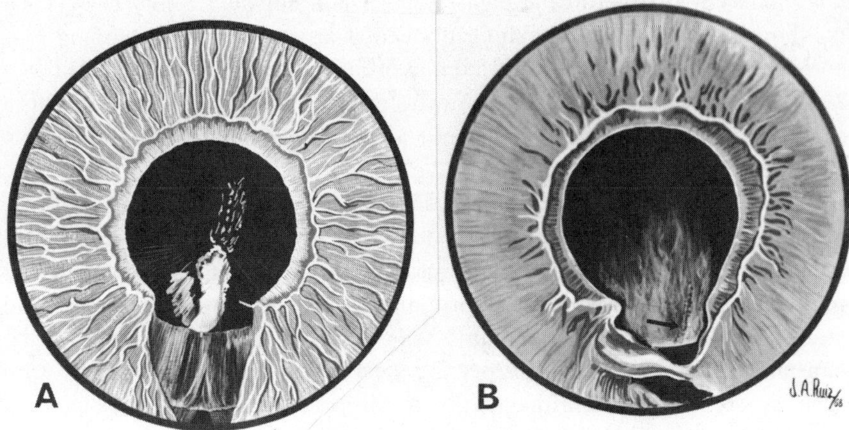

FIG. 11.A. Coloboma of choroid, lens, iris, and suspensory ligaments. B. Typical coloboma of iris with small strand bridging gap and row of pigment dots on lens (*arrow*).

affected side, i.e., a coloboma of the lens. Fig. 11A illustrates a coloboma of the choroid, lens, iris, and suspensory ligaments. Incomplete colobomata of the iris involve one or more, but not all, layers. The varieties include: (1) those cases in which both the stroma and pigment layers are defective

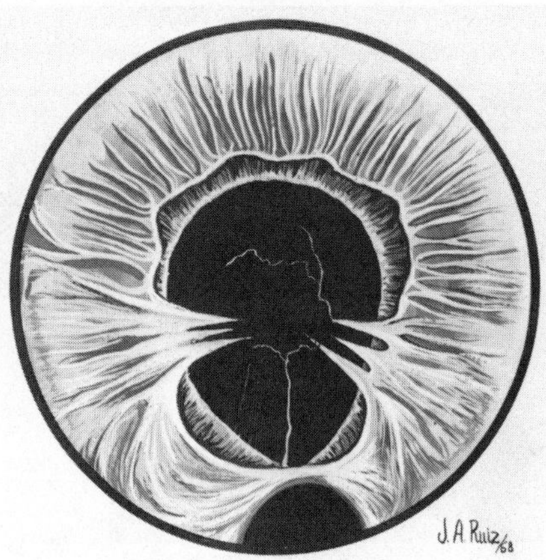

FIG. 12. Coloboma of iris with strand bridging gap and persistent pupillary membrane.

(bridge coloboma); (2) a defect in the stroma only and not in the pigment layer; and (3) a defect in the pigment layer and not the stroma. The typical coloboma is located in the inferior medial aspect of the developing eye, corresponding to the location of the choroidal fissure, and is inherited as a Mendelian recessive. Fig. 11B illustrates such a coloboma of the iris with a small strand bridging the defect and a row of pigment dots on the lens. Fig. 12 represents a coloboma of the iris with a strand bridging the gap, persistent pupillary membrane, and a persistent vessel on the lens opposite the defect. Colobomata appearing in locations other than the inferior medial aspect are termed atypical, and usually result from a persistence of mesoderm associated with the embryonic vascular system. As the fetal blood vessels pass over the margin and into the optic cup, depressions appear in the cup margin. Should the vessels persist, a variety of malformations may arise such as iris atrophy, aniridia and atypical colobomata.

An arrest in differentiation of the margin of the optic cup at the 70- to 85-mm stage (Fig. 13) results in aniridia. Other iris abnormalities arising early in embryologic development include polycoria, in which case there is an actual duplication of the pupil and sphincter muscle (Fig. 14). Polycoria is transmitted as an autosomal dominant so that a heterozygote would transmit

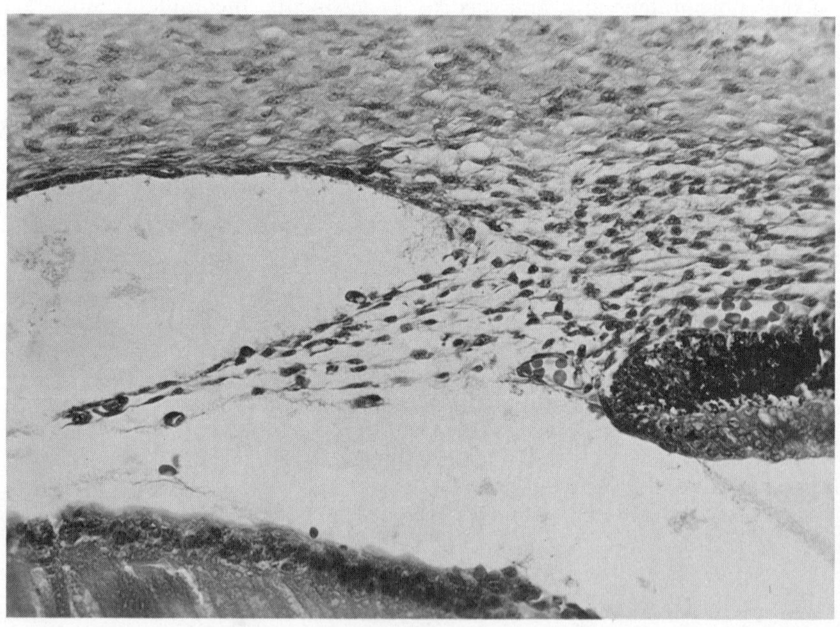

FIG. 13. Fetal eye at 85-mm stage. X 308. Margin of optic cup is beginning to differentiate. Structures of anterior segment are now evident.

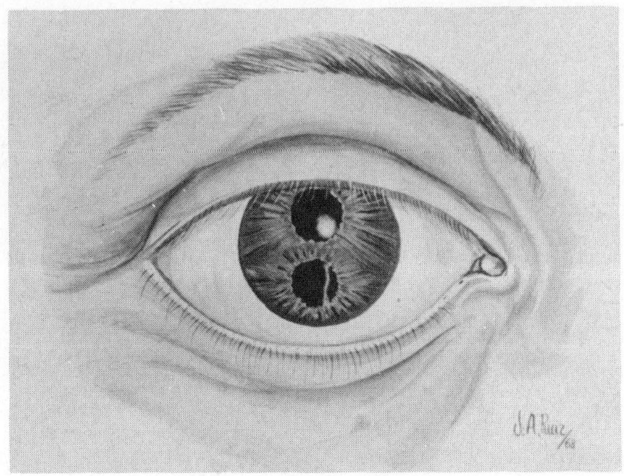

FIG. 14. Polycoria with duplication of the pupil and sphincter muscle. (Modified from Jaffe and Knie. **Am. J. Ophthalmol.** 35:253, 1952.)

this condition to 50 percent of his offspring. The iris may be also deformed due to dehiscence (splitting open) in iris tissue, or a diastasis (separation) at the iris root (Fig. 15). The two abnormalities may appear together in the

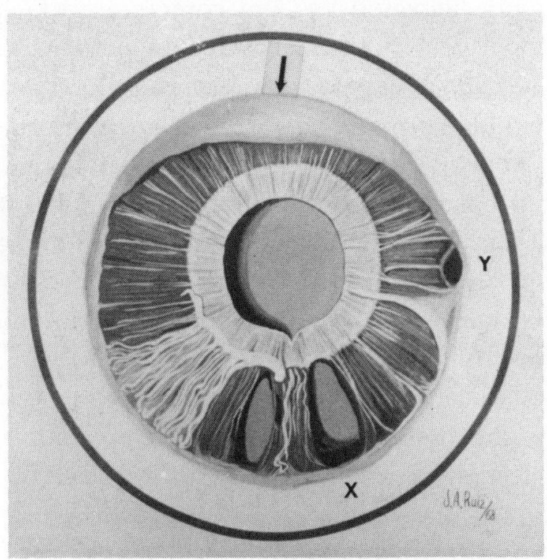

FIG. 15. Iris dehiscence (X) and diastasis (Y). The peripheral cornea is opacified (*arrow*).

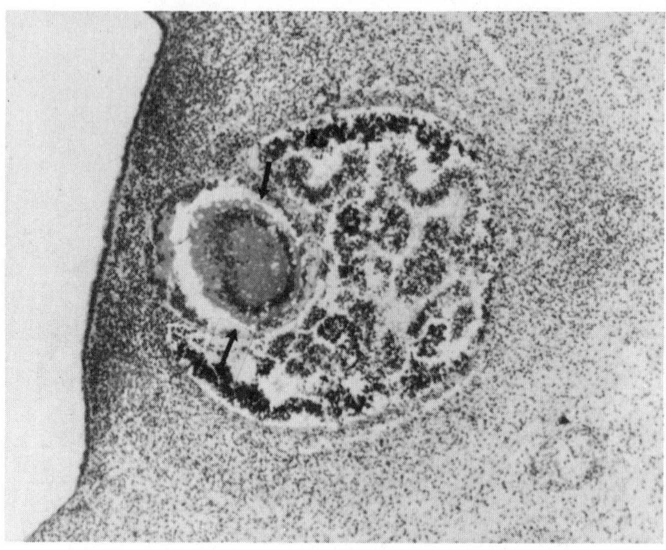

FIG. 16. Fetal eye at 22 mm, showing lens vesicle (*arrows*). X 60.

same eye, associated with peripheral corneal opacification as seen in the illustration.

Other iris abnormalities include anisocoria, which is transmitted as an autosomal dominant characteristic, and corectopia, which has a dominant hereditary tendency. The pigment epithelium of the iris is derived from neural ectoderm germinal tissue. Since the color of the iris depends upon the pigmentation of the stromal layer, underdevelopment of stromal tissue leads to an increase in translucency so that the ectodermal pigment and the sphincter muscle become visible. With hypoplasia of the peripheral stroma, Brushfield's spots may be seen. These defects consist of discrete white spots located at the junction of the middle and outer thirds of the iris. It is a common finding in mongolism (Down's syndrome). Albinism, an autosomal recessive trait, results from an insufficient production of the enzyme tyrosinase so that melanin pigment is not produced from tyrosine. The choroid, macula, and iris show retarded development. Heterochromia, a condition in which one eye is blue and the other brown is caused by either a defective sympathetic innervation on the side of the blue eye or an arrest in the development of iris pigmentation.

The retina is developed from the layers of the optic cup. The outer stratum of the cup persists as a single layer of cells that assume a columnar

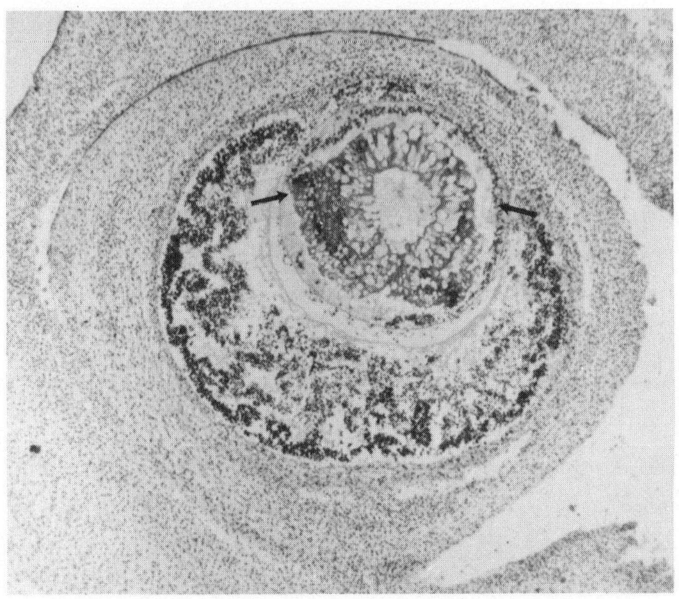

FIG. 17. Fetal eye at 35 mm, showing lens vesicle (*arrows*). X 48.

shape, acquire pigment, and form the pigmented layer of the retina, the pigment first appearing in the cells near the edge of the cup. The cells of the inner stratum proliferate, forming a layer from which nervous elements and supporting fibers of the retina, together with a portion of vitreous body, are developed. The inner stratum of that part of the cup which overlaps the lens does not differentiate into nervous elements. It persists as a layer of columnar cells that, together with the corresponding part of the pigmented layer, forms the pars ciliaris and pars iridica retinae.

The lens is developed from the lens vesicle which recedes within the margin of the optic cup and becomes separated from the overlying ectoderm by mesenchyme. Fine protoplasmic processes connecting the posterior surface of the lens vesicle to retinal cells of the optic cup are present at this early stage. The vesicle which at first fills a large part of the optic cup develops at a slower rate than the latter so as to remain proportionally smaller (Figs. 16 and 17). This allows the ciliary tract to come into relationship with the equator of the lens, while the margin of the optic cup which corresponds to the primitive iris comes to lie between the periphery of the cornea and the anterior border of the lens. The bundle of Drault contains fibers from the anterior portion of the developing vitreous which disappears

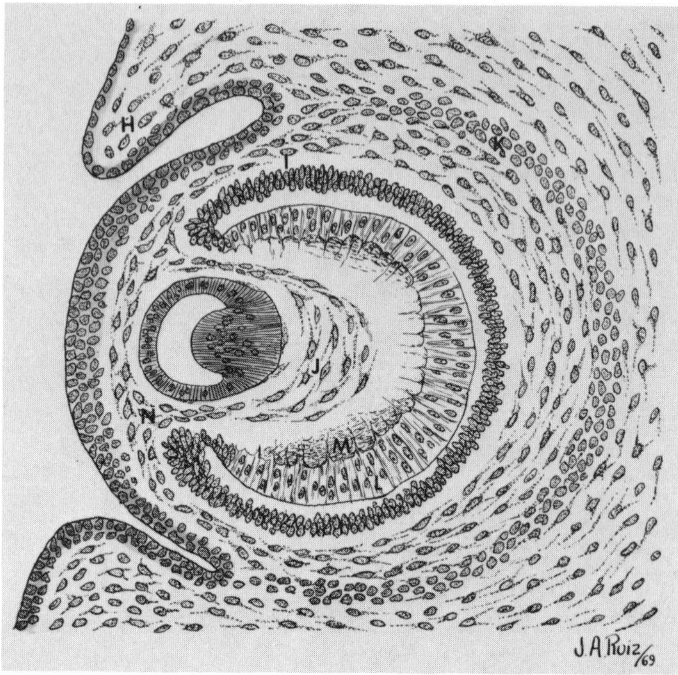

FIG. 18. Sagittal section through eye of human embryo about six weeks old. (H) Upper lid; (I) pigmented layer of retina; (J) mesenchymal part of vitreous body; (K) rudiment of sclera; (L) nervous layer of retina; (M) ectodermal part of vitreous body; (N) mesenchyme.

when the zonular fibers make their appearance.

The lens vesicle at first contains desquamated surface epithelial cells called epitrichial cells. The cells of the posterior wall of the lens vesicle, under the influence of the surrounding vascular network and proximity of the optic cup, thicken and elongate to form the primary lens fibers which grow into and fill the cavity of the vesicle (Figs. 18 and 19). The cells forming the anterior wall retain their cellular character and form the epithelium on the anterior surface of the fully developed lens. Once the lens capsule is laid down, the protoplasmic connections disappear. Fibers continue to be laid down in the periphery of the lens throughout intrauterine life and for some time after birth. The fibers are laid down in a disproportionate manner, thus changing the shape of the lens. As the cells elongate anteriorly and posteriorly, they fuse—giving rise to the Y suture. This takes place about the seventh week of intrauterine life. The development of lens fibers is most marked at the equator. It is from cells in this

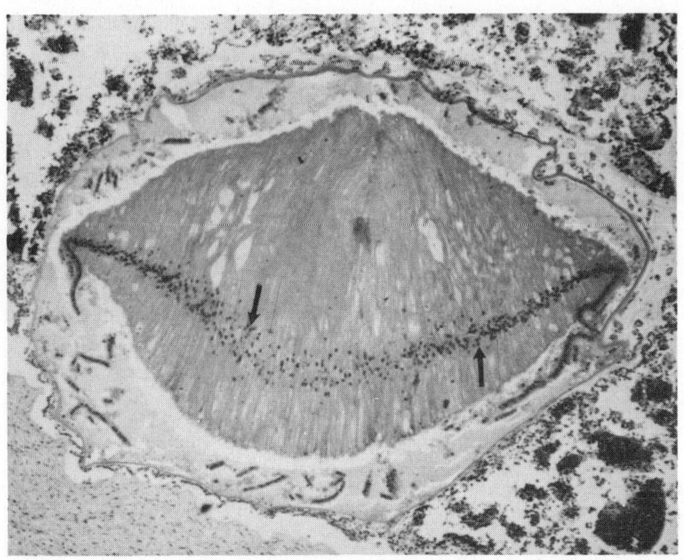

FIG. 19. Thirteen-week-old fetus, showing primary lens fibers (*arrows*). 110 mm. X 60.

region that the secondary lens fibers arise that form the bulk of the lens fibers in the adult (Fig. 20). As they develop and extend to each extremity, the Y suture becomes more complicated as the various cells are accommodated. The anterior lens surface may stretch and protrude, forming a cone (lenticonus). This condition occurs more commonly in males. Adhesions between the lens and iris may also be seen. During the fifth to the sixth month, the lens is spherical in shape. Further development may be arrested at this stage, resulting in microphakia or spherophakia. In this case the lens is small and spherical in shape, the anteroposterior axis being increased in size. The condition is often bilateral.

Any opacity of the crystalline lens is defined as a cataract. The inner portion, being the oldest, may be subjected to more adverse intrauterine conditions than the outer younger fibers. Because the lens grows continuously throughout life, almost all cataracts can be considered developmental in origin. In all cases, these are aberrations of development and not arrests. They may be an inherited result from some abnormality in intrauterine life, e.g., rubella (Fig. 21). When the lens nucleus fails to develop, it shrinks and calcifies, thus preventing the outer fibers from developing normally. Should a number of secondary lens fibers fail to reach the Y suture either anteriorly or posteriorly, a depression, called an umbilication, will result on the lens surface.

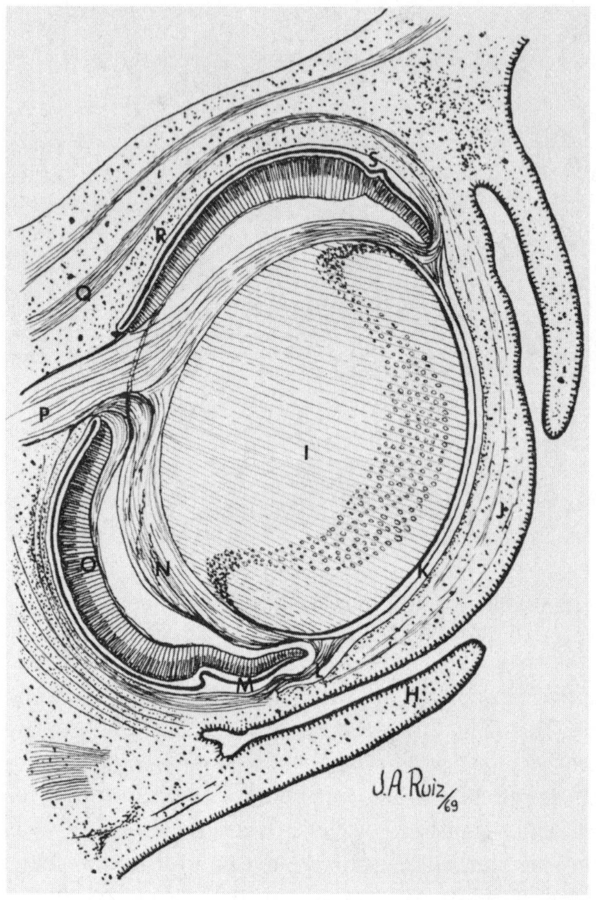

FIG. 20. Section through eye of rabbit embryo, about 18 days old. X 23. (H) eyelid; (I) lens; (J) cornea, (K) membrana pupillaris; (L) iris; (M) pars ciliaris and pars iridica retinae; (N) vitreous body (shrunken); (O) retina; (P) optic nerve; (Q) rectus muscle; (R) rudiment of choroid; (S) pigmented layer.

An example of cataracts developing in the postnatal period occurs in galactosemia. The child is unable to convert galactose to glucose so that the condition becomes evident in the first few weeks of life. The infant exhibits abdominal swelling and lens changes and shows evidence of malnutrition. The transmission is recessive.

The choroid and sclera are derived from the mesenchyme surrounding the periphery of the optic cup. The anterior part of the choroid is modified to form the ciliary body and ciliary processes. Marfan's syndrome is known

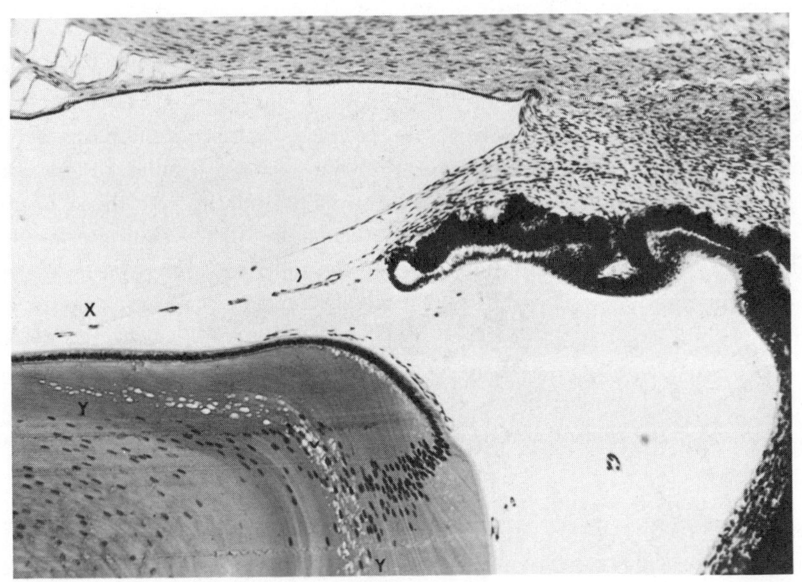

FIG. 21. Three-month fetus aborted from mother who suffered from rubella during first trimester. (X) Pupillary membrane; (Y) vacuolation of lens fibers. (Courtesy of D. A. Rosen.)

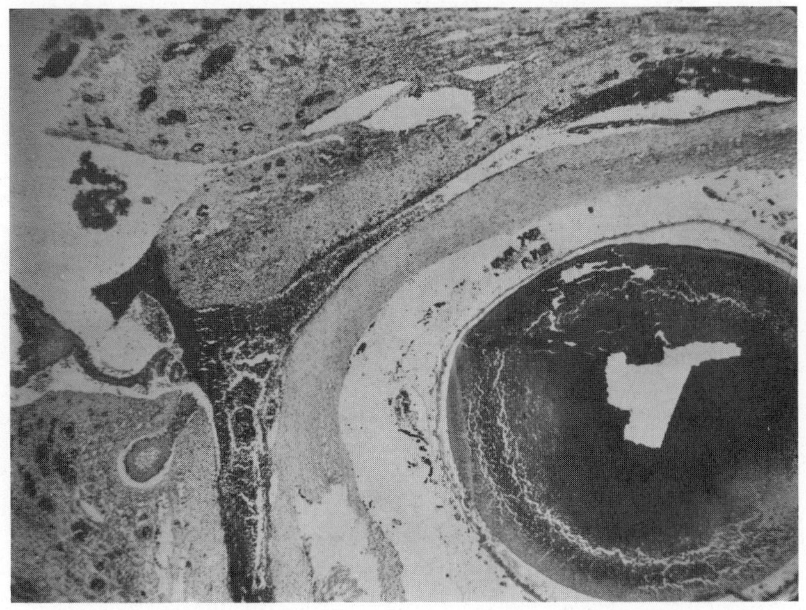

FIG. 22. Fetus at 160-mm stage, illustrating extraocular blood supply. X 27.

to be associated with an abnormal structure and arrangement of ciliary processes which is frequently associated with ectopia lentis. The origin of this abnormality may be during this period of embryological development. Dislocation of the lens—as seen in homocystinuria, Weill-Marchesani's syndrome, and Ehlers-Danlos syndrome—may have a similar origin. The fibers of the ciliary muscle are derived from mesoderm, but those of the sphincter and dilator pupillae are of ectodermal origin. The sphincter muscle of the iris is normally differentiated during the fourth to sixth month, before the dilator muscle makes its appearance. Therefore lack of a sphincter muscle as an isolated anomaly is very rare since a defect in the neural ectoderm at this early stage is usually associated with widespread abnormalities. An arrest in the last phase of neural ectoderm differentiation results in an absence of the dilator muscle alone, as the sphincter is already developed. The result is microcoria or congenital miosis.

According to Mann the hyaloid artery breaks up into branches and forms the fetal intraocular vascular system, which consists of two main sets of blood vessels. The first set forms a network on the posterior surface of the lens and drains forward around the equator into the annular blood vessel. The second set of blood vessels ramifies in the vitreous and anastomoses with the first set anteriorly.

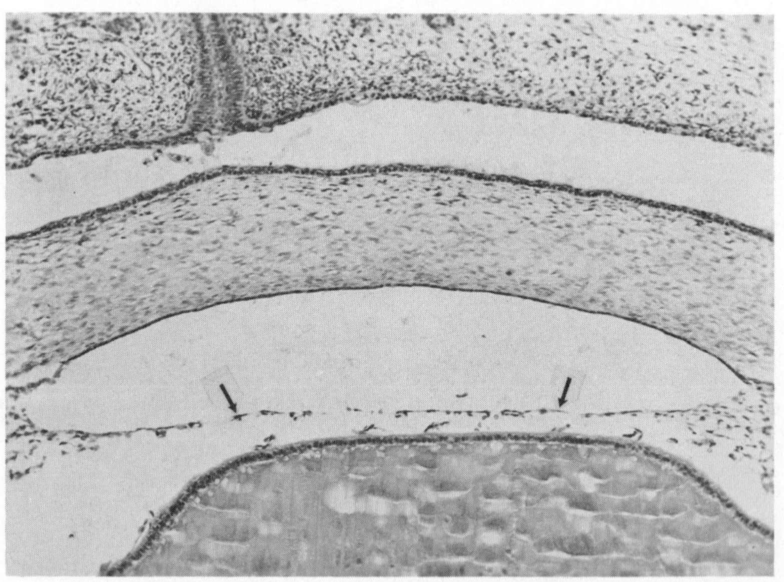

FIG. 23. Pupillary membrane in 85-mm fetal eye (*arrows*). X 98.

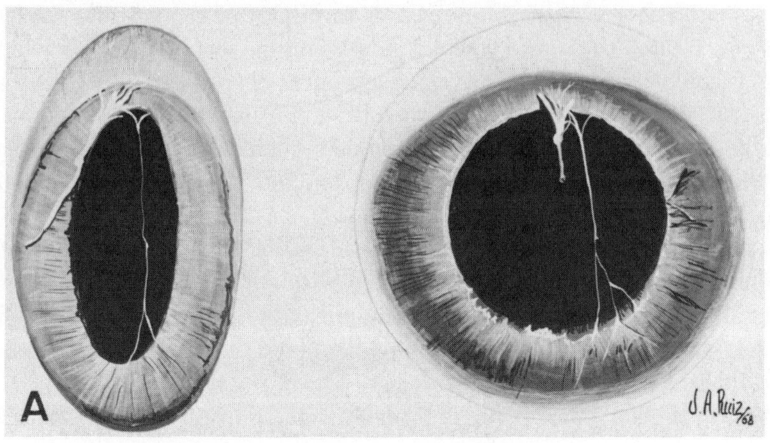

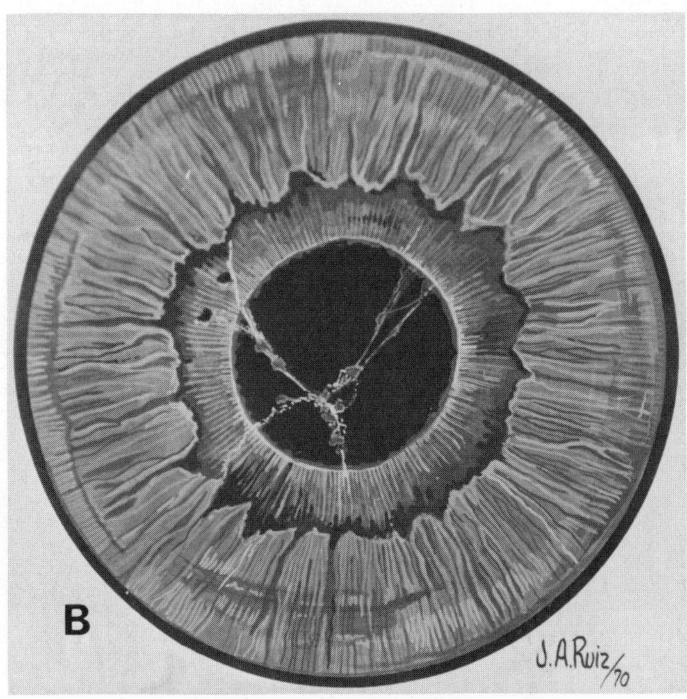

FIG. 24.A. Pupillary membrane, front view and profile. Superior corneal margin is scleralized. **B.** Pupillary membrane. Fine pigmented filaments cross the pupil. Anterior segment is otherwise normal.

The first or anterior blood vessels form part of the vascular capsule of the lens termed the tunica vasculosa lentis and the second or posterior blood vessels are known as the vasa hyaloidea propria.

After the 10-mm stage, the vascular arrangement of the embryonic eye can be divided into the extraocular blood system, which includes the vessels of the orbit and the primitive choroid, and the intraocular system, which consists of the hyaloid artery and its branches and the resulting vascular capsule of the lens. The extraocular blood system forms the rudiment of the definitive extraocular blood supply and with certain modifications persist. Fig. 22 illustrates an eye at the 160-mm stage in which the extraocular blood system is shown. The intraocular blood supply (derived from the hyaloid artery) atrophies.

The pupillary membrane is formed by the portion of embryonic tissue covering the anterior lens surface (Fig. 23). During the sixth month of development the central arcades that make up the pupillary membrane partly atrophy, leaving a minor vascular circle to supply the iris. These arcades and the associated mesodermal membrane may persist in a variety of forms that are collectively called persistent pupillary membrane. They appear as a nonpigmented strand of obliterated vessels that cross the pupil and find secondary attachments to the lens or cornea (Fig. 24A and B). The blood vessels supplying the posterior part of the lens capsule are derived from the

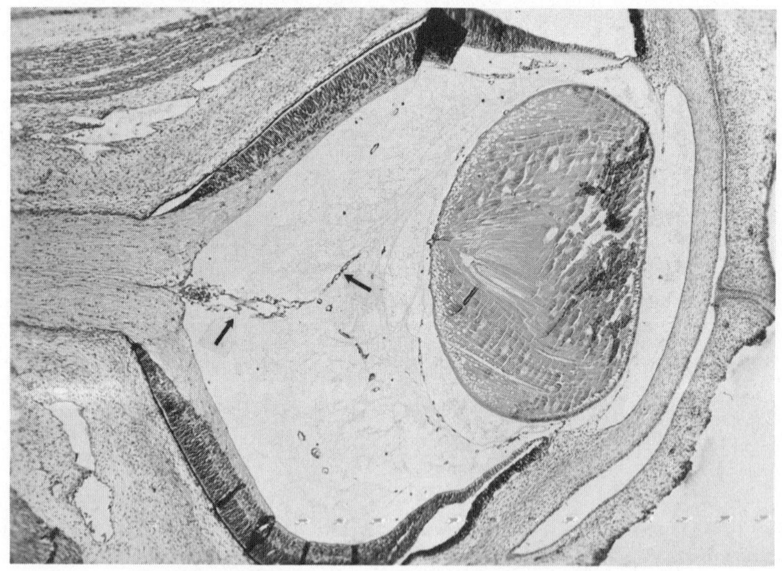

FIG. 25. Hyaloid artery in 60-mm fetal eye (*arrows*). X 52.

hyaloid artery. A triangular area of primitive mesenchyme located between the margin of the optic vesicle and anterolateral surface of the crystalline lens contains the vessel that will later constitute the major arterial circle of the iris. The anterior ciliary artery, which also originates in this area, contributes to the vascular membrane and supplies the anterior portion on the lens capsule. There is ample evidence to show the interdependence which exists between related structures. For example, should the hyaloid system fail to develop naturally, the vitreous body and retina are affected and microphthalmos may result even though other structures may develop normally.

By the second month of intrauterine life, the lens is invested by a vascular mesenchymal capsule. During the fourth month, the hyaloid artery (Fig. 25) gives off retinal branches and runs directly through the vitreous to the posterior surface of the lens where it breaks up into several nutrient blood vessels forming part of the tunica vasculosa lentis. A fragment of this fetal attachment may persist and adhere to the adult lens without impairment of vision. However, abnormal lens fiber development may take place secondary to this remnant–leading to a posterior polar cataract. An arrest in development causing a failure to atrophy may take place at the third month, leaving a part of the vascular tunic of the lens. It is quite

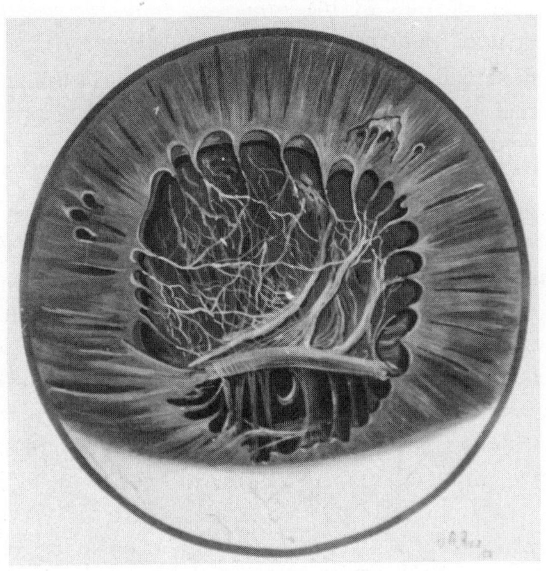

FIG. 26. Congenital atresia of pupil.

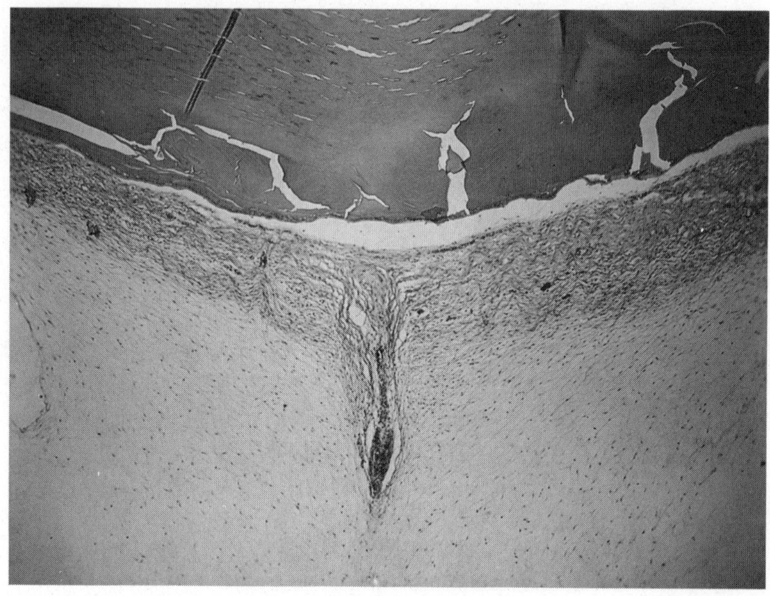

FIG. 27. Persistent hyperplastic primary vitreous.(A.F.I.P. Acc. Neg. 943372). (Courtesy of the Registry of Ophthalmic Pathology of the Armed Forces Institute of Pathology.) X 52.

common for some portion of the otherwise transient vascular system to persist either as patent blood vessels or strands of tissue.

If the hyaloid artery atrophies normally, the only remnant in the adult is the central canal of the vitreous (Cloquet's canal) but the proximal portion persists as the central retinal artery. In the newborn, the canal extends in a horizontal direction from the optic disc to the posterior aspect of the lens. With the loss of its blood supply, the tunica vasculosa lentis disappears, except for portions of the pupillary membrane that persist at birth, sometimes giving rise to the condition termed congenital atresia of the pupil (Fig. 26). The central hyaloid artery, even if it fails to atrophy, rarely remains in its entirety. Should the glial tissue persist, a plug of neuroepithelial tissue known as Bergmeister's papilla may be found on the optic disc. On rare occasions part or all of the hyaloid artery and vascular tunic on the lens remains. A condensation of primary vitreous may be present, giving rise to a fibrous retrolental mass termed persistent hyperplastic primary vitreous (Fig. 27).

The interrelationship of various parts of the eye may be seen in myopia, which may be due to faults in the cornea, depth of the anterior chamber, refractive power of the lens, or length of the eye.

The Anterior Chamber

Clefts and spaces that appear between various solid constituents and layers depend largely upon the degree of shrinkage that takes place. The fresher the specimen, the better the fixation and the fewer and smaller are the spaces that appear artifactitiously. According to Duke-Elder, the time and manner that the anterior chamber first makes its appearance is open to controversy because it is difficult to interpret fixed histologic specimens of a delicate tissue, although the structure is known to be present before the rim of the optic cup grows forward and inward to form the ciliary body and iris.

The anterior chamber is generally thought to be formed from the ingrowth in stages of the mesoderm that lies between the rim of the optic cup and the surface ectoderm. Ectoderm from the surface and neural ectoderm layers provide laminae that act as a scaffolding, which subsequently becomes permeated with mesoderm. The first ingrowth of mesoderm forms the corneal endothelium just before the 12-mm stage and a second ingrowth determines the corneal stroma. At the 18-mm stage a third wave of mesoderm forms the iris stroma and the pupillary membrane, extending axially posterior to the endothelium and anterior to the lens. The iris rudiment ends in the marginal sinus of von Szily. The cleft between the

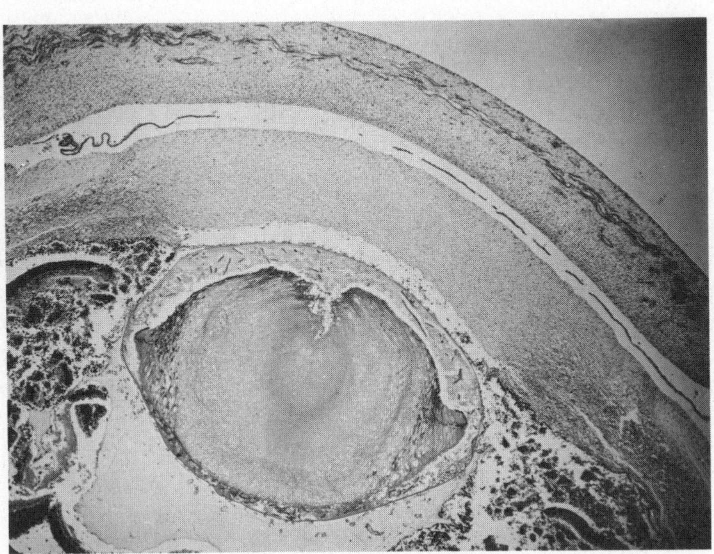

FIG. 28. Fetal eye at 160 mm, showing anterior chamber. X 24.

first and third mesodermal ingrowth is the anlage of the anterior chamber, which develops into a larger space as a result of the rapid growth of the anterior segment of the globe after the fifth month. Fig. 28 illustrates the anterior chamber of the 160-mm fetus.

At the seventh month of intrauterine life the pupillary membrane forms a relatively strong impermeable membranous structure, completely separating the posterior from the anterior chamber. Although resistant to tangential forces, it is readily broken when touched with glass microneedles. The vascular loops of the pupillary membrane contain blood and the intervascular webbing is covered by an endothelial layer which is continued directly onto the iris surface to the major collarette. The anterior chamber is temporarily free of fluid while the pupillary membrane remains intact, according to Worst. The intervascular webbing of the membrane disintegrates with maturation of the anterior segment, allowing an entry of free fluid from the posterior cavity—which may be a factor in deepening the anterior chamber.

Since vessels appear at an early stage of embryologic development and lie in intimate relationship with the primitive anterior chamber, fluid derived as a transudate from these primitive blood vessels may be noted in the anterior chamber before disintegration of the pupillary membrane takes place.

While the lens vesicle is separating from surface ectoderm, mesoderm migrates forward to form a single layer of cells called Descemet's mesothelium. Mesoderm then grows in from either side. The cells differentiate, forming lamellae which are laid down in a crosshatched manner. The epithelium of the cornea and conjunctiva is of ectodermal origin, derived from the superficial ectoderm where it closes over the lens vesicle. The principal portion of the cornea is of mesodermal origin and it is at this stage of development that deformities such as cornea plana and sclerocornea arise. In embryos of 20 to 30 mm the cornea measures 0.80 mm, while the opening of the optic vesicle measures 0.73 mm. By the end of the third month, the cornea measures 2.9 mm while the opening of the vesicle measures 2.8 mm. The pupillary opening during the third month is thus the

TABLE 1

CORNEAL TRANSPARENCY

	Cornea	Sclera
26th Day	moderate opaque	moderate opaque
Term	moderate opaque	moderate opaque
10 Days	almost translucent	opaque
18 Days	translucent	dense opaque

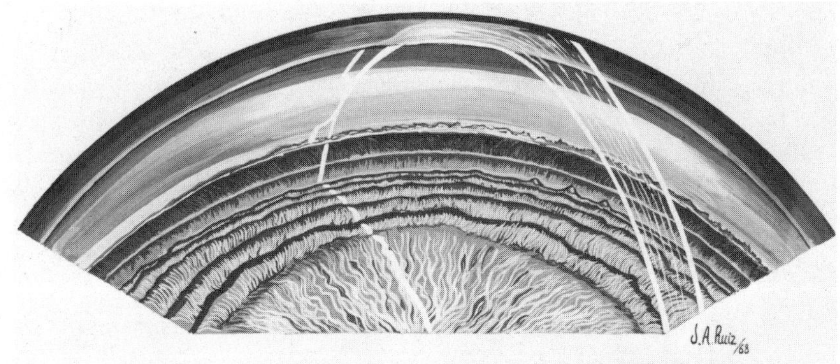

FIG. 29. Gonioscopic view of megalocornea. Features include deep anterior chamber, broad ciliary body band, unusually prominent scleral spur.

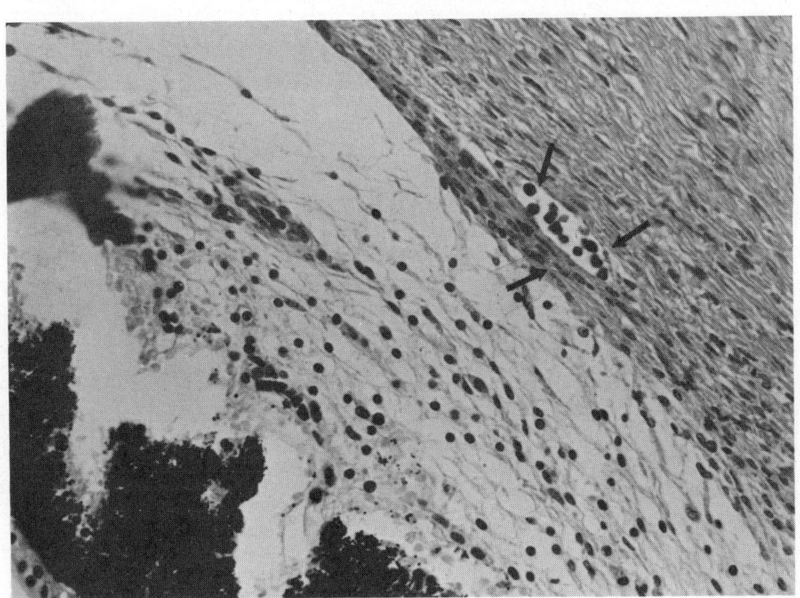

FIG. 30. Fetal eye at 135 mm. Red blood cells are evident in Schlemm's canal (*arrows*). X 270.

same size as the cornea. Disproportionate growth of the cornea leads to megalocornea (Fig. 29), which is usually associated with abnormalities in associated structures such that the ciliary ring is also enlarged.

Both the cornea and sclera are moderately opaque during early intrauterine life. As the fetus ages, the cornea becomes transluscent while the sclera becomes densely opaque (Table 1). The opening of the eyelids plays no role in determining the transparency of the cornea. Complete absence of the cornea occurs in conjunction with cryptophthalmos, in which case the skin of the forehead covers the eyes completely.

Keratoconus develops slowly after birth when there has been a failure of mesoderm to migrate to the central area of the cornea during embryonic life. The hereditary tendency is recessive or irregularly dominant. In the same way marked astigmatism may occur.

Angle of The Anterior Chamber

DEVELOPMENT. During the latter part of the third lunar month of gestation the canal of Schlemm makes its first appearance as a small plexus of venous channels within the fibers of the corneoscleral condensation, on the scleral side of the immature trabecular meshwork. At this time it is level with the deepest part of the angle of the anterior chamber and not in front of it, as in the term fetus. By the fifteenth week red blood cells may be seen in the canal (Fig. 30). However, according to Wulle, it is not until the fifth to sixth lunar month of gestation that aqueous humor begins to flow through the filtration system.

Wulle studied three human fetuses at the fourth lunar month and one premature infant at the eighth lunar month of gestation. The filtration angles were examined with the electronmicroscope. At the fourth month the canal consists of small branching vessels with a narrow lumen. Most of the endothelial cells lining the vessel (Fig. 31A) have a rather broad cytoplasmic body. The vessel wall is two layers thick in some places (Fig. 31B) and exhibits neither pores nor gaps. A material of low electron density, similar to basement membrane, exists at the base of the endothelial cells. Fibroblasts and fibrils of immature collagen lie close to the vessel both on its scleral and trabecular sides.

The cytoplasm contains a small amount of predominantly smooth surfaced endoplastic reticulum (Fig. 31C), many free ribosomes, a few lysosomes, and some small mitochondria with poorly developed cristae. Frequently large and small vacuoles—either empty or containing a flocculent material—are found in the cytoplasm of the cells (Fig. 31D). The junctional regions often show lap joints (Fig. 31E).

At about the fifth month a triangular wedge of dense scleral condensation appears immediately behind the canal of Schlemm, continuous with the longitudinal fibers of the ciliary muscle; it gradually consolidates to form the scleral spur, the full development of which is not achieved until birth. The filtration angle becomes evident two months after the canal of Schlemm has become visible or at about the sixth month. During development of the eye from the 120-mm stage to its adult size, the cross-sectional area of the angle increases more than six times, while the volume increase between the two stages is 35 times. As the angle gradually deepens, the mesoderm lying between the canal of Schlemm and the root of the iris consists of a solid mass of cells and fibers. With differentiation this tissue becomes laminated and ultimately forms the scleral and uveal portions of the trabeculum. As the angle deepens further, so as to lie in the mesodermal tissue between the corneoscleral condensation and the mesoderm forming the iris, the mutual relationship of the canal of Schlemm, the uveoscleral trabeculum, and the scleral spur remains fairly constant. Nevertheless, their position with regard to the angle of the anterior chamber changes continuously as the developing angle shifts posteriorly. At the same time an elongation of the innermost trabecular fibers takes place, contributing to the deepening of the anterior chamber. Thus by the sixth month (Fig. 32) the angle is level with the anterior border of the trabeculum. By the seventh month it lies above the middle of the trabecular fibers, with the canal of Schlemm and the scleral spur behind it. By the eighth month an outflow path already exists connecting Schlemm's canal with the scleral veins. At this time, according to Wulle, Schlemm's canal has a wide lumen throughout its whole circumference. The endothelial cells are thin (Fig. 33A), allowing apical and basal cell membranes to almost touch in some places. A basement membrane is not present. The low-density material at this stage is either situated some distance from the base of the cells and arranged in a band-shaped manner or equally distributed between the endothelium and the first layer of fibroblasts of the trabeculum. The canal no longer contains areas made up of two layers of endothelial cells as was seen in the fourth month; instead, its wall is formed by a single endothelial cell layer. The cytoplasm of the endothelial cells contains many pinocytotic vesicles (Fig. 33B) with about the same small amount of endoplasmic reticulum that was present at the fourth month. However, the mitochondria are larger and have more and better developed cristae. Large lysosomes and fine filaments are located in the cytoplasm (Fig. 33C). In junctional areas,

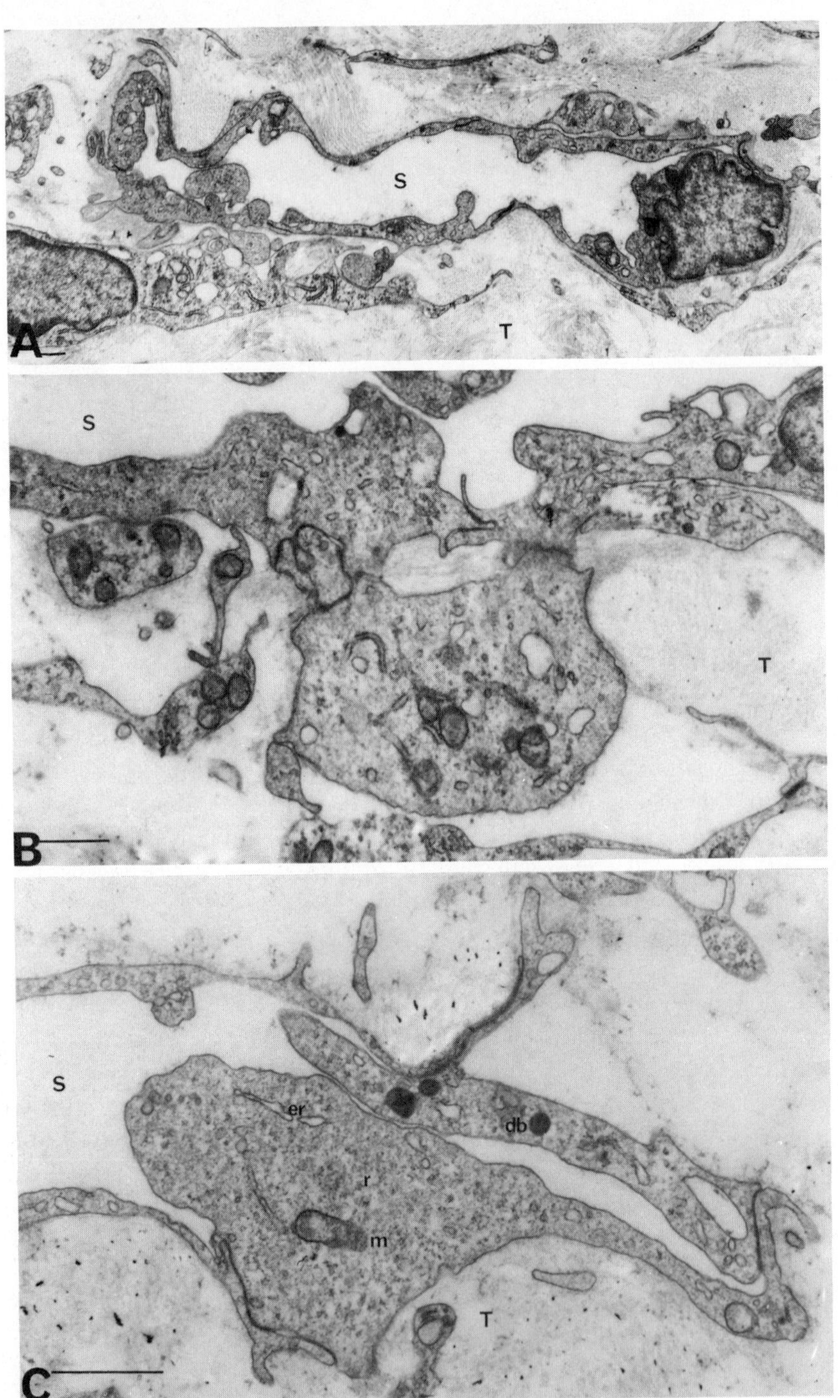
S
T
A
S
T
B
S
er
db
r
m
T
C

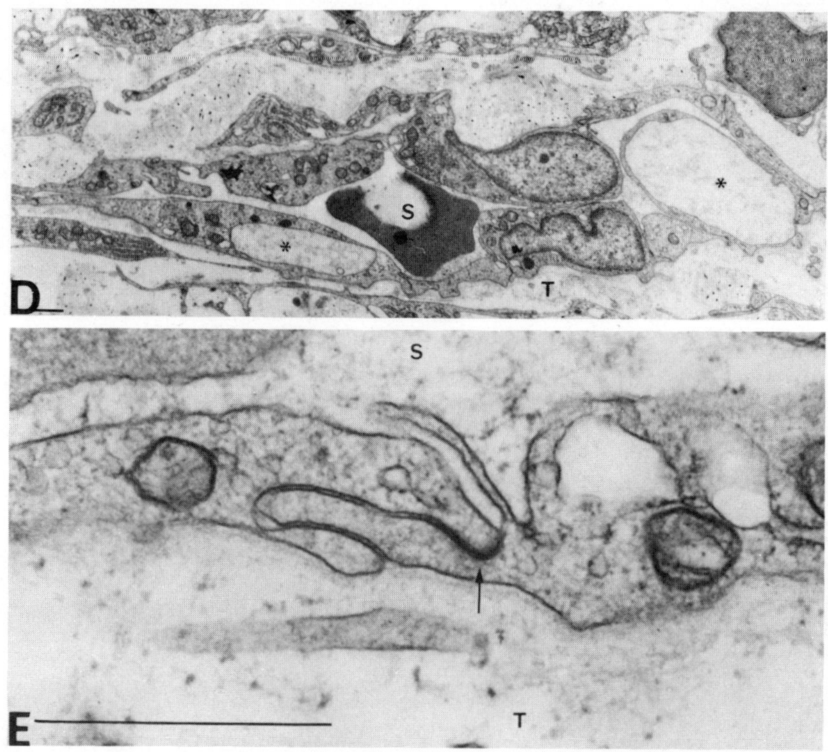

FIG. 31.A. Fourth month. Vessel of plexus forming Schlemm's canal. (S) Lumen of Schlemm's canal; (T) trabecular side of Schlemm's canal. Line shown in figure represents 1 μ. X 5,850. **B**. Fourth month. Double-layered endothelial wall of Schlemm's canal. (S) Lumen of Schlemm's canal; (T) trabecular side of Schlemm's canal. Line shown in figure represents 1 μ. X 10,800. **C**. Fourth month. Cytoplasmic organelles in endothelial cells lining Schlemm's canal. Smooth-surfaced endoplastic reticulum (er), mitochondrium (m), dense bodies (db), and free ribosomes (r) are visible. (S) Lumen of Schlemm's canal; (T) trabecular side of Schlemm's canal. Line shown in figure represents 1 μ. X 15,750. **D**. Fourth month. Vacuoles (*) in endothelial cells lining Schlemm's canal. (S) Lumen of Schlemm's canal; (T) trabecular side of Schlemm's canal. Line shown in figure represents 1 μ. X 5,400. **E**. Fourth month. Junctional complex (↑) between endothelial cells lining Schlemm's canal. (S) Lumen of Schlemm's canal; (T) trabecular side of Schlemm's canal. Line shown in figure represents 1 μ. X 40,500. (From Wulle. **Trans. Am. Acad. Ophthalmol. Otolaryngol.** 72:765, 1968.)

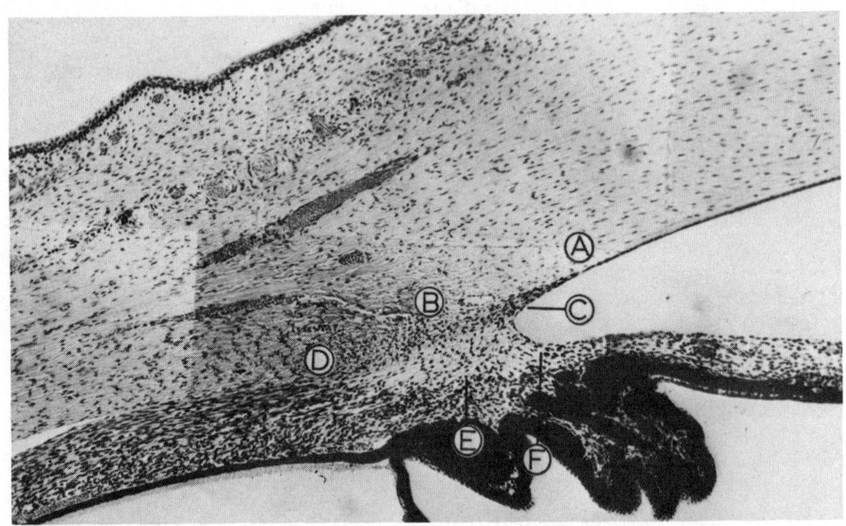

FIG. 32. Chamber angle of 5-month-old embryo. (A) Schwalbe's line; (B) Schlemm's canal; (C) trabeculum; (D) ciliary body; (E) ciliary processes; (F) iris root. (Courtesy of J. G. F. Worst.) X 52.

cell processes do not overlap as frequently as at four months and they often touch end to end (Fig. 33D). Frequently, the intercellular space at these junctions is obliterated, producing a well-developed tight junction. Gaps are noted in the endothelial lining of Schlemm's canal with a diameter of about 0.6μ (Fig. 33E), providing a direct short connection between the juxtacanalicular connective tissue and the lumen of Schlemm's canal. The size of the gaps noted in this study is in general agreement with that reported in other studies. Wulle also observed giant vacuoles (Fig. 33F) in the inner wall and in the outer scleral wall of the canal itself which bore no relationship to the endothelial gaps. In contrast to the vacuoles seen in the fourth month these vacuoles were shown to have an opening into the subendothelial space. They are therefore not strictly a "vacuole" but rather an extension of the intracellular space into the cytoplasm which almost completely envelops it.

Wulle made the following conclusions regarding the changes that occur in Schlemm's canal between the fourth and eighth fetal months, that is, after the flow of aqueous humor begins. First, the inner wall of the canal decreased in thickness by virtue of the fact that by the eighth month it was formed by a single, very thin cell layer. Second, the low-density material which covered the entire base of the endothelial cells in the early stages was only occasionally seen close to the base by the eighth month. Third, with increasing age there was a significant increase in the number of pinocytotic vesicles and intracytoplasmic filaments in the intracellular cells. Fourth, the large intracellular vacuoles observed in the fourth month have openings into the subendothelial space by the eighth month. Fifth, the continuous cell layer making up the endothelium of the canal noted at the fourth month developed gaps by the eighth month.

At birth (Fig. 34), the angle has reached a posterior or basal position to the meshwork with the scleral spur and canal of Schlemm well in front. The marked inequality of growth in this region is demonstrated by the fact that the major circle of the iris is anterior to the level of Schlemm's canal while the latter is first developed, but in the adult eye it has arrived at a point behind the scleral spur. Probably the most important factor causing this change in topographical relationship and contributing to the formation of the angular cleft is the development of the ciliary muscle. As this structure grows and develops it has the effect of forcing the ciliary processes and the root of the iris progressively farther from the trabecular region in an axial direction. The result is that the ciliary tissues formerly resting against the uveal trabeculae are pulled away, thus helping to extend the periphery of the anterior chamber outward and backward.

Faulty differentiation in the development of the chamber angle leads to the persistence of connecting fibers between the iris and peripheral cornea. This may be evidenced as large pectinate fibers (Fig. 35), Axenfeld's syndrome (Fig. 36) or a trabecular zone and Schwalbe's line visible through the peripheral cornea (Fig. 37).

Gross Examination of Angle Structures

CHAMBER ANGLE OF THE PREMATURE EYE. The anterior chamber of the premature eye is shallow owing to the relatively large size of the lens which projects into the anterior chamber covered by the iris. The most striking feature according to Worst is a broad band of highly transparent gray tissue made up of loosely meshed sheets arranged in layers, filling the angle from Schwalbe's line to the root of the iris. The scleral spur is thus obscured.

The amount of tissue present in the angle varies from case to case. In some eyes only a few sparse sheets are present, while in others the chamber angle may be completely filled. The tissue is more abundant in the horizontal meridian, sometimes filling the angle as far as Schwalbe's line so that a crescent of grayish tissue may be observed at the 9 and 3 o'clock

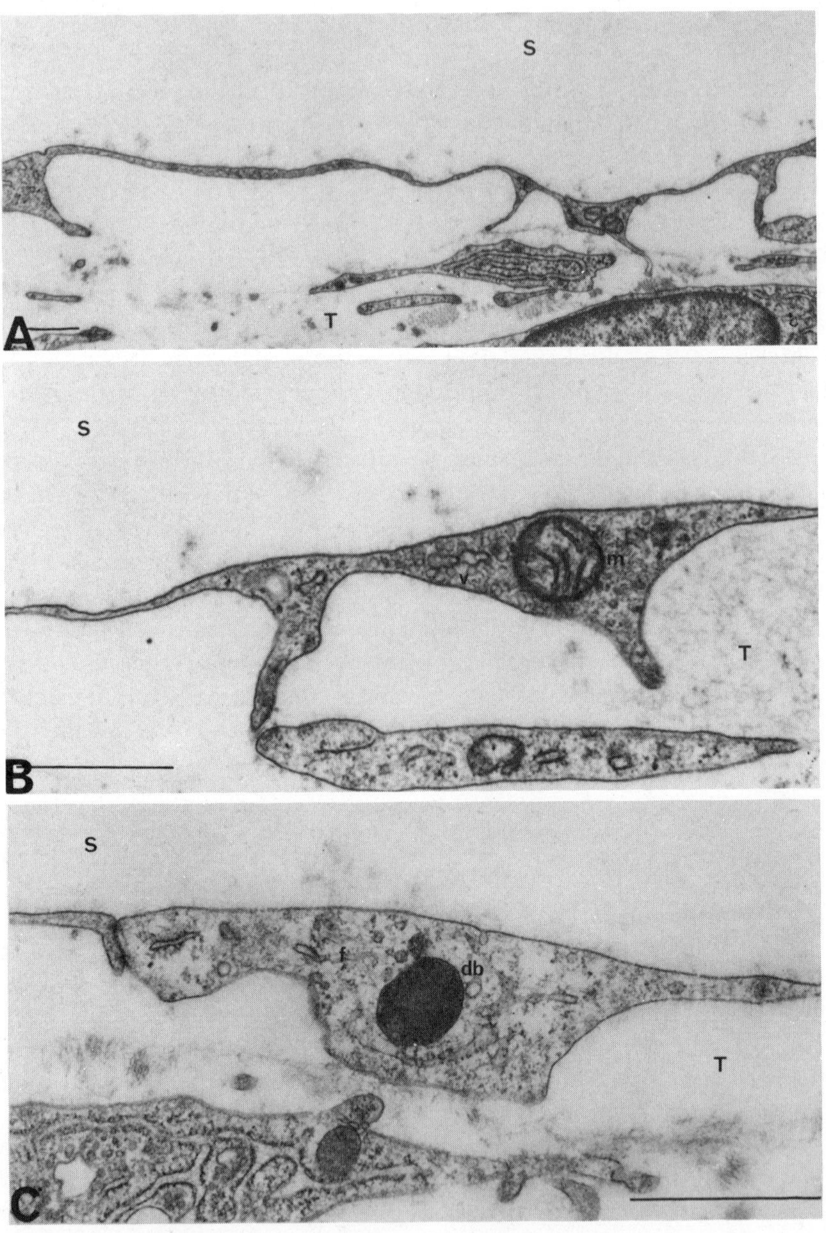

FIG. 33.A. Eighth month. Thin endothelial cells lining Schlemm's canal. (S) Lumen of Schlemm's canal; (T) trabecular side of Schlemm's canal. Line shown in figure represents 1 μ. X 8,100. (From Wulle. **Trans. Am. Acad. Ophthalmol. Otolaryngol.** 72: 765, 1968.)

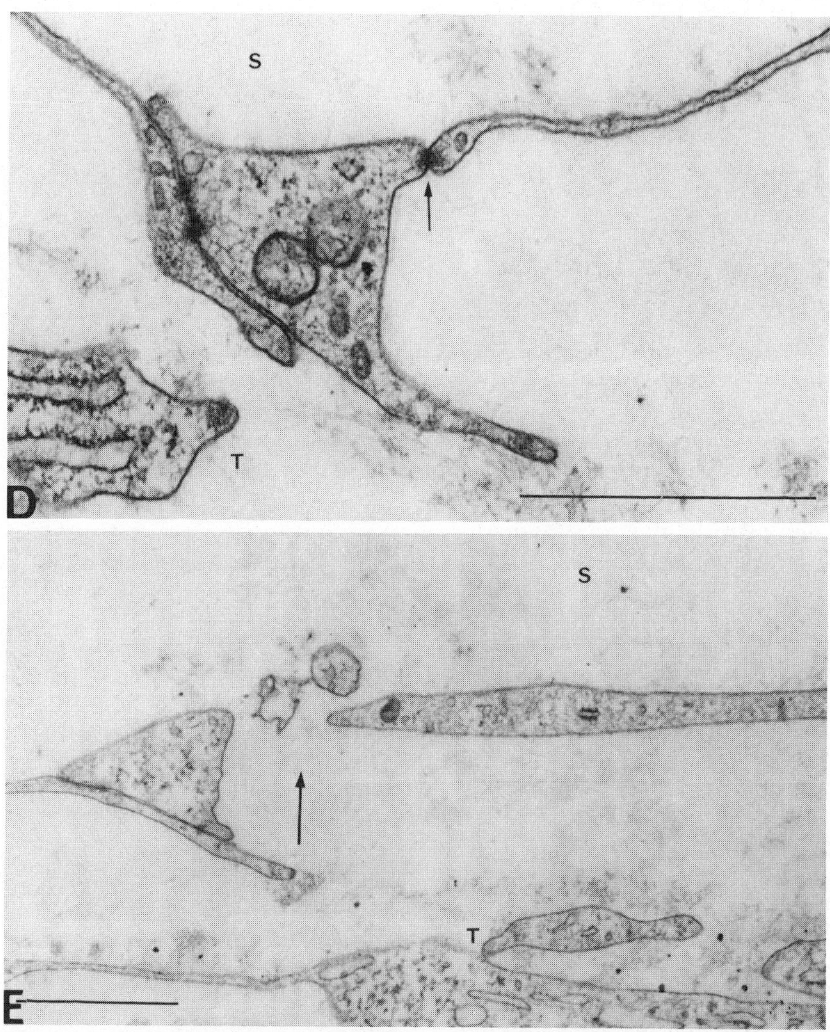

FIG. 33. (Cont.) B. Eighth month. Endothelial cell lining Schlemm's canal with large number of pinocytotic vesicles (v) and well developed mitochondria (m). (S) Lumen of Schlemm's canal; (T) trabecular side of Schlemm's canal. Line shown in figure represents 1 μ. X 21,600. C. Eighth month. Endothelial cell of Schlemm's canal containing large dense body (db) and fine filaments (f). (S) Lumen of Schlemm's canal; (T) trabecular side of Schlemm's canal. Line shown in figure represents 1 μ. X 26,100. D. Eighth month. Junctional complexes between endothelial cells lining Schlemm's canal. Cells touching end to end are combined by tight junction (↑). (S) Lumen of Schlemm's canal; (T) trabecular side of Schlemm's canal. Line shown in figure represents 1 μ. X 40,500. E. Eighth month. Gap (↑) in endothelial lining of Schlemm's canal providing direct short connection between lumen of canal (S) and extracellular space of trabecular meshwork. Two cell processes are cut in cross section inside gap. (S) Lumen of Schlemm's canal; (T) trabecular side of Schlemm's canal. Line shown in figure represents 1 μ. X 22,500.

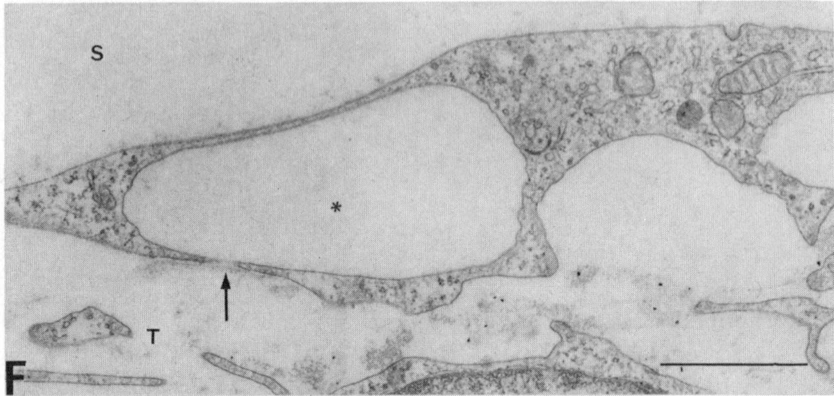

FIG. 33 (Cont.) F. Eighth month. Vacuole (*) in endothelial cell lining Schlemm's canal with opening into subendothelial space (↑). (S) Lumen of Schlemm's canal; (T) trabecular side of Schlemm's canal. Line shown in figure represents 1 μ. (From Wulle. **Trans. Am. Acad. Ophthalmol. Otolaryngol.** 72:765, 1968.) X 17,100.

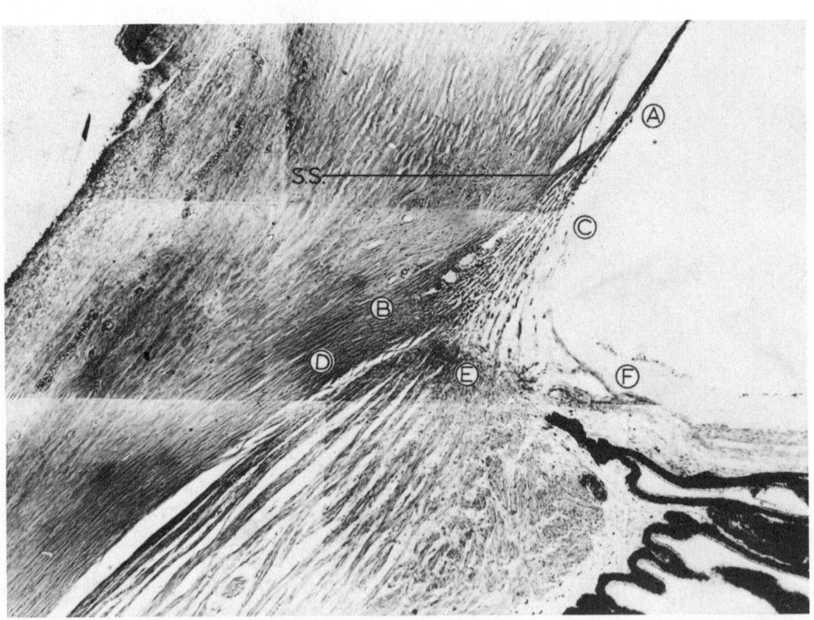

FIG. 34. Filtration angle in newborn. (A) Schwalbe's line; (B) scleral spur; (C) trabeculum; (D) sclera; (E) ciliary body; (F) iris; (S S) upper extent of trabeculum. (Courtesy of J. G. F. Worst.) X 56.

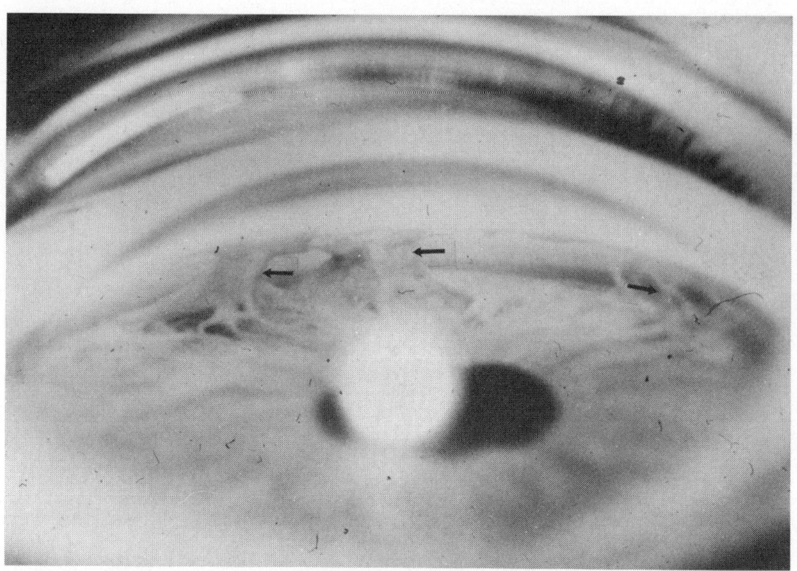

FIG. 35. Pectinate fibers in filtration angle (*arrows*). (Courtesy of N. S. Jaffe.)

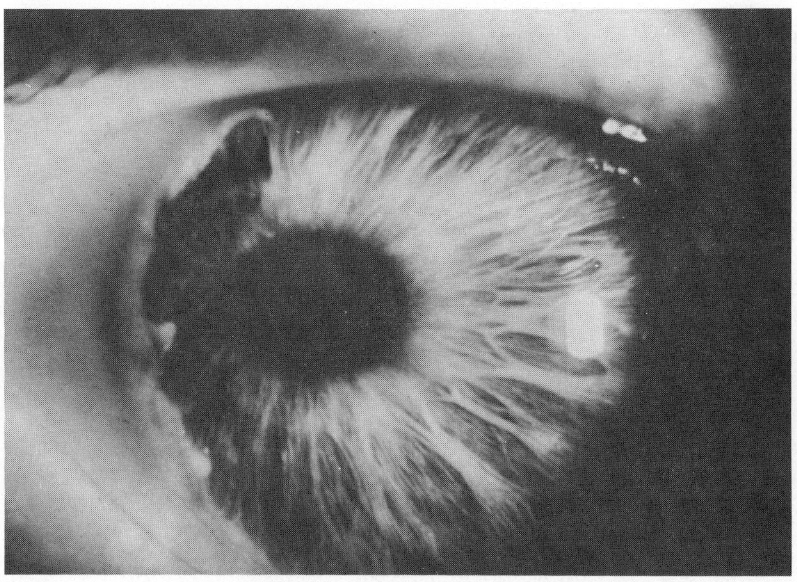

FIG. 36. Axenfeld's syndrome. (Courtesy of J. S. Speakman.)

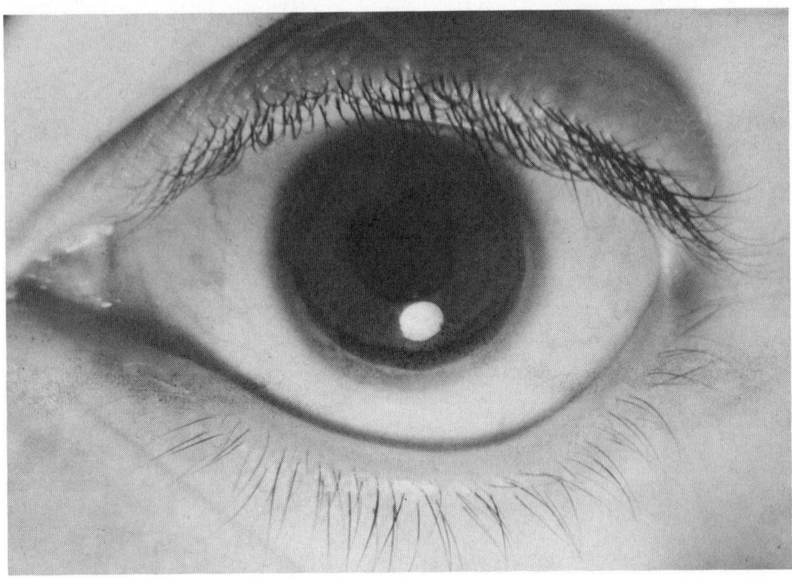

FIG. 37. Visible ring of Schwalbe and trabecular zone. (Courtesy of A. H. Katz.)

positions at the far corneal periphery.

When traction is exerted on the iris base, the ciliary muscle separates from the scleral spur region, leaving only a narrow band of longitudinal

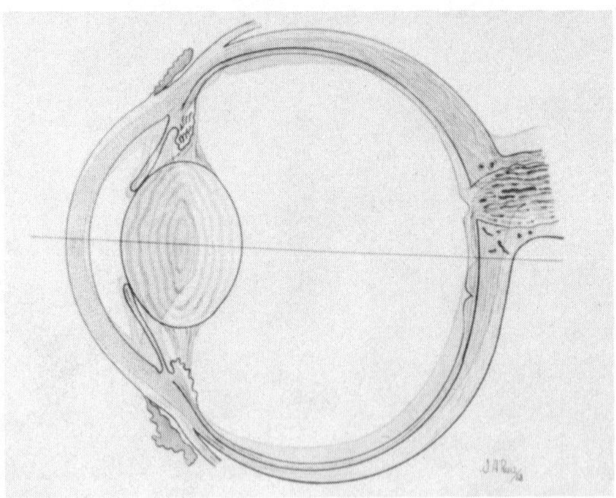

FIG. 38. Infant eye superimposed on adult eye (*shaded*).

muscle bundles attached. The block of transparent tissue sheets remains attached to the base of the separated ciliary body, which would suggest that it is composed of uveal meshwork fibers. If the tissue were part of the corneoscleral system it should remain attached to the scleral spur.

The iris has a typical deep blue color as light reflected from the pigment is filtered through the fine underdeveloped stromal layer. The iris root ends in a wavy scalloped line in front of the chamber angle, at the foot of the tissue in the angle. The iris vessels course toward the angle and disappear behind the band of gray tissue.

CHAMBER ANGLE OF THE NEWBORN EYE. A shallow chamber angle is still present and the iris stroma, although further developed, is still thin–resulting in the peculiar deep blue color usually seen at birth. The scalloped line (the transition point of the iris root and uveal meshwork) has receded toward the chamber angle but no angle recess is present (Fig. 34). A highly transparent sheet of tissue is present in the chamber angle to a varying degree. Schlemm's canal is situated nearer to the iris insertion than in older eyes. Large pectinate ligaments may be present in the angle but disappear during the early years so that they are almost completely absent after the fifth year. In cases where the angle fails to develop normally the ligaments may persist indefinitely (Fig. 35). (See Chap. 3.)

Upon traction of the iris root in older eyes, the ciliary muscle does not detach from the scleral spur as described in the premature eye, and the iris tends to form an iridodialysis, indicating the development of a firm union between the ciliary muscle and the scleral spur.

The pupillary membrane is usually seen as strands of tissue arising a short distance from the pupillary edge and extending to the lens or across the pupil to the opposite margin. The fibers are usually white and opaque, although blood vessels are occasionally observed (Fig. 24).

CHAMBER ANGLE AFTER FIVE YEARS OF AGE. The filtration angle now has a recess and the highly transparent sheet of tissue that is seen in earlier stages is absent. There is little pigmentation present, so that the corneoscleral trabeculum still appears as a highly transparent structure. Schlemm's canal, when filled with blood, is visible as a bright red line. In older eyes it is seen as a faint red band because the light is filtered through the semiopaque trabeculum. With advancing age the anterior segment undergoes numerous changes. The anterior aspect of the lens becomes flatter while the difference of curvature between the cornea and sclera becomes more pronounced. At birth the eye is about 66 percent of its adult diameter and lengthens approximately 8 mm by general enlargement (Fig. 38) to reach adult size.

CHAMBER ANGLE OF CONGENITAL GLAUCOMA. Worst has noted several features with some minor individual variations.

THE IRIS. Crypts are notably absent, resulting in a flat appearance of the iris (Fig. 39). The stromal layer is hypoplastic and the posterior pigment layer is exposed in local areas, producing deep blue patches in the otherwise gray-blue iris. The iris seems to be covered by a fine whitish cellophane-like layer which has been compared by Lister to morning mist. This "morning mist," which sometimes begins at the major collarette, may be complete and evenly distributed or may be irregular and patchy. It may be finely delicate or quite dense, filling the space in front of the chamber angle where it often displays a spongy appearance.

The iris vessels are all more or less exposed, stretched, and form a typical spoke wheel pattern of red lines, radiating outward from the lesser arterial circle toward the major arterial circle. In advanced cases the major circle is seen as a conspicuous sinuous red cord in the depth of the "morning mist," often obscured in the horizontal meridian. About 74 radial iris vessels are usually present, corresponding to the ciliary processes. A true pathologic type of vascularization also occurs as a fine network of mainly horizontally arranged vascular loops running parallel to the iris root. This peripheral rubeosis signifies a very grave prognosis.

THE IRIS BASE. The iris ends in a scalloped line and appears to be lifted upward in continuity with the chamber angle tissues. The iris periphery may actually present a moth-eaten appearance. The major arterial circle that runs along the base of the iris may be obscured by peripheral synechiae and large

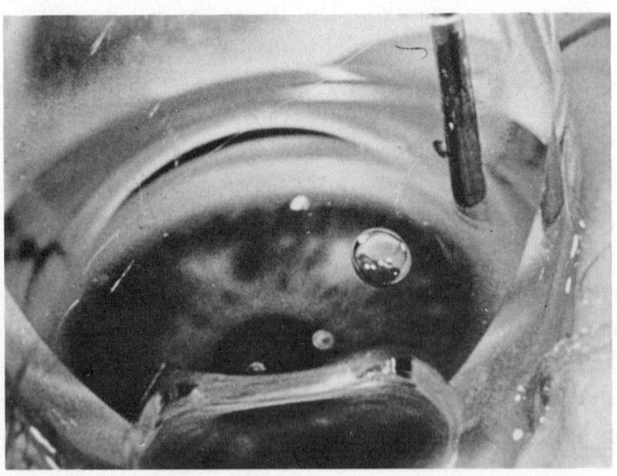

FIG. 39. Filtration angle and iris in congenital glaucoma.

pectinate ligaments with only incidental loops appearing above the iris root. The pectinate ligaments may be quite numerous. Some are short and some extend as far as Schwalbe's line. The abnormal tissue frequently fills the iris spaces between these processes and follows the concavity of the filtration angle.

THE CHAMBER ANGLE. The angle of congenital glaucoma is about 1 mm in width but the characteristics vary widely from case to case. The recess of the chamber angle is conclave and forms a right angle with the plane of the iris, reaching upward toward the cornea and ending at Schwalbe's line—which it often obscures as there appears to be a structural continuity with Descemet's membrane. The angle shows the following features: (1) a shagreened glistening surface with fine horizontal laminations seen with oblique light; (2) the angle has a wavy aspect with pillarlike folds at regular intervals where the iris root is lifted, leaving crypts between the folds; and (3) a space is present behind the surface of the angle recess which contains sheets of highly transparent tissue and vascular loops that run meridianally away from the major arterial circle and into the ciliary body. Many of these vascular loops form a continuation of the radial iris vessels. The corneoscleral junction is often poorly defined and clear cornea only gradually emerges from the sclera. The conjunctival insertion is often easily seen through the cornea as a semiopaque veil marked by stretched limbal vessels. Grant and Walton noted that the uveal meshwork appeared somewhat less transparent than the normal, but sufficiently transparent to identify the scleral spur and ciliary band behind it. Schlemm's canal can usually be filled with blood.

References

Alfano, J. E. Experiences with congenital glaucoma, Eye, Ear, Nose, Throat Mon., 47:274, 1968.

Allen L., Burian, H. M., and Braley, A. E. A new concept of the development of the anterior chamber angle. Arch. Ophthalmol., 53:783, 1955.

Burian, H. M. and Braley, A. E. The anterior border ring of Schwalbe and pectinate ligament. Arch. Ophthalmol., 53:799, 1955.

Andrew, W. Microfabric of Man. Year Book, Chicago, 1966.

Araki, Acta Soc. Ophthalmol. Jap., 61:1485, 1957. Cited by Duke-Elder, W. S. System of Ophthalmology, Vol. 3, Pt. 1, Henry Kimpton, London, 1963, p. 171

Arey, L. B. Developmental Anatomy. Saunders, Philadelphia, 1965.

Ashton, N. The role of the trabecular structure in the problem of simple glaucoma, particularly with regard to the significance of mucopolysaccharides. In Glaucoma, Transactions of the IV Conference, F. W. Newell, ed. J. Macy Foundation, New York, 1959, pp. 89-140.

Barber, A. Embryology of the Human Eye. Mosby, St. Louis, 1955.

Bartelmez, G. W., and Dekban, A. S. The early development of the human brain. Carnegie Contributions to Embryology, Vol. 37, 1962, pp. 13-32.

and Blount, M. P. The formation of neural crest from the primary optic vesicle in man. Carnegie Contributions to Embryology, Vol. 35, 1954, pp. 55-71.

Bielschowsky, A. Lectures on Motor Anomalies. Dartmouth College Publications, 1943.

Blechschmidt, E. Die vorgeburtlichen Entwicklungsstadien des Menschen (Atlas). Basle, Karger, 1961.

The Human Embryo. Stuttgart, Schattauer, 1964.

Vom Eizum Embryo. Stuttgart, Deutsche Verlagsanstalt, 1968.

Differenzierunglen im kinetischen Feld. Acta Anat. (Basel), 1971.

Blessig, E. Fall einer seltenen missbildung der augen. symblepharon totale congenitum palp. sup. oc. dextri, ankyloblepharon totale congenitum, kryptophthalmos oc. sinistri. Klin. Monatsbl. Augenheilk., 38:652, 1900.

Burian, H. M., Braley, A. E. and Allen, L. A new concept of the development of the angle of the anterior chamber of the human eye. Arch. Ophthalmol., 55:439, 1956.

Braley, A. E., and Allen, L. External and gonioscopic visibility of the ring of Schwalbe and the trabecular zone. Trans. Amer. Ophthalmol. Soc., 52:389, 1954.

and Allen, L. Histologic study of the chamber angle of patients with Marfan's syndrome. Arch. Ophthalmol., 65:323, 1961.

Cogan, D. G. Neurology of the Ocular Muscles, 2nd ed. Thomas, Springfield, Ill., 1956.

Corner, G. W., and Smelser, G. K. The Embryology of the Eye (a motion picture). Produced by Sturgis-Grant Productions, Inc., for the American Academy of Ophthalmology and Otolaryngology in co-operation with the Department of Embryology of the Carnegie Institution of Washington, Baltimore, 1950.

Costenbader, F. D., and Kwitko, M. L. Congenital glaucoma. Clin. Proc. Child. Hosp. (Wash.), 17:100, 1961.

and Kwitko, M. L. Congenital glaucoma, an analysis of seventy-seven consecutive eyes. J. Ped. Ophthalmol., 4:9, 1967.

Crisp, W. H. Devleopment of the anterior chamber in the human eye. Am. J. Ophthalmol., 1:46, 1918. Abstract of Sullo sviluppo della camera anteriore nell'occhio umano, Speciale-Cirincione, Ann. Ottal Clin. Ocul., 161, 1917.

Davson, H. The Eye. Academic Press, New York, 1962.

Dejean, C., Hervouet, F., and Leplat, G. L'Embryologie de L'Oeil et sa Teratologie. Bull. Soc. Opht. Paris, p. 392, 1958.

Donaldson, D. D. Atlas of External Diseases of the Eye: Bull. Soc. Opht. Congenital Anomalies and Systemic Diseases, Vol. 1, Mosby, St. Louis, 1966.

Duke-Elder, W. S. Systems of Ophthalmology: Vol. 3, Normal and Abnormal Development, Part 2, Congenital Deformities. Henry Kimpton, London, 1964.

Systems of Ophthalmology: Vol. 3, Pt. 1, Embryology. Henry Kimpton, London, 1963.

Feeney, L., and Wissig, S. Outflow studies using an electron dense tracer. In: Symposium: contributions of electron microscopy to the understanding of the production and outflow of aqueous humor. Trans. Am. Acad. Ophthalmol. Otolaryngol., 70:791, 1966.

Fine, B. Observations on the drainage angle in man and rhesus monkey: a concept of the pathogenesis of chronic simple glaucoma, a light and electron microscopic study. Invest. Ophthalmol., 3:609, 1964.

Structure of the trabecular meshwork and the canal of Schlemm. In: Symposium: contributions of electron microscopy to the understanding of the production and outflow of aqueous humor. Trans. Am. Acad. Ophthalmol. Otolaryng., 70:777, 1966.

Ford, F. R. Diseases of the Nervous System in Infancy, Childhood and Adolescence, ed. 5. Thomas, Springfield, Ill., 1966.

Francois, J. Heredity in Ophthalmology. Mosby, St. Louis, 1961.

Geeraets, W. J. Ocular Syndromes. Lea & Febiger, Philadelphia, 1965.

Grant, W. M., and Walton, D. S. Distinctive gonioscopic findings in glaucoma due to neurofibromatosis. Arch. Ophthalmol., 79:127, 1968.

Hamilton, W. J., Boyd, J. D., and Mossman, H. W. Human Embryology. Williams & Wilkins Co., Baltimore, 1962.

Hogan, M. J., and Zimmerman, L. E. Ophthalmic Pathology, An Atlas and Textbook, 2nd ed. Saunders, Philadelphia, 1962.

Holmberg, A. The fine structure of the inner wall of Schlemm's canal. Arch. Ophthalmol., 62:956, 1959.

Schlemm's canal and the trabecular meshwork: an electron microscopic study of the normal structure in man and cenkey (ecrcopithecus ethiops). Docum. Ophthalmol., 19:339, 1965.

Ide, C. H., and Wollschlaeger, P. B. Multiple congenital abnormalities associated with cryptophthalmia. Arch. Ophthalmol., 81:638, 1969.

Jaffe, N. S., and Knie, P. True polycoria. Am. J. Ophthalmol., 35:253, 1952.

Jauw, S. H. Een Geval van Cryptophthalmus. Med. Mndbl., 3:356, 1950.

Johnson, T. B., and Whillis, J. Gray's Anatomy. Longmans, Green and Co., London, 1949.

Jordan, E. H., and Kindred, J. E. Textbook of Embryology, Appleton-Century-Crofts, New York, 1948.

Kayes. J. Pore structure of the inner wall of Schlemm's canal. Invest. Ophthalmol., 6:381, 1967.

Kawai, K. An embryological study on the Schlemm's canal. Acta. Soc. Ophthalmol. Jap., 59:1834, 1955.

Keeney, A. H. Chronology of Ophthalmic Development. Thomas, Springfield, Ill., 1951.

Keibel, F., and Mall, E. P. Manual of Human Embryology. Lippincott, Philadelphia, 1912.

Kestenbaum, A. Applied Anatomy of the Eye. Grune & Stratton, New York, 1963.

Kronfeld, P. C. The Human Eye in Anatomical Transparencies. Bausch and Lomb Press, Rochester, N. Y., 1943.

Kwitko, M. L. Genetic aspects of the anterior chamber cleavage syndrome. Exerpta Medica. No. 154, Amsterdam, p. 80. Exerpta Medica Foundation, 1967.

Anterior segment anomalies: a clinical pathologic report of conditions simulating congenital glaucoma. Can. J. Ophthalmol., 3:120, 1968.

Congenital glaucoma: a clinical study. Can. J. Ophthalmol., 2:91, 1967.

Last, R. J., and Wolf, E. Anatomy of the Eye and Orbit. Saunders, Philadelphia, 1961.

Lieb, W. A., and Stark, N. Zur phylogenese und morphologie der kammerbucht. Klin. Monatsbl. Augenheilk., 144:1, 1964.

Lopashov, G. V. Developmental Mechanisms of the Vertebrate Eye Rudiments. Pergamon Press, Oxford, New York, 1963.

Mann, I. Developmental Abnormalities of the Eye. The University Press, Cambridge, England, 1957.

The Development of the Human Eye. The University Press, Cambridge, England, 1964.

Maumenee, A. E. The pathogenesis of congenital glaucoma: a new theory. Trans. Am. Ophthalmol. Soc., 56:507, 1958.

Missotten, L. L'ultrastructure des tissus oculaires., Bull. Soc. Belg. Ophthalmol., 136:3, 1964.

Nishimura, H. In 3rd International Conference on Congenital Malformations. The Hague, 1969.

Patten, B. M. Human Embryology. McGraw-Hill, New York, 1953.

Pearson, A. A., Eidemiller, L. R., Keane, J. M., Stuart, R. J., Rich, L. F., and Sauter, R. W. The Development of the Eye. Am. Acad. Ophthalmol. and Otolaryngol., Rochester, Minn., 1967.

Potter, E. L. Pathology of the Fetus and Infant. Year Book, Chicago, 1961.

Pathology of the Fetus and the Infant. Year Book, Chicago, 1962.

Prince, J. H. Comparative Anatomy of the Eye. Thomas, Springfield, Ill., 1956.

Smelser, G. K. The structure of the eye, in International Congress of Anatomists. Academic Press, New York, 1961.
Sorsby, A. Ophthalmic Genetics, 2nd ed. Appleton-Century Crofts, 1970.
Speakman, J. S. Drainage channels in the trabecular wall of Schlemm's canal. Br. J. Ophthalmol., 44:513, 1960.
and Leeson, T. S. Pathological findings in a case of primary congenital glaucoma compared with normal infant eyes. Br. J. Ophthalmol., 48:196, 1964.
Stark, N. Experimentelle Untersuchungen uber die physio-patholo- gische Bedeutung der Kammerwinkelstrukturen fur den Kammerwasserabfluss. Med. Diss., Frankfort Main, 1961.
Streeter, G. L. Developmental Horizons in Human Embryos. Carnegie Contributions to Embryology, Nos. 197, 199, 211: 1942, 1945 and 1948.
Vegge, T. The fine structure of the trabeculum cribriforme and the inner wall of Schlemm's canal in the normal eye. Z. Zellforsch., 77:267, 1967.
Waardenburg, P. J., Franceschetti, A., and Klein, D. Genetics and Ophthalmology. Thomas, Springfield, Ill. 1961.
Wachtel, J. G. The ocular pathology of Marfan's syndrome. Arch. Ophthalmol., 76:512, 1966.
Walls, G. L. The Vertebrate Eye and Its Adaptive Radiation. Cranbrook Institute of Science, Bloomfield Hills, Mich., 1942.
Whitnall, S. E. The Anatomy of the Human Orbit and Accessory Organs of Vision. Oxford Univers., New York, 1932.
Windle, W. F. Physiology of the Fetus. Saunders, Philadelphia, 1940.
Worst, J. G. F. The Pathogenesis of Congenital Glaucoma. Royal Vangorcum, Assen. Netherlands, 1966.
Wulle, K. G. Zelldifferenzierungen im Ciliarepithel wahrend der menschlichen Fatalentwicklung und ihre Beziehungen zur Kammerwasserbildung. Graefe Arch. Ophthalmol., 172:170, 1967.
Electron microscopic observations of the development of Schlemm's canal in the human eye. Trans. Am. Acad. Ophthalmol. Otolaryngol., 72:765, 1968.
Yamashita, T., and Rosen, D. A. Electron microscopic study of trabecular meshwork: in clinical and experimental glaucoma with anterior chamber hemorrhage. Am. J. Ophthalmol., 60:427, 1965.
Zimmerman, L. E. Demonstration of hyaluronidase sensitive acid mucopolysaccharide: in trabecular and iris in routine paraffin sections of adult human eye. Am. J. Ophthalmol., 44:1, 1957.
Zinn, S. Cryptophthalmia. Am. J. Ophthalmol., 40:219, 1955.

3

Normal and Abnormal Development of the Irido-Corneal Angle

The angle anomaly which results in primary infantile glaucoma is generally regarded to be genetically determined and exhibits a recessive inheritance pattern in most cases, even though several children of a family may be affected. In hydrophthalmia both parents are usually heterozygous carriers and may not have the disease. One-quarter of their children should be homozygous normal, one-half should be heterozygous carriers, and one-quarter will have congenital glaucoma (homozygous). The reservoir of this gene in the general population is small, amounting to only 2.34 to 2.80 percent, which would account for its rarity in clinical practice. Although sex linkage is not common in the inheritance pattern, more boys are affected by congenital glaucoma than girls.

Many recessive genes that are potential disease producers are held in check by the companion dominant gene. For this reason consanguineous matings will increase the probability of homozygous recessive combinations. Duke-Elder states that consanguinity is a factor in 10 percent of cases of congenital glaucoma.

Alfano has noted that local steroid drops administered to a child's eye could result in a condition simulating congenital glaucoma This subject is discussed in Chapter 11. Recent experiments using corticosteroid drops on patients with open-angle glaucoma and their children have caused a reassessment of the role that heredity plays in open-angle glaucoma. The role corticosteroid drops play in elucidating the manner of transmission of congenital glaucoma is still unknown. At the present time, as judged by steroid testing of parents of children with infantile glaucoma, the genetic abnormality in this disease is different from that of primary open-angle glaucoma. However, children of parents with open-angle glaucoma do show significant changes.

Marked increases in intraocular pressure can be produced when corticosteroid drops are administered for a period of time to adult patients with open-angle glaucoma. When the same drops are given to the children of open-angle glaucoma patients there is a similar response in over 90 percent of cases. When normal volunteers are tested, a rise in pressure is noted in about 35 percent. Open-angle glaucoma can therefore be considered to be homozygous with two recessive genes. If the mate of such a patient is heterozygous with one normal and one abnormal gene, 50 percent of the children will be homozygous and eventually develop glaucoma. If the mate has no abnormal gene, all the children will be heterozygous carriers and will be steroid responsive but will not develop glaucoma. While the normal parents of patients with infantile glaucoma are carriers of the disease, topical corticosteroids do not identify the carrier state. This is unlike the situation in primary open-angle glaucoma.

GENERAL CONSIDERATIONS

Physiologic Factors

Aqueous Secretions

Aqueous humor is a relatively cell-free, protein-free, clear fluid secreted by the ciliary epithelium into the posterior chamber. It passes through the pupil into the anterior chamber and leaves through the trabecular meshwork to Schlemm's canal and the venous system. During its passage through the eye, its composition is altered by diffusional exchange with the blood, by the metabolism of the ocular tissues, and by active transport processes. Compared with plasma concentrations, the aqueous humor of the human and monkey eye has an excess of hydrogen and chloride ions and a deficit of bicarbonate ions. In the rabbit eye, bicarbonate is in excess, and hydrogen and chloride are in deficit. Several other species have large excesses of ascorbate and lactate in the aqueous humor.

Microscopically, each ciliary process consists of a double layer of epithelium covering a connective tissue stroma rich in thin-walled capillaries. The outer, pigmented epithelial layers rest on a typical basement membrane, while the membrane covering the nonpigmented epithelial layer (the internal limiting membrane) is more complex. The apical surfaces of the two cell layers abut directly upon one another and are united at numerous points by junctional complexes. At the inner, free surfaces of the nonpigmented epithelium, multiple-microvillous processes project from one cell to another, producing a series of complex interdigitations, each covered by the internal limiting membrane. These multiple-membrane folds are characteristic of cells involved in salt and fluid transport, and are probably of considerable importance in aqueous production, according to Becker and Kolker. Aside from the membrane folds, the most striking feature of the cells, especially in the nonpigmented layer, is the large number of mitochondria found in the cytoplasm. Other cytoplasmic organelles present include the Golgi complex and endoplasmic reticulum. These are less well developed and not as numerous as the mitochondria. The secretion of aqueous humor is an energy-requiring process which is temperature dependent and requires oxygen. Several transport systems have been demonstrated or postulated to explain the composition and rate of production of aqueous humor. Friedenwald postulated a barrier between the epithelium and stroma of the ciliary body, with an electron transport system across the barrier. The bicarbonate system serves as a buffer on both sides of the barrier and requires the enzyme carbonic anhydrase. The inhibition of this enzyme would be expected to reduce aqueous production, according to Becker, and Kinsey and Reddy.

Another speculative approach supposes that carbonic anhydrase plays a direct role in the transport process. On this basis, it is postulated that hydrogen ions (in the human eye) or bicarbonate ions (in the rabbit eye), produced from carbon dioxide and water in the presence of carbonic anhydrase, are transported into the aqueous humor.

Bonting postulated that the enzyme sodium-potassium adenosine triphosphatase, present in the ciliary epithelium, resulted in the transport of sodium across the ciliary-epithelial cell wall into the aqueous humor, carrying water with it.

There are at least 5 other transport systems into the eye, including those for ascorbate, sugars, neutral amino acids, basic amino acids, and acidic amino acids. Other systems transport substances out of the eye, including iodide, amino acids, and several larger organic anions.

Little is known about the details of metabolic, hormonal, vascular, neurogenic, and psychogenic factors which alter the secretory rate. This rate decreases with age, with a particularly sharp decline after 60 years of age, and is intermittently decreased in glaucomatous eyes. Several drugs, including carbonic anhydrase inhibitors, epinephrine, and cardiac glycosides, significantly reduce aqueous production. The rate is also reduced in carotid occlusion and uveitis, and temporarily reduced by ocular surgery and retinal detachment.

Aqueous Flow and Vascular Influences

Methods for measuring aqueous flow include turnover of test substances, the determination of steady state chemistries, fluorescein appearance time, tonography, and the suction cup. While each of these methods is subject to considerable error, there is reasonably good agreement suggesting a rate of flow in the normal human eye of 1.5–2.5 μl/min. This rate is subject to both spontaneous and induced alteration. Aqueous flow in the ocular system is governed by Poiseuille's law, which can be expressed in a simplified formula as $F = (\Delta P)/R$. It must be remembered that aqueous flow varies spontaneously in a diurnal fashion, resulting in fluctuations in intraocular pressure. Given the rate of flow F and the fall in pressure ΔP between two points in the stream, it is possible to calculate the resistance R.

Approximately 30 collector channels conduct aqueous humor to the scleral venous plexus, which is in communication with the vascular system outside the eye. There is a pressure drop in the normal eye of 5 to 10 mm Hg across this barrier.

A rise in intraocular pressure may therefore result from an increase in volume flow per minute, an increase in the resistance, or an increase in episcleral venous pressure. Significant increases in the rate of flow for any length of time are exceptionally rare, and practically irrelevant in the case of primary glaucoma once the ciliary body has reached maturity. When changes in the rate of flow take place in experimental animals with no other ocular abnormalities, compensatory alterations in resistance result so that a normal intraocular pressure is maintained. Increase in episcleral venous pressure causing a rise in intraocular pressure has been reported in a case of an arteriovenous aneurysm between the carotid and the jugular. Therefore, raised intraocular pressure in primary glaucoma is the result of an increased resistance in the outflow pathway between the anterior chamber and the episcleral net of veins.

Neural Influences

Afferent nerves in the uveal tract are known to react to changes in intraocular pressure. Duke-Elder has demonstrated the presence of axon reflexes in the vascular mechanism of the eye. Local trauma or any other process which liberates histamine (or histamine-like substances) affects these reflexes causing a reaction which includes capillary dilatation, increased permeability, and edema, which is not locally confined but is spread by nervous agencies all over the globe. Raised intraocular pressure may be another feature.

By mechanically stimulating the peripheral end of the transected fifth cranial nerve of rabbits, Thomas produced a number of ocular changes similar to those produced by Duke-Elder. A marked vasodilatation of the conjunctival vessels took place followed by a dilatation of the iris blood vessels, which was associated with an influx of protein, as evidenced by the presence of an aqueous flare. Miosis and a rise in the intraocular pressure was noted within 5 minutes of the stimulation. This effect lasted 10 to 30 minutes. Interruption of the third cranial nerve did not modify the response nor did prior systemic or topical atropinization. These observations were previously noted by Perkins. The activating hypertensive substance was thought to be irin, a biologically active compound isolated from rabbit irises. The agent was thought to be released by the intraocular fibers of the fifth cranial nerve.

Perkins recorded increased temperature in the region of the ciliary body following stimulation of the fifth cranial nerve, indicating an increased blood flow and presumably an increased blood volume. Thomas was able to prevent the hypertensive effect by applying epinephrine bitartrate (2 percent) 3 times at 3-min intervals.

In addition, other alpha-adrenergic substances used in this experiment such as 10 percent phenylephrine, applied topically, consistently blocked the glaucomatous reaction and the miosis that accompanied it. Retrobulbar anaesthesia was also effective in preventing glaucoma, implying neural rather than vascular influences. Complete iridectomies effectively reduced the rise in ocular pressure, suggesting that the glaucoma resulted from the release of an intraocular hypertensive miotic substance. Thomas concluded that this substance was atrophine-resistant, had miotic and vasodilator qualities, but was distinct from histamine although similar in physiologic effects. It may be present in other ocular tissue but the primary focus appeared to be the iris, where it was intimately associated with fibers of the fifth cranial nerve. The agent diminishes aqueous outflow at an unknown site unrelated to angle closure by the iris. Its physiologic and pathologic effects appear to be antagonized by alpha-adrenergic agents such as phenylephrine.

Intraocular Pressure

The intraocular pressure (P_O in mm Hg) varies directly with the rate of secretion of aqueous humor (F in μl/min) and inversely with the facility of outflow (C):

$$P_O = F/C + P_V$$

where P_V is the episcleral venous pressure (mm Hg).

In the normal eye, variations in aqueous secretion related to diurnal fluctuations, endocrine disturbances, hydration, drugs, surgery, and so on, result in alterations in intraocular pressure. These are usually small and are accompanied by what appear to be compensatory adjustments in outflow facility, which maintain a relatively constant intraocular pressure.

Tonometry

INDENTATION TONOMETRY. In Schiotz tonometry a standardized instrument is applied to the cornea, and the depth of indentation of the cornea by the plunger under a given weight is determined. Friedenwald postulated that change in ocular volume (ΔV_s) varied as a log function of intraocular pressure in the living eye. When P_o is raised to P_t by applying the tonometer, the volume of corneal indentation (V_c) is assumed equal to the distention of the sclera (ΔV_s):

$$\log(P_t/P_o) = E\Delta V_s = EV_c$$

where E = coefficient of ocular rigidity, or

$$\log P_t - \log P_o = EV_c$$

Using a mean value for E of 0.0215 and experimentally measuring V_c and P_t, tables of P_o have been calculated.

APPLANATION TONOMETRY. In applanation tonomery, the intraocular pressure is measured directly as the force required to flatten a standard area of cornea (3.06 mm diameter). The method is not dependent upon alterations in ocular rigidity, since the tonometer does not displace much fluid or significantly increase the pressure in the eye. Applanation tonometry gives the most accurate estimation of intraocular pressure, and the measurements agree well with those obtained by direct cannulation of the eye.

Outflow Facility

Outflow facility can be measured in several ways, most of which have certain built-in assumptions and sources of error. These methods have been reviewed by Becker and Kolker.

PERFUSION. Fluid is perfused through the eye at different pressure levels, and inflow pressure P_I (mm Hg) is plotted against inflow I (μl/mm). From the slope of such a plot a measurement of C is obtained. For human eyes, mean values of approximately 0.28 μl/mm/mm Hg are obtained by in vitro perfusion.

PERFUSION BY ABRUPT RISE IN PRESSURE. The introduction of a known volume of fluid into the eye produces a sudden rise in intraocular pressure. The time course of the decrease in pressure which follows this disturbance of equilibrium can be utilized to estimate outflow facility.

FLUORESCEIN STUDIES. This method involves the turnover of intravenously administered fluorescein in the anterior chamber aqueous humor. Values for outflow facility in normal human eyes average 0.33.

TONOGRAPHY. At the present time this is the most commonly used method for estimating the outflow facility in adults. A Schiotz tonometer is placed on the eye for a period of 4 min resulting in progressive indentation of the cornea by the plunger. The pressure decay curve is recorded. During the 4 min interval while the tonometer is resting on the eye, a volume of fluid (ΔV) is expressed from the eye. The rate at which this occurs is a measure of the outflow facility (C).

$$C = \Delta V/4\,(P_{tav} - P_o)$$

where P_{tav} is the average intraocular pressure during tonography. The change in volume, ΔV, is the sum of the decrease in ocular distention (ΔV_s) and the increase in corneal indentation (ΔV_c) during the 4 min of tonography. Studies by Linner have demonstrated an average increase in venous pressure of about 1.25 mm Hg during tonography. Taking these studies into account, the above formula becomes

$$C = (\Delta V_s + \Delta V_c)/4[P_{tav} - (P_o + 1.25)]$$

CONSTANT PRESSURE TONOGRAPHY. P_t and ocular distention (ΔV_s) are kept constant during tonography and all volume changes are estimated from corneal indentation (ΔV_c). Errors induced by variations in ocular rigidity and pressure-decay artifacts are, hopefully, eliminated by this method.

SUCTION CUP. Occluding the outflow with a suction cup set at -50 mm Hg pressure for 15 min raises the intraocular pressure. After the cup is removed, intraocular pressure is measured at frequent intervals to determine the rate at which it returns to its steady state. This figure can be converted to volume of aqueous leaving the eye, and an estimate of outflow facility obtained.

These various methods as they apply to young infants and children are discussed in Chapter 7.

Animal Studies

Smelser and Ozanics studied the embryological development of the macaque embryo. The histologic sections were embedded in *Epon* which provides a firm support for the delicate ocular tissues. Gestation requires 160 to 162 days in this species. At the 60-day stage we have approximately the

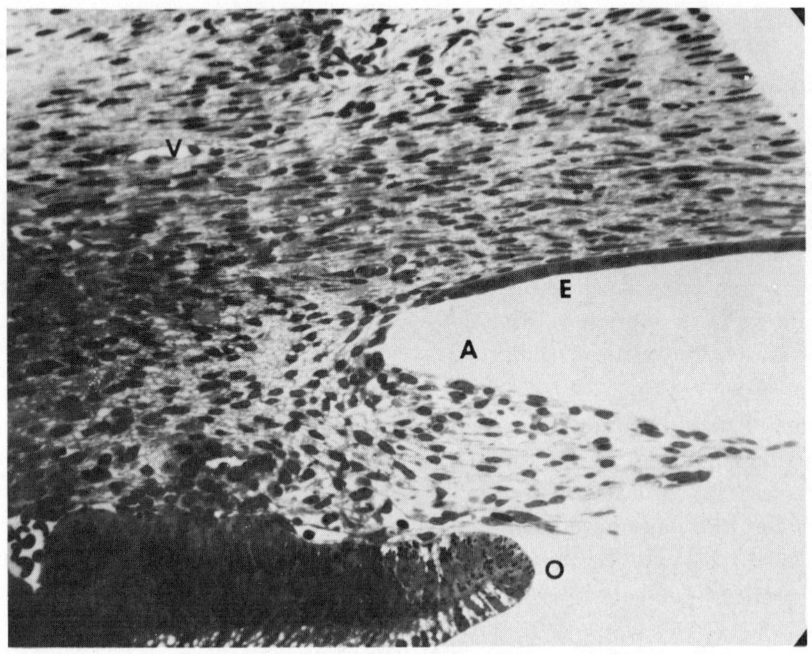

FIG. 1. Anterior chamber angle of a 60-day monkey embryo. There is no obvious Schlemm's canal and the angle is filled with loose reticular mesenchyme cells. The corneal endothelium consists of cuboidal cells. (A) Anterior chamber; (E) endothelium; (O) optic cup; (V) scleral vessel. (From Smelser and Ozanics. **Am. J. Ophthalmol.** 71:366, 1971.) X 30 μm.

equivalent in development with a 4-month human embryo. At this stage the iris epithelium has reached little more than the level where one might suppose that Schlemm's canal would arise (Fig. 1). Sections of the lumina of vessels, which might represent the canal, may be seen. The angle tissue appears spongy. The cells in this area are active, shown by large nucleoli in each nucleus. The corneal endothelium is composed of thick cuboidal cells and ends at the apex of the anterior chamber in a clump of cells. The earliest indication of a ciliary process is apparent as a buckling of both layers of the optic cup. The future ciliary vessel nests in this fold. The iris stroma appears to be rapidly growing. The 65-day chamber angle is slightly more developed and sections of Schlemm's canal and/or vessels containing erythrocytes, which could drain the anterior chamber, are visible. The corneal endothelium still ends at the chamber angle which is filled by a very loose spongy or porous mesenchyme. A group of polygonal, cytoplasm-rich cells is seen in

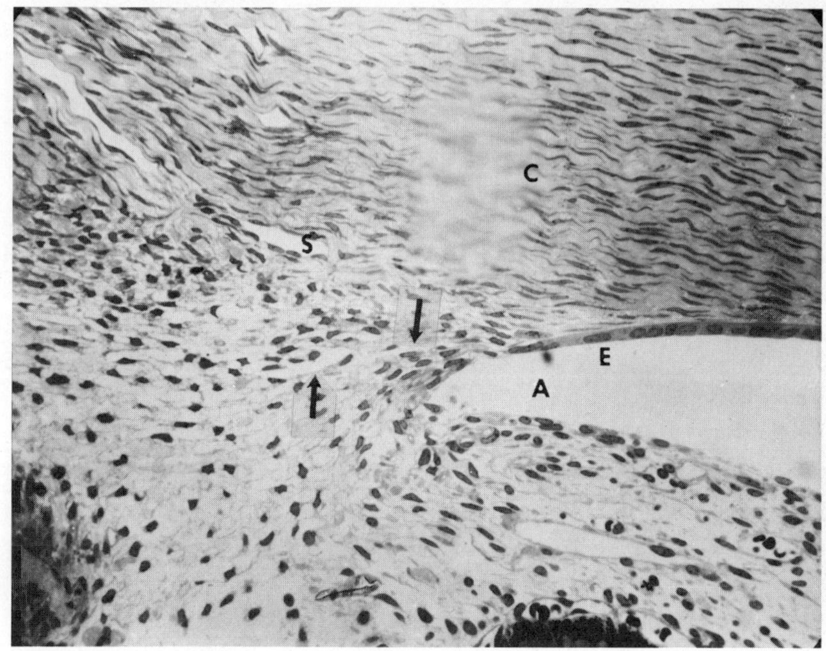

FIG. 2. Anterior chamber angle of an 84-day monkey embryo. A precursor or exit channel of Schlemm's canal is in the inner aspect of the sclera. The angle mesenchyme is loose and rarefaction which could lead to an artifactious cleft is shown at the arrows. The angle is lined by cells, a mass of which are seen at the apex. (A) Anterior chamber; (E) endothelium; (S) Schlemm's canal; (C) cornea. (From Smelser and Ozanics. **Am. J. Ophthalmol.** 71:366, 1971.) X 30 μm.

the angle, a feature of regular occurrence. No evidence of cell death (e.g., pyknotic nuclei) is seen. On the contrary, synthetic activity as expressed by the presence of nucleoli is observed in all cells.

The 76-day stage is characterized by better organization of the mesenchyme of the iris stroma than of the angle. The future trabecular meshwork consists of cells arranged in a most irregular fashion. The anterior border of the iris seems to be covered by a definite layer of fusiform cells, and the sphincter muscle is formed. The ciliary processes each contains a vessel. Descemet's membrane is not yet visible. By the 84-day stage, Schlemm's canal and some of its excurrent vessels may be visible (Fig. 2). The angle tissue is very porous. Large, reticular-shaped spaces are seen between the cells but evidence of cell death is not obvious. What may be interpreted as cleavage may be illustrated by another section at this same

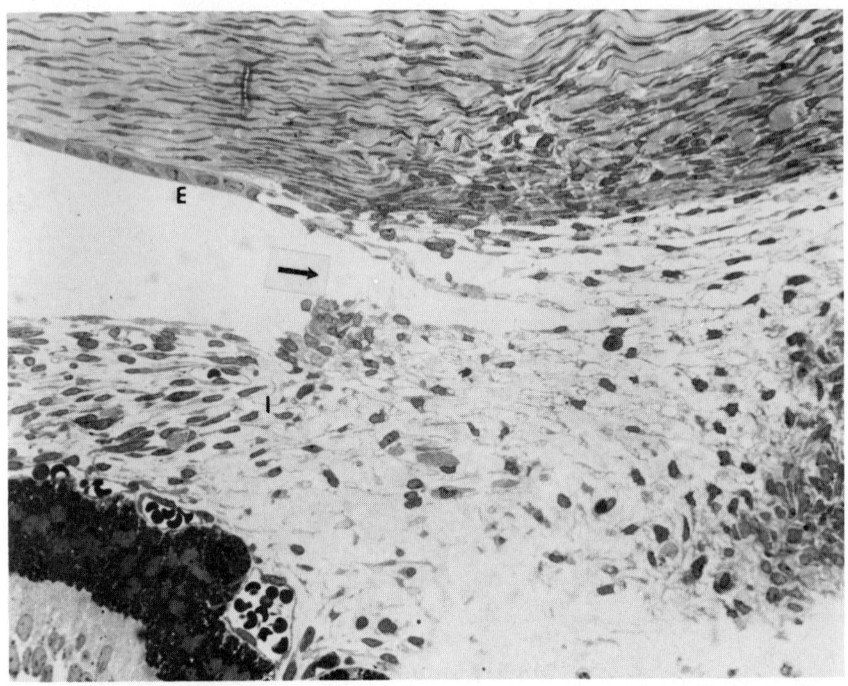

FIG. 3. Another section of the same eye shown in Fig. 2 reveals a cleft which is believed to be artifactual in origin (arrow). Below the cleft is a clump of polygonal cells which, in other sections, is continuous with the endothelium. Note the rarefaction evident in the angle mesenchyme. (E) Endothelium; (I) iris. (From Smelser and Ozanics. Am. J. Ophthalmol. 71:366, 1971.) X 30 μm.

stage (Fig. 3). This cleavage occurred anterior to what may be the terminus of the corneal endothelium. The separation of some of the endothelial cells from each other, and the isolation of some strands of angle mesenchyme suggest that mechanical factors may have been responsible. The chamber angle of a 90-day fetus is shown in Fig. 4. The mesenchyme-filled angle is loose and spongy or reticular in character. The nucleus of each cell has 2-3 nucleoli, indicating vigorous protein synthesis. The anterior chamber surface is covered by cells. Those lining the angle itself and forming a clump at its deepest portion are large, and resemble corneal endothelial cells more than those covering the anterior surface of the iris. Schlemm's canal is well dilated and for the first time some vesicles, which form part of the aqueous humor outflow system, can be found on the trabecular wall of the canal. This is also the first stage in which two types of mesenchyme cells appear in the angle.

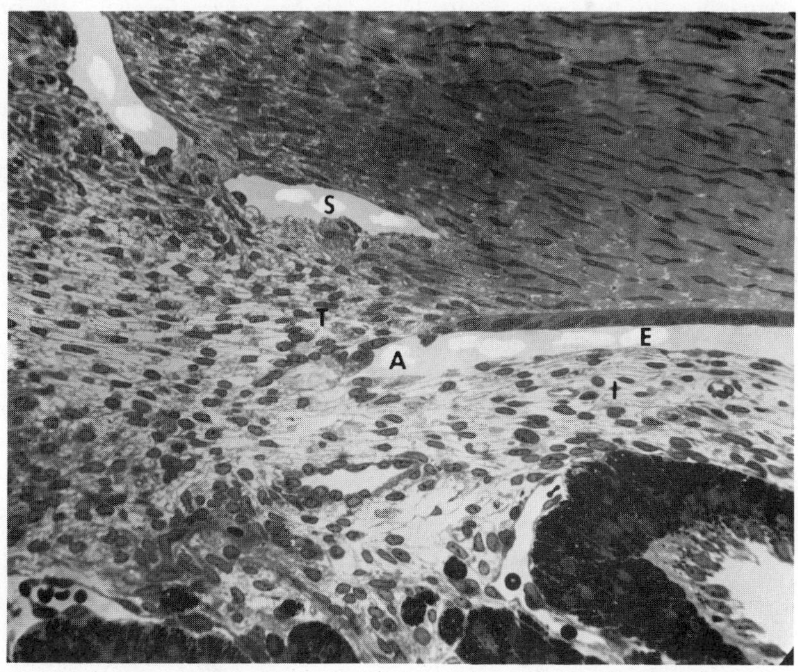

FIG. 4. The anterior chamber angle of a 90-day monkey embryo. Schlemm's canal is visible and the beginning of the trabecular meshwork may be seen below it. Note the nucleoli in most of the cells of the angle. (A) Anterior chamber; (E) endothelium; (I) iris; (S) Schlemm's canal; (T) trabecular meshwork. (From Smelser and Ozanics. **Am. J. Ophthalmol.** 71:366, 1971.) X30 μm.

Those adjacent to the sclera near the supposed canal of Schlemm are closer together and associated with more intercellular material than those nearer the ciliary body. The latter are the precursors of the trabecular meshwork. The mesenchyme below this is more regularly oriented than previously, so that the spaces are elongated in the meridional plane. The iris, at 90 days, is thinner at its root than centrally. Its anterior surface is covered by a regular endothelial-like layer of cells which is very tenuous in places.

By the 98-day stage the chamber angle seems deeper and more open than in the previous specimen at 90 days. The layer of densely stained cells, continuous with the corneal endothelium, apparently ends near the periphery of the chamber, as one or two thin cells rather than in a clump of cells. If this is the normal situation, the likelihood is greater that the cleft seen at 84 days (Fig. 3) is an artifact. The outstanding feature of the mesenchyme in the angle is its loose, spongy character with its large proportion of patent intercellular spaces. The mesenchyme seems to be composed of strands which lie in the meridional plane. The spaces between them are large and one can see how, if they become confluent, a cleft would suddenly appear. This arrangement of cells represents rarefaction of the tissue produced by cell rearrangement and was first noted at the 90-day stage (Fig. 4). The collagen core of trabeculae are beginning to develop in the area contiguous to Schlemm's canal or its emissary, but not in association with the mesenchyme adjacent to the ciliary body. The 100-day embryo is similar and is the first in which a Descemet's membrane can be discerned.

There is little change at the 121-day stage. The corneal endothelial layer is not interrupted, and ends abruptly, quite far from the apex of the chamber angle (the lining of which, from that point on, is composed of loose mesenchymatous cells). The apex of the chamber angle appears to be more

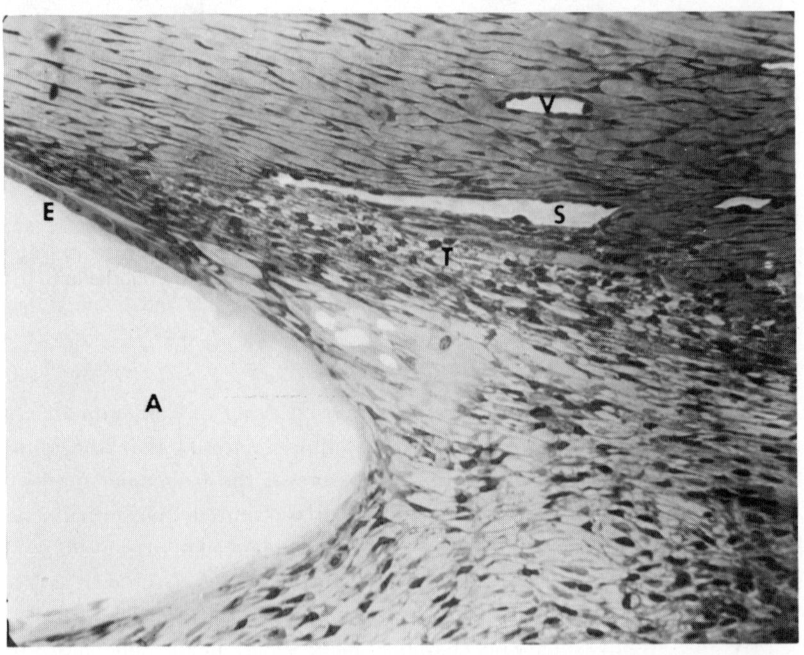

FIG. 5. The anterior chamber angle of a 121-day monkey embryo. The trabecular meshwork is well developed and its central portion is covered by the corneal endothelium and beginning Descemet's membrane. The loose angle mesenchyme is rarefied but the tissue lining the angle appears to be continuous. (A) Anterior chamber; (E) endothelium; (T) trabecular meshwork; (S) Schlemm's canal; (V) scleral vessel. (From Smelser and Ozanics. **Am. J. Ophthalmol.** 71:366, 1971.) X30 μm.

peripheral, but no cleft is apparent (Figs. 5 and 6). The tissue in the angle is extraordinarily loose and has a parallel arrangement, resembling trabecular formation in the adult. The spaces between cells are larger, and the tissue appears as if aqueous humor would readily "percolate" through it. There is no break in the continuous lining of the anterior chamber angle. However, elongated spaces are seen in the loose mesenchyme of both sections (indicated by arrows.) The longitudinal ciliary muscle fibers are well developed at this stage. They can be seen penetrating the trabecular meshwork area and ending in sclera, where as yet there is no distinct scleral spur.

Smelser and Ozanics also studied electron micrographs of the monkey embryo and noted that the cellular and tissue characteristics of all stages

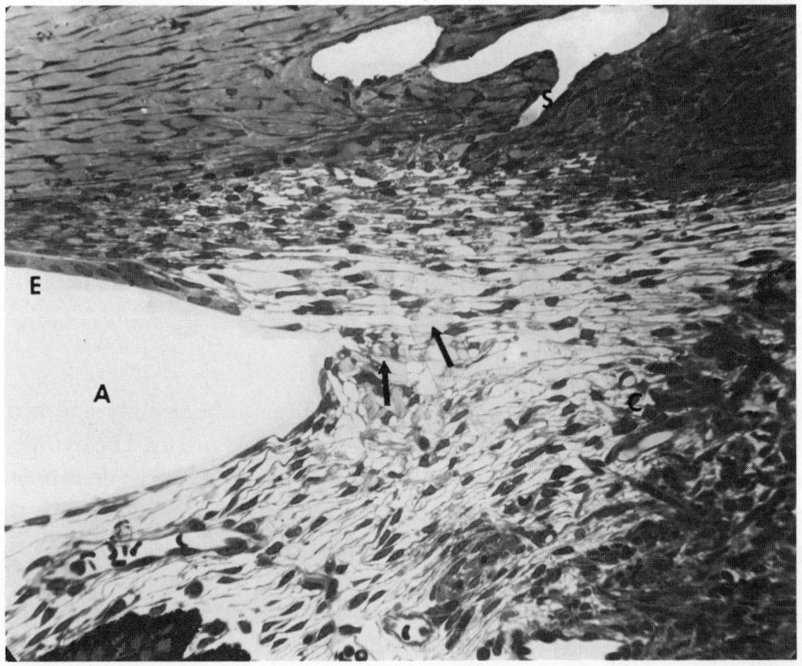

FIG. 6. Another section of the anterior chamber angle of the same eye as shown in Fig. 5, illustrating the variation in development of Schlemm's canal in different meridians. It appears that the Schlemm's canal (S) is just developing from a scleral vessel. The angle mesenchyme is continuous but merging of intercellular spaces has created elongated cavities (arrows) within the mass of angle tissue which could be converted into clefts by very slight rearrangement of the cellular processes. (A) Anterior chamber; (E) endothelium; (C) ciliary muscle; (S) Schlemm's canal. (From Smelser and Ozanics. **Am. J. Ophthalmol.** 71:366, 1971.) X 30 μm.

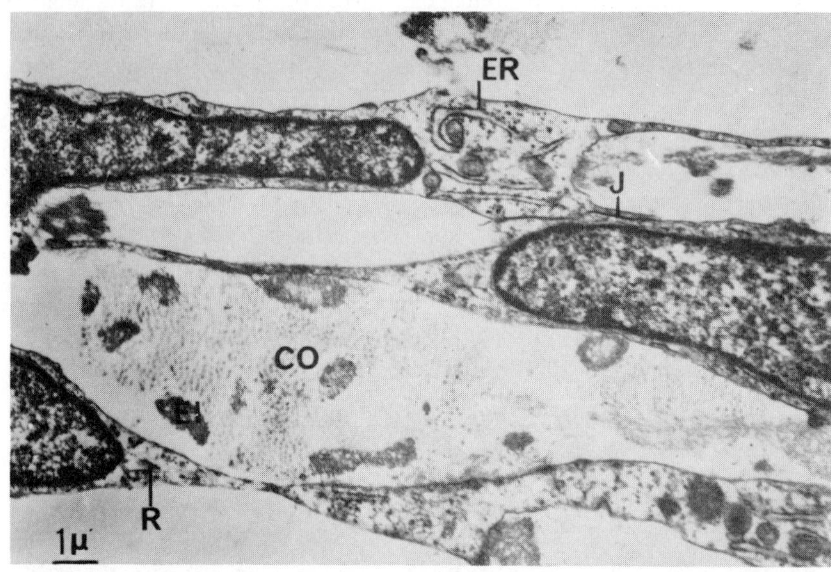

FIG. 7. Electron micrograph of trabeculae of a 121-day monkey embryo. Note the rough-surfaced endoplasmic reticulum (ER) and ribosomes (R) indicating protein synthesis. The cells are joined together by complexes which look like tight junctions (J). Collagen (CO) and elastic fibers (EL) are evident in the beams. (From Smelser and Ozanics. **Am. J. Ophthalmol.** 71:366, 1971.) X 1 μm.

have many features in common. The cells appear to be healthy and active. Nucleoli are demonstrable while lysosomes are rare or absent. The cytoplasm of the cells is rich in ribosomes and rough-surfaced endoplasmic reticulum (Fig. 7). The cells are extremely irregular or retricular in shape with their cytoplasm drawn out into extremely long, thin processes. These are so narrow that no organelles could be accommodated in them (Fig. 8). The large spaces of the meshwork are, therefore, bridged by these exceedingly fine cytoplasmic strands which are usually not associated with collagen fibers and are very delicate. Presumably tight junctions are evident. These are characterized by very narrow intercellular spaces and densification of adjacent cell membranes. Collagen and elastic fibers, forming the core of the trabecular beams, are well developed in 121-day-old embryos. The beams appear similar to those in the adult, but less compact. Often subendothelial empty areas are seen between the cells and the collagenous cores and between cells open to the intertrabecular spaces.

The 130-day embryo (Fig. 9) shows continuity of the tissue lining the

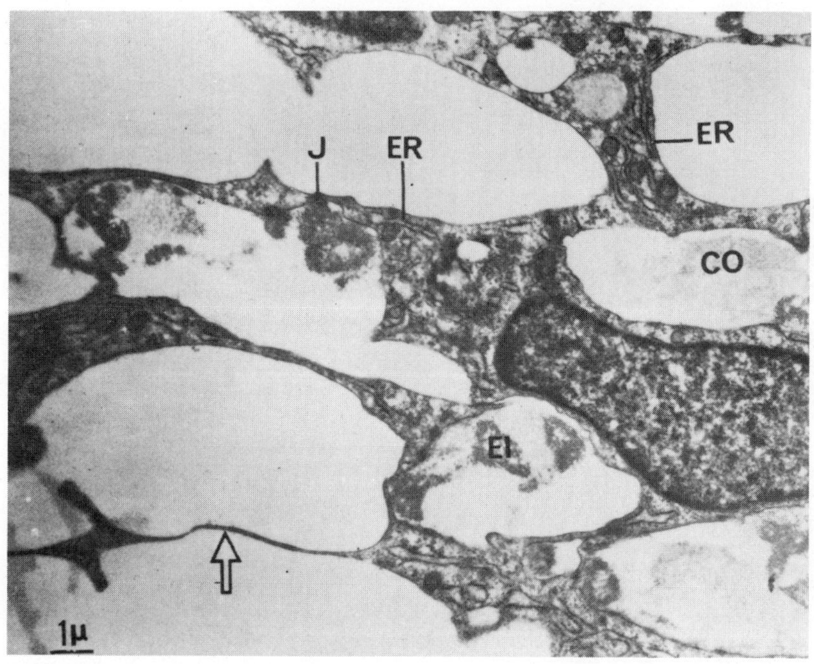

FIG. 8. Electron micrograph of the angle tissue in a 121-day monkey embryo. Note the evidence of synthetic activity, rough-surfaced endoplasmic reticulum (ER). The cells are joined together by apparently tight junctions (J). The trabecular beams are composed of both collagen (CO) and elastic (EL) fibers. The delicacy of the tissue is evident in the large amount of intercellular space and the extremely thin cytoplasmic strands (arrow) which connects the cells.(From Smelser and Ozanics. **Am. J. Ophthalmol.** 71:366, 1971.) X 1 μm.

anterior chamber angle. Schlemm's canal may be identified. The structure of the trabecular meshwork adjacent to the canal is more clearly differentiated than the loose tissue between it and the iris, but neither signs of atrophy (dying or dead cells) nor of a dramatic cleavage are noted. Sections of this eye show the collagen components of the trabecular beams to be well developed and for the first time a recognizable scleral spur is present. The apex of the anterior chamber angle, however, is still central to the ciliary muscles. Vesicles are seen in the trabecular wall of Schlemm's canal. indicating that the adult functional structure has been established. The meshwork of a 159-day-old embryo appears very loose or porous, but no signs of a cleavage or a split, or of cell death or atrophy are seen (Figs. 10 and 11). The apex of the angle is clearly more peripheral with respect to

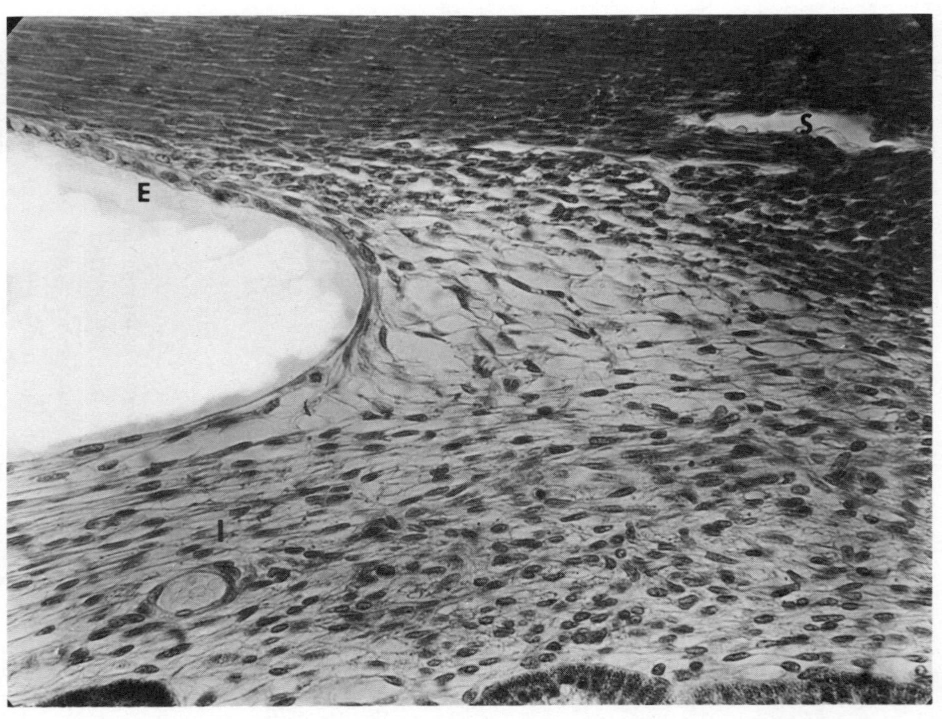

FIG. 9. A celloidin section, 12 μm thick, of a 130-day embryo. Schlemm's canal has vacuoles in its trabecular wall. The angle tissue is intact but rarefied. A continuous layer of cells lines the anterior chamber angle. (A) Anterior chamber; (E) endothelium; (S) Schlemm's canal; (I) Iris. (From Smelser and Ozanics. **Am. J. Ophthalmol.** 71:366, 1971.) X 30 μm.

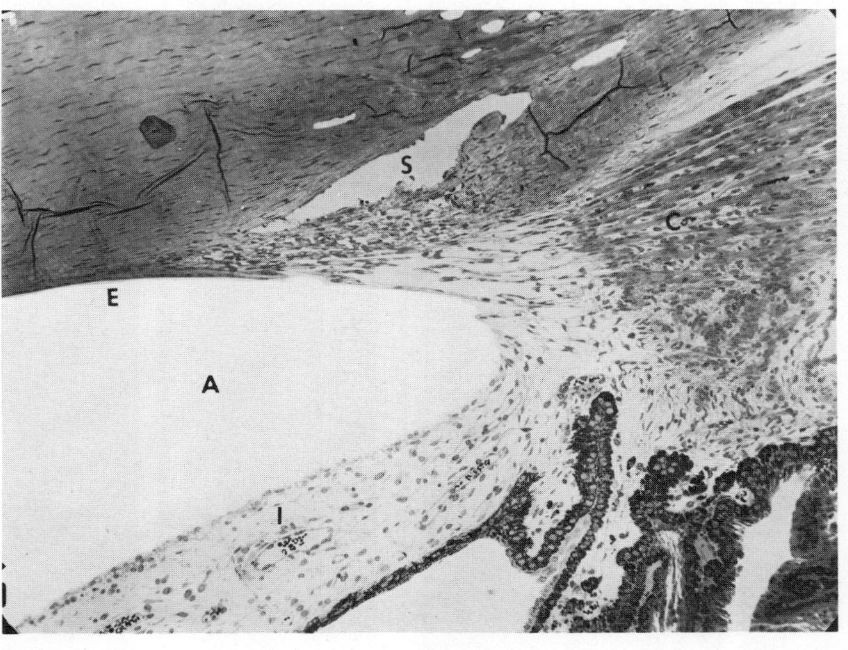

FIG. 10. The anterior chamber angle of a 159-day embryo, just a few days prior to birth. Rarefaction of the angle tissue has advanced greatly over earlier stages, but no simple cleft penetrates the angle opening it to the anterior chamber. (A) Anterior chamber; (E) endothelium; (S) Schlemm's canal; (C) ciliary muscle; (I) iris. (From Smelser and Ozanics. **Am. J. Ophthalmol.** 71:366, 1971.) X 60 μm.

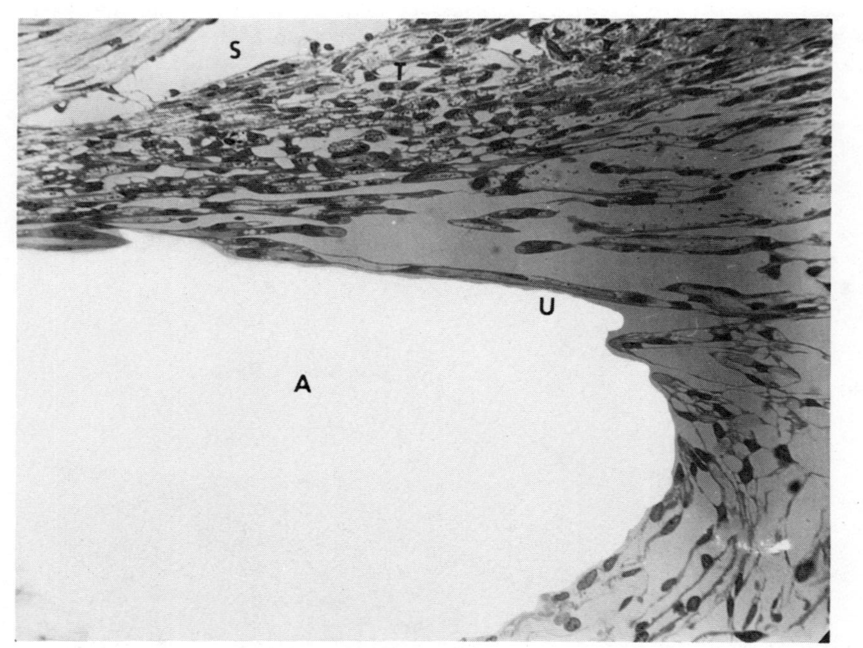

FIG. 11. A higher magnification of the section shown in Fig. 10. It is easy to see how the slightest tearing of the tissue during preparation could create a wedge-shaped opening. (A) Anterior chamber; (U) uveal trabecula; (S) Schlemm's canal; (T) trabecular meshwork. (From Smelser and Ozanics. **Am. J. Ophthalmol.** 71:366, 1971.) X 30 μm.

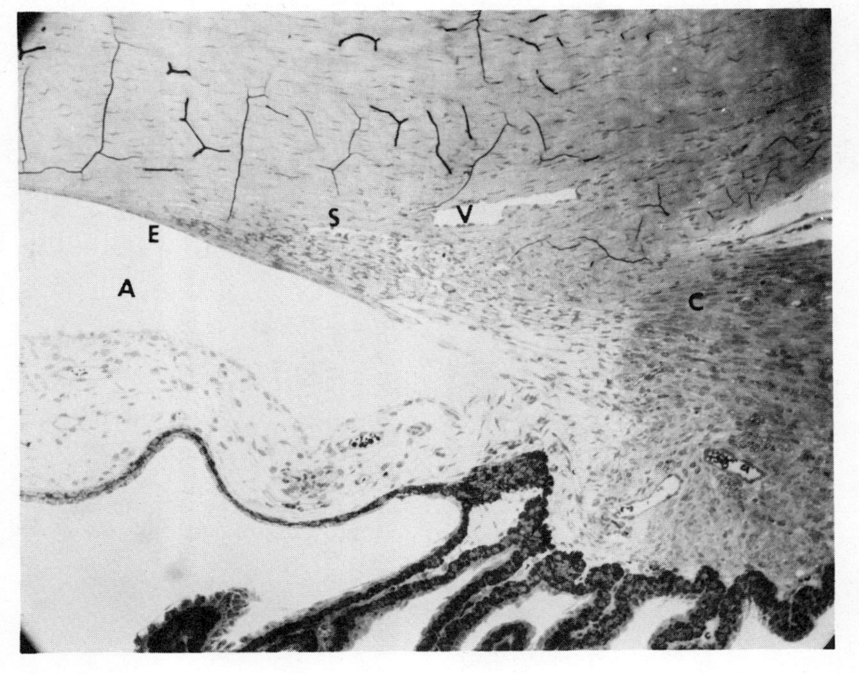

FIG. 12. This section of the eye of a two-day-old monkey infant shows that the angle tissue is decidedly more open than in Fig. 10. There is no evidence of cellular atrophy. (A) Anterior chamber; (E) endothelium; (S) Schlemm's canal; (V) scleral vessel; (C) ciliary muscle. (From Smelser and Ozanics. **Am. J. Ophthalmol.** 71:366, 1971.) X 60 μm.

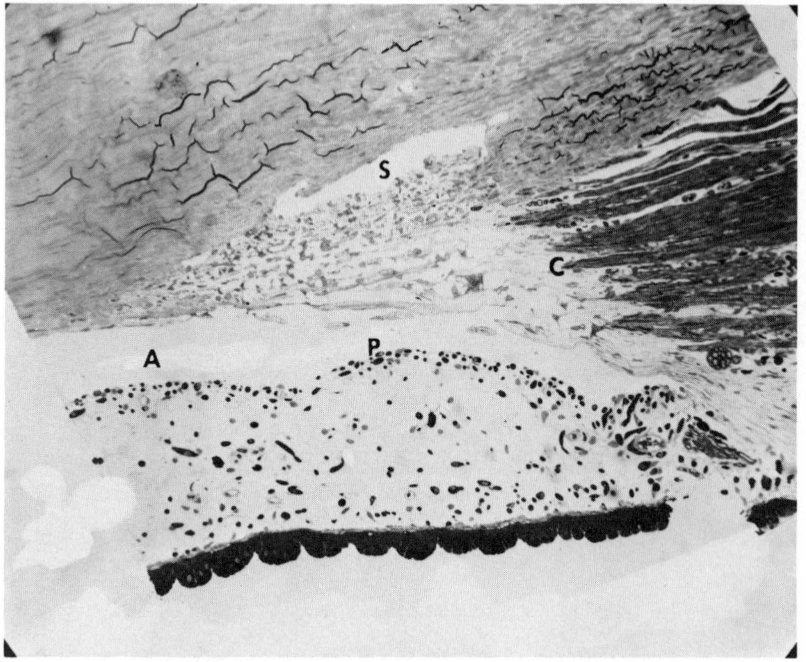

FIG. 13. This figure shows normal adult structure of the macaque monkey angle. The periphery of the anterior chamber is much more lateral to Schlemm's canal than it was at birth. (A) Anterior chamber; (P) pigment; (S) Schlemm's canal; (C) ciliary muscle. (From Smelser and Ozanics. **Am. J. Ophthalmol.** 71:366, 1971.) X 60 μm.

Schlemm's canal than before. Trabeculae appear more organized. The spaces between the uveal trabeculae are very large. The trabecular lying adjacent to the canal are much more organized than the others. Schlemm's canal itself is well developed, and the endothelial layer, on the trabecular side, contains vacuoles similar to those described in the adult, which are presumed to be a part of the outflow pathways. Development of the angle as a whole has not reached the adult form; thus the process continues after birth.

Fig. 12 shows the angle of a two-day postpartum macaque which exhibits a structure similar to the 159-day fetus, but rarefaction of the angle tissue has greatly progressed, thus deepening the concavity. The iris stroma is not yet pigmented.

The anterior chamber angle of an adult monkey (Fig. 13) is somewhat deeper than at birth but otherwise appears very similar. Beams of uveal meshwork, separated from each other by large spaces, may be seen.

Human Embryological Development

Vrabec noted that a fibrillar mesodermal substance fills the portion of the eye which is to form the anterior chamber in the first stages of embryological development following the 16-mm stage. Using *celodal* embedding, he demonstrated that at the 22-mm stage the anterior chamber is barely perceptible. The epithelium of the lens closely adheres to the corneal endothelium with only an insignificant layer of a slightly metachromatic substance between them. This metochromasia was seen in sections stained with cresyl violet. On the other hand, paraffin sections show the anterior chamber to be an obvious structure at this stage.

Therefore in the early stages of anterior chamber development, a true chamber angle is only present as a slitlike extension which is a virtual space, potentially present, but visible only after fixation fluids have artificially opened it. The endothelial elements migrate to the anterior chamber from the mesodermal tissue surrounding the anterior border of the optic cup. They are also formed by local mitotic divisions in the endothelial elements themselves. By the 45- to 55-mm stage the anterior chamber is present and contains a fibrinous coagulum. The corneoscleral junction is not yet clearly defined. A condensation of cells with darkly stained, spindle-shaped nuclei arranged in radial fashion is present at the peripheral edge of the corneal endothelium, and ends posteriorly in the inner layers of the scleral condensation. These cells are the anlage of the trabeculum and their insertion posteriorly is the anlage of the scleral spur. Therefore even at this stage trabecular cells may be differentiated from the looser mesodermal tissue which will form the ciliary body and root of the iris. On the other hand, the muscle bundles of the ciliary body cannot as yet be identified.

Reticulation

At the 26 mm stage and older, a striking change appears between the compact mesoderm, close to the anterior border of the optic cup, and the loose fibrillar stroma of the cornea. The mesodermal condensation near the border of the cup is highly cellular, and the nuclei are tightly packed. Fibrillogenesis is poor, and even at the 60-mm stage fibrils are quite rare in the scleral meshwork in comparison to the rich collagen bundles of the deep scleral and corneal layers. Fibrils of the uveal as well as the scleral meshwork are mostly impregnated in black by Gomori's method, while in the corneal and scleral tissue, collagen bundles are prevalent. According to Bolch, tissue demonstrates the property of transformation of compact tissue into open spongy tissue of the trabecular meshwork and anterior surface of the iris. Vrabec referred to this characteristic as "reticulation." This also includes the formation of reticular fibers. He noted that "reticulation" of the uveal meshwork and later of the scleral meshwork was evident in paraffin sections from the middle of the fourth month. In *celodal* sections of a 310-mm fetus, this "reticulation" was much less conspicuous. This could be explained by dehydration which takes place during the paraffin-embedding process, causing shrinkage of the cellular content.

Origin of Schlemm's Canal

In their study of the development of the chamber angle, Smelser and Ozanics proposed the following hypothesis on the origin of Schlemm's canal. The angle mesenchyme is very early clearly divisible into two distinct masses, one adjacent the sclera where Schlemm's canal can be expected to appear and the other, larger and more posterior, adjacent the ciliary body and root of the iris. The mass adjacent the sclera is triangular in shape, with its apex lying between the corneal stroma and its endothelium. The tissue is dense and the cells oriented parallel to the sclera. The area which forms the trabecular meshwork synthesizes considerable collagen and, in later stages, elastic fibers. The cells nearer the ciliary body are of a looser reticulum in which appreciable collagen does not develop during the embryonic stages.

Early in development, vessels in the sclera near the definitive position of the canal can be found. They are in the sclera, not between it and the developing meshwork. Their endothelial inner and outer walls are not differentiated as in the adult Schlemm's canal, and in some sections no trace of the vessel is seen. Extensions of the plexus of channels later become the aqueous veins. This is the classical concept. Thus, the ring-shaped canal would or could have several points of origin around the circumference of the eye and at early stages be present in some sections and absent in others. The blind ends of the collector channels would grow through the scleral tissue and anastomose with one another to form the circumferential canal between scleral tissue and the trabecular meshwork. Once in that position, differentiation of the endothelial lining to that characteristic of Schlemm's canal takes place. The section studies were compatible with this suggestion but direct anatomical proof was lacking.

Fourth and Fifth Month

The anterior chamber is still very shallow at the four-month stage (Fig. 14). The corneal endothelium reaches the apex of the anterior chamber angle where it ends in a clump of polygonal cells. There is no clear-cut differentiation of sclera from cornea. The supposed site of the future trabecular meshwork is composed of a wedge-shaped (in meridional sections) mass of mesenchyme with its apex between the corneal stroma and the endothelium. The iris, consisting of a short portion of the lips of the optic cup, is covered by mesenchyme, the future iris stroma, and pupillary membrane. The outer (anterior) layer of iris epithelium is pigmented but the layer lining the posterior chamber is not. There is no indication of iris muscles. More posteriorly both layers of the optic cup are slightly folded, indicating the beginning of ciliary processes. A ciliary vessel occupies the indentation of each fold (Fig. 15).

By the fifth month the anterior chamber tends to deepen. The filtration

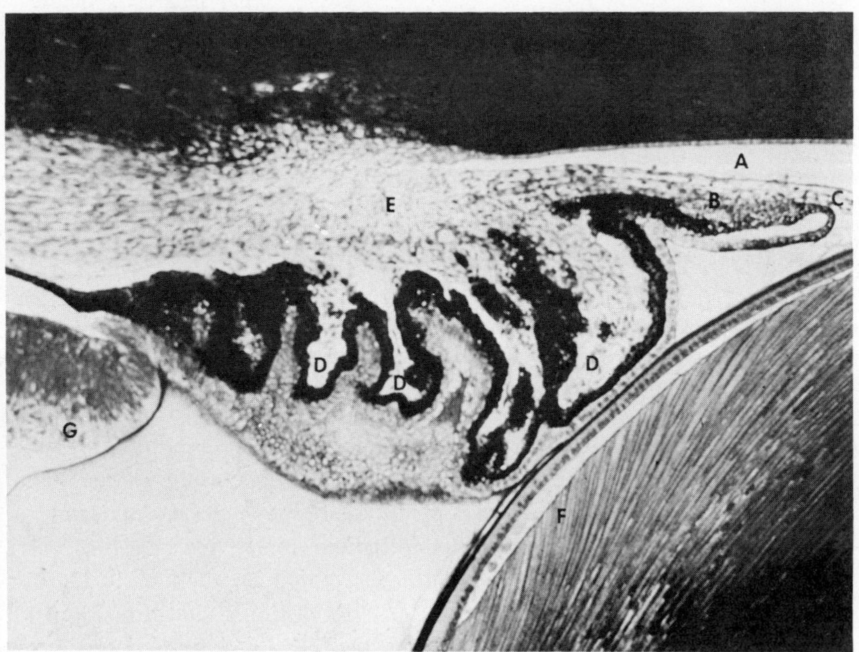

FIG. 14. Four-month-old human fetus. The anterior chamber (A) is still shallow. (B) Iris; (C) pupillary membrane; (D) ciliary processes; (E) ciliary body; (F) lens; (G) retina.

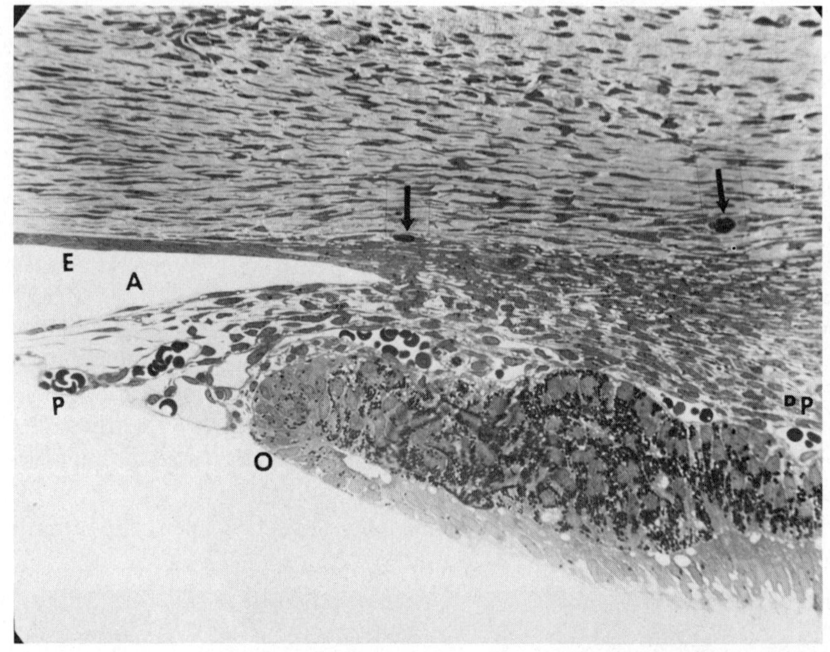

FIG. 15. Four-month-old human fetus. The corneal endothelium ends in a clump of polygonal cells. Scleral vessels (arrows) are present but no definite canal of Schlemm can be identified. The angle tissue is loose. A slight fold in the epithelium in which a blood vessel is lodged indicates the location of the ciliary processes. Compare with Fig. 2. (E) Endothelium; (A) anterior chamber; (P) pupillary membrane; (O) optic cup. (PP) ciliary process. (From Smelser and Ozanics. **Am. J. Ophthalmol.** 71:366, 1971.) X 30 μm.

angle recess is formed by a block of mesodermal tissue and consists of loosely meshed fibers which are a direct extension of the longitudinal portion of the primordial ciliary muscle and its primordial tendon. This area, by definition, is called the fetal pectinate ligament, according to Seefelder. The anterior chamber angle is rounded, lined by an unbroken string of attenuated cells from the corneal endothelium to the iris (Fig. 16). The periphery of the corneal endothelium covers about one-half of the future trabecular meshwork, where it faces the anterior chamber, and stops short of the apex of the angle. It has started to form a definite Descemet's membrane. The tissues in the angle have begun to differentiate into two types: a loose reticulum toward the iris and ciliary body and a more organized or oriented mass of cells, the future trabeculae adjacent the sclera. The primordial corneoscleral system forms part of the primitive scleral

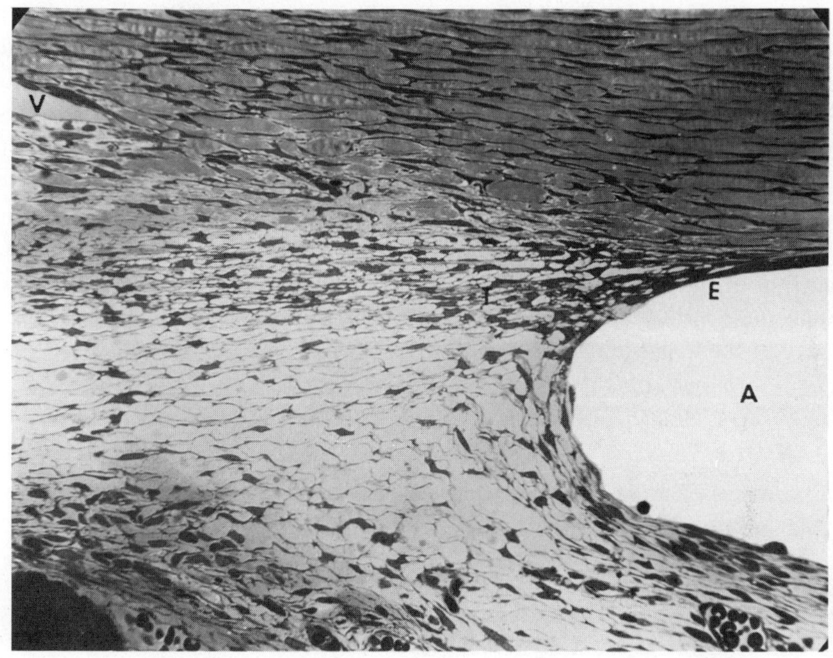

FIG. 16. Five-month-old human fetus. Schlemm's canal is not easily identifiable; however, an intrascleral vessel (V) may be seen. The tissue in the chamber angle is loose and reticular in nature; tissue adjacent the sclera appears to be organized in a more parallel pattern indicating the location of the future trabecular meshwork (T). (A) Anterior chamber; (E) endothelium. (From Smelser and Ozanics. **Am. J. Ophthalmol.** 71:366, 1971.) X 30 μm.

tissue. It is a fanlike extension situated at the end of the early Descemet's membrane formation. This primitive corneoscleral system lies side-by-side with the ciliary body—uveal meshwork complex. The ciliary body musculature (longitudinal portion) is inserted into the fetal uveal meshwork (fetal pectinate ligament). In other words, the uveal meshwork, as part of the uvea, forms the extension of the longitudinal muscle fibers. On microdisection these two groups (sclera-corneoscleral system and uvea-uveal meshwork system) are readily separated from each other. Definite ciliary processes are found at this stage and the iris possesses a well developed sphincter muscle, but the dilator is less easily distinguished. In summary, by the end of the fifth month (1) Schlemm's canal is present, lying between the sclera and the trabecular tissue, peripheral to the anterior chamber angle; (2) the anlage of the corneoscleral system is present but free spaces between its sheets are not yet in evidence; (3) cells which will develop into the circular muscle bundles can be recognized; (4) the trabecular fibers measure 0.23 mm; and (5) longitudinal fibers of the ciliary muscle are well developed and pass forward over a small blunted projection of collagen bundles located just posterior to Schlemm's canal, i.e., the anlage of the scleral spur. The fibers insert into the uveal meshwork. This fetal meshwork disappears in normal development but may persist, resulting in a permanent attachment (Fig. 17). In this event, the uveal meshwork fiber system represents in great part the tendon of insertion of the longitudinal muscle as pointed out by Henderson. This is reasonable since both the longitudinal muscle and trabecular meshwork come from the same mesodermal anlage. Goniotomy might therefore be called a tendonotomy of the longitudinal muscle.

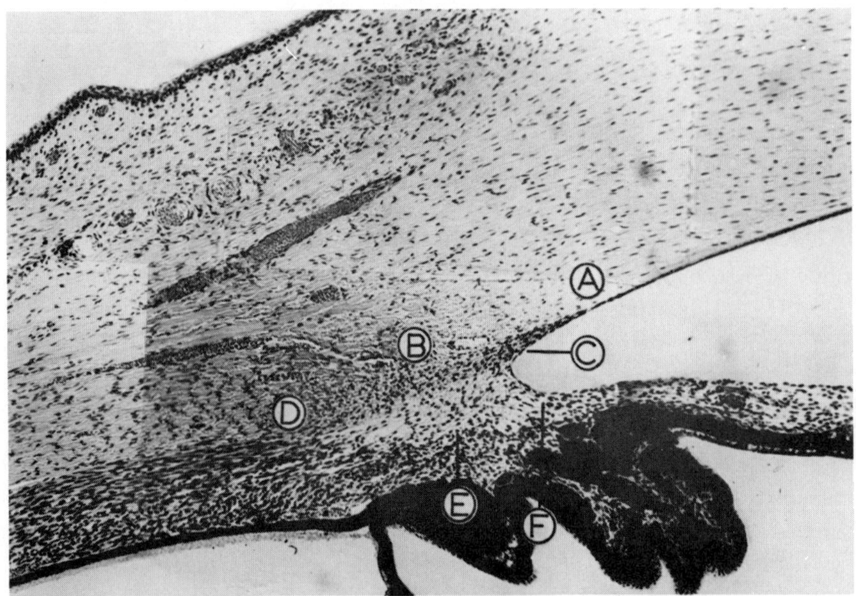

FIG. 17. Five-month-old human fetus. The corneoscleral meshwork begins to differentiate and the fetal pectinate ligament (C, D, E, F) or uveal meshwork is well developed. Schlemm's canal (B) is present but still in the fetal stage. The anlage of the corneoscleral system is present. The longitudinal fibers of the ciliary muscle insert into the uveal meshwork and have as yet no direct relationship with the scleral spur. Descemet's membrane fans out (A) into the corneoscleral primordium. The fetal pectinate ligament (C, D, E, F) may be subdivided into the ciliary portion (C, D, E) and the irideal portion (E, F, C). (Courtesy of J. G. F. Worst.)

The Artifact Factor

Forceful contraction and shrinkage of the ciliary muscle may occur during fixation. Kupfer studied a series of 20 eyes from fetuses ranging in age from 3 months of gestational age to birth. These eyes were fixed in 10 percent neutral formalin and processed through 95 percent alcohol. The eyes were then processed through celloidin and serial sections were cut at 18 μm thickness. The material was stained with hematoxylin and eosin, periodic acid-Schiff reagent and Mallory trichrome. He concluded that the concept of formation of the anterior chamber by cleavage appeared to be related to artifactual detachment of the ciliary body from the overlying scleral spur. This conclusion was based on two findings. Firstly, "cleavage" appeared and disappeared in different portions of the same angle, invariably associated with detachment of the ciliary body. Secondly, this appearance of cleavage was noted only in the 5-month-old fetus. In all subsequent ages, he found no evidence of "cleavage" whether or not there was artifactual detachment of the ciliary body. Kupfer felt that if "cleavage" were the mechanism for formation of the angle, it would be noted in subsequent age groups. It therefore appears that forces causing artifactual detachment of the ciliary body during fixation also cause the tissue in the angle to separate, suggesting a process of cleavage.

Another concept on the development of the filtration angle has been presented by Smelser and Ozanics. They concluded that the angle forms by a process of rarefaction of the reticular mesenchyme. The intercellular spaces enlarge throughout the angle area as the eye grows and the cells rearrange themselves. These enlarging spaces become confluent and more or less linear cavities, oriented in the meridional plane of the eye, appear within the tissue. These may, by slight tissue damage in processing, appear in sections as clefts or cleavage planes leading from the anterior chamber deep into the angle tissue. This concept, however, differs only slightly from the cleavage theory itself.

Further Development

As the embryo enters the sixth month (1) free spaces begin to develop between the corneoscleral meshwork layers which still form part of the sclera; (2) most of the longitudinal muscle fibers which are now clearly defined still insert into the fetal pectinate ligament, which has assumed a more fibrillar aspect, although some fibers are connected to the anlage of the scleral spur, a structure now easily identified; (3) mechanical traction has separated the outer layers of the uveal meshwork; (4) the ciliary processes have formed; and (5) the trabecular fibers measure 0.30 to 0.35 mm in length. Using the PAS and Best's carmine method it is possible to illustrate an important difference between the deeper scleral and corneal layers and the trabecular meshwork. A large amount of glycogen is found in the sclera of very young embryos and only a minimal amount in the trabecular meshwork and choroid. In later stages, when the fibers of the ciliary muscle are differentiating, the glycogen content appears to increase in the region of the ciliary muscle. This difference in glycogen content strongly supports the concept of a fundamental difference in the nature of the trabecular meshwork and scleral and corneal tissue (except the endothelium of the cornea).

The corneoscleral system fans out and its base (the scleral spur which is a true scleral structure) passes into the uveal meshwork and into the receding tendons (the fetal uveal meshwork) of the ciliary muscle. The scleral spur consists of circularly oriented collagen bundles on the anterior chamber side

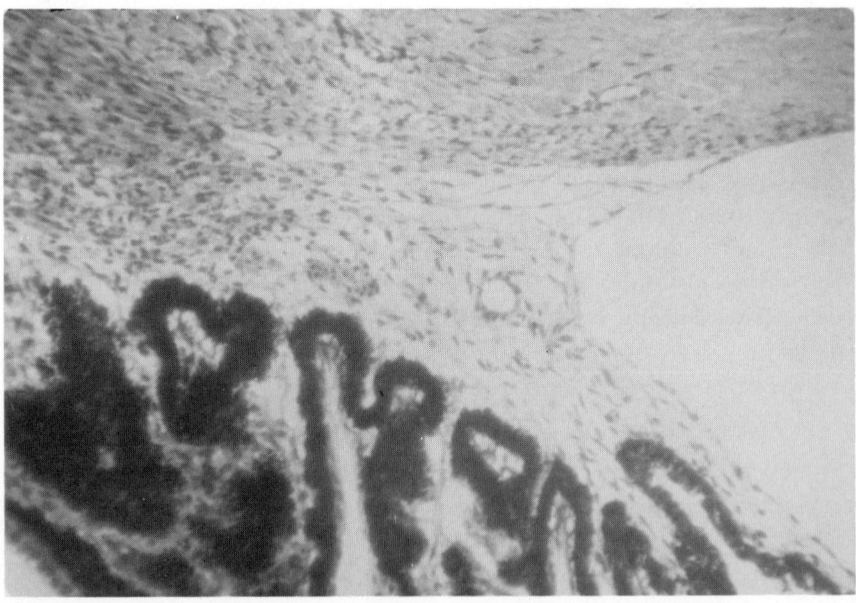

FIG. 18. Seven-month-old fetus. What appears to be a membrane envelops the filtration angle. (Courtesy of R. Bar Izchak.)

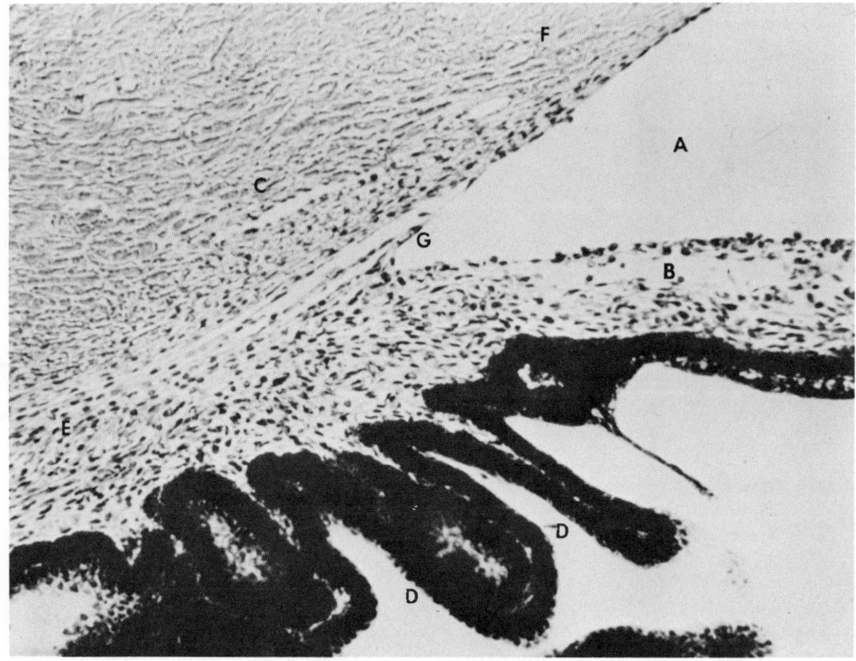

FIG. 19. Seven-month-old premature infant. The anterior chamber (A) is still shallow. (B) Iris; (C) Schlemm's canal; (D) ciliary processes; (E) ciliary body; (F) cornea; (G) pectinate fiber.

of the limbus, where scleral fibers having a relatively large radius of curvature abut with corneal fibers having a relatively smaller radius of curvature. The longitudinal muscle endings gradually become incorporated into the scleral spur attaching themselves to the lower side from the inside, outwards. Each ciliary muscle fiber sheet, which has found its "footing" on the scleral spur, means the loss of one sheet of fetal uveal meshwork. Therefore, the ingrowing scleral spur influences the gradual disappearance of the uveal meshwork. The further broadening of the scleral spur, which grows from the back forward and from within the scleral lamellae outward, spreads the base of the corneoscleral sheets, opening in this way the spaces which separate the sheets. If the scleral spur separation mechanism fails to occur, a certain amount of uveal meshwork will fill the chamber angle, according to Worst. The corneoscleral system at this stage is still underdeveloped in comparison with the relatively larger mass of the uveal meshwork.

During the transitional stages of the shift in relations between the ciliary muscle-uveal meshwork and the corneoscleral-scleral spur complex, a

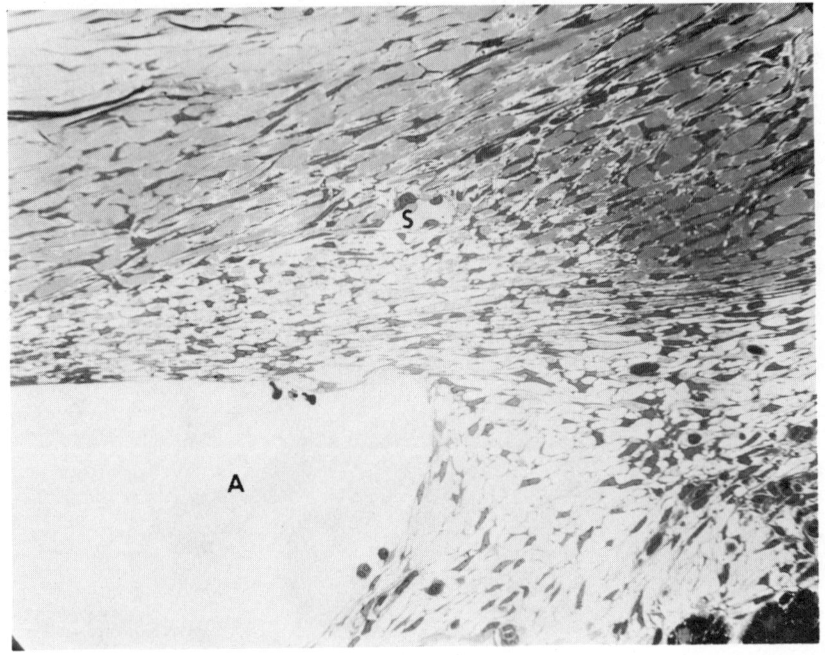

FIG. 20. Seven-month-old human fetus. The chamber angle is filled with loose reticular cells. The tissue lining the chamber angle appears to be intact. The future trabecular tissue has more substance than that adjacent the ciliary body. (A) Anterior chamber; (S) Schlemm's canal. (From Smelser and Ozanics. **Am. J. Ophthalmol.** 71:366, 1971.) X 30 μm.

regular layer of endothelial cells continuous with Descemet's endothelium covers the sinus formed by the iris base, the base of the uveal meshwork, and the top of the corneoscleral system (Fig. 18). This layer also covers the anterior surface of the pupillary membrane, which at this early stage separates the anterior chamber sac from the posterior chamber.

At the beginning of the seventh month the anterior chamber is still very shallow (Fig. 19). The trabeculae have developed collagenous cores and the edge of the anterior chamber is back as far as Schlemm's canal (Fig. 20). The uveal portion still resembles the loose reticulum of the fifth month. There is no cleft apparent but it is easy to see how it could develop, as shown in Fig. 21 of the same eye. Some of the intercellular spaces have become confluent and a potential cleft is obvious which, however, in this section does not reach the anterior chamber. The central extremity of the trabecular wedge is composed of dense, cell-rich tissue and almost every nucleus in this area has

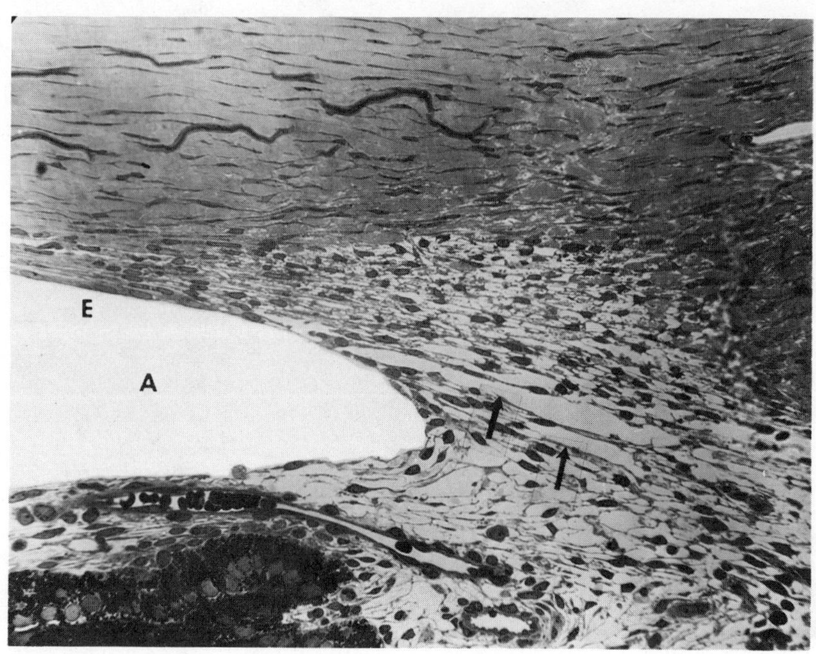

FIG. 21. Seven-month human fetus. This section is from the same eye as shown in Fig. 19. The trabecular meshwork is clearly differentiating. The spaces in the mass of reticular angle tissues are becoming confluent. In one or two places (arrows) slits or clefts have formed. (A) Anterior chamber; (E) endothelium. (From Smelser and Ozanics. **Am. J. Ophthalmol.** 71:366, 1971.) X 30 μm.

one or two nucleoli indicating their highly functional state. The corneal endothelium and Descemet's membrane cover the central half of the trabecular meshwork but do not reach the apex of the chamber angle.

The following histological features are noted in the premature infant: (1) the corneoscleral meshwork lacks normal spaces suggesting it to be still a scleral structure; (2) the scleral spur is obvious in relation to Schlemm's canal; (3) the circular and longitudinal muscle fibers of the ciliary body sweep up underneath Schlemm's canal and penetrate the looser trabecular tissue anterior and central to Schlemm's canal; and (4) Schlemm's canal is underdeveloped. It is obvious in some sections, but in others it appears deeply embedded in the sclera.

The 8-month fetus still shows an embryonic angle (Fig. 22) not much more advanced than that seen at the 7-month stage. Schlemm's canal is clearly shown in its adult relationship, and the trabecular wall contains

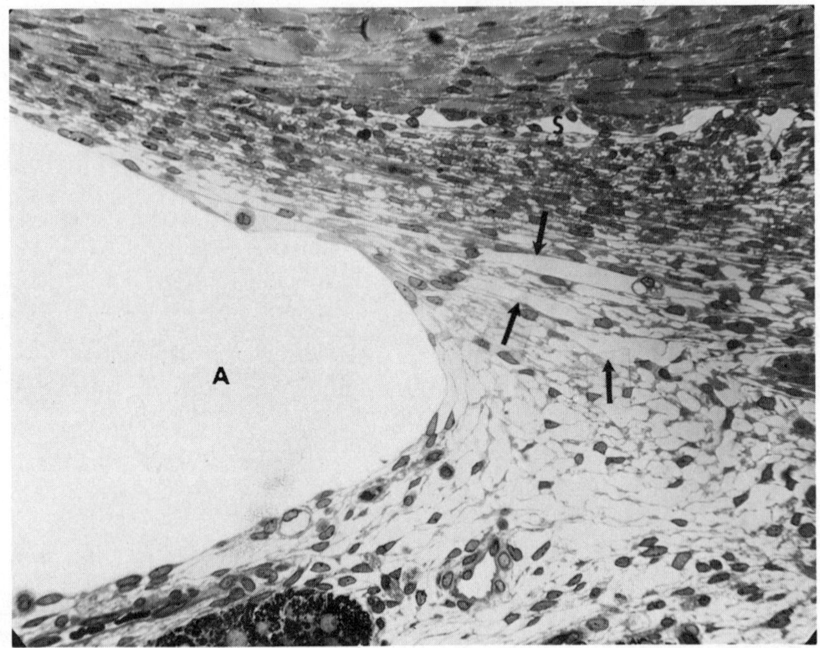

FIG. 22. Eight-month human fetus. Schlemm's canal (S) is well formed as are the trabecular beams. The wall of the chamber angle is intact and continuous. The extremely loose reticular mesenchyme cells of the angle exhibit nucleoli indicating protein synthesis. The intercellular spaces are occasionally enlarged and enlongated (arrows) but not open to the anterior chamber. (A) Anterior chamber. (From Smelser and Ozanics. **Am. J. Ophthalmol.** 71:366, 1971.) X 30 μm.

vacuoles indicating that it is functional. The trabeculae are more mature but the angle is closed by a continuous, unbroken strand of cells in which most of the nuclei appear active. There is also no break in the cellular lining of the anterior chamber. The spaces between the trabecular cells are large and some of them, having coalesced with others, are enormous and elongated (Fig. 22, arrow). The ciliary muscle reaches far into the trabecular tissue. Descemet's membrane is perhaps one-fifth the thickness of the endothelium and covers a portion of the trabecular mesenchyme at the periphery of the cornea.

The trabecular beams are very well developed in the 9-month fetus. Elastic fibers are evident as small black dots (Fig. 23). The intertrabecular spaces are open. The anterior chamber angle below the trabecular meshwork, however, is filled by a mass of loose reticular cells, not associated with appreciable intercellular connective tissue elements. These cells appear

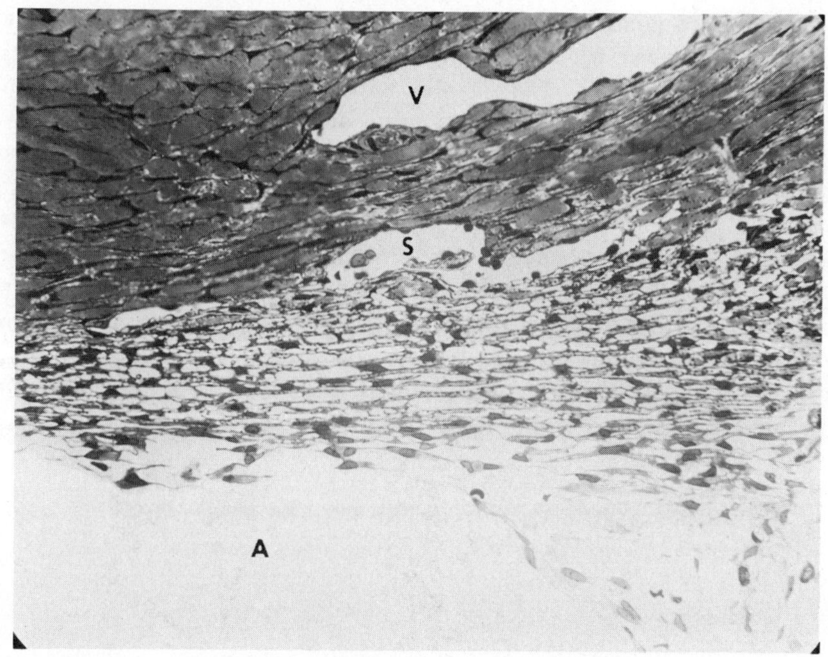

FIG. 23. Nine-month human fetus. The trabecular meshwork and Schlemm's canal (S) are well developed. Elastic fibers are demonstrated. The loose uveal tissue in the angle is still intact and composed of active cells. (A) Anterior chamber; (V) Scleral vein. (From Smelser and Ozanics. **Am. J. Ophthalmol.** 71:366, 1971.) X 30 μm.

healthy and engaged in synthetic processes as evidenced by their nuclear structure. The spaces between these cells are enormous. This embryo shows no evidence of a cleft but rarefaction is evident. Schlemm's canal seems to be complete and a good scleral spur is formed. The corneal endothelium still covers the central part of the trabecular meshwork. The longitudinal fibers of the ciliary muscle are well developed and come near the most peripheral part of the anterior chamber angle. Pigment cells are noted with greater regularity in the iris stroma and the dilator muscle is now present.

In the near-term fetus, Schlemm's canal lies at the level of the apex of the anterior chamber angle. Ciliary muscles sweep up to and past a well developed scleral spur and some enter the trabecular meshwork. The iris stroma now contains pigment cells in its most anterior superficial layers, which are the last to become pigmented. Dilator muscle fibers are well developed. The end of Descemet's membrane and the endothelium still cover some of the trabecular meshwork. The uveal trabeculae are well formed and the lining of the anterior chamber angle is no longer continuous. The very loose reticular tissue which filled the angle heretofore is confined to only its deepest part (Fig. 23). The circular muscle of the ciliary body often manifests itself late in the development of the fetus and is frequently difficult to find even at birth. It usually becomes evident during the first year of life. It is a matter of conjecture exactly when the excretory pathways open, but is seems plausible that this occurs in time with the onset of production of aqueous humor. For aqueous humor to leave the anterior chamber in fetal life, two barriers must have been removed: the pupillary membrane and the endothelial covering of the uveal meshwork. In addition to these barriers, other structures must have reached functional maturity, namely (1) the uveal meshwork; (2) the corneoscleral meshwork; and (3) Schlemm's canal.

THE FILTRATION ANGLE OF THE INFANT EYE

Gonioscopy

The angle of the infant anterior chamber differs from that in the adult in several ways. Firstly, the trabecular fibers appear more transluscent than they do in the adult so that one has the feeling of being able to see deeper into the tissue. Secondly, iris processes are found much more frequently than they are in the adult. In blond infants these appear as nonpigmented fiber bands extending from the surface of the peripheral iris to Schwalbe's line. In black infants they are heavily pigmented.

Barkan studied the appearance of the anterior chamber and described the changes that took place from infancy to adult life. At birth the normal infant eye still has a relatively shallow chamber. The iris inserts in a horizontal plane so that there is no ciliary sulcus (Fig. 24) as seen in the adult eye (Fig. 25); however, the anterior tip of the ciliary body may be seen. The angle is clothed by what appears to be an almost transparent membrane with a shagreened surface, which extends downward from the line of Schwalbe to the level of the scleral spur and then drops in a vertical plane over the trabecular zone. It covers the uveal meshwork, extends over the peripheral portion of the iris, and has been observed to cross a portion of a crypt as an isolated layer. It was Barkan's impression that this layer represented the endothelium noted in fetal life. In the months following birth, fenestrations in the shagreened membrane begin to appear. In older eyes the anterior chamber is deeper but the angle recess is still absent. The

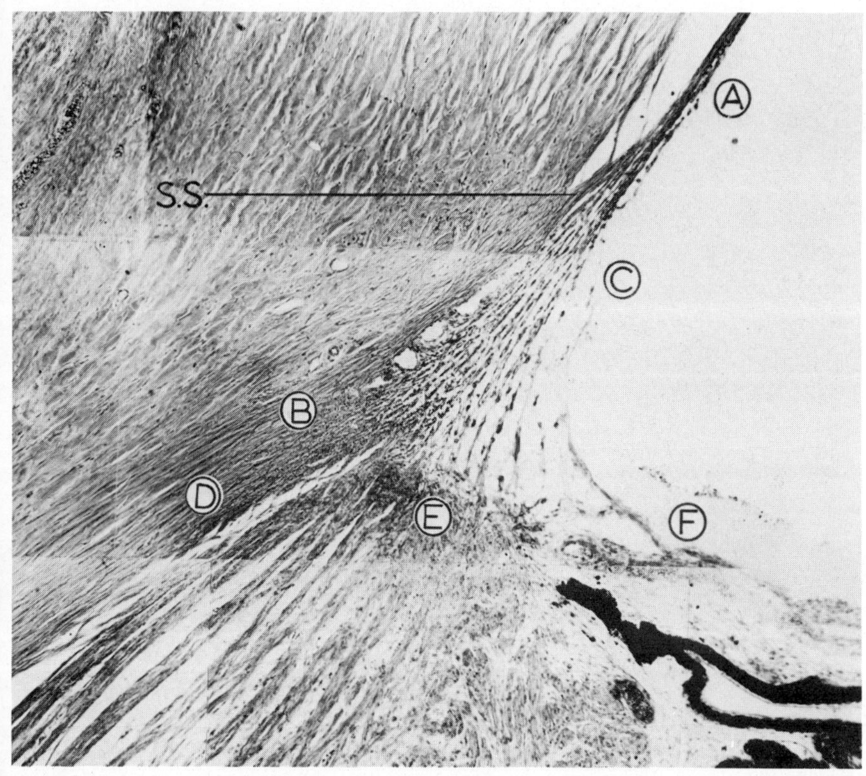

FIG. 24. Normal infant eye at birth. The iris inserts in a horizontal plane so there is no angle recess. (A) Schwalbe's line; (B) scleral spur; (C) pectinate ligament; (D) sclera; (E) ciliary muscle; (F) iris; (SS) Upper extent of trabecular meshwork. (Courtesy of J. G. F. Worst).

distance between the line of Schwalbe and the iris base is increased. The scleral spur is usually visible and Schlemm's canal approaches the adult position.

The changes in the gonioscopic appearance of the angle that occur with age caused Barkan to conclude that the filtration angle of the normal infant is still incompletely differentiated and that development is still taking place. It is generally agreed that full development is not reached until 2 to 4 years of age. The clinical application of this fact lies in the observation that although many cases of congenital glaucoma begin normal function in the first few days after surgery and some even immediately, other cases take several weeks to reach a normal intraocular tension.

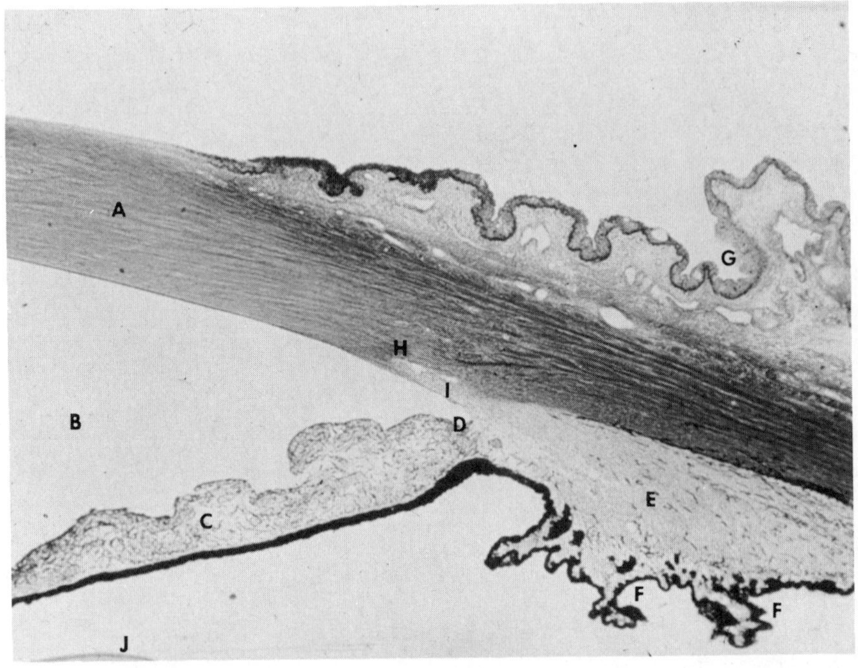

FIG. 25. Normal adult eye. (A) Cornea; (B) anterior chamber; (C) iris; (D) iris recess; (E) ciliary body; (F) ciliary processes; (G) conjunctiva; (H) Schlemm's canal, (I) trabeculum, (J) lens.

The Normal Filtration Angle

In the normal human eye, Schlemm's canal is located in the iridocorneal angle recess, in a corneoscleral groove called the internal scleral sulcus. The trabeculum which covers the canal takes the form of a triangle with the apex at Schwalbe's line and the base, the scleral spur. The inner and outer boundaries are made up of the anterior chamber and the inner wall of Schlemm's canal, respectively. In the trabecular meshwork of primates, 3 different zones can be distinguished. The first zone, or uveal portion, contains a wide network of collagenous strands. These fibers are surrounded with concentric layers of homogeneous substances and endothelial cells. The second zone, the so-called trabeculum corneosclerale, consists of lamellae with a central core of ground substance and a system of fibers completely covered by "glass membranes" and cells. The third zone is called the pore

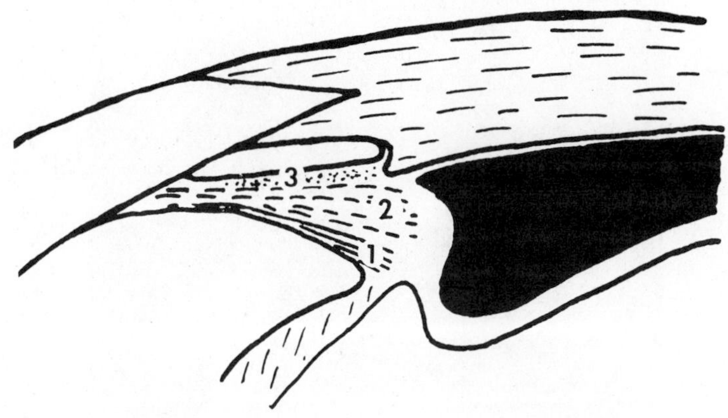

FIG. 26. Schematic drawing of chamber angle of primates showing 3 distinct parts in the trabecular meshwork area. (1) Uveal meshwork area; (2) trabeculum corneosclerale area; (3) inner wall or pore area, Schlemm's canal. (Modified from J. Rohen.)

area and comprises the inner wall of Schlemm's canal. This zone contains an argyrophilic fiber system which is embedded in a homogeneous interfibrillar

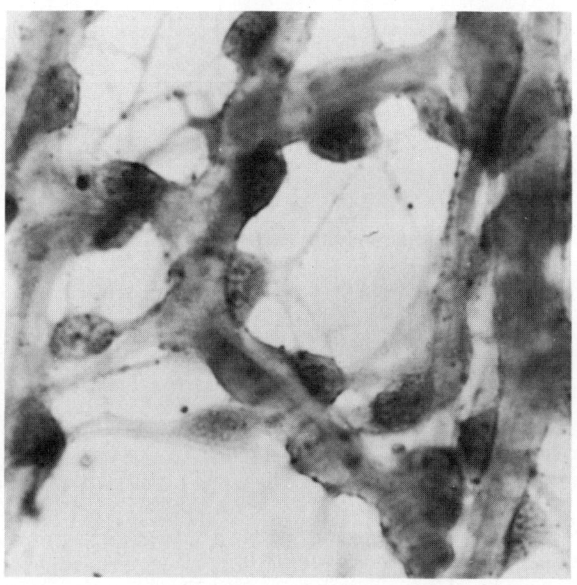

FIG. 27. Normal trabecular meshwork (18 months). Flat preparation of trabecular meshwork showing corneoscleral fibers. (Courtesy of J. S. Speakman.) Polychrome methylene blue X 400.

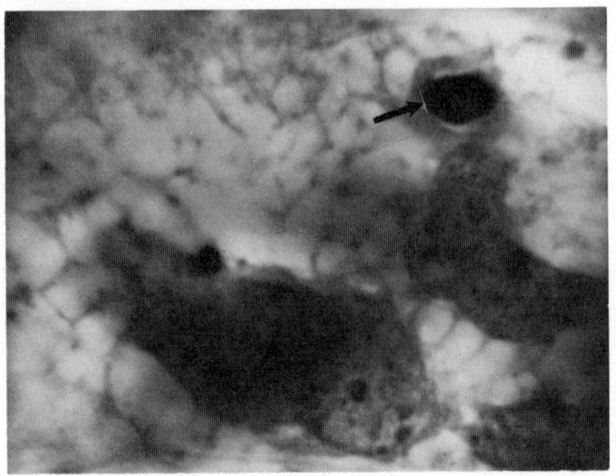

FIG. 28. Normal corneoscleral meshwork (5 months). Flat preparation showing spaces of varying sizes in the cytoplasm lying between lamellae. Clumps of pigment (arrow) and red blood cells are seen in these spaces. (Courtesy of J. S. Speakman.) Polychrome methylene blue X 1500.

ground substance rich in mucopolysaccharides (Fig. 26).

Speakman and Leeson examined the trabecular area of apparently normal infant eyes using the flat preparation technique and made the following observations.

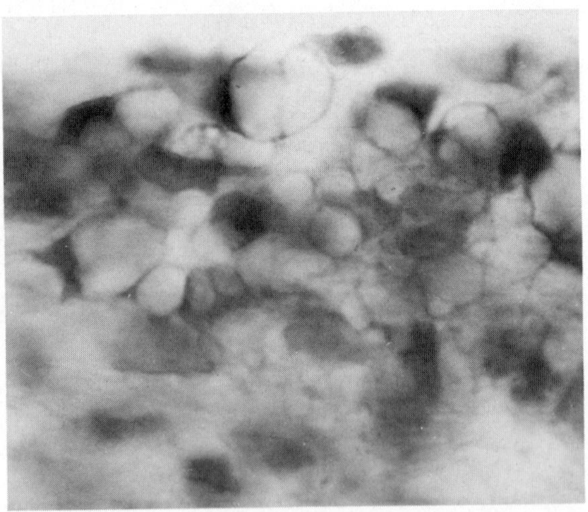

FIG. 29. Normal corneoscleral meshwork (3 months). Flat preparation of trabecular wall of Schlemm's canal showing spaces. (Courtesy of J. S. Speakman.) X 625.

Corneoscleral Meshwork

The corneoscleral meshwork consists of sheets of collagen lined by endothelial cells and perforated by many oval and spiral openings. The collagen lamellae are thinner near Schlemm's canal and the meshwork is more cellular. The gaps between lamellae are crossed by fine intercellular bridges and many of the spaces resemble vacuoles (Fig. 27). In the innermost layers near the uveal meshwork, oval and spiral defects lead from one intertrabecular space to the next. These larger openings are confined to the layers just beneath the uveal meshwork. The outer third of the meshwork consists of a mass of cells and fibers in which no definite lamellae can be identified (Fig. 28). Although fine spaces or vacuoles less than one micron in diameter are present, the majority are larger and occasionally contain pigment granules deposited on the cytoplasm or red blood cells in the clefts showing that bulk flow has occurred through these channels. In the adult the smaller vacuoles are absent.

The outermost portion of the meshwork (or the trabecular wall of Schlemm's canal) contains spaces developed to a remarkable degree (Fig. 29). The cytoplasm surrounds relatively enormous cavities and smaller

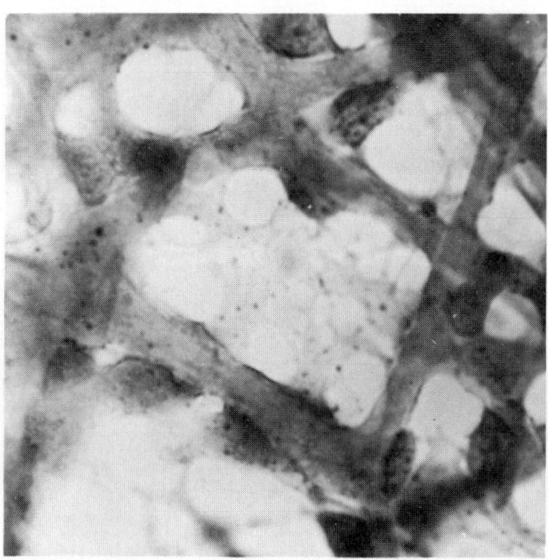

FIG. 30. Normal uveal meshwork (18 months). Flat preparation showing perforated membranes of cytoplasm stretching across gaps between fibers. Increased staining of fiber bundles forms thick bands. (Courtesy of J. S. Speakman.) Polychrome methylene blue X 400.

intercommunicating spaces are present in or between every cell. Similar spaces are found in the trabecular meshwork lying immediately below the wall of the canal, resulting in a communication system made up of irregular tunnels through the meshwork.

Uveal Meshwork

Flat preparations show long strands of fibers running in an antero-posterior direction from the root of the iris to Schwalbe's line (Fig. 30). The spaces between the fibers are divided into circular openings which are covered with thin sheets of cytoplasm that are frequently attenuated causing round perforations. In the adult the openings in the uveal meshwork are larger and the membranes of cytoplasm between the fibers are virtually absent.

THEORIES ON THE CAUSE OF CONGENITAL GLAUCOMA

Numerous theories and hypotheses have been postulated to explain the defect in the eye of infants and young children that leads to hydrophthalmia. These theories have implicated abnormal development of the chamber angle, physiologic abnormalities such as hypersecretion of aqueous as a result of a neurogenic disorder, endocrine disease, ocular inflammation including intrauterine uveitis, periphlebitis of the vortex and ciliary veins, and structural defects such as weakness of the sclera. Some of these latter factors have already been discussed in the early part of this chapter.

It is generally agreed that congenital glaucoma arises from an abnormality (some have called it an arrest) in development of mesoderm of the corneoscleral junction, resulting in a structural defect in the region of the filtration angle which causes an obstruction to the drainage of aqueous humor. Maumenee noted one specimen in which there was a very prominent Schwalbe's line and an almost complete failure of development of the angle of the anterior chamber. It was almost impossible to differentiate the cells and fibers in the iris and ciliary body from those in the trabecular fibers. In addition there was a total failure of the tissues to separate, beginning at Schwalbe's line. Schlemm's canal could not be identified. The appearance of the angle of the anterior chamber of this specimen was that of a 140-mm embryo. In most cases of congenital glaucoma, Schlemm's canal in one form or another is present, although eyes devoid of the canal have been reported. In cases where a canal is not found, rows of endothelial cells with-

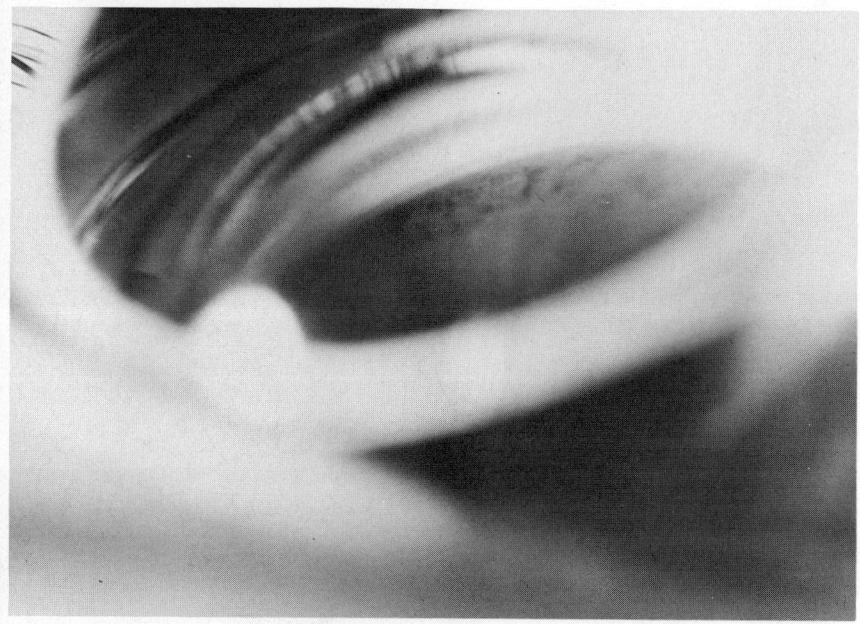

FIG. 31. Normal eye of child with uniocular buphthalmos. The trabecular zone is easily identified.

out any sign of a lumen have been observed in the region of Schlemm's canal, giving rise to the possibility of collapse from functional inactivity. Later there would be further distortion as the eye begins to distend. Anderson's survey concluded that closure of the canal was a secondary process. Barkan studied the gonioscopic appearance of the filtration angle in congenital glaucoma. He stated that there is more tissue or tissue which is more opaque overlying Schlemm's canal, as judged by the more subdued color and lesser definition of the blood-filled Schlemm's canal and by the thicker optical section. The so-called shagreened membrane is less transparent than in the normal eye and in the area of Schlemm's canal appears to represent the anomalously differentiated trabeculum which crosses the angle. The folds or tents of uveal tissue, which insert into the membrane, or anomalous trabeculum, from the anterior surface of the iris, are more definite and extend higher toward the line of Schwalbe.

The iris stroma is semitransparent so that one may see the reflection of the pigment epithelium from the ciliary body to the iris, leaving a narrow

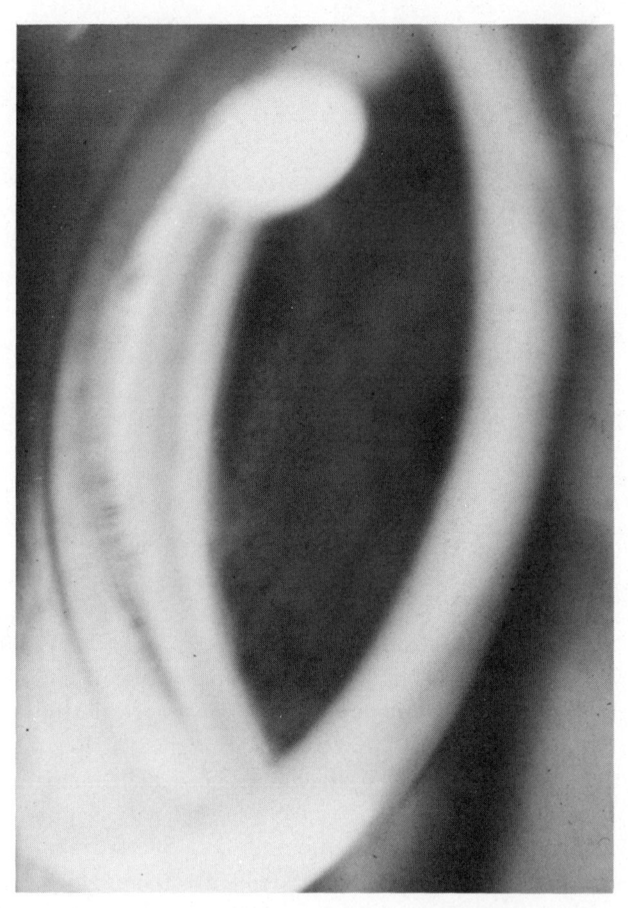

FIG. 32. Buphthalmic eye of same child as in Fig. 31.

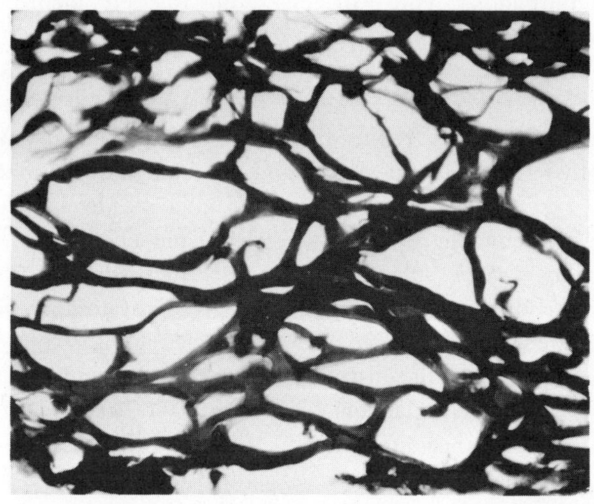

FIG. 33. Congenital glaucoma. Flat preparation showing large openings in uveal meshwork between short pectinate ligaments. (Courtesy of J. S. Speakman.) X 140.

peripheral zone of iris tissue with no pigment epithelium posteriorly.

Fig. 31 illustrates the filtration angle of the normal eye in a child with

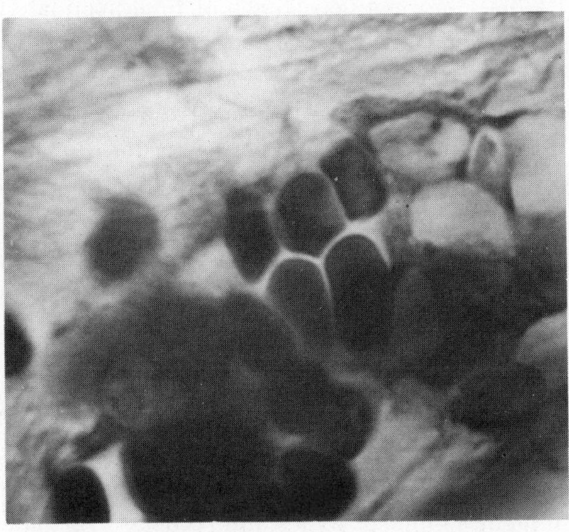

FIG. 34. Congenital glaucoma. Flat preparation of outer corneoscleral meshwork showing many small vacuoles in cytoplasm. (Courtesy of J. S. Speakman.) X 1250.

uniocular buphthalmos. The trabecular zone is easily identified. Fig. 32 shows the involved eye. No trabecular zone can be detected in the recess of the angle. Flat preparations of the uveal meshwork show large openings into the underlying layers but the length of the fibers running from iris root to Schwalbe's line is greatly reduced and the pectinate ligaments are more matted together (Fig. 33). Speakman and Leeson also noted that in contrast with normal eyes there are large numbers of much smaller spaces or vacuoles in the cytoplasm covering the beams (Fig. 34) and a noticeable reduction in cellularity. This feature also characterized the region of the canal of Schlemm where the spaces, although large, were not comparable in size to those seen in the wall of the canal of normal eyes.

Seefelder described the histological appearance of angle structures in infants with congenital glaucoma as follows: "There is an abnormal development in the trabeculum with insufficient differentiation of its outer layers. The root of the iris is inserted closer to the ring of Schwalbe than normal, at the same time sending a thick hook-like process toward the end of Descemet's membrane. The potential chamber angle is crossed by the anomalously differentiated or abnormally persisting trabeculum. Schlemm's canal plexus is narrowed and partially obliterated. The area of access to the lumina of Schlemm's canal which are placed behind the actual free angle is obstructed or narrowed by incomplete separation of the root of the iris from the posterior surface of the cornea." He summarized the changes found in congenital glaucoma as follows: (1) the rudimentary development of the scleral spur; (2) the abnormal persistence of fetal pectinate ligaments (also called abnormally abundant or persistant uveal meshwork or mesodermal tissue); (3) abnormal narrowing and backward displacement of Schlemm's canal; and (4) the retarded differentiation of the corneoscleral trabeculum. Other features include the insertion of a large part of the longitudinal muscle fibers into the uveal meshwork, and the close relationship of the circular muscle fibers with the more superficial sheets of the uveal meshwork.

The Cleavage Theory

Schlemm's canal appears about the latter part of the third lunar month of gestation. By the sixteenth week red blood cells may be seen in the lumen of the canal (Fig. 35). Allen et al. noted that the human anterior chamber opens during fetal development by a simple process of separation or cleavage of two dissimilar layers of mesodermal tissue (Fig. 36). This theory is an extension of the old concept of anterior chamber formation by splitting which rests on Kolliker's hypothesis. These two clearly defined groups of

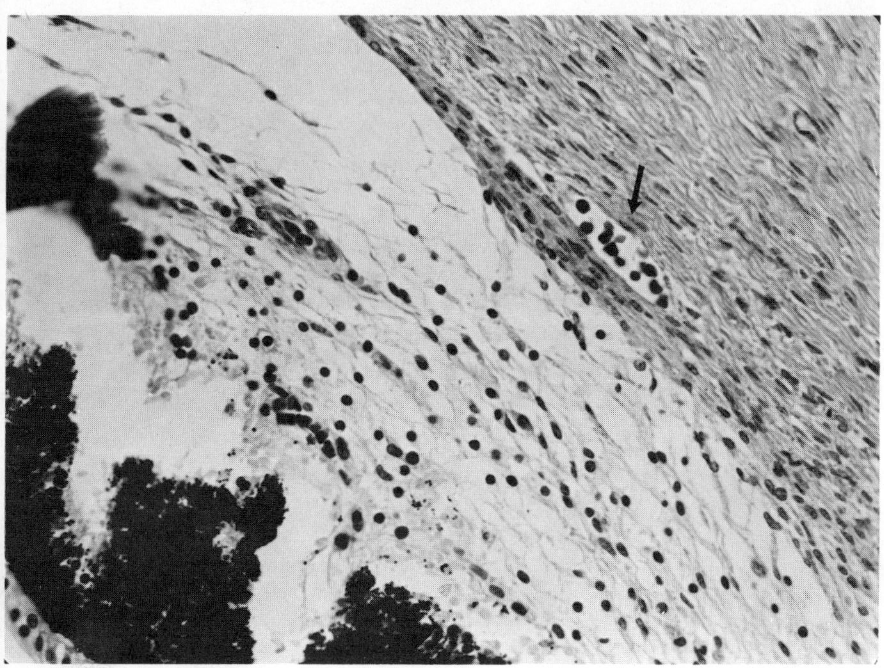

FIG. 35. Fetus (sixteenth week). Red blood cells fill Schlemm's canal (arrow). X 330.

cells are the anlage of the trabecular fibers on the one hand and the root of the iris and ciliary body on the other. Differential growth rate between the external, internal, and forward portions of the ciliary body is sufficient to account for cleavage which occurs along the line of the inner layer of uveotrabeculae (Fig. 37). Continuing growth of the ciliary muscle aids the process (Fig. 38). Allen et al. showed that the number of cell layers in the trabeculum of the adult filtration angle is about the same as in the fetal angle, implying that the volume of tissue is virtually the same in both the adult and the fetus. If atrophy took place there should be less tissue in the adult. Smelser and Ozanics noted that there was no evidence of atrophy or cell death. In fact, they noted cytologic evidence of active growth (nucleoli, ribosomes, and rough-surfaced endoplasmic reticulum). Allen et al. suggested that a retardation in this process of cleavage would leave the iris displaced anteriorly.

Based on the study of both human and monkey embryos, Smelser and Ozanics concluded that a gradual process of rarefaction of the reticular mesenchyme (akin to cleavage) explained the means of deepening and

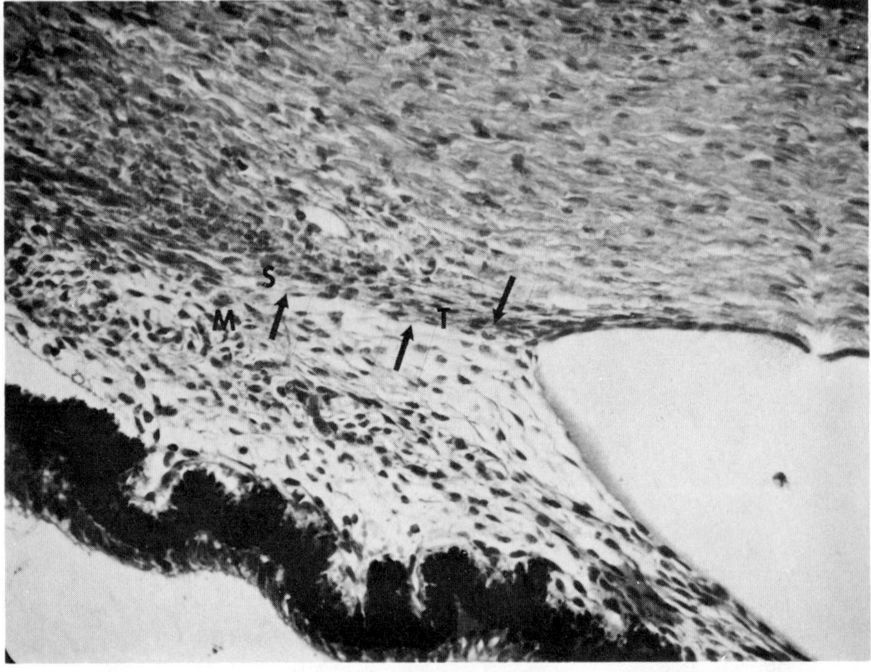

FIG. 36. Fetus (sixteenth week) showing the demarcation line between the two dissimilar layers of mesodermal tissue (arrows). The longitudinal muscle (M) of the ciliary body can be distinguished from the trabecular fibers (T) at the location of the anlage of the scleral spur (S). X 330.

extending the anterior chamber. The spaces in the spongy or reticular meshwork grow in size, become confluent, and the resulting fused areas also continue to grow. The cells are suspended in this space, together with the fibrous material which they have synthesized and on which they rest. The spaces form a continuum (as do those in a sponge) and later become continuous with the anterior chamber. The openings from one irregular space to another, or to the anterior chamber may be very small (on the order of 100 Å) but become larger and more clearly demonstrable in later stages.

The mass of open-textured tissue in the angle begins just lateral, or posterior, to the end of the layer of corneal endothelial cells. Where the angle tissue borders on the anterior chamber, these small spaces enlarge and eventually open into the anterior chamber (of which they then become a part) and its most peripheral portion, i.e., the angle. The process is one of rearrangement of cells throughout the entire angle tissue mass, not in just one plane, and not by simply splitting a mass of homogeneous mesenchyme

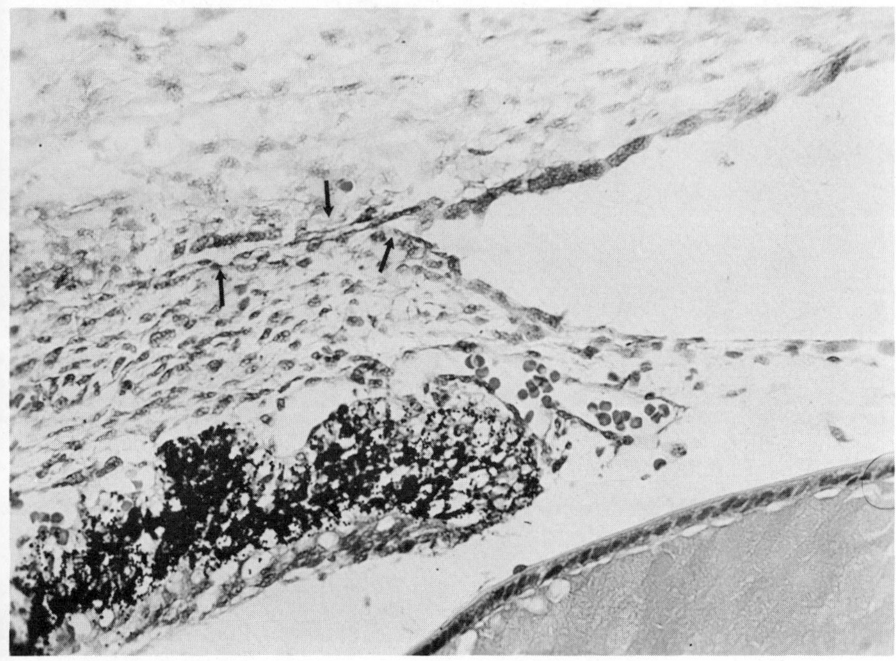

FIG. 37. Fetus (sixteenth week) showing cleavage taking place along the inner layer of the uveo-trabeculae (arrows). X 400.

cells into two portions, but by gradual enlargement of the innumerable intercellular spaces, until they become confluent with the anterior chamber. The chamber is thereby made wider, and the angle moved peripherally to its final location. This concept differs very slightly from the "cleavage" theory and only in that it substitutes tissue rarefaction or reorganization for a splitting of the mesoderm as a method of creating the angle.

Maumenee noted the following abnormalities in a large series of cases. (1) In congenital glaucoma there is a failure of the iris and ciliary body to separate from the trabecular fibers. This, however, does not account for the decreased facility of outflow in these eyes, firstly, because the adherence of these tissues to the trabecular fibers varies from an attachment to Schwalbe's line to an attachment just forward of the scleral spur, and secondly, because in eyes that had been recently operated upon (3 goniotomies and one sclerectomy with iridectomy) red blood cells were found between all but the outermost layers of the trabecular fibers, 180° from the operative site even where the iris and ciliary body were extensively adherent to the trabecular

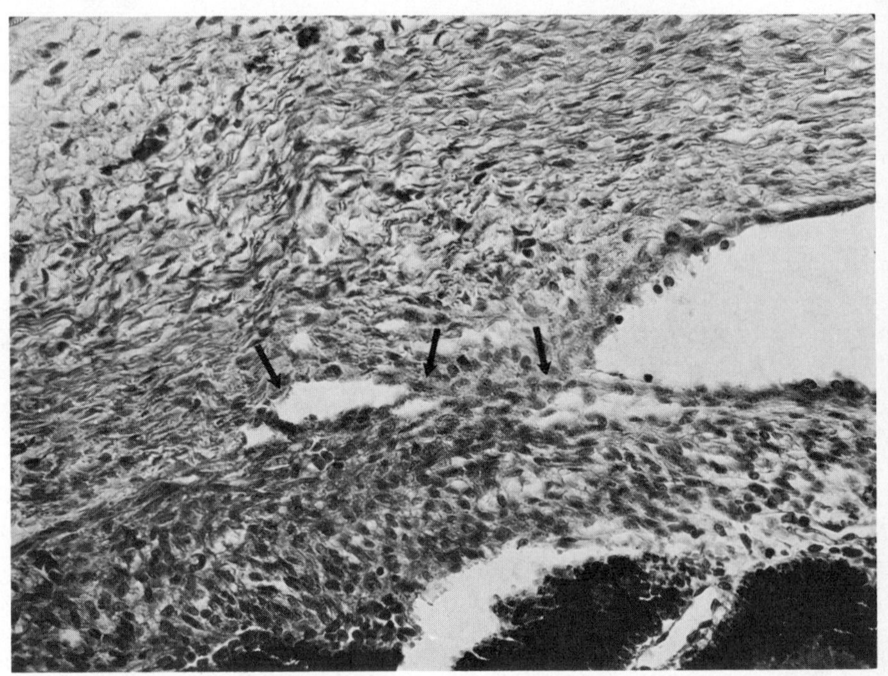

FIG. 38. Fetus (sixteenth week) showing the separation of tissue layers. X 300.

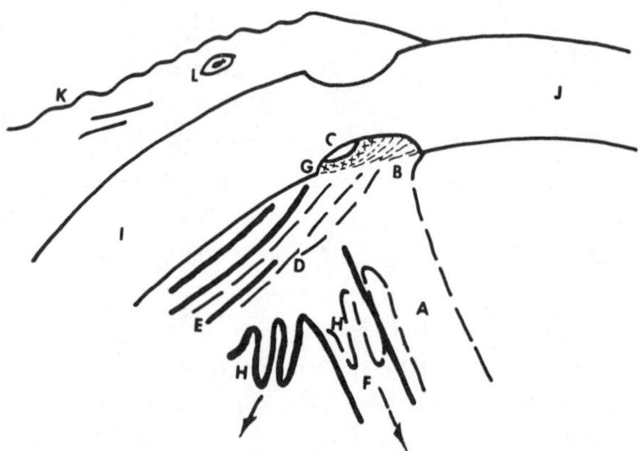

FIG. 39. Schematic drawing of the filtration angle to demonstrate the cleavage theory. The iris (A, broken lines) is displaced to a forward position. (B) Trabeculum; (C) Schlemm's canal. The longitudinal fibers (D) of the ciliary body (E) insert into the trabecular fibers. The unbroken heavier lines indicate the normal location of the iris (F), in which longitudinal fibers of the ciliary body insert into the scleral spur (G). (H) Ciliary processes; (I) scleral; (J) cornea; (K) conjunctiva; (L) conjunctival vessel.

fibers. (2) The ciliary processes and ciliary body are pulled centrally, possibly due to a microphakia or relative microphakia, so that the ciliary processes are central to an imaginary line that passes vertically through the posterior end of Schlemm's canal. (3) An endothelium-lined Schlemm's canal can be found in most specimens of early congenital glaucoma. In other eyes the canal may be collapsed in certain sections, possibly due to the anterior external position of the scleral spur. (4) The scleral spur is frequently difficult to see because of its displacement forward and externally. (5) The longitudinal and circular muscle fibers insert further forward and to a greater extent than normally into the corneoscleral portion of the trabeculae. In most instances, the longitudinal fibers extend forward beyond the anterior tip of the scleral spur, even up to the posterior one-fourth of Schlemm's canal. Since the circular muscle is attached to the inner surface of the trabecular fibers instead of at the ends of the fibers, it would not exert the normal spreading effect to open the trabecular spaces. This may in some way

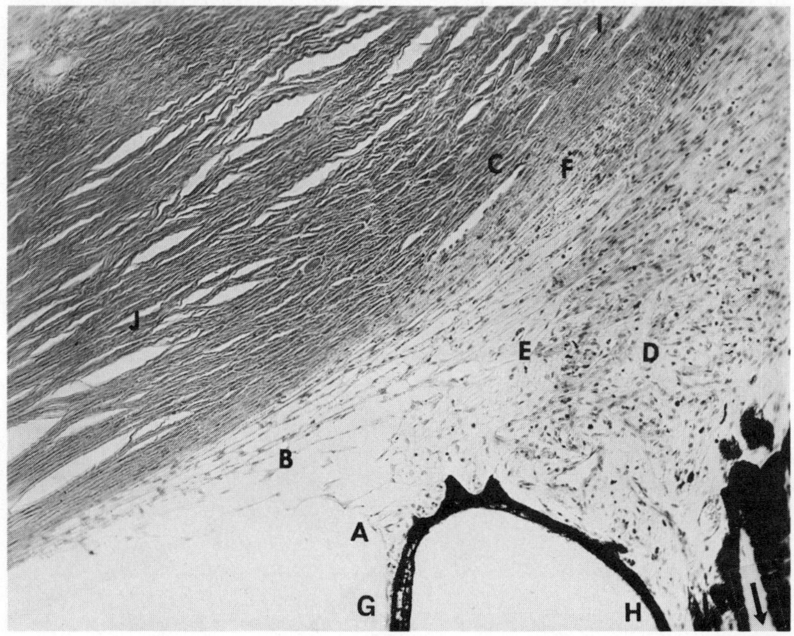

FIG. 40. Histological section of the filtration angle in congenital glaucoma. The iris is displaced to a forward position (A-B) and the longitudinal muscle fibers (E) of the ciliary body (D) reach centrally to insert into the trabeculum. (C) Schlemm's canal; (F) scleral spur; (H) ciliary processes; (I) sclera; (J) cornea.(A. F. I. P. Acc. No. 331614). (Courtesy of F. D. Costenbader and the Registry of Ophthalmic Pathology of the Armed Forces Institute of Pathology.) X 130.

be responsible for the decreased facility of outflow. In 3 eyes that had had a recent goniotomy and in one eye with a successfully functioning goniotomy, the base of the iris and ciliary body had been cleaved from the trabecular fibers. The longitudinal muscle of the ciliary body had been cut free from the trabecular fibers and an artificial scleral spur was created. This was thought to be the mechanism whereby goniotomy increased the facility of outflow in congenital glaucoma.

In the normal infant eye (Fig. 24) the longitudinal fibers of the ciliary body (E) insert largely into the scleral spur (B). Schlemm's canal is therefore directly exposed via the trabecular meshwork to the anterior chamber and aqueous humor flow. In the case of congenital glaucoma the angle is altered in such a way that aqueous humor may not reach the outflow channels, resulting in a retention of aqueous humor which gradually causes a pressure elevation and buphthalmia. Fig. 39 illustrates the anatomical configuration of a case of congenital glaucoma representing an arrest of the cleavage process. The iris (A, broken lines) is displaced to a more anterior position than is normal (F, dark lines). The longitudinal muscle fibers of the ciliary

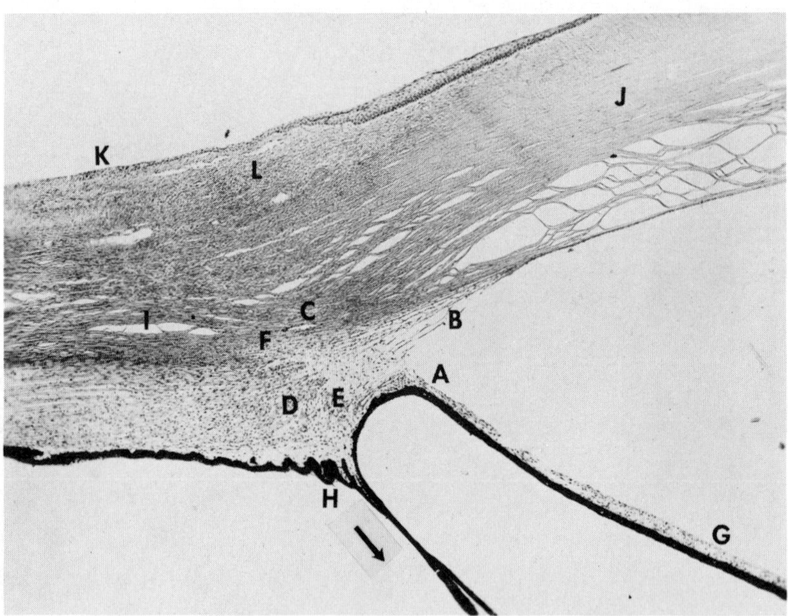

FIG. 41. Histological section of a case of congenital glaucoma. Same case as Fig. 40, under low power. A–B, Filtration angle; (C) Schlemm's canal; (D) ciliary body; (E) longitudinal fibers; (F) scleral spur; (G) iris; (H) ciliary processes; (I) sclera; (J) cornea; (K) conjunctiva; (L) conjunctival vessel. (A. F. I. P. Acc. No. 331614.) (Courtesy of F. D. Costenbader and the Registry of Ophthalmic Pathology of the Armed Forces Institute of Pathology.) X 50.

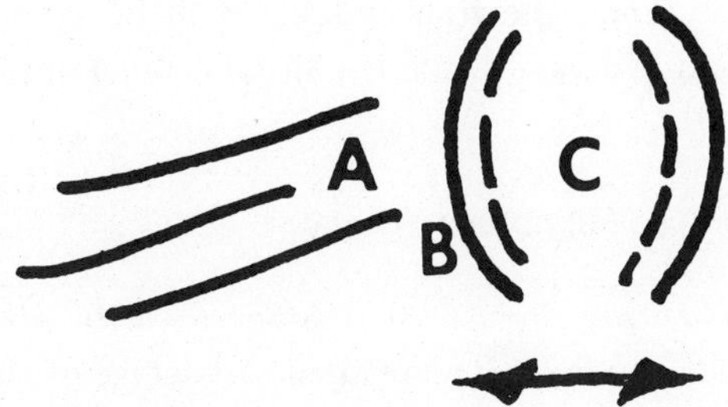

FIG. 42. In the normal eye the longitudinal fibers (A) of the ciliary body insert into the scleral spur (B). Contraction of the muscle opens the trabecular spaces (C) as an accordion would open if pulled at the handle.

body (D, thin lines) will therefore insert anteriorly to the scleral spur (G) directly into the trabecular fibers (B). In the normal infant these fibers (E, dark lines) insert largely into the scleral spur (G). The filtration angle of a case of congenital glaucoma is shown in Figs. 40 and 41. The longitudinal fibers (E) of the ciliary body (D) insert directly into the trabecular fibers anterior to Schlemm's canal (C), bypassing the scleral spur (F).

The functional results of this anatomical arrangement may now be illustrated. In the normal eye (Fig. 24) the longitudinal fibers of the ciliary body insert primarily into scleral spur (Fig. 42). Contraction of these muscle fibers (A) will therefore cause a posterior displacement of the scleral spur (B) and an opening of the trabecular spaces and Schlemm's canal (C). The oval openings in the meshwork become more rounded in shape as the trabecular fibers spread, increasing the filtration area. (Movement at (C) is in an outward direction.)

In the glaucomatous eye (Fig. 43) the longitudinal fibers of the ciliary muscle (A) appear to be attached to a greater extent than normal to the trabecular fibers and extend anterior to the scleral spur (B). With this arrangement, contraction of these ciliary body fibers would tend to flatten the scleral spur (B) externally and thus compress Schlemm's canal (C). The

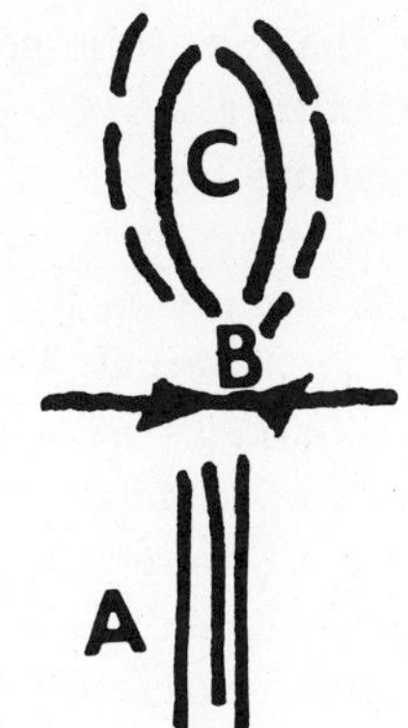

FIG. 43. According to the cleavage theory, insertion of the longitudinal fibers (A) of the ciliary body takes place in the trabeculum itself to a great extent. Contraction would compress the scleral spur and narrow Schlemm's canal. The effect on the trabeculum would be to close the spaces (C).

effect upon the trabeculum would be to close the spaces and reduce the filtration area. (Movement at (C) is in an inward direction.)

The Membrane Theory

A persistence of mesoderm with its covering surface layer is an essentially normal state at an early stage of chamber angle development. This surface membrane, which is probably of endothelial origin, normally breaks down with maturation of the angle in the same way that the pupillary membrane atrophies, leaving the uveal meshwork exposed to the aqueous humor. In congenital glaucoma the imperforate surface structure persists, covering the uveal meshwork and preventing its exposure to aqueous humor. This is in effect a persistence of the fetal condition. The insertion of the longitudinal muscle fibers into uveal meshwork also reflects the fetal condition of the chamber angle. In normal adult anatomy these fibers insert into the corneoscleral meshwork or its base formed by the scleral spur.

Barkan described the gonioscopic appearance of a transparent membrane with a shagreened surface, which he assumed to be endothelium, clothing the filtration angle in eyes of all infants. The membrane might not be observed histologically due to the techniques involved in preparation. In congenital glaucoma, the shagreened membrane was more opaque gonioscopically, representing the anomalously differentiated trabeculum in the region of Schlemm's canal. (Figs. 44–46). Fenestration may still occur spontaneously (Fig. 47).

Barkan listed the causes of congenital glaucoma as (1) decreased permeability of the tissue overlying Schlemm's canal (Fig. 48); (2) anterior insertion of the iris (Fig. 49); (3) anomalously picked-up folds of the anterior stromal layer of the iris (Figs. 50 and 51); and (4) exaggerated upturning of the scalloped ends of the pigment sectors (Fig. 52). It was stressed that the relative impermeability of the trabeculum was the main cause of congenital glaucoma with the abnormal anterior insertion of the iris being a contributing factor.

Worst has recently reemphasized this concept and described the filtration angle as covered by "mesodermal sheets" into which the ciliary muscle fibers are inserted. The sheets are covered by a membrane which Worst called "Barkan's membrane." (Fig. 53). The membrane concept is illustrated in Fig. 54. Maturation has evolved so that the iris plane lies in the normal position. However, the trabeculum is still obstructed by a membrane which sweeps up from the anterior surface of the iris to attach to the peripheral cornea. A triangle (dotted line) is thus formed by the membrane

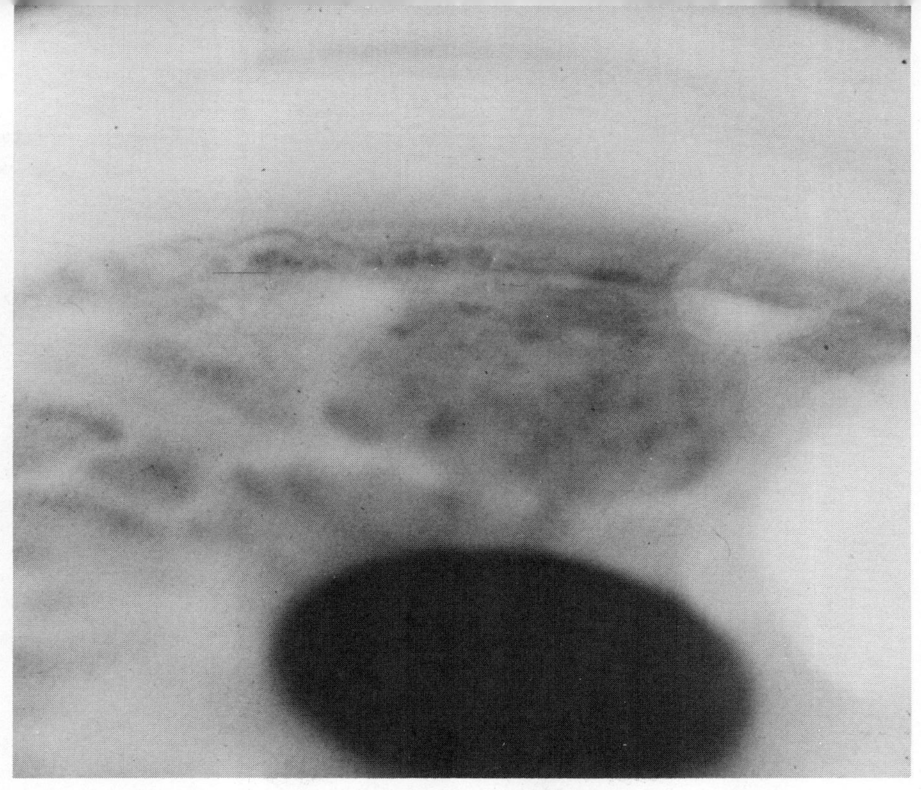

FIG. 44. Congenital glaucoma. The filtration angle is obscured by mesodermal tissue. (Courtesy of J. G. F. Worst.)

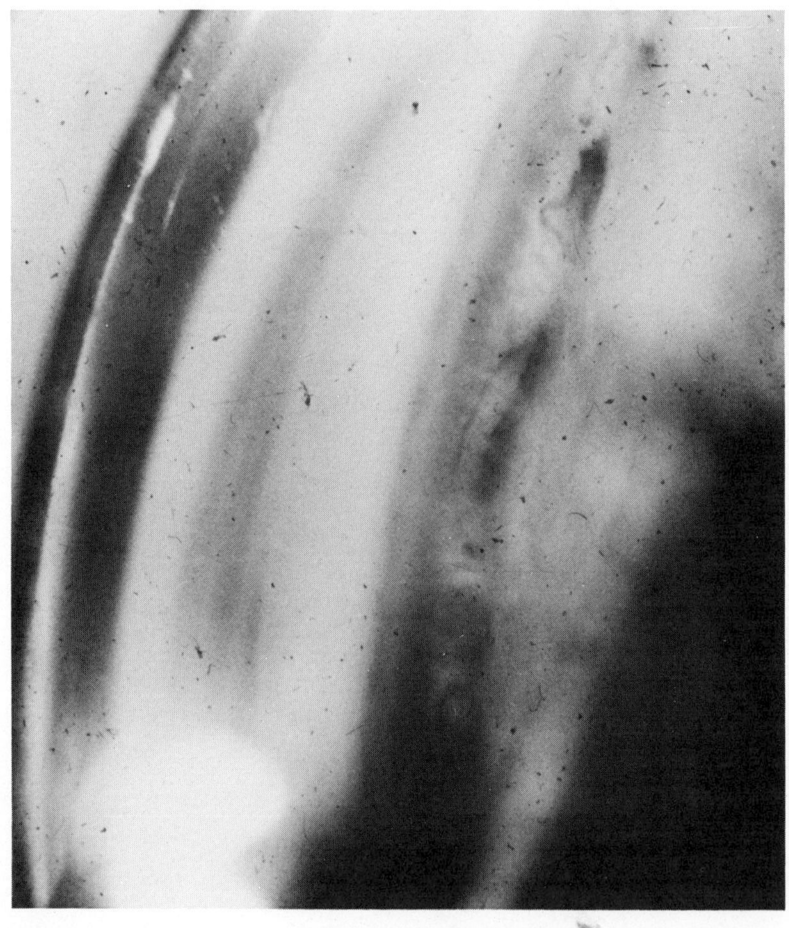

FIG. 45. Congenital glaucoma. The filtration angle is filled with tissue of mesodermal origin containing relatively large tortuous blood vessels. (Courtesy of J. G. F. Worst.)

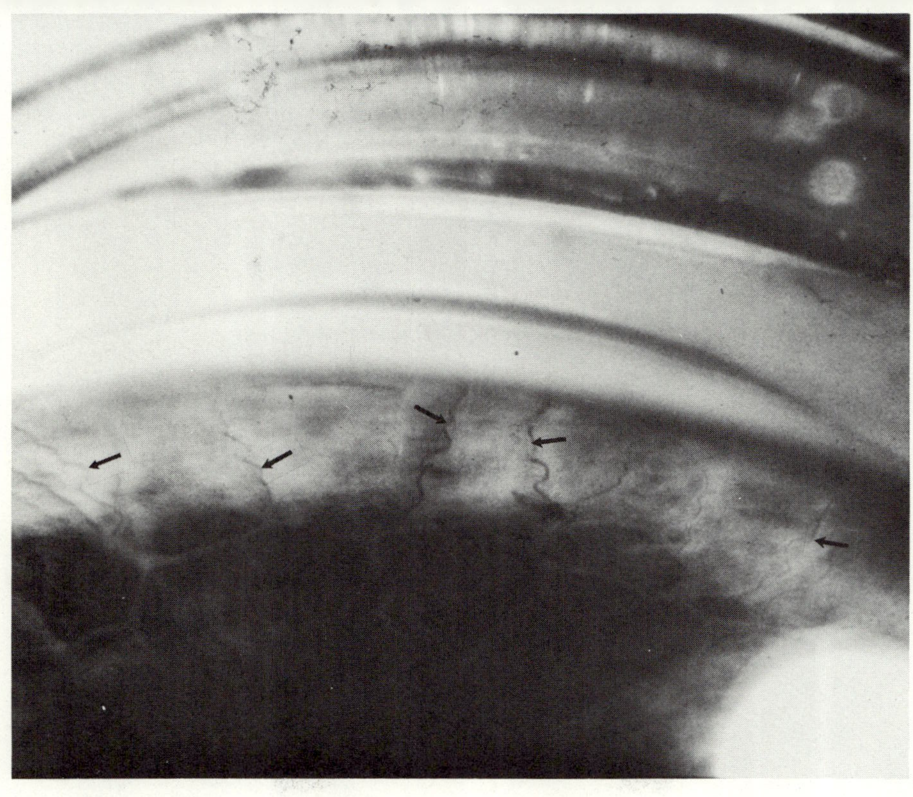

FIG. 46. Congenital glaucoma. Persistence of mesoderm in periphery of angle. Large radial blood extending into tissue (arrows).

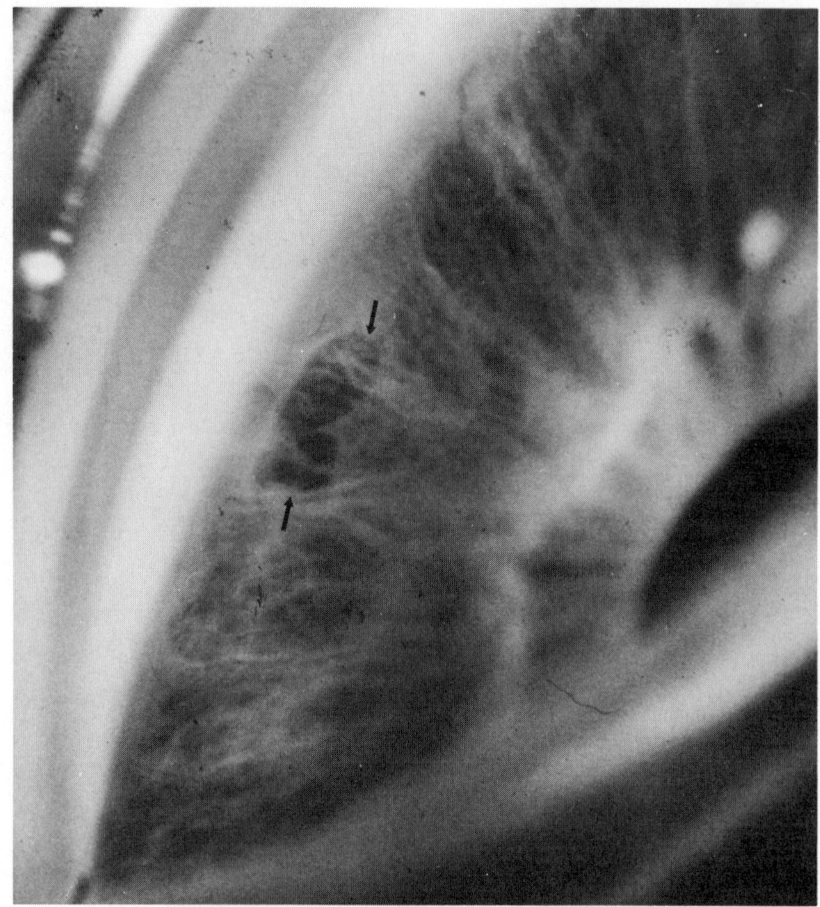

FIG. 47. Congenital glaucoma. Large defect (arrow) in shagreened surface clothing the filtration angle.

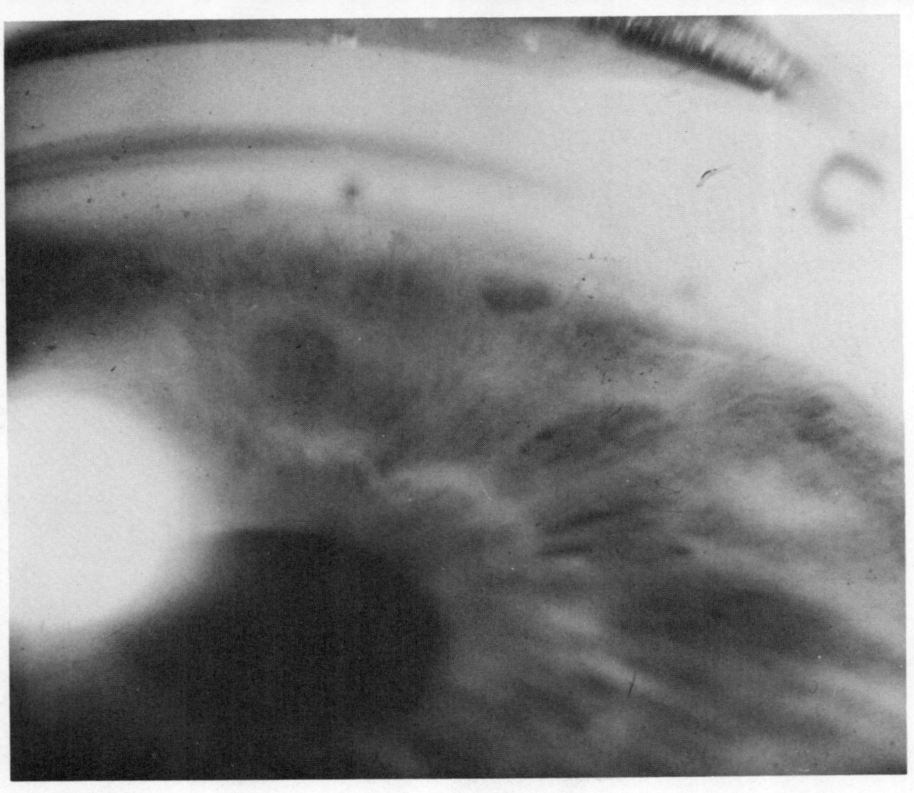

FIG. 48. Congenital glaucoma. Anterior sheet of mesoderm extending up toward Schwalbe's line.

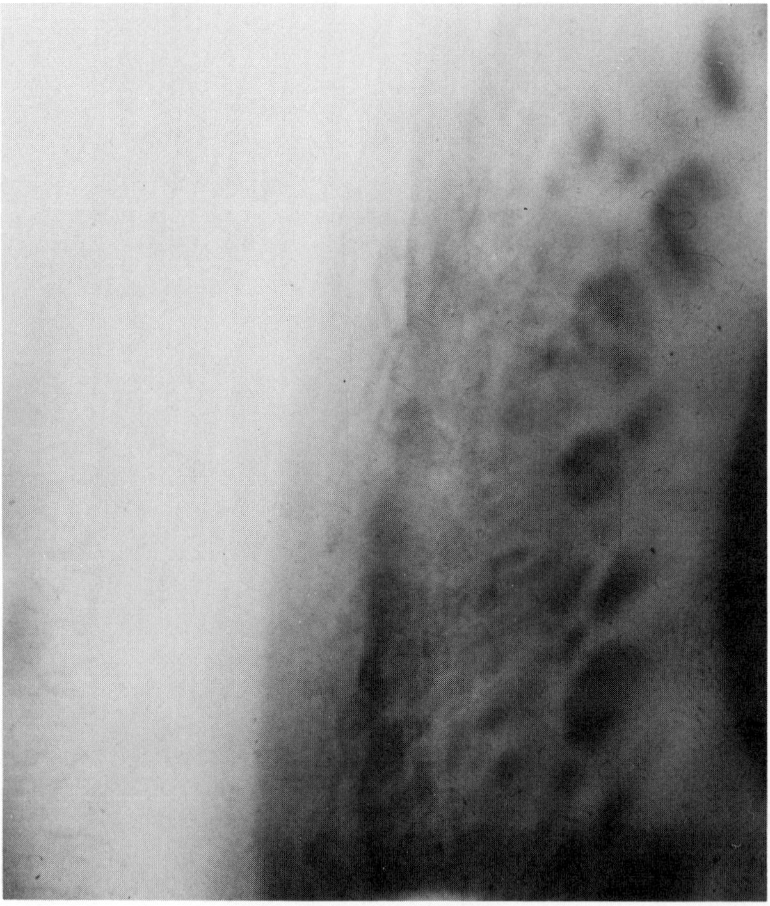

FIG. 49. Congenital glaucoma. High mesodermal "wall" or Barkan's membrane.

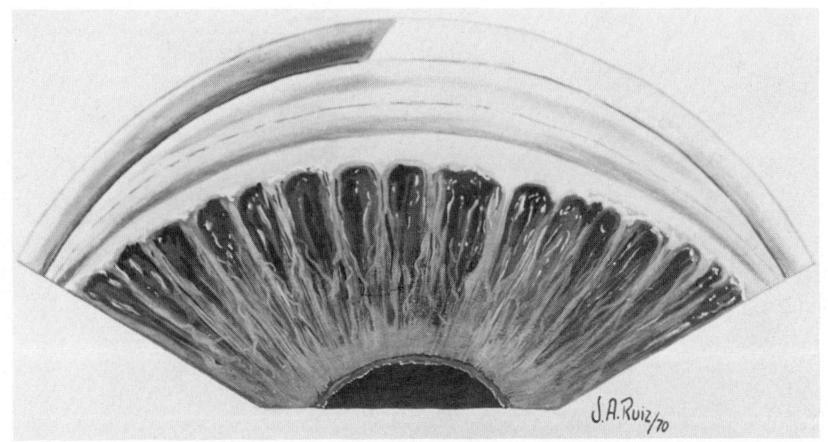

FIG. 50. Congenital glaucoma. Anomalously picked up folds of the anterior stromal layer of iris.

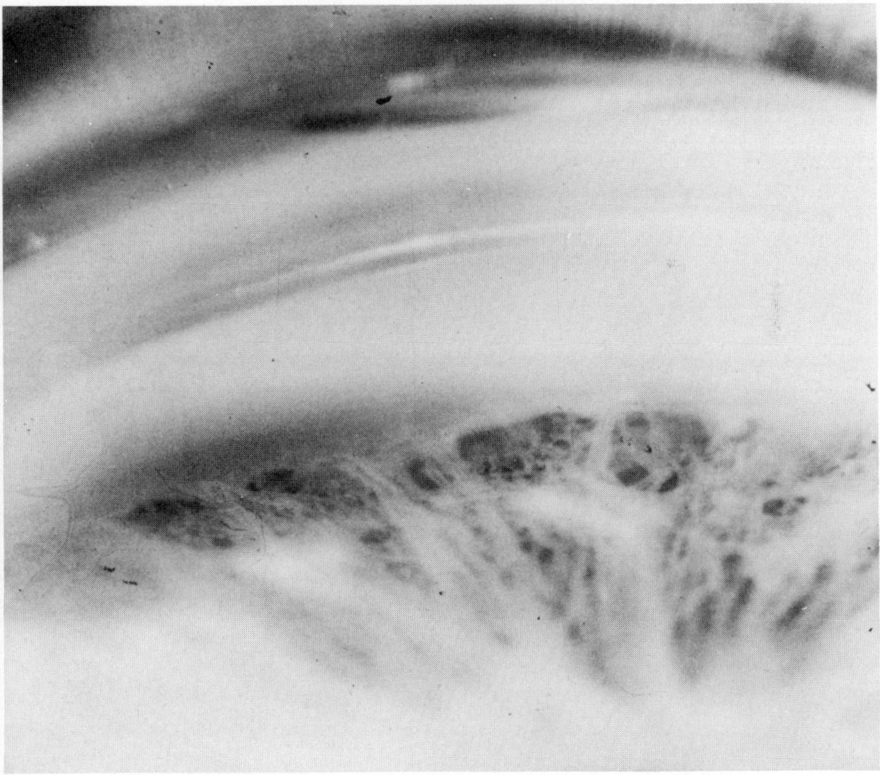

FIG. 51. Congenital glaucoma. Anomalously picked up folds with "morning mist" of Lister.

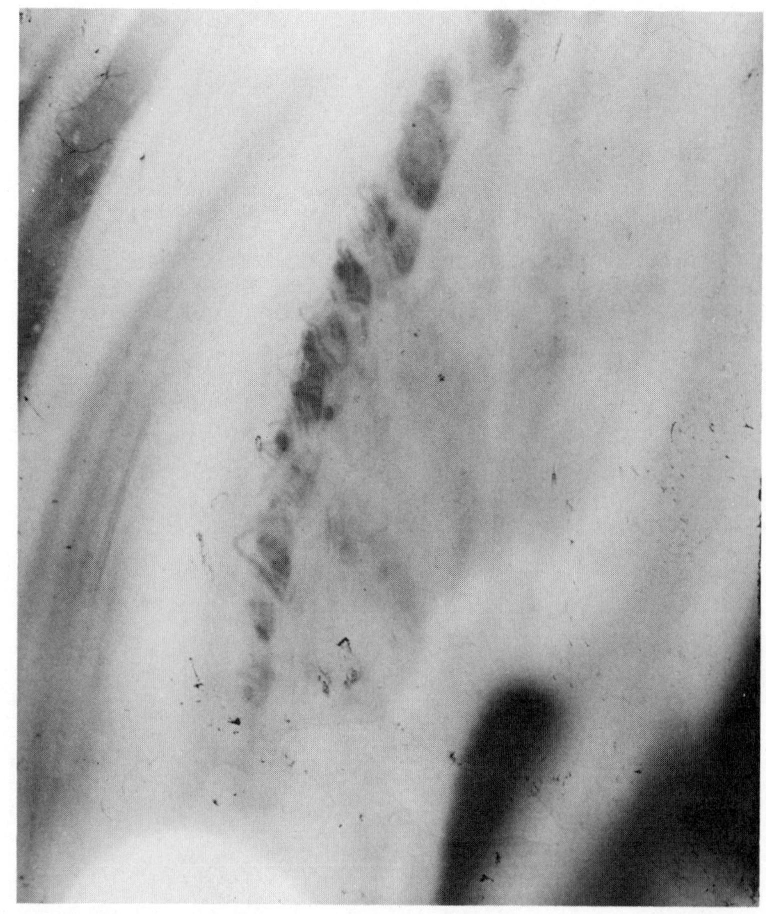

FIG. 52. Congenital glaucoma. Exaggerated upturning of scalloped ends of the pigment sectors.

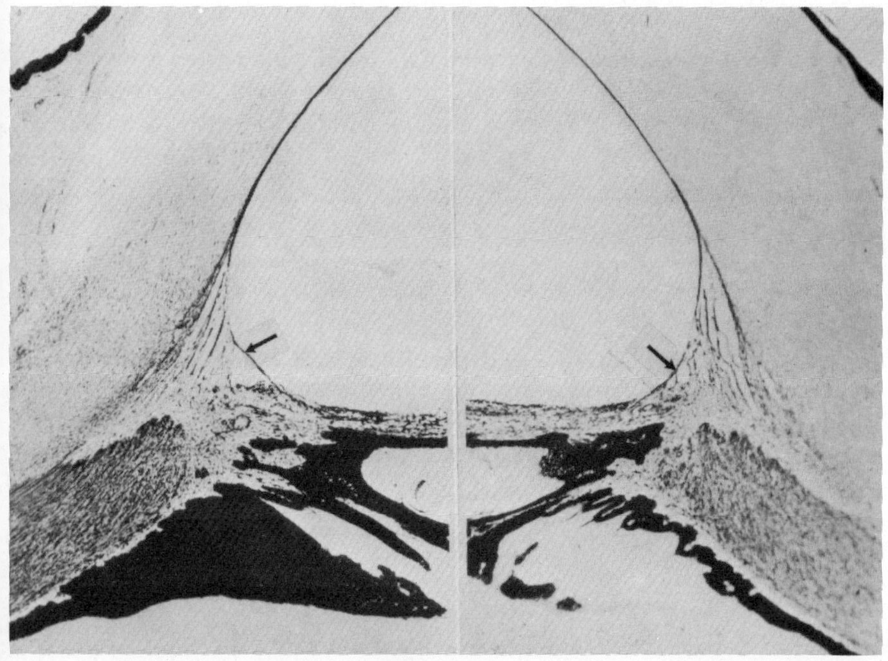

FIG. 53. Congenital glaucoma. Histological specimen demonstrating the structure referred to as Barkan's membrane (arrows) by Worst. (Courtesy of J. G. F. Worst and A. Castelli.)

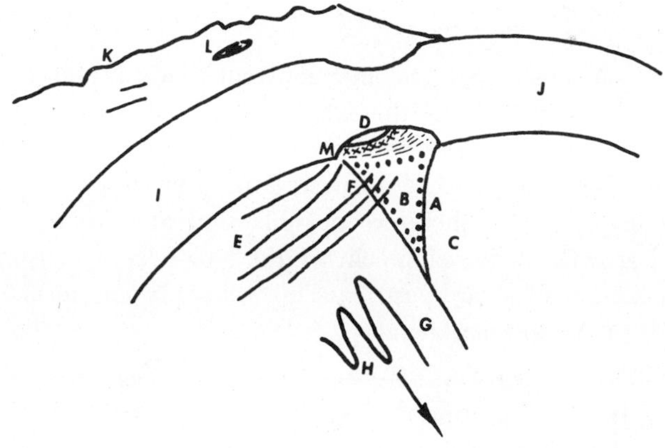

FIG. 54. Congenital glaucoma. Schematic drawing of the filtration angle to demonstrate the membrane theory. Barkan's membrane (A) and mesodermal "sheets" (B) obstruct the filtration angle (C) and Schlemm's canal (D). The ciliary muscle (E) is pulled forward and the longitudinal fibers (F) insert into the sheets. The iris (G) is lifted upward. Ciliary processes (H) reach centrally. (I) Sclera; (J) cornea; (K) conjunctiva; (L) conjunctival blood vessel; (M) scleral spur.

anteriorly, the anterior limiting membrane of the iris posteriorly, and the trabeculum. According to Worst this triangle is filled with loose mesodermal sheets. In a fashion not unlike that proposed by adherents to the cleavage theory, the ciliary muscle (E) is pulled forward and longitudinal fibers (F) insert into the mesodermal sheets (anterior to the scleral spur). The iris (G) is thus lifted upward and the ciliary processes (H) reach centrally.

Schlemm's canal and the trabecular apparatus are thus obstructed and as aqueous humor forms, the pressure rises. Two factors can vary the time of onset of the disease: (1) the membrane may be incomplete in the 360° circumference of the filtration angle and (2) aqueous humor production does not reach its full potential until several months after birth, since the ciliary body in the newborn may still be immature. Therefore, the intraocular pressure may be normal at birth. As the ciliary body reaches maturity, aqueous humor production begins to approach normal levels and the pressure begins to rise, resulting in classical signs and symptoms of congenital glaucoma. Goldenburg noted that the degree of abnormal development in congenital glaucoma varies, depending on the stage of arrest. Similarly, the histological appearance of the chamber angle of the buphthalmic eye may show involvement of various degrees and even include cases extending into the juvenile age limit. On the basis of this theory Barkan reintroduced the de Vincentiis operation.

Other Factors

LENS. Maumenee noted the apparent inward pull on the ciliary processes and ciliary body by the zonular fibers and observed the associated relative microphakia in cases of congenital glaucoma. Hess made a similar observation. Eyes with persistent hyperplastic primary vitreous demonstrate this same feature. It is therefore possible that at a transitional stage of embryonic growth, maldevelopment of the lens occurs, causing the ciliary body to remain in a forward position. This would prevent normal maturation of the angle of the anterior chamber.

PROMINENT SCHWALBE'S LINE. A prominent Schwalbe's line has been noted in cases of congenital glaucoma. The relationship between this finding and the failure of development of the angle of the anterior chamber is not known, but it should be pointed out that this is a constant feature in Axenfeld's syndrome or mesodermal dysplasia of the iris.

MECHANICAL OBSTRUCTION. Mechanical obstruction of the trabecular surface caused by a failure of the iris root to attach normally into the ciliary body has been observed by practically all authors working in this field. The actual relationship between this finding and aqueous humor obstruction is still unclear. Barkan noted that in some cases, the insertion of the iris is so far anterior that only a narrow area of the trabecular zone can be seen. He observed that this would obstruct or narrow Schlemm's canal, an interpretation held by Collins. Shaffer noted that a lack of angle cleavage causes the iris to insert directly into the trabeculum, covering it by as much as 50 percent in some cases. Worst has also observed a high insertion of the iris on the persistent uveal meshwork in about 10 percent of cases. Maumenee noted varying degrees of adherence of the iris and ciliary body to the corneoscleral trabecular fibers. The extent to which this occurs is extremely variable. In one case, almost the full extent of the trabecular fibers was covered. In another, the ciliary body was adherent only to the most posterior end of the trabeculae. However, it did not appear that these adhesions were sufficient to prevent aqueous from leaving the anterior chamber, for in 3 eyes that had been operated upon shortly before death, red blood cells permeated the trabecular fibers up to the inner wall of Schlemm's canal.

COMPACT TRABECULUM. Maumenee has noted a distinct compactness of the corneoscleral portion of the trabecular meshwork in several cases in his series. In some sections it was difficult to distinguish the trabecular meshwork from the scleral fibers. In one of these specimens red blood cells passed from the anterior chamber through the trabecular fibers to the inner wall of Schlemm's canal, suggesting that compact corneoscleral trabecular fibers would not inhibit aqueous outflow. This was shown by perfusing one of the enucleated eyes. An increase in the facility of outflow from 0.10 to 1.0 was produced by a goniotomy that did not incise the corneoscleral trabecular fibers.

Speakman and Leeson, in their study of congenital glaucoma, noted a marked reduction in the number of large spaces seen normally in the outer third of the meshwork in the region of Schlemm's canal. In addition, they observed a large number of small vacuoles in the cytoplasm covering the trabecular fibers and a failure of the uveal fibers to lengthen. There was a noticeable reduction in the cellularity of this region; the pectinate ligaments were more matted together.

In the early part of this chapter, it was noted that endothelial tissue demonstrates the property of transformation from compact tissue to open spongy tissue by a process called "reticulation." Although the significance of compact trabeculum is unknown as far as the cause of congenital glaucoma is concerned, its presence does represent an arrest in development of the fetal filtration angle at an early stage.

ATROPHY OF ANTERIOR CHAMBER MESENCHYME. Several

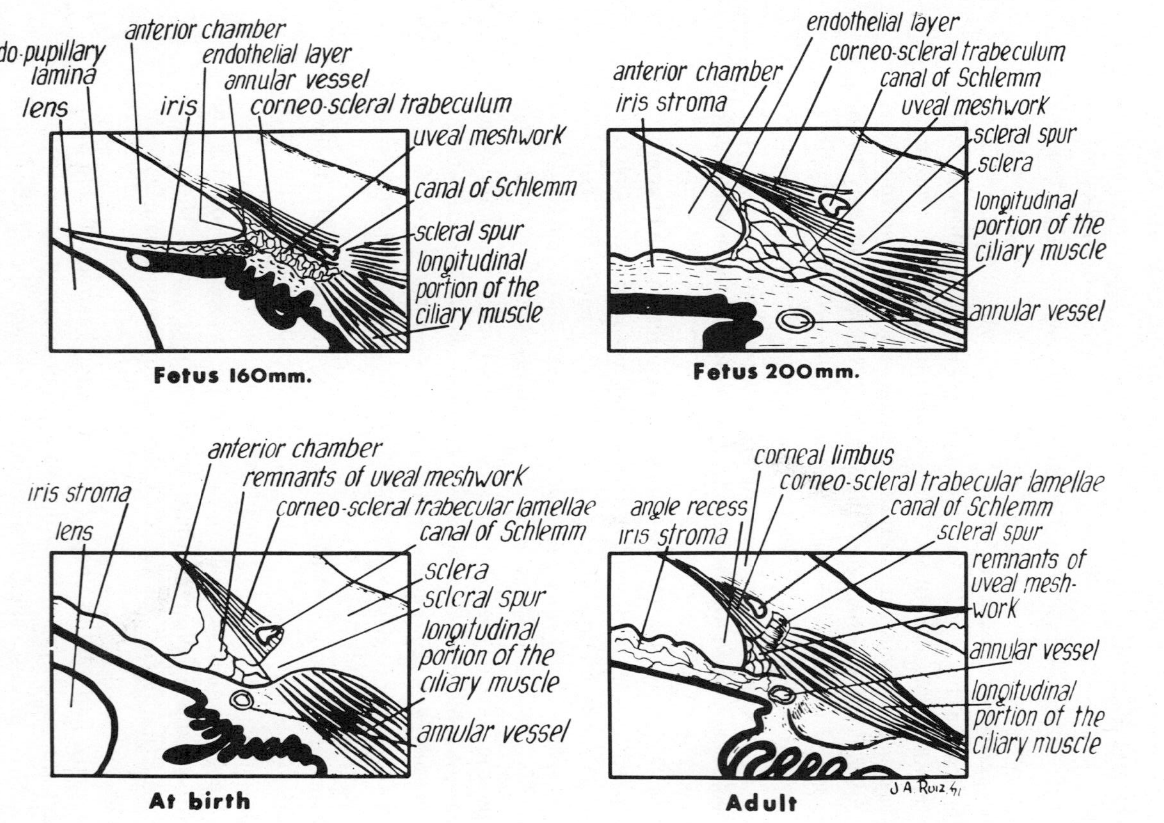

FIG. 55. Schematic illustration through the iridocorneal angle of the normal human eye (160 mm, 200 mm, birth and adulthood). A gradual change in the position of the canal of Schlemm in relation to the anterior chamber is noted. (According to A. Barber, T. Jerndal, and H. A. Hansson.)

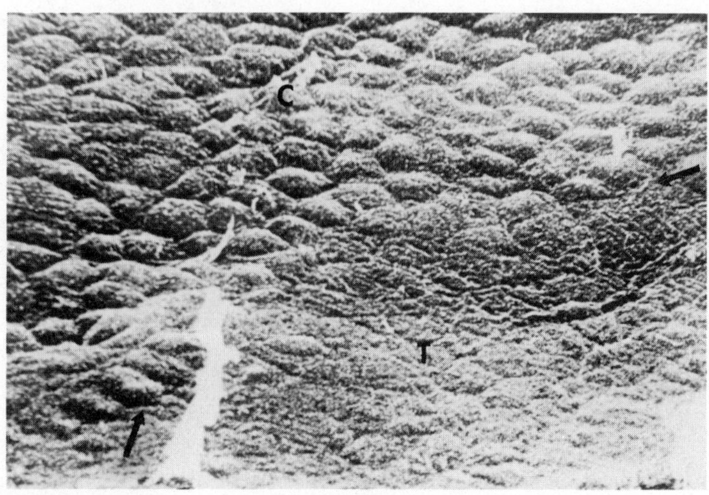

FIG. 56. Human fetus, crown-rump length 26 mm, estimated age 30 weeks. The corneal endothelium (C) above is made up of polyhedral cells distinguishing it from the corneoscleral trabeculum (T) below. Arrows mark the border between the two different cell types. (Courtesy of H. A. Hansson and T. Jerndal.) X 1,160.

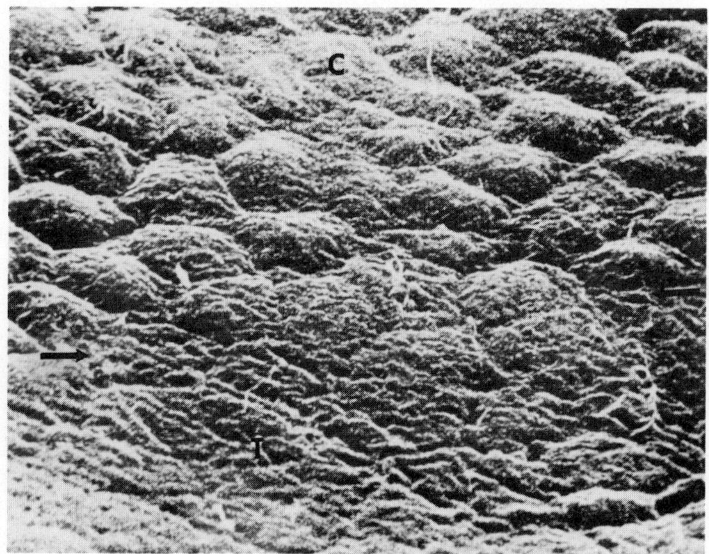

FIG. 57. Human fetus, crown-rump length 26 mm, estimated age 30 weeks (central area of Fig. 56). Arrows mark a fairly distinct border between the corneal endothelial cells (C) above and the trabecular endothelial cells (T) below. (Courtesy of H. A. Hansson and T. Jerndal.) X 2,350.

authors including Ida Mann have suggested that the anterior chamber and filtration angle form by atrophy of mesenchyme which in the early stages fills all but the central portion. As the mesenchyme atrophies–a process which implies cell death–the chamber enlarges and its periphery or "angle" comes to lie more and more laterally. The layer of mesenchyme over Schlemm's canal, which differentiates into the trabecular meshwork, is thus uncovered. Evidence to support this hypothesis has not been found. In fact there are definite indications of active cell growth in this area such as the presence of nucleoli, ribosomes, and rough-surfaced endoplasmic reticulum.

DISCUSSION

It has been shown that even at the present time there is still not complete agreement as to the exact nature of the cause of congenital glaucoma. Although all the current theories and contributing factors have been outlined above, present thinking centers on the membrane and cleavage theories. It should be appreciated that the contributing factors may also play a role in producing obstruction to aqueous outflow.

A variety of authors have described in a variety of ways the presence of tissue in the filtration angle of children suffering from congenital glaucoma, which Lister has likened to "morning mist."

Hansson and Jerndal used the scanning electron microscope to study the normal fetal filtration angle. Fig. 55 shows their schematic interpretation of the development of this area from the 160-mm through the 200-mm stage, to birth and adulthood. During the early stages of development (Figs. 56 and 57) the iridocorneal angle is covered by a continuous, thin monolayer of endothelial cells that may be observed in premature infants up to about 8 months of gestational age. These cells become flattened and more irregular in the iridocorneal angle, thereby distinguishing them from those on the corneoscleral trabeculum. All of the endothelial cells in the iridocorneal angle show short processes along their border, interdigitated with those of neighboring cells. A small number of microvilli are observed. The initially polygonal cell thus acquires a multipolar or star-shaped cell body with no structural resemblance to the other endothelial cells lining the anterior chamber.

The continuous covering of endothelial cells splits along the border between neighboring cells (Figs. 58–60). The size and number of these slits increases rapidly, although no signs of degeneration or cell death are noted. These developmental changes are not advanced to the same degree in various locations of the iridocorneal angle nor are they uniformly present in eyes of

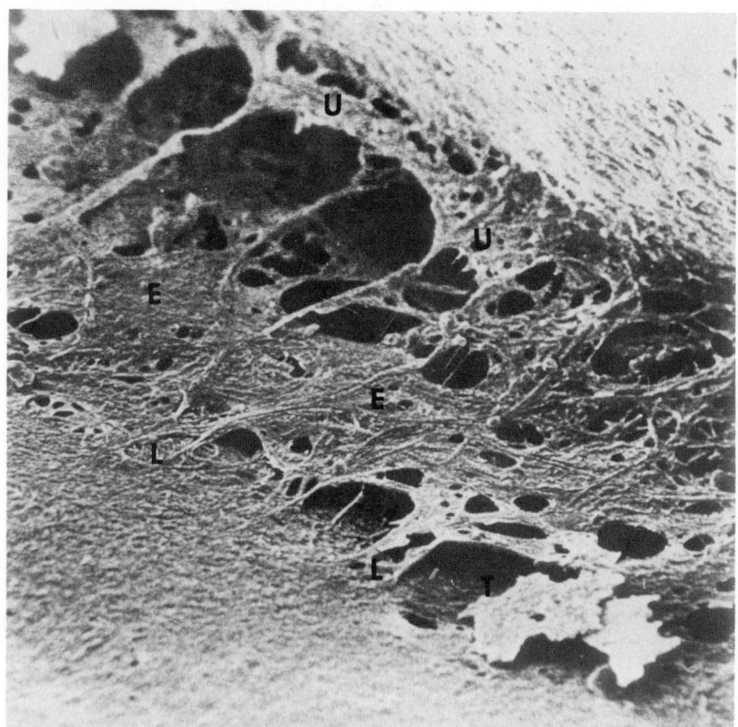

FIG. 58. Human fetus, estimated age 38 weeks. The endothelial cells (E) in the iridocorneal angle are seen as a membranous structure. The cells are arranged in several layers, partly covering the uveal meshwork (U) and the corneoscleral trabecular meshwork (T). The endothelial cells insert into the cornea in the region of Schwalbe's line (L) below. (Courtesy of H. A. Hansson and T. Jerndal.) X 350.

the same age. At birth the iridocorneal angle is covered by endothelial cells which form a discontinuous layer of cells at different depths.

Kupfer determined by perfusion studies that the mean value of the facility of outflow in normal fetuses between the ages of 22 to 28 weeks was 0.16 μl/min/mm Hg. In fetuses 31 weeks or older the mean value of the facility of outflow was 0.24 μl/min/mm Hg. He has observed that the angle of the anterior chamber in fetuses younger than 28 weeks gestational age had a more or less continuous layer of cells from the iris base to corneal endothelium covering the trabecular meshwork. This correlates with the lower facility of outflow. In eyes from fetuses older than 31 weeks, a loss in continuity of the covering cell layer took place resulting in the appearance of openings in the cellular lining. This correlates with a higher facility of outflow.

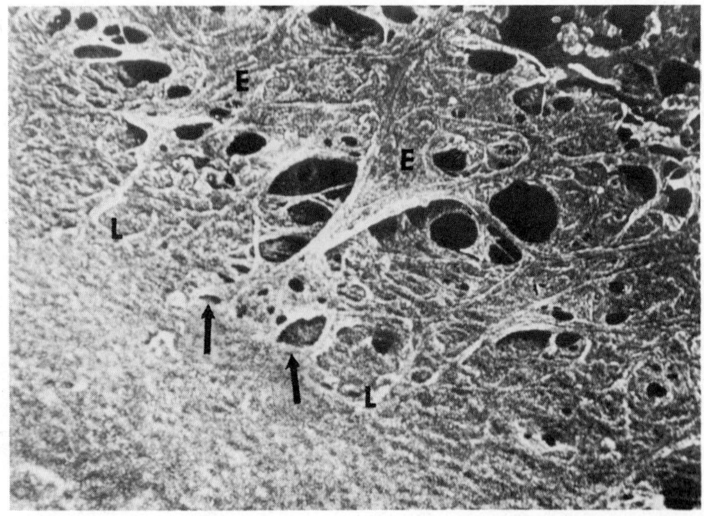

FIG. 59. Human fetus, estimated age 38 weeks (opposite eye of Fig. 58). The iridocorneal endothelial membrane (E) maturates into processes, separated by large open impressions (arrow) which reach Schwalbe's line (L). (Courtesy of H. A. Hansson and T. Jerndal.) X 350.

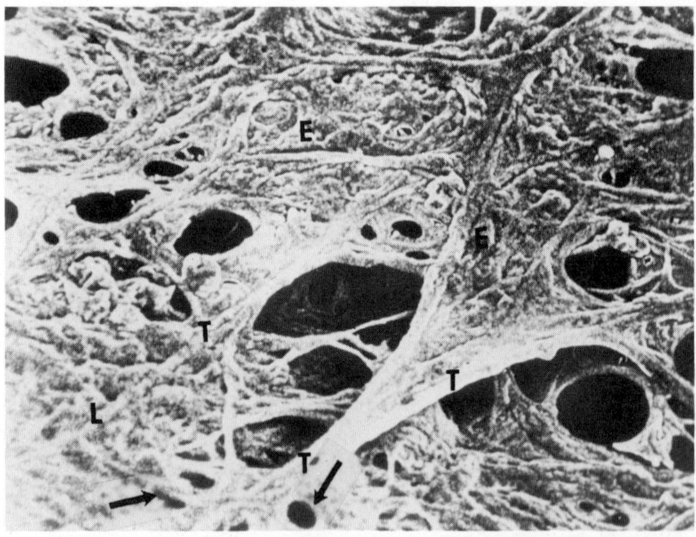

FIG. 60. Human fetus, estimated age 38 weeks (opposite eye of Fig. 59). The region of Schwalbe's line (L) appears as open meshwork partly covered by endothelial cells (E). The trabeculae (T) consists of fibers surrounded by endothelial cell processes. (Courtesy of H. A. Hansson and T. Jerndal.) X 860.

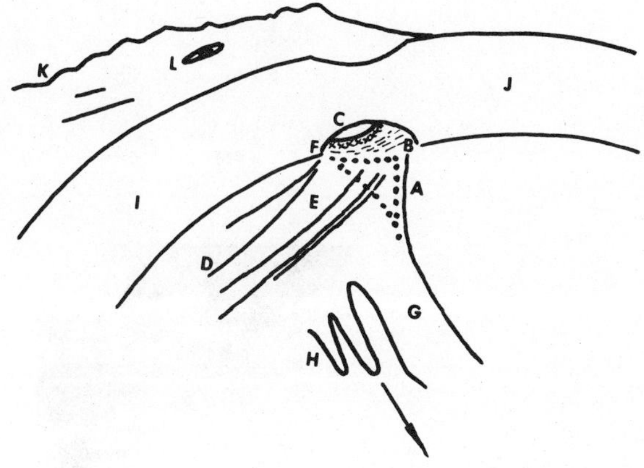

FIG. 61. Congenital glaucoma. Schematic drawing of the filtration angle to demonstrate the cleavage theory. The drawing is based on Fig. 40. The iris (G) is displaced to a forward position. (A) Anterior limiting membrane of the iris; (B) trabeculum; (C) Schlemm's canal. The longitudinal fibers (E) of the ciliary body (D) insert into the trabecular fibers. (H) Ciliary processes; (F) scleral spur; (I) sclera; (J) cornea; (K) conjunctiva; (L) conjunctival vessel.

Sugar states, " . . . in nearly all such eyes (congenital glaucoma) there is a persistence of an abnormally great amount of mesodermal meshwork." Alfano has described abnormal tissue in the chamber angle of a case where congenital glaucoma formed part of the rubella syndrome. Smith et al. have noted the presence of a thin, grayish, nearly transluscent membrane covering the trabeculum in a case of congenital glaucoma associated with the Pierre Robin syndrome. Kluyskens believes that it is actually abnormal mesodermal tissue lying on top of the iris which gives the gonioscopic appearance of an anterior insertion of the iris root.

Shaffer has stated that the so-called semitransparent membrane described by Barkan, which veils the peripheral anterior surface of the iris and continues over the trabeculum, is really the uveal portion of the trabeculum and not abnormal mesoblastic tissue. He commented further that there is a relative impermeability of the trabeculum in congenital glaucoma, an opinion held by Barkan himself. Maumenee's argument against the membrane concept includes the fact that breakage of the membrane should leave some remnants which up to the present time have not been found on histological examination. Worst's interpretation of Maumenee's histological description is that the increased pressure causes a thinning of the sclera in the limbal area. "This backward stretching of the outer coats has pulled the

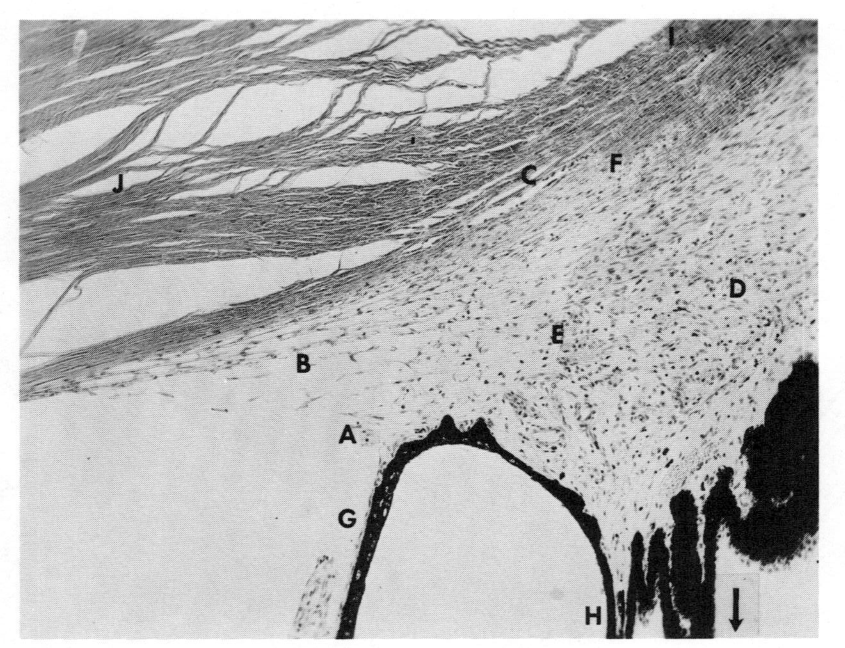

FIG. 62. Congenital glaucoma. (A) anterior surface layer of iris; (B) trabeculum; (C) Schlemm's canal; (D) ciliary body; (E) longitudinal fibers of the ciliary body; (F) scleral spur; (G) iris; (H) ciliary processes; (I) sclera; (J) cornea (A. F. I. P. Acc. No. 331614). X 115. (Courtesy of F. D. Costenbader and the Registry of Ophthalmic Pathology of the Armed Forces Institute of Pathology.)

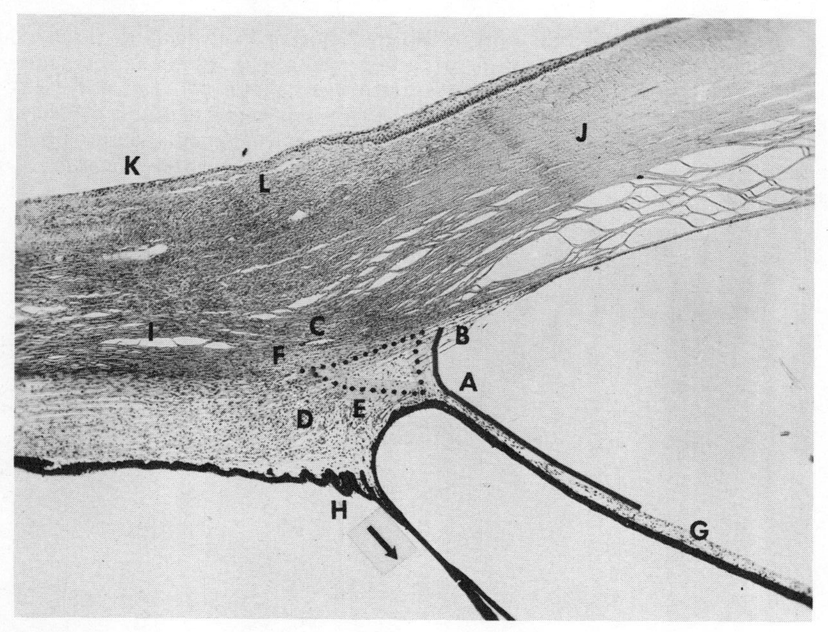

FIG. 63. Congenital glaucoma, modified to show anterior surface layer of iris. The triangle outlined corresponds to the triangle in Fig. 61. (A–B) anterior surface layer of iris; (C) Schlemm's canal; (D) ciliary body; (E) longitudinal fibers of the ciliary body; (F) scleral spur; (G) iris; (H) iris processes; (I) sclera; (J) cornea; (K) conjunctiva; (L) conjunctival vessel. The ciliary processes reach centrally (A. F. I. P. Acc. No. 331614) (Courtesy of F. D. Costenbader and the Registry of Ophthalmic Pathology of the Armed Forces Institute of Pathology.) X 50.

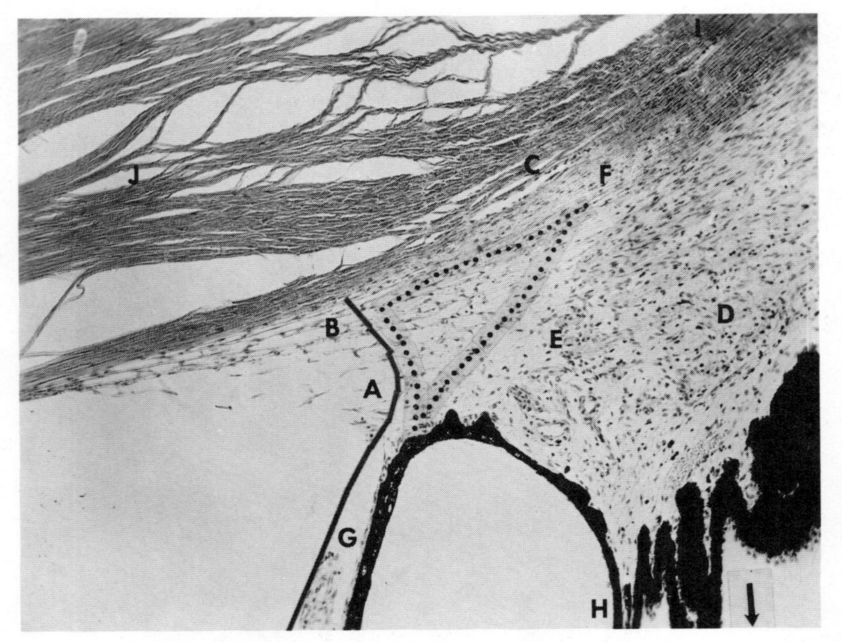

FIG. 64. Congenital glaucoma, modified to show anterior surface layer of iris. The triangle outlined corresponds to the triangle in Fig. 61 and 63. (A–B) anterior surface layer of iris; (C) Schlemm's canal; (D) ciliary body; (E) longitudinal fibers of the ciliary body; (F) scleral spur; (G) iris; (H) ciliary processes; (I) slcera; (J) cornea. The ciliary processes reach centrally (A. F. I. P. Acc. No. 331614). (Courtesy of F. D. Costenbader and the Registry of Ophthalmic Pathology of the Armed Forces Institute of Pathology.) X 115.

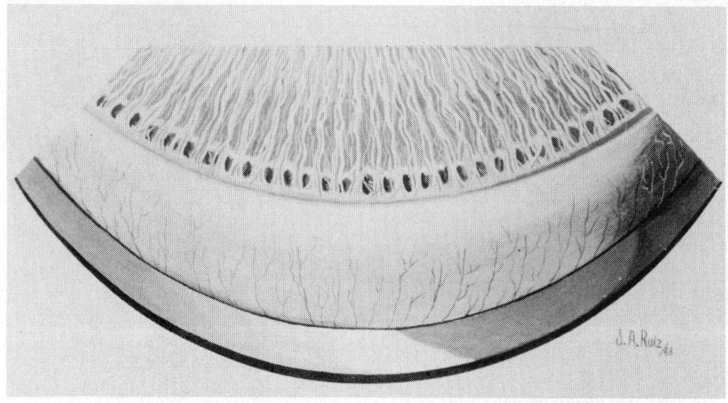

FIG. 65. Congenital glaucoma. Drawing illustrates the surface layer of the iris as it sweeps upward toward Schwalbe's line.

ciliary muscle relatively forward. This has erroneously been called an anterior insertion of the iris." He stated further that red blood cells may enter the trabeculum through the goniotomy puncture site, and then pass circumferentially around the eye deep to the membrane so that at 180 degrees away from the puncture, blood may be found in the trabecular meshwork. On the other hand, Maumenee observed a patient where only an iridectomy was performed (not a goniotomy), and here, too, blood could be seen in the trabeculum that obviously came from the anterior chamber. "If blood can pass through this meshwork, certainly aqueous could also."

In their study of human embryos, Smelser and Ozanics observed a gradual enlargement of innumerable intercellular spaces in the filtration angle which became confluent with the anterior chamber as the fetal membrane clothing the filtration angle broke down. There are other similarities between the two theories.

A dotted triangle has been outlined on Fig. 54, used to demonstrate the membrane theory. The sides consist of Barkan's membrane anteriorly, the anterior limiting membrane of the iris posteriorly, and the trabeculum above. This same triangle has been outlined on Fig. 61 demonstrating the cleavage theory showing a forward displacement of the iris. The triangle in this case consists of the border layer of the iris anteriorly, iris stroma posteriorly, and the trabeculum above.

Although Fig. 61 is a simplified version of Fig. 39 (used to describe the cleavage theory), the configurations of anterior chamber structures are also in keeping with Fig. 54 (used to illustrate the membrane theory). By altering

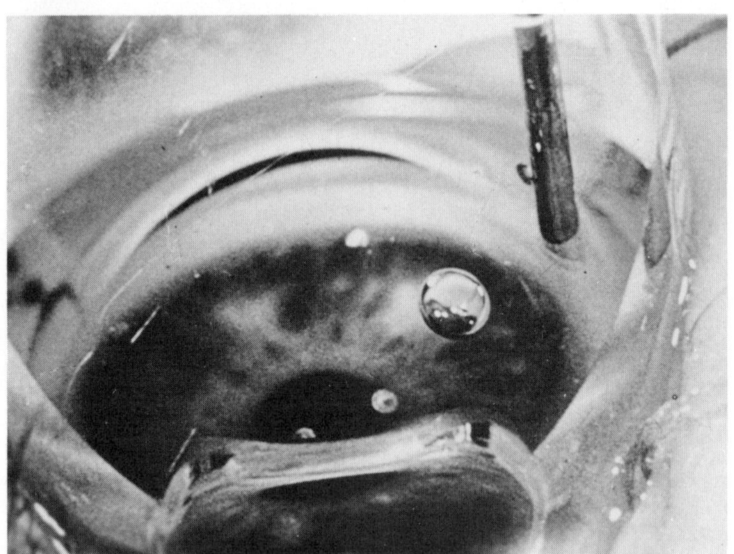

FIG. 66. Congenital glaucoma. The anterior surface of the iris viewed through the goniolens.

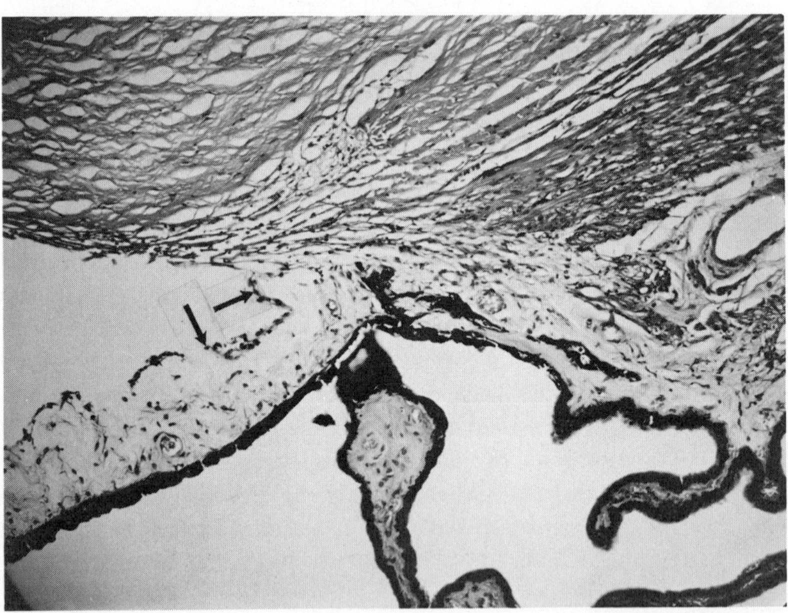

FIG. 67. Congenital glaucoma. The anterior border layer of the iris (arrows) appears to envelop the filtration angle as it sweeps up toward the peripheral cornea. The longitudinal fibers of the ciliary body insert largely into the trabecular fibers.

the nomenclature, the anterior limiting membrane of the iris assumes the position of Barkan's membrane (A) and a forward displacement of the iris (G) is achieved. There is no further disagreement since the longitudinal fibers (E) of the ciliary muscle (D) pass through the mesodermal sheets which are, in reality, iris stroma (mesodermal origin) on their way toward the trabeculum (B) anterior to the scleral spur (F) while other fibers insert directly into the scleral spur itself. The ciliary muscle (D) is thus pulled forward, and the iris (G) is lifted upward and the ciliary processes (H) reach centrally.

Fig. 62 represents a photomicrograph used by Maumenee to advance the cleavage theory. The triangle outlined on the drawing (Fig. 61) has been placed on Figs. 63 and 64. In this way it can be shown that the membrane of Barkan is really the anterior surface of the iris which has maintained its embryonic appearance. The surface layer sweeps upward toward the peripheral cornea (Figs. 65 and 66). Fig. 67 represents the angle of a case of congenital glaucoma which illustrates features common to both the membrane and cleavage theories. The longitudinal fibers of the ciliary body musculature insert largely into the trabecular fibers, bypassing the scleral spur, while the anterior limiting membrane of the iris appears to be continuous with a membrane which attaches to the peripheral cornea.

Profusion studies have shown that a goniotomy as small as 1.0 to 1.5 mm could improve the facility of outflow from 0.10 to 1.0. The goniopuncture operation of Scheie produces a small fistula in the filtration angle that extends under the conjunctiva. Whether this fistula produces active permanent filtration has still not been determined. The success of this operation may simply be due to the goniotomy alone as small as it may be. Maumenee reported a case in which a goniotomy that severed the longitudinal muscle from the trabecular fibers increased the facility of outflow from approximately 0.10 to 1.0. However, the fact that red blood cells from the anterior chamber may be found in the trabecular fibers 180° away from the goniotomy site would be evidence supporting the presence of an obstructing surface which had been disrupted. This disruption, however small, could result in the passage of red blood cells and by the same token, aqueous humor.

References

Adams, S. T., Grant, W. M., and Smith, T. R. Congenital glaucoma (possibly Lowe's syndrome). Arch. Ophthalmol., 68:191, 1962.

af Ursin, K. V. The fate of infantile and juvenile glaucoma patients. Acta Ophthalmol. (Kbh.), 25:345, 1947.

Alfano, J. E. Ocular aspects of the maternal rubella syndrome. Trans. Am. Acad. Ophthalmol. Otolaryngol., 70:235, 1966.

Steroid induced glaucoma simulating congenital glaucoma. Am. J. Ophthalmol., 61:922, 1966.

Allen, L., Burian, H. M., and Braley, A. E. A new concept of the development of the anterior chamber angle. Arch. Ophthalmol., 53:783, 1955.

The anterior border ring of Schwalbe and pectinate ligament. Arch. Ophthalmol., 53:799, 1955.

Allen, T. D., and Ackermann, W. G. Hereditary glaucoma in a pedigree of three generations. Arch. Ophthalmol., 27:139, 1942.

Ambache, N. Properties of irin, a physiological constituent of the rabbit's eye. J. Physiol. (Lond.), 135:114, 1957.

Anderson, J. R. Hydrophthalmia or Congenital Glaucoma. Its Causes, Treatment and Outlook. Cambridge Univ. Press, London, 1939.

Ashton, N. Anatomical study of Schlemm's canal and aqueous veins by means of neoprene casts. Br. J. Ophthalmol., 35:291, 1951.

Brini, A., and Smith, R. Anatomical studies of the trabecular meshwork of the normal human eye. Br. J. Ophthalmol., 40:257, 1956.

Badtke, G. Zu Sondermann's These von der Entwicklung des Schlemmschen Kanals und Ciliarfortsätze. Graefe's Arch. Ophthamol., 145:321, 1943.

Bailliart, P. Le glaucome infantile a l'institution nationale des jeunes aveugles. Ann. Ocul. (Paris), 180:257, 1947.

Barkan, O. Goniotomy for relief of congenital glaucoma. Br. J. Ophthalmol., 32:701, 1948.

Surgery of congenital glaucoma. A review of 196 eyes operated by goniotomy. Am. J. Ophthalmol., 36:1523, 1953.

Pathogenesis of congenital glaucoma, gonioscopic and anatomic observations of the angle of the anterior chamber in the normal eye and congenital glaucoma. Am. J. Ophthalmol., 40:1, 1955.

Goniotomy. Trans. Am. Acad. Ophthalmol. Otolaryngol., 59:322, 1955.

Becker, B. Carbonic anhydrase and the formation of aqueous humor. Am. J. Ophthalmol., 47:342, 1959.

and Friedenwald, J. S. Clinical aqueous outflow. Arch. Ophthalmol., 50:557, 1953.

and Kolker, A. Vision and its Disorders, Glaucoma. NINDB Monogr. No. 4, U. S. Dept. Health, Education, and Welfare, Bethesda, Md. 1967, p. 87.

Bentley, M. D. Congenital abnormalities of the eyeball accessible to external examination. J. Mich. State Med. Soc., 59:1837, 1960.

Bentzen, C. F., and Leber, T. Filtration of the anterior chamber in normal and glaucomatous eyes. Graefe's Arch. Ophthalmol., 41(III):208, 1895.

Berg, F. Erbliches jungendliches Glaukom. Acta Ophthalmol. (Kbh.), 10:568, 1932.

Birò, J. Notes on the hereditary of glaucoma. Ophthalmologica, 98:43, 1939.

Recent observations upon the occurrence of hereditary glaucoma. Ophthalmologica, 138:161, 1959.

Bolch, F. Die Endotheliome. Thieme, Lipsig, 1952.

Boles Carenini, B. Contributo alla conoscenza del cosidetto glaucoma giovanile. Ann. Ottalmol. Clin. Ocul., 91:140, 1965.

Bollack, J., Voisin, J., et Camps, S. Sur une form particuliere de glaucome infantile. Malformation de l'angle irido-cornéen, integrite fonctionnelle. Bull. Soc. Ophthalmol. Fr., 127:1938.

Bonting, S. L. Na-K activated ATPase and active cation transport. In J. DeGraeff and B. Leijnse (Eds.), Water and Electrolyte Metabolism II. Elsevier, Amsterdam, 1964, p. 35.

Burian, H. M., Braley, A. E., and Allen, L. External and gonioscopic visibility of the ring of Schwalbe and the trabecular zone. Trans. Am. Ophthalmol. Soc., 52:389, 1954.

Braley, A. E., and Allen, L. Visibility of the ring of Schwalbe and the trabecular zone. Arch. Ophthalmol., 53:767, 1955.

Braley, A. E., and Allen, L. A new concept of the development of the angle of the anterior chamber of the human eye. Arch. Ophthalmol., 55:439, 1956.
Busacca, A. Examen gonioscopique d'un cas d'hydrophthalmie. Ann. Ocul. (Paris), 181:627, 1948.
Elements de Gonioscopie Normal, Pathologique et Experimentale. Sao Paulo, 1945.
Castelli, A. Contributo alla conoscenza della anatomia pathologica e della eziologia dell 'irdroftalmo congenito. Ann. Ottalmol. Clin. Ocul., 68:801, 1940.
Chandler, D. A., and Grant, W. M. Lectures on Glaucoma. Macmillan, Toronto, 1965.
Charnay, C. Glaucoma de l'adulte jeune par anomalie de l'angle irido-cornéen. Thèse, Bordeaux, 1962.
Clark, W. B. (Ed.). Symposium on Glaucoma. Mosby, St. Louis, 1959.
Collins, T. Anatomy and congenital defects of ligamentum pectinatum. 9th International Ophthalmol. Congress, Utrecht, 1899.
Researches into Anatomy and Pathology of the Eye. Lewis, London, 1896.
Cosmettatos, G. F. Sur la genese de l'hydrophthalmie congenitale. Ann. Ocul. (Paris), 165:752, 1928.
Coulombre, A. J. The role of the intraocular pressure in the development of the chick eye. Arch. Ophthalmol., 57:250, 1957.
Cross, F. R. Congenital hydrophthalmos. Trans. Ophthalmol. Soc. U. K., 16:340, 1895.
Dalsgaard-Nielsen, E. A survey of buphthalmic patients admitted to the eye clinic of the Rigshospital in the period of 1910–1943. Acta Ophthalmol. (Kbh.), 23:49, 1945.
de Buen, S. Nuevos datos sobre la histologia y probable functionamiento del plexo epiescleral del ojo humano su relacion con el glaucoma. Anal. Soc. Mexico Oftalmol., 38:121, 1965.
Dejean, C. Embryologie des diverses parties de l'appareil oculaire. I. Développement de corps vitré et de la zonule de Zinn. II. Développement du cristallin. Traité Ophtalmol., 1:128, 1939.
Hervouet, F., et Leplat, G. L'embryologie de l'oeil et sa teratologie. Soc. Franc. Ophtalmol., 1958.
de Lapersonne, A. Hydrophalmie et troubles cardiovasculaires. Arch. Ophtalmol., 22:565, 1902.
de Vincentiis, M. Incisione del l'angolo irideo nel glaucoma. Ann. Ottalmol. Clin. Ocul., 22:540, 1893.
de Vries, M. S. Les veines aqueses. Visibilité, incidence, morphologie. Bull. Mem. Soc. Fr. Ophtalmol., 62:184, 1949.
Dollfus, M. A. Le glaucome infantile, a propos de deux cas recemment observes. Le Nourrisson, 17:287, 1929.
Duke-Elder, W. S. Textbook of Ophthalmology, Vol. 3. Mosby, St. Louis, 1932.
Textbook of Ophthalmology, Vol. 3. Mosby, St. Louis, 1938, pp. 1295 and 1297.
The blood-aqueous barrier. Trans. Ophthalmol. Soc. U. K., 68:413, 1948.
System of Ophthalmology, Vol. 3. Kimpton, London, 1964, pp. 548–551.
Erickson, L. A. Twenty-four hourly variations of the aqueous flow. Examination with perilimbal suction cup. Acta Ophthalmol. (Suppl.) (Kbh.), 50:1, 1958.
Falls, H. F. A gene producing various defects of the anterior segment of the eye. Am. J. Ophthalmol., 32:41, 1949.
Fischer, F. Entwicklungsgeschichtliche und Anatomische Studien ueber den Skleral-sporn im Menschlichen Auge. Graefe's Arch. Ophthalmol., 131:318, 1933.
Flocks, M. The pathology of the trabecular meshwork in open angle glaucoma. Meeting of the Am. Acad. Ophthalmol. Otolaryngol., 1957.
and Zweng, H. C. Studies on the mode of action of pilocarpine on aqueous flow. Am. J. Ophthalmol., 44:380, 1957.
Fortin, E. P. Contributions to solutions of problems of glaucoma. Arch. Oftalmol. B. Aires, 6:219, 1931.

Fralick, F. B. Symposium: Office management of the primary glaucomas. Trans. Am. Acad. Ophthalmol. Otolaryngol., 64:105, 1960.

Franceschetti, A. Kurzes Handbuch der Ophthalmologie. Springer, Berlin, 1930, p. 712.

François, J. La gonioscopie. Soc. Belge Ophtalmol., 1948.

De la persistance d'un tissu mesodermique embryonnaire dans l'angle irido-corneen des yeux atteints de glaucome congenital ou d'autres malformations. Ann. Ocul. (Paris), 186:804, 1953.

La gonioscopie et therapeutique oculaire. Ann. Ther. Ophthalmol., 1953, p. 359.

Le glaucome juvenile existe-t-il? Acta 17th Conc. Ophthalmol. Canada-U. S. A., 1954, p. 1145.

Friedenwald, J. S. Contribution to the theory and practice of tonometry. Am. J. Ophthalmol., 20:985, 1937.

The formation of the intraocular fluid. Am. J. Ophthalmol., 32:9, 1949.

Standardization of tonometers. Decennial Report of the American Academy of Ophthalmology and Otolaryngology, Rochester, Minn., 1954.

Gabrielides, A. J. Recherches sur l'embryogenie et l'anatomie comparée de l'angle de la chambre anterieure chez le poulet et chez l'homme. Arch. Ophtalmol. (Paris), 15:176, 1895.

Gallenga, R. Dell 'irdroftalmo congenito. Ann. Ottalmol., 14:1885, cited by Castelli.

and Matteucci, P. Idroftalmo. Relazione al 39th congresso della Societa Italiana di Oftalmologia Torino, Oct. 9., 1952.

Gallois, J. A propos de deux cas d'hypertension oculaire juvenile, verification et compairson des tonometres, champ visuel peripherique absolu. Bull. Soc. Ophtalmol. Fr., 13:1948.

Gelzer, A. I., Guber, D., and Sears, M. L. Ocular manifestations of the 1964-1965 rubella epidemic. Am. J. Ophthalmol., 63:221, 1967.

Gillespie, F. D. Congenital glaucoma, juvenile glaucoma, chronic simple glaucoma, all in one family. Virginia Med. Monthly, 90:556, 1963.

Glucksmann, A. Zur entwicklung der Vorderen Augenkammer beim Menschen. Graefe's Arch. Ophthalmol., 132:51, 1934.

Goldenburg, M. Discussion of paper. Hereditary juvenile glaucoma simplex, Courtney, R. H., and Hill, E. J. A. M. A., 97:1609, 1931.

Goldmann, H. Zur Technik der Splatlampenmicroscopie. Zur Untersuchung des Kammerwinkels mit der Spaltlampe (Spaltlampengonioscope). Ophthalmologica, 96:90, 1938.

Abflussdruck, Minutenvolumen und Widerstand der Kammerwassertromung des Menschen, Ophthalmologica, 5–6:278, 1951.

Un nouveau tonomètre à applanation, Bull. Soc. Fr. Ophthalmol., 67:474, 1954.

Goldstein, J. E., and Cogan, D. G. Sclerocornea and associated congenital anomalies. Arch. Ophthalmol., 67:761, 1962.

Gorin, G. Developmental glaucoma. Am. J. Ophthalmol., 58:572, 1964.

Grant, W. M. Clinical measurements of aqueous outflow. Arch. Ophthalmol., 46:113, 1951.

Tonographic method for measuring the facility and rate of aqueous flow in human eyes. Arch. Ophthalmol., 44:204, 1950.

Gros, E. L. Etude sur l'hydrophtalmie ou glaucome infantile. Thèses, Paris, 1897.

Gross, B. H. Glaucome sur des jeunes sujets. Ann. Ocul. (Paris), 180:366, 1947.

Haag, C. Das Glaukom der Jugendlichen, Klin. Monatsbl. Augenheilkl., 54:133, 1915.

Hagedoorn, A. The early development of the endothelium of Descemet's membrane, the cornea, and the anterior chamber of the eye. Br. J. Ophthalmol., 12:479, 1928.

Beitrag zur Entwicklungsgeschichte des Auges. Arch. Augenheilkd., 102:33, 1929.

Comparative anatomy of the eye. Arch. Ophthalmol., 16:783, 1936.

Congenital anomalies of the anterior segment of the eye. Arch. Ophthalmol., 17:223, 1937.

Hambresin, L., and Schepens, C. Glaucome familial. Bull. Mem. Soc. Fr. Ophtalmol., 59:219, 1946.

Hansson, H. A. Ultrastructure of the surface of the iris in rat eye. Z. Zellforsch., 110:192, 1970.

and Jerndal, T. Scanning electron microscopic studies on the development of the iridocorneal angle in human eyes. Invest. Ophthalmol., 10:252, 1971.

Henderson, T. The cribriform ligament of the ciliary muscle. A demonstration of the comparative anatomy of the angle of the anterior chamber in man and monkeys. Trans. Ophthalmol. Soc. U. K., 41:465, 1921.

Hess, L. Pathogenesis of glaucoma and "glaucomatous" atrophy of the optic nerve. Arch. Ophthalmol., 37:324, 1947.

Hogan, M. J., and Zimmerman, L. E. Ophthalmic Pathology. Saunders, Philadelphia, 1962.

Holmberg, A. S. Ultrastructure of the ciliary epithelium. Arch. Ophthalmol., 62:935, 1959.

Schlemm's canal and the trabecular meshwork. An electron microscopic study of the normal structure in man and monkey (*Cercopithecus ethiops*) Doc. Ophthalmol., 19:339, 1965.

Holmes, W. J. Congenital buphthalmos complicated by dislocation of lens and hemorrhage into vitreous with complete recovery of central vision. Arch. Ophthalmol., 20:757, 1938.

Holm-Pederson, E. Juvenile glaucoma, adult glaucoma, juvenile glaucoma in three successive generations. Nord. Med., 39:1615, 1948.

Iwanoff, A. Mikroscopische Anatomie des Uvealtractus und der Linse. 1st der Ubealtractus, Graefe-Saemisch Hand. I., 1:265, 1874.

Jaendelize, P., Drouet, P. L., Thomas, C., et Bardelli, Tension oculaire, glaucome et hypophyse. Bull. Mem. Soc. Fr., Ophthalmol., 1:478, 1938.

Jaensch, P. A. Anatomical and clinical investigations of the pathology and therapy of hydrophthalmos congenitus. Graefe's Arch. Ophthalmol., 118:21, 1927.

Jeannatulos, P. Recherches embryologiques sur la mode de formation de la chambre antérieure chez les mannifères et chez l'homme. Arch. Ophthalmol., 16:529, 1896.

Jerndal, T. Goniodysgenesis and hereditary juvenile glaucoma. Acta Ophthalmol. (Suppl.) (Kbh.), 107, 1970.

Johnson, W. B. Buphthalmia, an interesting series of cases occurring in the same family. Trans. Am. Ophthalmol. Soc., 8:308, 1898.

Kalt, M. L'hydrophtalmie congénitale altérations anatomiques. Bull. Mem. Soc. Fr. Ophtalmol., 45:317, 1932.

L'hydrophthalmie congénitale. Ann. Ocul. (Paris), 170:97, 1933.

Kapuscinski, W. Uber die Beeinflussung des Augendruckes Jugenlichen Glaukomformen. Graefe's Arch. Ophthalmol., 138:673, 1938.

Kaye, G. I., Cole, J. D., and Donn, A. Electron microscopy. Sodium localization in normal and ouabain-treated transporting cells. Science, 150:1167, 1965.

Kindt, P. Ein fall von Spontan Geheiltem Hydrophthalmus Congenitus. Acta Ophthalmol. (Kbh.), 15:333, 1937.

Kinsey, V. E., and Reddy, D. V. N. Chemistry and dynamics of aqueous humor. In J. H. Prince, (Ed.), The Rabbit in Eye Research. Thomas, Springfield, Ill., 1964, p. 218.

Kluyskens, J. Le glaucome congénital. Bull. Soc. Belge Ophtalmol., 94:3, 1950.

Le Glaucome Congenital. Imprimerie. Medicale et Scientifique, Bruzzelles, 1950.

Le glaucoma congénital. Arch. Ophtalmol., NS11:574, 1951.

Glaucome congénital tardif. Bull. Soc. Belge Ophtalmol., 118:328, 1955.
Knapp, A. A. A case of corectopia. Am. J. Ophthalmol., 13:141, 1930.
Koeppe, L. Die Microscopie des lebenden Kammerwinkels im fokalen Lichte der Gullstrandschen Nernstspaltlampe. Graefe's Arch. Ophthalmol., 101:48, 1919.
Die Microscopie des Kammerwinkels etc. Graefe's Arch. Ophthalmol., 101:238, 1920.
Korte, W. Beitrage zur Erblichkeit des Glaukoms. Klin. Monatsbl. Augenheilkl., 102:664, 1939.
Kronfeld, P. C. Tonography. Lecture at San Francisco Ophthalmological Round Table, Oct. 1953, quoted by Shaffer. Trans. Am. Acad. Ophthalmol. Otolaryngol., 59:297, 1955.
McGarry, H., and Smith, H. Gonioscopic studies of the canal of Schlemm. Am. J. Ophthalmol., 25:1163, 1942.
Kupfer, C. The relationship of ciliary body, meridional muscle and corneoscleral trabecular meshwork. Arch. Ophthalmol., 68:818, 1962.
A note on the development of the anterior chamber angle. Invest. Ophthalmol., 8:69, 1969.
and Ross, K. Outflow resistance in the developing human eye. Thirtieth Clinical Meeting, Wilmer Residents Assoc., the Wilmer Ophthalmological Institute, April 23, 1971.
and Ross, K. The development of outflow facility in human eyes. Invest. Ophthalmol., 10:513, 1971.
Kwitko, M. L. Congenital glaucoma, a clinical study. Can. J. Ophthalmol., 2:91, 1967.
Lagrange, F. Rapport sur le traitment du glaucome infantile. Bull. Mem. Soc. Fr. Ophtalmol., 38:1, 1925.
Lange, O. Zur Anatomie des Auges des Neugeborenen. II. Suprachoroidalraum, Zonula Zinii, Ora Serrata und Sog. Physiologische Excavation der seh Nervenpapille. Klin. Monatsbl. Augenheilkd., 39:202, 1901.
Langham, M. E. Aqueous humor and control of intraocular pressure. Physiol. Rev., 38:215, 1958.
and Maumenee, A. E. The diagnosis and treatment of glaucoma based on a new procedure for the measurement of intraocular dynamics. Trans. Am. Acad. Ophthalmol. Otolaryngol., 68:277, 1964.
Lehrfeld, L., and Reber, J. Glaucoma at the Wills Hospital. Arch. Ophthalmol., 18:612, 1937.
Leplat, G. Embryologie de l'appareil oculaire, developpement général de l'appareil visuel. Traité Ophthalmol., 1:87, 1939.
Levinsohn, G. Beitrag zur Pathologischen Anatomie und Pathogenese des Glaukoms. Arch. Augenheilkd., 62:131, 1909.
Leydhecker, W. Glaukom. Ein Handbuch. Springer, Berlin, 1960, p. 168.
Lindner, K. Zur Klinik des Glaskorpers. Graefe's Arch. Ophthalmol., 135:333, and 135:462, 1936.
Linner, E. Episcleral venous pressure during tonography. Acta 17th Concilium Ophthalmologicum (1954). 3:1532, 1955.
Lister, A. Surgery of congenital glaucoma. Trans. Ophthalmol. Soc. Aust., 11:39, 1952.
Some aspects of congenital glaucoma. Trans. Ophthalmol., Soc. U. K., 79:163, 1960.
Lohlein, W. Glakom als Erbleiden in Gutt's Hb. d. Erkrankeiten, Vol. 5. Theime Ed., Leipzig, 1938, p. 35.
Maggiore, L. Struttura, comportamento e significato del canale di Schlemm nell 'occhio umano in condizione normali e pathologische. Ann. Ottalmol. Clin. Ocul., 40:317, 1917.

Magitot, A. Étude anatomique sur le glaucome infantile. Ann. Ocul. (Paris), 147:241, 1912.

La tension pathologique. Traité Ophtalmol., 6:161, 1939.

Thalamus et glaucome. Ann. Ocul. (Paris), 180:1, 1947.

Mann, I. Development of the Human Eye, ed. 3. Cambridge Univ. Press, London, 1964.

Developmental Anomalies of the Eye. Cambridge Univ. Press, London, 1957.

Manschot, W. A. Ocular anomalies in osteogenesis imperfecta. Ophthalmologica, 149:241, 1965.

Histology of congenital glaucoma. Ophthalmologica, 160:326, 1970.

Mansheim. B. J. Aqueous outflow measurements by continuous tonometry in some unusual forms of glaucoma. Arch. Ophthalmol., 50:580, 1953.

Maschimo, M. Ein Beitrag zur Kenntnis der Angeborenen Hornhauttrubungen. Klin. Monatsbl. Augenheilkd., 71:184, 1923.

Matteucci, P., Vannini, A. Il Tessuto Mesodermico dell' angolo iridocorneale nell 'irdroftalmo. Communicazione alla Soc. Oftalmol. Lombarda, March 16, 1932.

Sull 'innervazione simpatica e sulla regolazione neuro-vegetativa dell 'uvea. Rass. Ital. Ottalmol., 15:161, 1946.

Maumenee, A. E. The pathogenesis of congenital glaucoma. A new theory. Trans. Am. Ophthalmol. Soc., 56:507, 1958; Am. J. Ophthalmol., 47:827, 1959.

Further observations on the pathogenesis of congenital glaucoma. Trans. Am. Ophthalmol. Soc., 60:140, 1962; Am. J. Ophthalmol., 55:1163, 1963.

Discussion of J. G. F. Worst. The cause and treatment of congenital glaucoma. Trans. Am. Acad. Ophthalmol. Otolaryngol., 68:766, 1964.

Mauthner, L. Lehrbuch der Ophthalmoscopie. Tender, Wien, 1868.

Mawas, J. Les cellules nerveuses ganglionnaires de la choroide chez l'homme. Bull. Soc. Ophtalmol. Fr. (Paris), 21:172, 1936.

Meisner, V. Hydrophthalmus und Angeborene Hornhauttrubunger. Graefe's Arch. Ophthalmol., 112:433, 1923.

Meller, J. Hydrophthalmus als Folge einer Entwicklungsanomalie der Iris. Graefe's Arch. Ophthalmol., 92:34, 1917.

Augenarzliche eingriffe. Wien, 1921.

Moses, R. A., and Becker, B. Clinical tonography. The scleral rigidity correction, Am. J. Ophthalmol., 45:196, 1958.

Musini, A. Morganti, G. Contributo allo studio della trasmissione ereditaria del glaucoma giovanile. Attisoc. Ophthalmol., 11, 1949.

Newell, F. W. (Ed.) Glaucoma: Transactions of the First, Second, Third, Fourth and Fifth Conferences, New York, 1956–60, Josiah Macy, Jr., Foundation.

Pashby, T. J., and Halliday, J. A. Congenital glaucoma. Trans. Can. Ophthalmol. Soc., 7:159, 1956.

Paufique, L. Le glaucoma congénital. Contexte clinique et indications thérapeutiques. Ann. Ocul. (Paris), 189:27, 1956.

et Etienne, r. Examen clinique d'un glaucoma infantile. Indications thérapeutiques. Ann. Ocul. (Paris), 187:305, 1954.

Penzani, B. Eredità nel glaucoma giovanile tardivo. G. Ital. Ottalmol., 8:54, 1954.

Perkins, E. S. Glaucoma in the younger age groups. Arch. Ophthalmol., 64:882, 1960.

Influence of the fifth cranial nerve on the intraocular pressure of the rabbit eye. Br. J. Ophthalmol., 41:247, 1957.

Peters, A. Ueber Angeborene Defektbildung der Descemetschen Membran. Klin. Monatsbl. Augenheilkd., 1:27, and 1:105, 1906.

Hornhautveranderungen bei Buphthalmus. Klin. Monatsbl. Augenheilkd. 79:544, 1927.

Plocher, R. Beitrag zum Juvenilen Familiaren Glaukom. Klin. Monatsbl. Augenheilkd., 60:592, 1918.
Purtscher, E. Fetaler Hydrophthalmus bei Amniogener Mibbildung der Orbita. Graefe's Arch. Ophthalmol., 142:453, 1940.
Radnot, M., Follmann, P., and Musci, G. Neuroendocrine factors in the etiology of primary glaucoma. Acta Chir. Acad. Sci. Hung., 9:423, 1968.
Rasmussen, D. H., and Ellis, P. P. Congenital glaucoma in identical twins. Arch. Ophthalmol., 84:827, 1970.
Redslob, M. E. Dedoublement et developpement de la membrane de Descemet. Bull. Mem. Soc. Fr. Ophthalmol., 46:216, 1933.
Reed, H., Briggs, J. N., and Martin, J. K. Congenital glaucoma, deafness, mental deficiency, and cardiac anomaly, following attempted abortion. J. Pediatr., 46:182, 1955.
Reeh, M. J. Bilateral congenital glaucoma. Trans. Am. Acad. Ophthalmol. Otolaryngol., 65:178, 1961.
Reese, A. B., and Ellsworth, R. M. The anterior chamber cleavage syndrome. Arch. Ophthalmol., 75:307, 1966.
Reis, W. Untersuchingen zur Pathologische Anatomie und zur Pathogenese des Angeborenen Hydrophthalmus. Graefe's Arch. Ophthalmol., 60:1, 1905.
Rochon-Duvigneaud, A. Recherches anatomiques sur l'angle de la chambre antérieure et le canal de Schlemm. Arch. Ophthalmol., 12:732, 1892.
Rohen, J. W. Morphology and pathology of the trabecular meshwork. In G. K. Smelser (ed.), The Structure of the Eye. Academic Press, New York, 1961, p. 335.
(Ed.). Das Auge und seine Hilfsorgane. In J. W. Rohen, Handbuch der mikroskopischen Anatmoi des Menchen. Springer-Verlag, Berlin, 1968.
Lutjen, E., and Bárány, E. The relation between the ciliary muscle and the trabecular meshwork and its importance for the effect of miotics on aqueous outflow resistance. A study of two contrasting monkey species, *Macaca irus* and *Cercopithecus aethiops*. Graefe's Arch. Klin. Exp. Ophthalmol., 172:23, 1967.
Rosetti, D., Betetto, G. Glaucoma familiare e quadri malformativi multipli. Ann. Ottalmol., 82:139, 1956.
Roussy, G. et Mosinger, M. Le complexe hypothalamo-hypophysaire, neurocrinie, neuricrinie et orocrinie. Rev. Neurol. (Paris), 77:281, 1945.
Royer, J. Les glaucomes congéitaux chez l'enfant. Conf. Lyonn. Ophthalmol., 71:1, 1958.
Rytkölä, T. Über die Entwicklung des Kammerwinkels der menschlichen Feten. Suomalaisen Tiedeakatemian Toimituksia Annales Academiae Scientiarum Fennicae. Suomalanen Tiedakatemia, Helsinki, 1952, p. 68.
Saltzmann, M. The Anatomy and Histology of the Human Eyeball in the Normal State. Its Development and Senescence. Translated by E. V. L. Brown, Univ. of Chicago Press, Chicago, 1912, p. 112.
Die Ophthalmoskopie der Kammerbucht. Z. Augenheilkd., 31:1, 1914, 34:26, 1915.
Sampaolesi, R. New gonioscopic signs in congenital glaucoma of late onset. In Modern Problems in Ophthalmology, Vol. 6. Karger, Basel, 1968, p. 106.
Sautter, H. Eine Spatform des Juvenilen Glaucoms? Ber. Dtsch. Ophthalmol. Ges., 63:342, 1960.
Scheerer, O. Demonstration klinischen falles. Klin. Monatsbl. Augenheilkd., 89:829, 1932.
Scheie, H. G. Infantile and juvenile glaucoma. Trans. Am. Acad. Ophthalmol. Otolaryngol., 67:458, 1963.
Schieck, F. II. Die spezielle Pathologie der Cornea. A. Die anomalien der Hornhautgestalt. 1. Die angeborenen Anomalien der Grobe und der Wolbung der Cornea. Kurzes. Hand. Ophthalmol., 4:236, 1931.

Seefelder, R. Klinische und Anatomische Untersuchungen zur Pathologie und Therapie des Hydrophthalmus Congenitus. Graefe's Arch. Ophthalmol., 63:205, and 63:481, 1906.

Demonstration Mikroskopischer Praeparate. Ber. Dtsch. Ophthalmol. Ges., 36:308, 1910.

Das verhalten der Kammerbucht und ihres Gerustwerkes bis zur Geburt. Graefe-Saemisch Hand., Abt., 50:1, 1910.

Pathologische-anatomische Beitrage zur Frage der Angeborenen zentralen Defektbildung der Hornhauthinterflache. Klin. Monatsbl. Augenheilkd., 65:539, 1920.

Hydrophthalmus als Folge einer Entwicklungsanomalie der Kammerbucht. Graefe's Arch. Ophthalmol., 103:1, 1920.

Die Entwicklung des Menschen Auges in Kurzes Handbuch der Ophthalmologie. Edited by F. Schieck, and A. Bruckner. Springer-Verlag, Berlin, 1930, Fig. 38, p. 503.

und Wolfrum, R. Zur Entwicklung der vorderen Kammer und der Kammerwinkels beim Menschen nebst Bemerkingen uber ihre Enstehung bei Tieren. Graefe's Arch. Ophthalmol., 63:430, 1906.

Shaffer, R. N. Pathogenesis of congenital glaucoma. Gonioscopie and microscopic anatomy. Trans. Am. Acad. Ophthalmol., Otolaryngol., 59:297, 1955.

Manual of Gonioscopy. Mosby, St. Louis, 1962.

and Weiss, D. I. Congenital and Pediatric Glaucomas. Mosby, St. Louis, 1970.

Shirley, S. Y. Congenital glaucoma without megalocornea. Trans. Can. Ophthalmol. Soc., 10:51, 1958.

Simon, K. A., and Bonting, S. L. Possible influences of cardiac glycosides in treatment of glaucoma. Arch. Ophthalmol., 68:227, 1962.

Smelser, G. K., and Ozanics, V. The development of the trabecular meshwork, in primate eyes. Am. J. Ophthalmol., 71:366, 1971.

Smith, J. L., and Stowe, F. R. The Pierre-Robin syndrome. A review of 39 cases with emphasis on associated ocular lesions. Pediatrics, 27:128, 1961.

Cavanaugh, J. J. A., and Stone, F. C. Ocular manifestations of the Pierre-Robin syndrome. Arch. Ophthalmol., 63:984, 1960.

Sondermann, R. Ueber Entwicklung, Morfologie und Funktion des Schlemmschen Kanals. Acta Ophthalmol. (Kbh.), 11:280, 1933.

Ueber Physiologie und Pathologie des Augendrucks. Klin. Monatsbl. Augenheilkd., 112:113, 1947.

Speakman, J. S. The structure of the trabecular meshwork in relation to the pathogenesis of open angle glaucoma. Can. Med. Assoc. J., 84:1066, 1961.

The development and structure of the normal trabecular meshwork. Proc. R. Soc. Med., 52:72, 1959.

and Crawford, J. S. Congenital opacities of the cornea. Br. J. Ophthalmol., 50:68, 1966.

and Leeson, T. S. Pathological findings in a case of primary congenital glaucoma compared with normal infant eyes. Br. J. Ophthalmol., 48:196, 1964.

Speilberg, S. Contribution to the pathogenesis of hydrophthalmus congenitus. Klin. Monatsbl. Augenheilkd. 49:313, 1911.

Spenser, W. H., Alvarado, J., and Hayes, T. L. Scanning electron microscopy of human ocular tissue: trabecular meshwork. Invest. Ophthalmol., 7:651, 1968.

Stein, L. Linkbuphthalmus mit Gleichseitiger Hemihypertrophie der Entsprechenden Geisichtschalfte. Klin. Monatsbl. Augenheilkd., 102:541, 1939.

Stieve, R. Anatomischer anzeiger. Zentralbl. Wiss. Anat., 97:69, 1949.

Stimmel, F., and Rotter, F. Contributions to the pathology and therapy of hydrophthalmus congenitus. Z. Augenheilkd., 28:114, 1912.

Stokes, W. H. Hereditary primary glaucoma. Arch. Ophthalmol., 24:885, 1940.

Sugar, H. S. Gonioscopy and glaucoma. Arch. Ophthalmol., 25:674, 1941.
Concerning the chamber angle. I. Goniotomy. Am. J. Ophthalmol., 23:857, 1940.
The congenital or infantile glaucomas. Am. J. Ophthalmol., 33:1679, 1950.

Terry, C. C., Paton, R. T., and Katzin, M. H. Primary degeneration in the vicinity of the chamber angle. Am. J. Ophthalmol., 40:619, 1955.

Theobald, G. Schlemm's canal. Its anastromoses and anatomic relations. Trans. Am. Ophthalmol. Soc., 32:574, 1934.

Theodore, F. H. Congenital opacities of the cornea. Arch. Ophthalmol., 31:138, 1944.

Thomas, R. P. Experimental transient glaucoma in animals. Arch. Ophthalmol., 75:92, 1966.
Neurohumeral factors in experimental glaucoma. Am. J. Ophthalmol., 65:729, 1968.

Thomassen, T. L. The venous tension in eyes suffering from simple glaucoma. Acta Ophthalmol., (Kbl.), 25:221, 1947.

Thompson, A. The filtration angle. The anatomy and function of its parts together with certain suggestions bearing on their association with the production of glaucoma. Ophthalmoscope, 9:470, 1911.

Troncoso, M. A Treatise on Gonioscopy. Davis, Philadelphia, 1947.

Valude and Duclos. Opening of the angle of eyes. Ann. Ocul. (Paris), 119:98, 1898.

Verhoeff, F. Discussion of paper by R. H. Courtney, and E. Hill. Hereditary juvenile glaucoma simplex, J. A. M. A., 97:1609, 1931.

Vogelsang, V. Zur erbbegutachtung des Hydrophthalmus. Klin. Monatsbl. Augenheilkd., 102:587, 1939.

von Hippel, E. Ueber Hydrophthalmus Congenitus nebst bemerkingen uber die Verfarbung der Cornea durch Blutfarbstoff. Graefe's Arch. Ophthalmol., 44:539, 1897.
Ueber angeborene defektbildung der Descemetschen Membran. Klin. Monatsbl. Augenheild., 2:1, 1906.

Vos, T. A. Geheilte Netzhautablosung bei Hydrophthalmus. Graefe's Arch. Ophthalmol., 140:691, 1939.

Vrabec, F. Sur la question de l'endothelium de la surface antérieure de l'iris humain. Ophthalmologica, 123:20, 1952.

Vrabec, F. The endothelium of the anterior chamber angle of the eye. In G. K. Smelser (Ed.), The Structure of the Eye. Academic Press, New York, 1961, p. 311.

Waardenburg, P. J. Beobachtungen uber vererbung im Grezgebiete zwischen Jugendlichem und Alters Glaukom sowie zwischen Kindlichem und Jugendlichem Glaukom. Graefe's Arch. Ophthalmol., 140:662, 1939.

Weekers, L., et Weekers, R. Contribution à la pathogenie du buphthalmos. Ophthalmologica, 120:285, 1950.

Weekers, R., and Delmarcelle, Y. Pathogeneses of intraocular hypertension in cases of arteriovenous aneurysm, Arch. Ophthalmol., 48:338, 1952.
Priojot, E., Delmarcelle, Y., Lavergne, G., Watillon, M., Gougnard, L., Gougnard-Rion, C., et Gustin, J. Le diagnostic précoce du glaucome débutant. Bull. Soc. Belge Ophtal., 121:140, 1959.
et Watillon, M. Glaucome congénital sans mégalocornée. Ophthalmologica, 133:37, 1957.

Wessely, K. Einige besondere Probleme aus der Pathologie des Glaukoms. Graefe's Arch. Ophthalmol., 148:111, 1947.

Westerlung, E. On the hereditary of congenital hydrophthalmus. Acta Ophthalmol. (Kbh.), 21:331, 1943.

Wexler, D., and Kornzweig, A. Bupthalmos in a six-month premature infant. Arch. Ophthalmol., 37:318, 1947.

Worst, J. G. F. Microforceps and microscalpels. Nature (Lond.), 170:1129, 1952.

Goniotomy, an improved method for chamber angle surgery in congenital glaucoma, Am. J. Ophthalmol., 57:185, 1964.

The cause and treatment of congenital glaucoma. Trans. Am. Acad. Ophthalmol. Otolaryngol., 68:766, 1964.

Le phénomène du réflux de sang dans le canal de Schlemm. Bull. Mem. Soc. Fr. Ophtalmol., 77:219, 1964.

The Pathogenesis of Congenital Glaucoma. Thomas, Springfield, Ill, 1966.

and Otter, K. Low vacuum diagnostic contact lenses. Am. J. Ophthalmol., 51:527, 1961.

Wulle, K. G. Elektronenmikropische Befunde zur Entwicklung des menschlichen Trabekelwerks. Dtsch. Ophthalmol. Ges. Ber., 69:425, 1968.

Young, R. L. Congenital bilateral glaucoma. Am. J. Ophthalmol., 34:1040, 1951.

Zimmerman, L. E. Demonstration of hyaluronidase-sensitive acid mucopolysaccharide in trabecula and iris in routine paraffin sections of adult human eyes. Am. J. Ophthalmol., 44:1, 1957.

Further histochemical studies of acid-mucopolysaccharides in the intraocular tissues. Am. J. Ophthalmol., 45:299, 1958.

Zimmerman, L. E., et al. Symposium: Contribution of electron microscopy to the understanding of the production and outflow of aqueous humor. Trans. Am. Acad. Ophthalmol. Otolaryngol., 70:737, 1966.

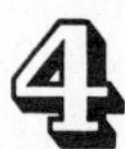

The Infant Eye

A study of the development of the eye must not end with the birth of the fetus. The eye of the newborn does not in every particular way resemble that of the adult so that one must consider that "development" continues throughout the whole of life. Birth places the human eye in a new environment and exposes it for the first time to its so-called adequate stimulus, that is, light. Birth also allows the application of in-vivo and in-situ methods of examination and measurements that yield correlations with anatomical data. Understandably, therefore, birth has been considered a milestone in the development of the human eye. There is a distinct parallel between the postnatal growth of the eye and that of the brain. Thus from birth to adulthood the eye grows 3.25 times and the brain 3.76 times. The body volume and weight, on the other hand, increases 21.36 times. Therefore the basic structure of the infant eye differs markedly from that of the adult, resulting in the difference in response of the globe when subjected to an elevation in the intraocular pressure.

GENERAL CONSIDERATIONS

No single anatomical description of the orbit, eyeball, and adnexa will apply to all ages of infancy and childhood. Fortunately, however, the problem is simplified by the precocious development of the visual organs. That is, the eye is almost fully grown by the end of the second year of extrauterine life and the child of eight already possesses a well-formed orbit. The appearance of the eye is characteristic in babies owing to the fact that the palpebral aperture is almost as long at birth as in the adult while the vertical lid opening is only half the width. Therefore less of the sclera is visible than in the adult.

Perhaps the most striking feature of the newborn infant eye is one that is readily appreciated without any detailed knowledge of ophthalmology—that is, the baby does not appear to be able to see. Two main factors combine to produce this somewhat vacant stare of the newborn. First, the development of the macula is not completed until several months after birth, and secondly the infant has not yet gained those cumulative postural and tactile experiences which contribute so largely to sensations accepted as purely visual by the unsophisticated observer. However, a completely vacant gaze that persists beyond the first few weeks of life is always of serious importance, signifying either mental retardation or visual defect. Sometimes both handicaps are operative as exemplified by cases in which the optic nerves are implicated in widespread cerebral trauma, so that stunted mental development is found associated with bilateral optic atrophy. Other obvious features of the newborn are the small size of the pupil and the uniform texture of the iris stroma compared with the elaborately decorated surface of the adult iris.

It will be remembered that the adult eye is almost a perfect sphere, with the qualification that the anterior one-sixth representing the cornea bulges forward with a slightly sharper convexity than that of the rest of the globe. The eye of early infancy, on the other hand, is less of a sphere. The horizontal diameter is slightly greater than the sagittal while the reverse is the case in the adult. The eye's anteroposterior diameter varies from 12.5 to

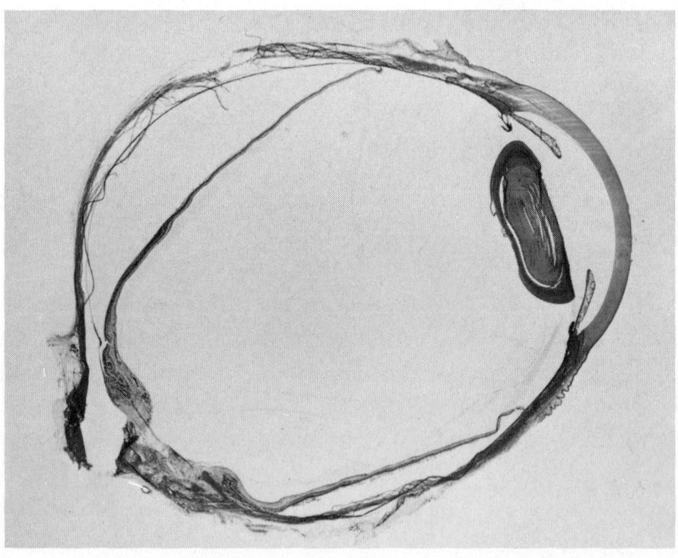

FIG. 1. One-month-old infant eye. (Courtesy of R. J. Schneider.) X 3

17.9 mm, the vertical diameter from 14.5 to 17.3 mm, and the transverse diameter from 16.0 to 18.4 mm, according to different authors (Fig. 1). Growth is rapid in the first year of life, with the vertical diameter growing faster so that the eye becomes more nearly spherical. The rate then decreases until puberty when it again becomes more rapid until the early twenties. To offset the comparative shortness of the infant eye, which would make it exceedingly hypermetropic, the media are more highly refractive than in the adult, the seat of the excess of refractivity being located in the lens. Retinoscopy of the infant's eye practically always shows between +3 and +6 diopters of hypermetropia. This hypermetropia, which is the normal refractive state during infancy and early childhood, entails no appreciable disability in the majority of cases and the condition appears to be easily overcome. When a small child is found to be free of hypermetropia, subsequent examination at intervals will often reveal the onset of myopia before growth has ceased. It would seem that the type of eye is developmentally or even genetically determined long before the associated refractive error appears. For the next few years, the amount of hypermetropia tends to diminish steadily as the eye attains its full anteroposterior length. The increase in axial length would result in excessive myopia were it not for another factor, that is, flattening of the lens.

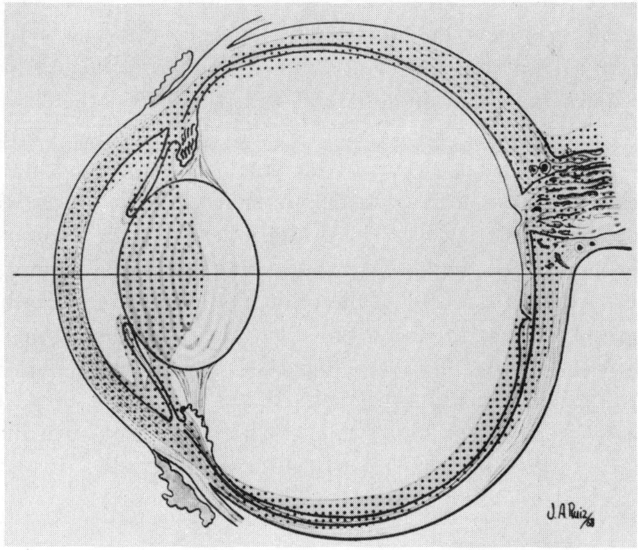

FIG. 2. Adult eye (*shaded*) and infant eye both enlarged to same size.

The conjunctiva is thin and there is no subepithelial adenoid tissue until some weeks after birth. The lacrimal gland is very small and does not function fully for about six weeks.

The shape and the outside diameters of the eyeball reach a steady state around the age of 14 years. The same may be said for most of the anatomic and histologic characteristics of the ocular tissue with the exception of the ciliary body and the crystalline lens which continue to change grossly throughout life and thereby affect the fluid spaces around them, particularly the depth of the anterior chamber. These differences in shape are shown diagrammatically in Fig. 2, which represents the eyes of a newborn child and of an adult magnified to approximately the same size and superimposed. It is obvious that the differences are most marked in the anterior part of the globe.

THE ORBIT

The fetal skull has a large cranium (orbital roof) and a small face. (Fig. 3). The orbit margin is sharp and well ossified at birth, which affords the eye protection from stress and injury during parturition. It becomes less sharp with age. Since the eye is relatively large in relation to the orbit and in an advanced stage of development at birth such protection is desirable. The rarity of birth injuries to the globe in cases of unassisted delivery attests to this protection. In the newborn the form of the orbit is that of an ellipse—higher on the lateral side than on the medial side. This changes with age so that the orbit on coronal section behind the orbital margin becomes that of a quadrilateral with rounded corners.

The orbital fissures are relatively large in the child owing to the narrowness of the orbital surface of the greater wing of the sphenoid. The interorbital distance at birth is small but increases with the growth of the frontal and ethmoidal air cells. The orbital process of the zygomatic malar bone may almost reach the lacrimal fossa and this condition may persist up to ten years. At birth the roof of the orbit is relatively much larger than the floor compared with adult proportions. The fossa for the lacrimal gland is shallow but the accessory fossa is well marked. The optic canal has no length at birth so that it is actually a foramen. At one year it measures 4 mm. The periosteum or periorbita is much thicker and stronger at birth than in the adult. The size of the orbit changes little after seven years.

THE AQUEOUS VEINS

The aqueous veins of Ascher are exit channels for aqueous fluid and

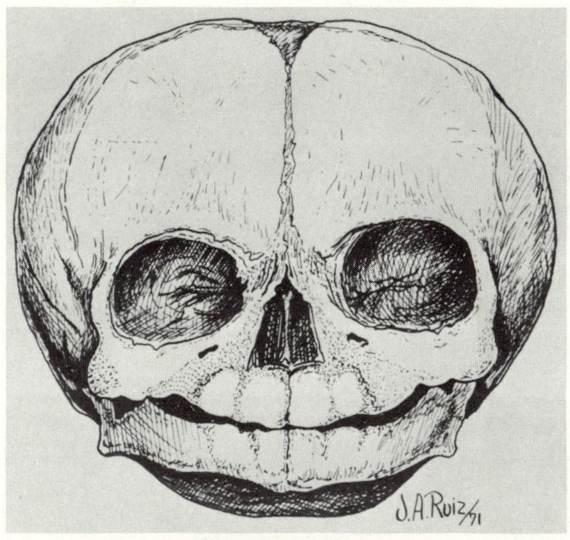

FIG. 3. Infant skull.

these vessels vary in size from 0.01 to 0.1 mm in diameter. While they are usually seen with a slitlamp, the largest can be made out with a loupe. They are found about 2 mm from the limbus most often inferonasally and often commencing in a hook-shaped bend where they arise from the sclera. They contain a clear fluid or very diluted blood and run a short course from 0.1 to just over 1.0 cm. They join the episcleral venous system, the blood of which is thus altered. It may become more diluted, or clear fluid and blood may run side by side unmixed—forming a laminated vein of Goldmann. Sometimes a clear central stream is flanked by a blood column on either side. Ashton has traced one of these vessels into the canal of Schlemm.

THE ANTERIOR CHAMBER

The anterior chamber at birth is 2.3 mm to 2.7 mm deep—shallower than in the adult. This is due to the steeper curve of the anterior surface of the lens which lifts the iris forward (Fig. 4). In spite of this, however, the angle of the anterior chamber is deeper and more widely open at birth (Fig. 5).

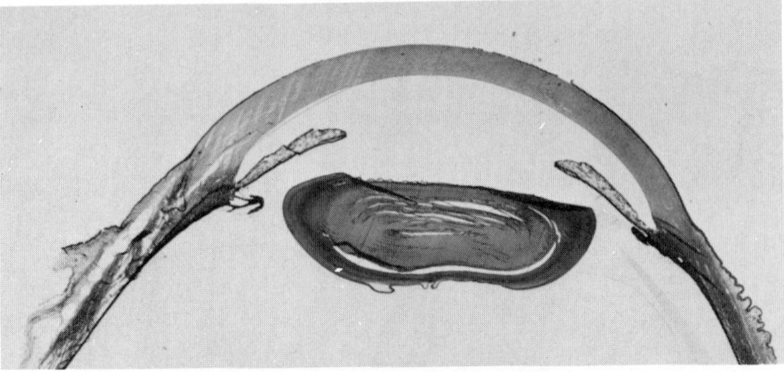

FIG. 4. One-month-old infant eye, anterior chamber. (Courtesy of R. J. Schneider.) X4.5.

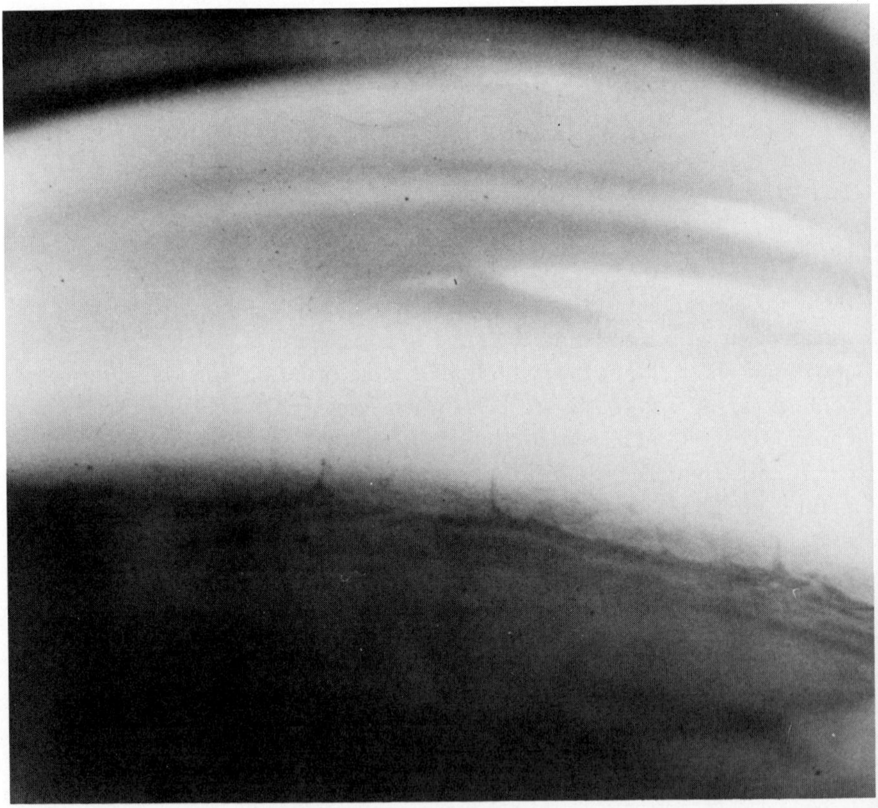

FIG. 5. Filtration angle of normal Negro infant. Remnants of uveal meshwork are still present. (Courtesy of J. G. F. Worst.)

THE UVEAL TRACT

Most babies belonging to the white race are born with blue eyes. The reason is that the dark pigment on the posterior aspect of the iris seen through the translucent stroma, which as yet has no mesodermal pigment cells of its own, appears blue just as the veins look blue through skin, although the blood in them is of a port wine color. In addition the stroma is more cellular than in the adult and the iris vessels as yet have no adventitia so the blood is partly visible through their wall. In deeply pigmented races a certain number of pigment cells are present at birth and the vessel walls are thicker so that the iris may look blue or hazel or even brown. Pigment is deposited in the anterior limiting layers of the stroma in the first few days of life; varying with the amount so laid down, the color changes. If little is deposited the eye remains blue or gray, if much is laid down the eye becomes brown and in some cases to such a degree that details of structure may be entirely hidden. The change is gradual and spreads over periods of varying length in different subjects. As a rule, the change is considerable within the few weeks after birth. The so-called sculpturing of the iris (radial striations) seen in life in blue and gray eyes is due to the visibility of the vessel walls and occasionally, as seen under magnification, the blood column itself, the intervening stroma being quite transparent. In light blue eyes with good illumination and magnification (of 24 X or more) it is often possible to actually make out two or sometimes three layers of vessels which may cross at acute angles, the deeper ones running to the pupillary margin and the superficial ones anastomosing at the lesser circle. The stroma of brown eyes is no longer transparent and vessels cannot be seen except those which may be in relief on the iris surface. The sphincter pupillae muscle is well developed but the dilator is not entirely functional at birth so that the pupil is small and does not dilate fully.

The stroma of the uveal tract has no pigment except possibly posteriorly near the optic nerve. The stroma of the ciliary body is highly cellular but the various muscles can be recognized, especially the meridional fibers. The pars plana is short. Some ciliary processes are still in contact with the iris. The choroid is slightly thicker and more cellular but otherwise resembles that of the adult. The line of demarcation between the retina and the ciliary body is obvious but does not reach adult relationships until about seven years. As the ciliary processes are displaced backward the angle of the anterior chamber widens to adult size between two and four years. There is no muscle of Muller present at birth. It is only after the fifth year that the ciliary muscle and thus the whole ciliary body takes on a triangular form. The amount of connective tissue in the uveal tract increases, the ciliary body thickens and the circumlental space diminishes.

THE LENS

The infant lens is more spherical than in the adult. The curvature of the anterior surface is exaggerated in the newborn, increasing the total refractive power of the eye, an increase rendered necessary by the fact that the anteroposterior diameter of the eye measures only about 17 mm compared with a corresponding dimension of 23.5 mm in the adult. The lens occupies a disproportionately large area in the infant and is much rounder, resulting in a shallower anterior chamber (see Fig. 2). The lens grows rapidly in the first years of life and becomes flatter. Growth and development continue throughout life (Table 1).

TABLE 1

THE LENS

	Newborn (mm)	Adult (mm)
Equatorial diameter	6.7	9.1
Anteroposterior diameter	3.76	3.6
Anterior radius	5.0	10.0
Posterior radius	4.0	6.0

AQUEOUS HUMOR

The fluid content of the eye consists of vitreous humor, which is static, and aqueous humor, which is constantly changing. Aqueous is secreted by the ciliary body into the posterior chamber. After entering the anterior chamber through the pupil it transverses the trabecular meshwork to reach Schlemm's canal. Approximately 30 collector channels conduct aqueous to the scleral plexus. There is a pressure drop in the normal eye of 5 to 10 mm Hg across this barrier. Obstruction to aqueous outflow occurs somewhere in the drainage pathway between the anterior chamber and episcleral plexus in the glaucomatous state. (Fig. 6).

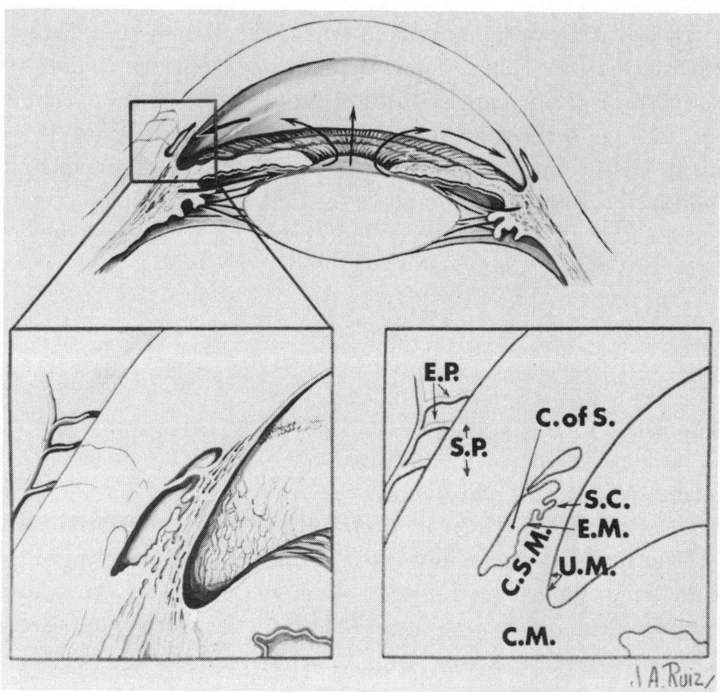

FIG. 6. Pathways through which aqueous humor passes upon leaving the anterior segment of the eye. (C M) Ciliary muscle; (C of S) canal of Schlemm; (C S M) corneoscleral meshwork; (E M) endothelial meshwork; (E P) episcleral plexus; (S P) scleral plexus; (S C) Sondermann's canal; (U M) uveal meshwork. (Modified from Speakman. **Canad. Med. Asso. J.** 84:1066, 1961.)

VITREOUS CAVITY

At birth Cloquet's canal extends horizontally from a point a little below and to the nasal side of the posterior pole of the lens backward to the optic disc. The exteme anterior end of the main trunk of the hyaloid artery extends horizontally backward from the lens capsule along the first part of the canal. After birth this vascular remnant undergoes further atrophy and gradually drops until it comes to hang down perpendicularly from the lens. It also becomes curled into a spiral form. At the same time, the walls of Cloquet's canal become very lax and the whole structure tends to sag down so that its anterior open mouth, instead of pointing straight backwards, comes to lie well below the posterior pole of the lens and finally on a level with the lower border of the dilated pupil. It is thus not obvious in the living eye when a person is in the upright position, although the backward slope of the vitreous face as seen with the slitlamp is an indication of the canal's continued presence in the lower part of the eye. Its walls remain extremely slack and in the adult it can be made to float up and assume its embryonic position for a short time by use of appropriate movements of the head and eyes.

THE CORNEA

The cornea is one of the most advanced ocular structures, having already attained more than three-quarters of its adult diameter at birth. Postnatal growth occurs and the cornea's adult diameter is attained variably between six months to five years (Fig. 7). The dividing line between micro-, normal, and megalocornea is not fixed, but rather a flowing transition. The literature is in agreement, however, that megalocornea has a horizontal diameter of greater than 12.5 mm and that microcornea measures under

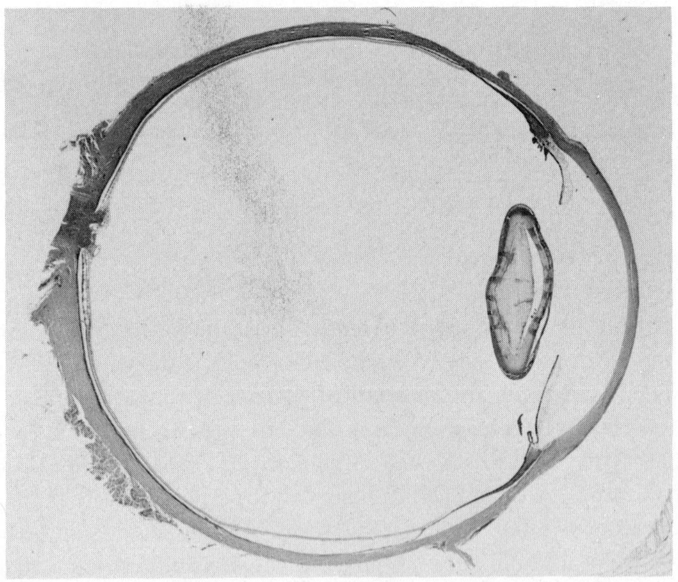

Fig. 7. Normal eye of young child enucleated because of glioma of optic nerve. X 2. (A. F. I. P. Neg. 939387.) (Courtesy of the Registry of Ophthalmic Pathology of the Armed Forces Institute of Pathology.)

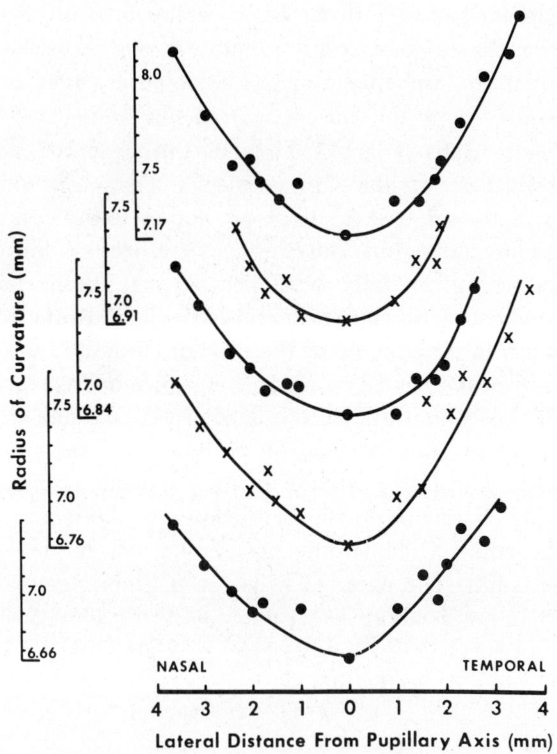

FIG. 8. Contours for horizontal meridian of five infant corneas. (Adapted from R. B. Mandell. **Arch. Ophthalmol.** 77:345, 1967.)

10 mm. The adult cornea is closely approximated by a section at one end of an ellipsoid; the pole of which nearly corresponds to the geometric center of the cornea. The radii of curvature in any meridian increase as a function of the distance from the geometric center, although there is significant variation.

Mandell studied corneal contour in the human infant by using a photokeratoscope of his own design. He found that the radii of curvature at the central corneal position are about 1 mm less than those of adults, but that the general contour is geometrically similar; that is, the cornea is more curved at the periphery than at its center. He concluded that the eye of the newborn was structured so that it partially corrects for ocular spherical aberration and thereby contributes to maximum visual acuity (Fig. 8). These findings are in contrast to those of Merkel and Orr, who reported that the cornea of the infant had radii of curvature which decrease as a function of the distance from the geometric center, that is, the cornea is nearly spherical. This suggests that the asphericity of the adult cornea may be induced by long-term pressure from the lids or extraocular muscles.

The cornea is relatively large at birth, measuring approximately 9.4 mm across. The refraction of the cornea is high, being approximately 50.5 diopters while in the adult it is about 43 diopters. The corneal corpuscles appear to be more numerous, but this may be because the fibrils of the substantia propria are not fully developed, so that the nuclei look closer together. The medial rectus muscle is relatively closer to the cornea than in the adult. Corneal measurements of the newborn and the adult vary widely, as summarized by Wilmer and Scrammon and shown in Table 2. The external diameter of the horizontal base in the newborn is 10.0 mm compared with 11.8 mm in the adult. External diameter of the corneal arc is 14.0 mm in the newborn and 18.2 mm in the adult. The internal diameter of the corneal arc is 5.4 mm greater in the adult. Mean thickness is 0.8 mm compared with 0.9 mm in the adult. Oblique thickness is 1.1 mm in the newborn and 1.6 mm in the adult. The external height is 0.4 mm greater in the adult. Internal height in the newborn is 1.1 mm and in the adult 2.7 mm. Average radius of corneal curvature in the newborn is between 6.6 and 7.44 mm, as opposed to the adult 7.4 to 8.4 mm.

TABLE 2

CORNEAL MEASUREMENTS OF THE NEWBORN AND ADULT EYE

	Newborn (mm)	Adult (mm)
External diameter of horizontal base	10.0	11.8
External diameter of corneal arc	14.0	18.2
Internal diameter of corneal arc	11.0	16.4
Mean thickness	0.8	0.9
Oblique thickness	1.1	1.6
External height	3.0	3.4
Internal height	1.1	2.7

From data of H. A. Wilmer and R. E. Scammon.

The increase in size during the first years of life affects mainly the anterior segment, that is, the cornea and the sclera up to the insertions of the muscles. Thus the cornea reaches adult size at about two years or earlier. With age the cornea flattens but more in the vertical than in the horizontal meridian.

THE SCLERA

The expansile qualities of the infant eye and the eye of an adult have been analyzed by Squire and are outlined in Table 3. Squire's study showed that the thickness of the scleral sac of the adult was 2.4 times that of a three-day-old infant. With use of strips of sclera 5 mm wide by 1 mm thick, it was shown that adult material was 1.7 times stronger than material taken from an infant. In addition, the adult eye was shown to have an overall strength with respect to collapse of about four times that of the infant. The bright blue color that is often evident in the baby's sclera is an optical effect attributable to the thinness of the sclera, which sets off the screen of its pigment lining. The sclera later becomes thicker and more rigid. There is a tendency for the deposition of fat that changes the color from white to yellow.

TABLE 3

COMPARISON OF THE ELASTIC PROPERTIES OF AN ADULT EYE AND A THREE–DAY–OLD INFANT EYE

Thickness of scleral sac		
1. Adult average thickness		1.09 mm
2. Infant average thickness		0.45 mm
Adult material		2.4 times thicker
Coefficient for stretching (strip 5-mm wide by 1-mm thick)		
1. Adult	4.6 dynes/cm	
2. Infant	2.7 dynes/cm	
Adult material		1.7 times stronger

From data of C. Squire.

THE RETINA

The retina is not fully differentiated at birth. The nuclei are closer together and more numerous. The cones are still short and stumpy. The macula is not fully developed, the macula cones being still undifferentiated. A depression is just visible. The fovea is not completely developed until one month after birth. The distance from the disc to the macula is the same as in the adult, indicating a relatively advanced condition of the fundus in the neighborhood of the posterior pole. The medial part of the eye is thus slightly less well advanced than the lateral. Rapid development during the first year of life and to a less extent during the second year renders the globe spherical. A detailed description of the infant retina is beyond the scope of this book.

THE OPTIC NERVE

On ophthalmoscopic examination, the optic nerve head is somewhat pale while the major retinal blood vessels are well developed. Richardson reviewed 483 randomly selected normal newborn infants who were examined within the first 96 hrs of life. He found that only 11 (2.3 percent) of this large series displayed optic cup asymmetry of any degree. Snydacker found that in an adult series of 500 randomly selected patients, 15 showed asymmetry. In 3 of the 11 asymmetrical infant cups, the asymmetry involved depth alone, the cup areas being similar. Marked asymmetry of the optic cups occurred in only 3 infants (0.6 percent). There were 14 normal infants (3.0 percent) in whom one or both cups were greater than one-third disc diameter. Marked asymmetry occurred in 4 of these 14 infants (29 percent) who showed either or both cups greater than one-third disc diameter in size as compared with 0.6 percent in the total series. In other studies it has been found that between 3 to 10 percent of normal infant eyes demonstrated cups greater than one-third disc diameter and about 3 percent have some asymmetry. Only 10 percent had cupping. The conclusion is that optic cups in newborn infants are normally symmetrical. The method of comparative ophthalmoscopy is therefore of great significance in evaluating the functional status of infantile glaucoma patients, as those individuals are prone to follow a more asymmetrical course than adults with glaucoma.

Myelinization of nerve fibers of the optic nerve descends to reach the lamina cribosa a few weeks after birth, but the nerve is thinner (0.8 to 1.1 mm diameter) than in the adult (1.34 to 4.5 mm). After the eyes have been exposed to light for about 10 weeks, myelination is complete, but the process normally stops short of the optic disc. Opaque nerve fibers signify the continuation of myelination beyond the optic disc and is, of course, never visible immediately after birth. In those animals in which the eyes are not opened at birth it has been shown that the stimulus of light hastens myelinization. Thus a premature baby will have its myelinization farther advanced by the time it reaches the ninth month than a newborn term infant.

References

Ascher, K. W. Aqueous veins. Am. J. Ophthalmol., 25:1174, 1942; 25:1301, 1942.

and Spurgeon, W. M. Compression tests on aqueous veins of glaucomatous eyes. Am. J. Ophthalmol., 32:239, 1949 (Pt. II).

Barany, E., and Kinsey, V. E. The rate of flow of aqueous humor. Am. J. Ophthalmol., 32:177, 1949 (Pt. II); 32:189, 1949 (Pt. II).

Barats, V. G. Growth of the Eye and its Various Properties in Infants. A. V. Orloff, St. Petersburg, 1902.

Berg, F. Vergleichende Messungen der Form der Vorderen Hornhautflache mit Ophthalmometer und mit Photographischer Method. Acta Ophthalmol., 7:386, 1929.

Christensen, R. E., and Garai, M. H. Developmental glaucoma. Am. J. Ophthalmol., 71:490, 1971.

Cogan, D. G. Applied anatomy and physiology of the cornea. Trans. Am. Acad. Ophthalmol. Otolaryng., 55:329, 1951.

Dekking, H. M. Zur Photographie der Hornhautoberflache. Arch. Ophthalmol., 74:708, 1930.

De Vries, F. Remarques de la Cornée. Soc. Neerlandaise d'Ophtalm., 1900.

Dieckmann, H. W. Beitrage zur Anatomie und Physiologie des neugebornen Auges. F. Sommering, Marburg, 1896.

Doggart, J. H. Diseases of Children's Eyes. Mosby, St. Louis, 1947.

Druault, A., and Druault, S. Oeil du nouveau ne. Ann. Ocul., 179:375, 1946.

Duke-Elder, W. S. The blood-aqueous barrier. Trans. Ophthamol. Soc. U. K., 68:413, 1948.

and Wybar, K. C. The Anatomy of the Visual System, in Duke-Elder, S. W. System of Ophthalmology, Mosby, St. Louis, 1961, p. 94.

Francois, J. Les informations gonioscopiques particulierement dans l'etude et le traitement du glaucome. Bull. Soc. Belge d'Opht., 88:3, 1948.

Friedenwald, J. S. Some problems in the calibration of tonometers. Am. J. Ophthalmol. 31:935, 1948.

Goldmann, H. Abflub des Kammerwassers beim Menschen. Ophthalmologica, 111:146, 1946.

Weitere Mitteilung uber den Abflub des Kammerwassers beim Menschen. Ophthalmologica, 112:344, 1946.

Studien uber den Abflubdruck des Kammerwassers beim Menschen. Ophthalmologica, 114:81, 1947.

Grod, A. Uber die Dauerresultate der Operationen bei augenborenem Star mit Besonderer Berucksichtigung der Wachstumverhaltnisse. Arch. Augenheilk., 67:251, 1910.

Gullstrand, A. Anatomical description of the eye, in von Hemholtz, Handbuch der Pysiologischen Optik. Voss, Hamburg and Leipzig, 1909.

Hymes, C. The postnatal growth of the cornea and palpebral fissure and the projection of the eyeball in early life. J. Comp. Neurol., 48:415, 1929.

Johnson, G. J., Corey, P. N., and Morin, J. D. Tonography in infants and children. Can. J. Ophthalmol., 6:24, 1971.

Johnston, T. B., and Whillis, J. Gray's Anatomy. Longmans, Green, London 1949, p. 1193.

Kaiser, J. H. Die Grosse und das Wachstrum der Hornhaut im Kindesalter. Arch. Ophthalmol., 116:288, 1926.

Kinsey, V. E., Grant, M., and Cogan, D. G. Water movement and the eye. Arch. Ophthalmol., 27:242, 1942.

——— and Barany, E. The rate of flow of aqueous humor, II. derivation of rate of flow and its physiologic significance. Am. J. Ophthalmol., 32:189, 1949 (Pt. II).
Knoll, H. Corneal contours in the general population as revealed by the photokeratoscope. Am. J. Optom., 38(7):389, 1961.
Koeppe, L. Die Mikroskopie des lebenden Kammerwinkels im focalen Lichte der Gullstrandschen Nernstspaltlampe. Graefes Arch. Ophthalmol., 101:48, 1919.
Kronfeld, P. C., McGarry, H. I., and Smith, H. E. Gonioscopic studies on the canal of Schlemm. Amer. J. Ophthal., 25:1163, 1942; Arch. Ophthalmol., 29:684, 1943.
Last, R. J. Eugene Wolff's Anatomy of the Eye and Orbit. Saunders, Philadelphia, 1968.
Mandell, R. B. Corneal contour of the human infant. Arch. Ophthalmol., 77:345, 1967.
Mann, I. The Development of the Human Eye. Butler and Tanner, London 1969.
Merkel, F., and Orr, W. Das Auge des Neugeborenen an einem schematischen Durchschnitt erlautert. Anat. Hefte, 1:273, 1892.
Meyer, B. Incidence of anisocoria and difference in size of palpebral fissures in 500 normal subjects. Arch. Neurol. Psychiat., 57:464, 1947.
Ortlepp, J. Messung des Hornhautdurchmessers und Krummungsradius als Beitragzur Klarung der Speziellen Struktur des Glaukomauges. Graefes Arch. Klin. Exp. Ophthal., 169:194, 1966.
Pendse, G. S., Bhave, L. S., and Dandekar, V. M. Refraction in relation to age and sex. Arch. Ophthalmol., 52:404, 1954.
Peyton, W. T. A topographic study of the orbit and bulbus oculi during a part of the growth period. Anat. Rec., 76:343, 1940.
Redslob, E. Anatomie du globe oculaire, disposition general de l'appareil visuel. Trait d'Opht., 1:369, 1939.
Richardson, K. T. Optic cup symmetry in normal newborn infants. Invest. Ophthalmol., 7:137, 1968.
——— and Shaffer, R. N. Infant ophthalmoscopy and gonioscopy. Arch. Ophthalmol., 73:55, 1965.
Salzmann, M. The Anatomy and Histology of the Human Eyeball. Univers. Chicago Press, Chicago, 1912.
Shaffer, R. N. New concepts in infantile glaucoma. Trans. Ophthal. Soc. U. K., 87:581, 1967.
Smelser, G. K., and Ozanics, V. Distribution of radioactive sulfate in the developing eye. Am. J. Ophthalmol., 44:102, 1957.
Smith, P. On the size of the cornea in relation to age, sex, refraction and primary glaucoma. Trans. Ophthal. Soc. U. K., 10:68, 1890.
Snydacker, D. The normal optic disc, ophthalmoscopic and photographic studies. Am. J. Ophthalmol., 58:958, 1964.
Speakman, J. S. The structure of the trabecular meshwork in relation to the pathogenesis of open angle glaucoma. Can. Med. Assoc. J., 84:1066, 1961.
——— and Leeson, T. S. Pathological findings in a case of primary congenital glaucoma compared with normal infant eyes. Br. J. Ophthalmol., 48:196, 1964.
Squire, C. Cited by Girard, L. J., Neely, W., and Sampson, W. G. The use of alpha chymotrypsin in infants and children. Am. J. Ophthalmol., 54:95, 1962.
Stone, J. The validity of some existing methods of measuring corneal contour compared with suggested new methods. Br. J. Physiol. Opt., 19:205, 1962.
Thomas, C. I. The Cornea. Thomas, Springfield, Ill., 1955.
Thomassen, T. L. On aqueous veins. Acta Ophthalmol., 25:369, 1947.
Thomson, A. The Anatomy of the Human Eye. Clarendon Press, Oxford, 1912.
Troncoso, M. U. Gonioscopy and its clinical application. Am. J. Ophthalmol., 8:433, 1925.

Tscherning, M. Optique physiologique. G. Carre y c Naud, Paris, 1898.
von Reuss, A. Untersuchung uber den Einfluss des Lebensalters auf die Krummung der Hornhaut nebst einigen Bermerkungen uber die Dimension der Lidspalte, Arch. Ophthal., 27:27, 1881.
Wolff, E. The Anatomy of the Eye and Orbit. McGraw-Hill, New York, 1951, p. 375.
Wilmer, H. A., and Scrammon, R. E. Growth of the components of the human eyeball. Arch. Ophthalmol., 43:599, 1950.

5

Classification of Glaucoma in Infancy and Childhood

The factors concerned with the production of an elevated intraocular pressure are the formation, circulation, and outflow of aqueous humor. The most important factor in congenital glaucoma is the obstruction to aqueous humor outflow that is present in the anterior chamber filtration angle. The various theories concerning the pathogenesis of this obstruction have already been reviewed in Chapter 3. For the purpose of classification, the exact origin of the obstruction is less important than the nature of the blockage itself. In other words, the degree and extent of the involvement of the filtration angle greatly influence the manner of onset of the symptoms. Also important is the maturity of the aqueous-humor-producing organ, for even an impaired excretory mechanism at Schlemm's canal may adequately accommodate a low aqueous production rate.

In secondary infantile glaucoma, the circulation may very well be blocked with inflammatory debris, red blood cells, and a host of other materials depending upon the cause. In the infant eye malformed by some embryologic aberration, again the circulation of aqueous humor may be obstructed, the extent depending on the degree of involvement of the filtration angle.

It is difficult to find unanimity among authors as to the ideal classification for any condition. However, some type of organization is essential with the provision that changes will be necessary as knowledge increases. The following classification for primary congenital glaucoma based on age of onset appears to satisfy most criteria since the degree of severity, the number of surgical procedures, and the final outcome are strongly correlated with the age of onset of the condition. It must be remembered that the age limits are taken entirely arbitrarily and that cases in one group flow easily into the prior and following groups. However, for the most part, the age of onset allows us to make certain predictions as to treatment, course, and prognosis.

The broad title "Anomalies associated with infantile glaucoma" classifies glaucoma in infants and children when it is associated with obvious local abnormalities in the anterior segment, sometimes related to a variety of syndromes and clinical manifestations.

Secondary glaucoma includes those conditions in which an elevated intraocular pressure in a young infant or child is the by-product of the primary insult to the eye or occurs secondarily in the eye as a result of the child's suffering from a generalized condition.

The basic flaw in this classification is that certain conditions have been placed arbitrarily under one heading at the expense of another. On the other hand, conditions related to lens anomalies and lens-induced glaucoma are classified in two places. By virtue of our present knowledge, however, this appears to be a reasonable organization of the manner in which an elevated intraocular pressure may appear in the infant eye. As knowledge in this field expands, changes will have to be made and this inherent need for improvement is acknowledged.

PRIMARY CONGENITAL GLAUCOMA

Infantile glaucoma

(1) birth to five days (newborn congenital glaucoma)
(2) five days to six months
(3) six months to thirty-six months

Juvenile glaucoma

(1) true juvenile glaucoma
(2) neglected infantile glaucoma
(3) presenile glaucoma
(4) angle-closure glaucoma

ANOMALIES ASSOCIATED WITH INFANTILE GLAUCOMA

Corneal Anomalies

(1) sclerocornea
(2) microphthalmos
    microcornea
    pure microphthalmos or nanophthalmos
    microphthalmos with cyst (congenital cystic eyeball)
    microphthalmos with anomalous development of surface ectoderm, cryptophthalmos
    microphthalmus associated with multiple ocular defects

(3) cornea plana
(4) adhesions between iris and cornea and associated anomalies
    anterior chamber cleavage syndrome
    Peter's anomaly, mesodermal dysgenesis of the cornea
    goniodysgenesis
    Reiger's disease
        Reiger's anomaly
        Reiger's syndrome
    Axenfeld's syndrome

Iris Anomalies

(1) aniridia
(2) coloboma of the iris
(3) persistent pupillary membrane
(4) iridodiastasis and iridodehiscence
(5) hyperplasia of the iris layers
    anterior layer of the iris stroma
    pigment border of the iris (flocculi)
(6) corectopia
(7) congenital microcoria
(8) polycoria
(9) essential iris atrophy

Lens and Related Anomalies

(1) congenital aphakia
    primary aphakia
    secondary aphakia
(2) congenital cataract
    inflammatory
    genetic
(3) subluxation and dislocation of the lens
    Ehlers-Danlos syndrome (EDS)
    mandibulofacial dysostosis of Franceschetti
(4) anterior lenticonus, lentiglobus
(5) microspherophakia
(6) persistent hyperplastic primary vitreous (PHPV)
(7) other syndromes
    Conradi syndrome (dysplasia epiphysealis punctata)
    Werner's syndrome
    syndrome of Francois
    Hallerman-Streiff syndrome (mandibulooculofacial dysmorphia)

Phacomatosis

(1) neurofibromatosis (von Recklinghausen's disease)

(2) retinocerebellar angiomatosis (von Hippel-Lindau's disease)
(3) oculodermalmelanocytosis (Blue nevus of Ota)
(4) encephalooculofacial hemangiomatosis (Sturge-Weber's syndrome)

Mesodermal Anomalies

(1) systemic hypoplastic mesodermal dystrophy (Marfan's syndrome)
(2) systemic hyperplastic mesodermal dystrophy (Weill-Marchesani syndrome)

Metabolic Disease

(1) oculocerebrorenal syndrome (Lowe's syndrome)
(2) homocystinuria
(3) sulfite oxidase deficiency

Other Genetically Determined Diseases

(1) Turner's syndrome
(2) hereditary oculodentoosseous dysplasia
(3) Pierre Robin syndrome
(4) mongolism (Down's syndrome)

Other Conditions

(1) hemangioma of the choroid
(2) pigmentary glaucoma
(3) thalidomide
(4) Rubenstein's syndrome, broad thumb syndrome

SECONDARY GLAUCOMA IN INFANCY AND CHILDHOOD

Inflammation

(1) chemical
(2) infection (syphilis, tuberculosis, other bacteria, sinus disease, protozoal infection, metazoan infection, parasitic cysts of the eye)
(3) rubella and other viral diseases
(4) nonspecific inflammatory diseases

Trauma

(1) nonpenetrating wounds
(2) penetrating wounds
(3) phacoanaphylactic endophthalmitis
(4) foreign bodies
(5) sympathetic ophthalmia

Carotid-cavernous sinus fistula

Tumors

(1) retinoblastoma

(2) neuroblastoma
(3) diktyoma
(4) leiomyoma

Retrolental fibroplasia

Juvenile xanthogranuloma

Metabolic disorders

Dietetic disorders

Lens-induced glaucoma

Norrie's disease

Spontaneous rupture of the eyeball

Administration of steroids

PRIMARY CONGENITAL GLAUCOMA

The symposium on congenital glaucoma held by the American Academy of Ophthalmology and Otolaryngology classified congenital glaucoma into two groups: (1) infantile glaucoma, in which onset took place prior to thirty-six months and (2) juvenile glaucoma, in which the disease occurred after this time. This classification was based on the concept that for the most part the eye loses its expansile qualities after the age of three. The symposium further divided the infantile group into those cases in which signs and symptoms began before six months and after six months of age. Costenbader and Kwitko described a series of patients in whom the disease was noted in the newborn nursery during the first five days of life. The five-day period was taken because this is the average hospital stay of the neonate. The characteristics, management, and final outcome of these eyes differed from those of the other groups enough to suggest that these cases formed a distinct group within the classification of congenital glaucoma (newborn glaucoma).

Infantile Glaucoma

Intraocular pressure depends upon the integrity of the outflow apparatus and the rate of production of aqueous humour at the ciliary body. The ciliary body is immature at birth, so the rate of production of aqueous humour at this time is low. If the outflow apparatus is completely defective, e.g., absence of Schlemm's canal, glaucoma will be evident at birth. This is the group that Costenbader and Kwitko have defined as "newborn glaucoma." If the outflow mechanism is only partially defective, it may be adequate to excrete the amount of aqueous humour produced at that time. However, at a later time in life when normal production takes place, the signs and symptoms of glaucoma would become evident depending on the degree of involvement of the filtration angle. This group of cases is arbitrarily divided into the following subgroups: birth to five days, five days to six months, and six months to thirty-six months.

Birth to five days

When the diagnosis of congenital glaucoma is made in the newborn nursery the ophthalmologist faces perhaps the most serious problem. The condition is usually bilateral. In the author's series eight out of nine patients had both eyes affected. The corneas are often opaque. Surgical intervention must therefore be performed under the most trying conditions. In the author's series of 16 eyes, 55 surgical procedures were performed, an average of 3.4 operations per eye. The final outcome of these cases is often grave, as shown in Chapter 14.

Fig. 1A and B illustrates one eye of a bilateral case of newborn congenital glaucoma. Five surgical procedures (one goniotomy, two goniotomies with goniopuncture, and two iridectomies with scleral cautery) were carried out on each eye. The intraocular pressure remained elevated until the second iridectomy with scleral cautery (Scheie procedure) was performed, after which the tension fell to within normal limits. The left cornea then showed progressive clearing over the next three months until only a small portion in the central area remained cloudy. The right cornea remained opaque.

Five Days to Six Months

When the symptoms of congenital glaucoma appear after the neonatal hospital period, the condition is likely to be somewhat less severe than the newborn case. The aqueous outflow pathways must be functioning to some degree, otherwise the condition would have been present at birth. Therefore the cornea will likely be clear enough to allow the surgeon to perform a successful goniotomy under direct visualization. In addition the condition need not be bilateral. In the author's series only 14 out of 24 patients had both eyes involved. It was also found that 68 surgical procedures were necessary to treat a series of 37 eyes or an average of 1.8 operations per eye.

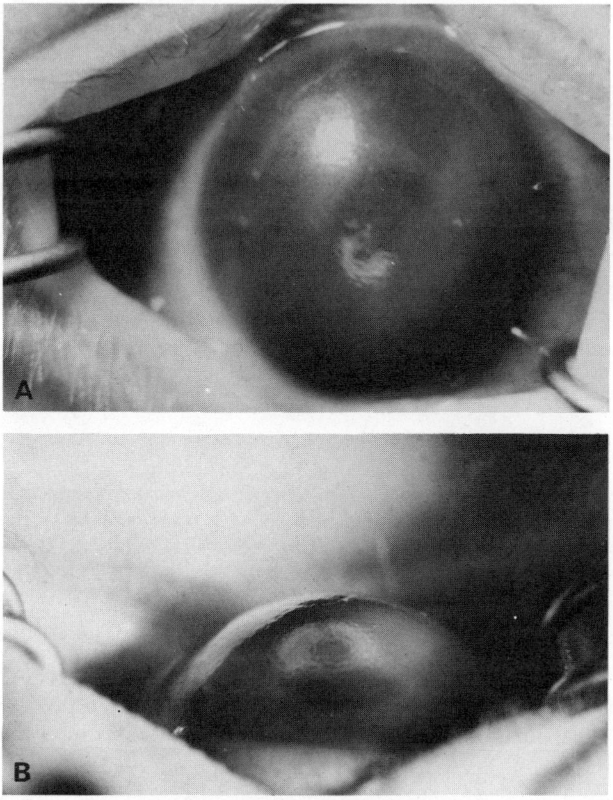

FIG. 1.A. Newborn glaucoma (birth to five days). Both corneas were opaque at birth. **B.** Profile of a case of newborn glaucoma.

Fig. 2 illustrates a bilateral case in which the condition was first noted at the fourth month of life. The corneas had been hazy at birth but there was no tearing, redness, or evidence of pain. The iris and pupils had never been seen by the mother. On examination the corneas were opaque, the anterior chamber structures were not visible, and there was no fundus reflex. The right cornea measured 12.5 mm in the horizontal diameter and the left cornea measured 13 mm. The initial intraocular pressure measurement was 13 mm Hg in each eye. It was tentatively thought to be a case of congenital idiopathic corneal opacification or a formes fruste of Hurler's syndrome. On a later examination the intraocular pressure was measured at 50 mm Hg in each eye. A goniotomy was performed in the right eye without success. Later, bilateral iridectomies with scleral cauterization were

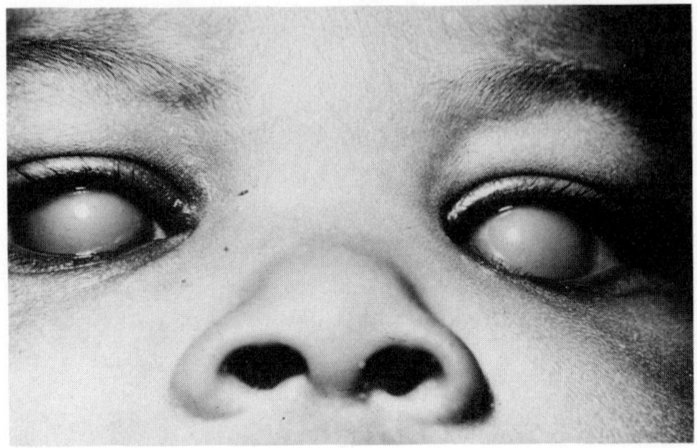

FIG. 2. Bilateral infantile glaucoma (child showed cloudy corneas from birth but intraocular pressure was not elevated until four months). (Courtesy of C. M. Alexander.)

performed on each eye, which controlled the pressure. The corneas began to clear at the periphery leaving only a central opacification. Fig. 3A, B, and C illustrates a unilateral case of infantile glaucoma. The cornea began to enlarge at the fourth month of age. Haziness of the cornea, photophobia, and tearing soon became evident. The child underwent two goniotomies which resulted in a normalization of intraocular pressure and a complete subsidence of all other signs and symptoms.

Six Months to Thirty-Six Months

When the diagnosis of congenital glaucoma is made after the sixth month, a less severe condition is usually present. The eye already has a filtration facility that has functioned to some degree for a considerable period of time. The condition is usually unilateral. In the author's series only 6 out of 14 patients had both eyes affected. In addition 34 procedures were performed on 20 eyes, or an average of 1.7 operations per eye. Fig. 4 illustrates a case of bilateral infantile glaucoma in which the onset of symptoms took place after the sixth month of life. Goniotomies were performed on both eyes. The intraocular pressure remained elevated in the left eye and a Scheie procedure was performed. At the time the photograph was taken, the right eye was free of symptoms. Fixation ability was maintained and central. The intraocular pressure was 15 mm Hg and the corneal diameter was 12.5 mm in the horizontal meridian. The left eye

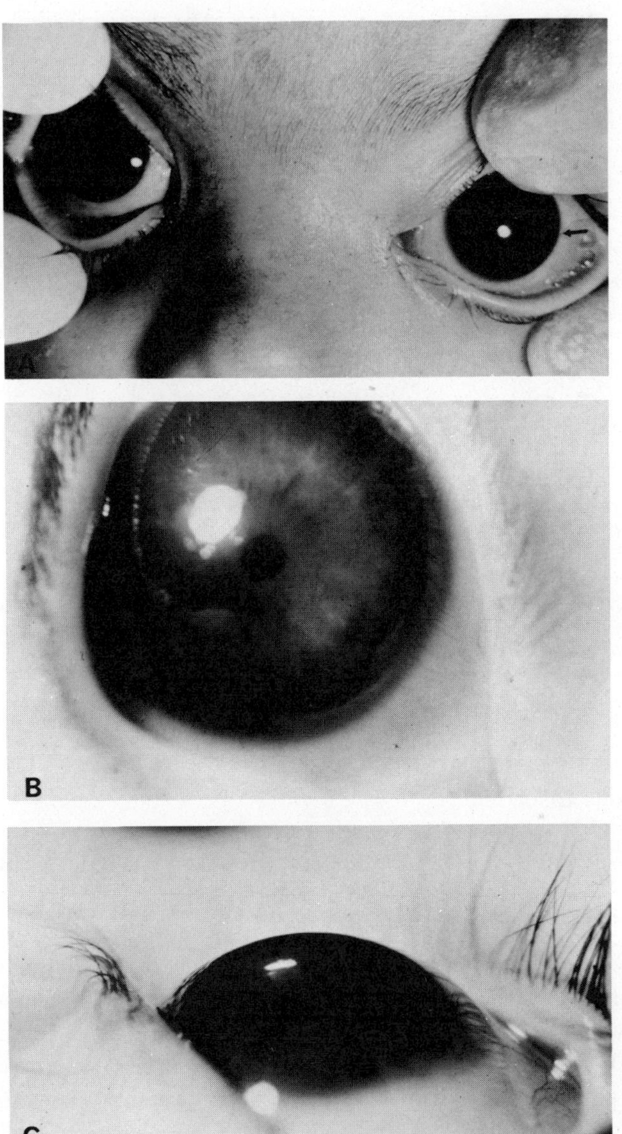

FIG. 3.A. Unilateral glaucoma (five days to six months). Cornea began to enlarge after fourth month (*arrow*). B. Infantile glaucoma. C. Profile of eye with infantile glaucoma.

displayed clouding of the cornea. The pupil was oval and an iridectomy was present. The anterior chamber was shallow and peripheral anterior synechiae

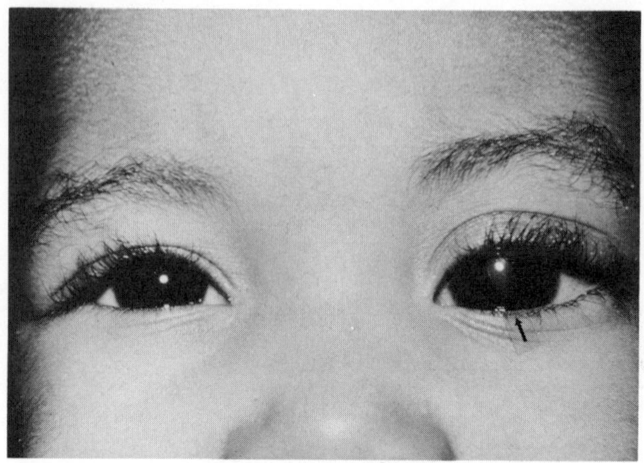

FIG. 4. Bilateral infantile glaucoma (six to thirty-six months). Onset after sixth month. Left eye (*arrow*) failed to respond to treatment.

were observed on gonioscopic examination. The bleb did not appear to be functioning. The intraocular pressure was 60 mm Hg and the corneal diameter measured 14.5 mm in the horiziontal meridian. The optic nerve was cupped.

Juvenile Glaucoma

Sorsby noted the description of juvenile glaucoma as outlined by Löhlein. Drawing mainly on cases recorded in the literature, he observed that juvenile glaucoma was a clinical entity because in the group as a whole, extending from the artificial limits of 5 to 35 years, about 40 percent occurred between the ages of 16 and 20. In addition, 50 percent of the patients were myopic, and there was a familial occurrence in some 20 percent. He held that this type of condition occurs most often in men. For the purpose of classification, the term juvenile glaucoma is used to describe that group of cases in which an elevation in intraocular pressure is noted after the thirty-sixth month of life. It is based on the assumption that after the age of three the sclera loses much of its expansible qualities so that an enlarged globe is less likely to be seen clinically. This is true only to some degree, as Scheie and other authors have noted an enlarged globe even in teenagers. It is in juvenile glaucoma that the hereditary factor may appear most evident. Numerous authors including Allan and Ackerman,

Stokes, Löhlein, Scheerer, Côté et al., Berg and Derby have described pedigrees of up to six generations in which ocular hypertension was noted in one of the parents, as well as in the siblings and offspring at various ages from birth to adolescence. Juvenile glaucoma probably represents a group of cases as categorized below.

True Juvenile Glaucoma

The outflow mechanism has functioned well up to the age of three probably because aqueous humor has been produced at a diminished rate due to a retardation in development of the ciliary body. After three, production of aqueous reaches its full potential, which embarrasses the impaired outflow facility. Since stretching of ocular tissues does not occur to the same degree as in the infant or the intraocular pressure is simply insufficient to produce enlargement, blepharospasm, tearing and photophobia are not a feature and the patient may run a symptom-free course similar to adult open-angle glaucoma. The variations that take place in aqueous humor production in the face of an impaired outflow will cause low pressure measurements at certain times and elevated spikes of pressure that can cause transient corneal edema. Therefore some patients may experience periodic episodes of hazy vision with halos.

Because of continued development, the gonioscopic appearance of the angle after five years differs somewhat from that of the infant, although features characteristic of congenital glaucoma are observed. The trabecular meshwork is thinner but still a highly transparent structure. The "morning mist" of Lister has all but disappeared so that there is less of the thick spongy appearance of infancy.

Extensive damage to the optic nerve can occur before the parents realize that there is a visual problem. Detailed ophthalmoscopy to observe abnormal cupping of the optic disc together with careful tonometry and tonography are essential in these patients. The visual field examination is difficult to perform satisfactorily in a young patient because cooperation is often poor. Therefore it is wise to do the test at varied distances so as to rule out emotional factors. In the early stages of the disorder, progressive cupping is possible in the young patient without a corresponding visual field defect. After pressure normalization the cup may disappear as in infantile glaucoma unless a field defect has appeared.

The young patient with advancing high myopia must be regarded as a potential candidate for glaucoma. The cribriform plate is located in a more anterior position so that cupping is shallower and therefore less obvious than in the hyperopic eye. Such eyes have a lowered ocular rigidity which may result in a mistaken low reading of the intraocular pressure taken with a Schiötz type indentation tonometer. The applanation tonometer is a more reliable instrument in such a case.

The ophthalmologist must be careful to rule out secondary causes for the elevated intraocular pressure. For example, a traumatic hyphema in a young child may resolve leaving a recession angle deformity which is not recognized at the time of injury because of the difficulty in performing satisfactory gonioscopy. Years later the child may appear with elevated intraocular pressure, a deep anterior chamber, and optic nerve cupping.

Neglected Infantile Glaucoma

Even at the present time a parent, through ignorance or neglect, may fail to notice the steady enlargement of one or both eyes of a young child. Deterioration of the eye may be so insidious that some patients do not come under medical observation until visual loss is far advanced. When expansion of the globe takes place in the posterior portion of the eye, the cornea and anterior segment may remain unaffected for a prolonged period, giving rise only to minimal symptoms. The case may even be confused with the large eye of unilateral myopia (Fig. 5). The diagnosis is made only after the intraocular pressure is measured or a chance ophthalmoscopic observation that the optic nerve shows abnormal cupping. One patient was referred to the author when the general practitioner noted pulsation of the central

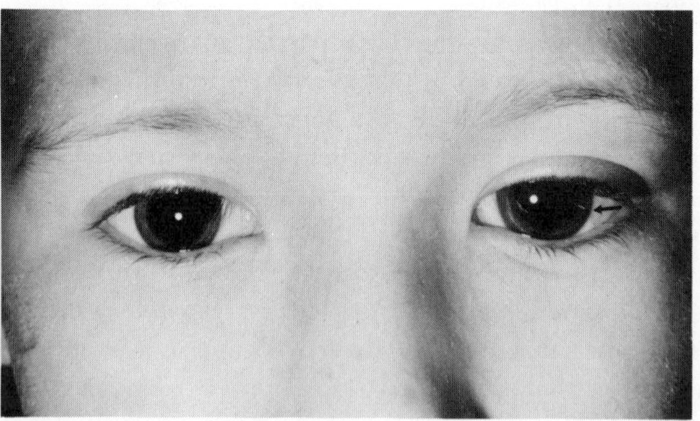

FIG. 5. Large cornea in unilateral case of high myopia (*arrow*).

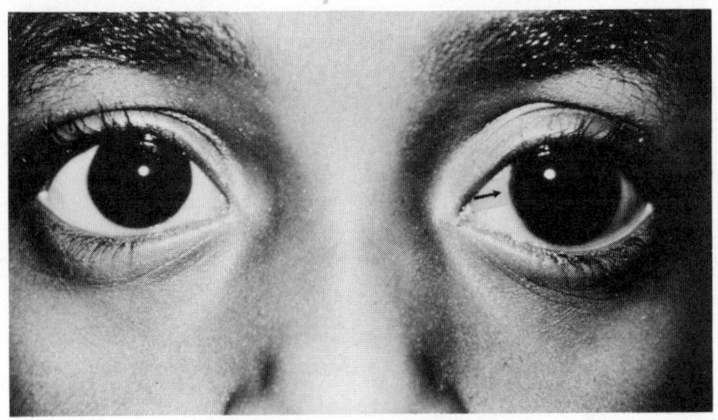

FIG. 6. Juvenile glaucoma (neglected case) in left eye (*arrow*); megalocornea right eye. (Courtesy of C. M. Alexander.)

retinal artery in one eye. On examination the cornea was enlarged and the optic nerve markedly cupped with nasal displacement of the retinal vessels and extensive visual field loss. The opposite eye was normal. The mother failed to appreciate the obvious corneal enlargement until it was demonstrated to her in detail.

Fig. 6 illustrates a case classified as juvenile glaucoma because the patient was first examined by an ophthalmologist at five years of age. However, the history revealed that the left eye had been increasing in size since birth and had undergone intermittent episodes of corneal clouding. On examination a visual acuity of 20/20 and an intraocular pressure of 17 mm Hg was noted in the right eye. The corneal diameter measured 13.5 mm in the horizontal meridian. The optic disc was normal and on gonioscopy the filtration angle was open to the ciliary body throughout the 360° circumference. This probably represented a case of megalocornea. The left eye had light perception vision. The intraocular pressure was 47 mm Hg and the corneal diameter was 15 mm. The optic disc was deeply cupped. On gonioscopic examination the filtration angle was obstructed by aberrant tissue with only the nasal trabeculum exposed. Fig. 7A illustrates an example of infantile glaucoma which was first treated when the child was seven. Fig. 7B shows the left eye which was satisfactorily controlled with an iridencleisis operation. However, by this time the optic nerve was already cupped (Fig. 7C). Figure 8A illustrates the profile of a neglected case of congenital glaucoma which was never treated. The cornea (Fig. 8B) shows breaks in Descemet's membrane and extensive enlargement.

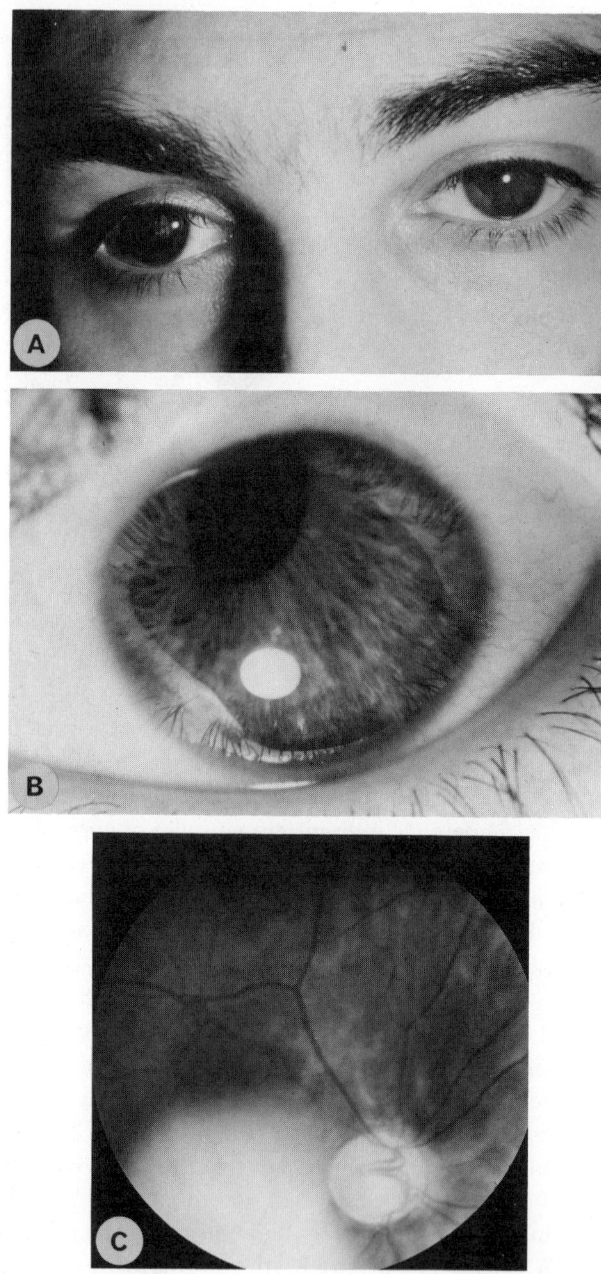

FIG. 7.A. Juvenile glaucoma. **B.** Left eye of case of juvenile glaucoma showing iridencleises site. **C.** Optic nerve cupping in juvenile glaucoma.

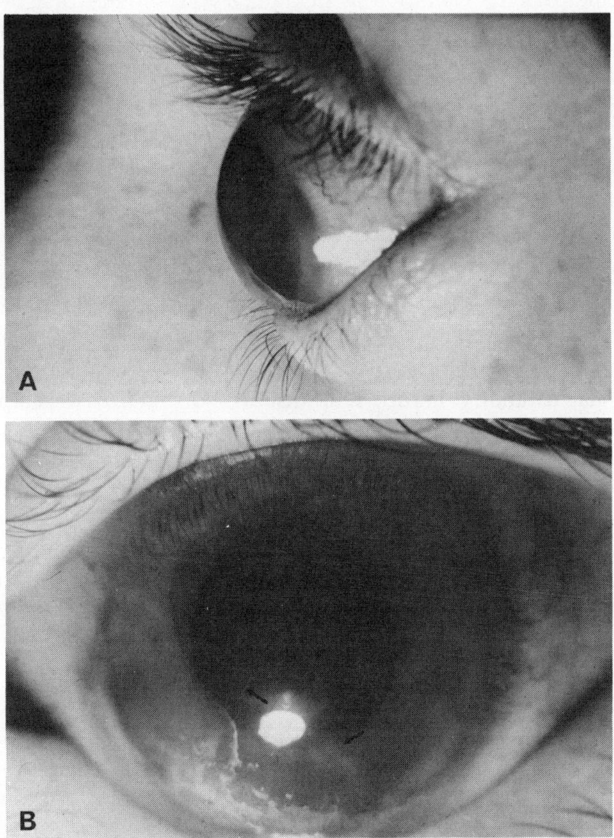

FIG. 8.A. Juvenile glaucoma (neglected case). **B.** Cornea shows breaks in Descemet's membrane (Haab's stria, *arrow*).

Presenile Glaucoma

Patients with presenile glaucoma are often under 30 years when the disorder is first diagnosed, frequently presenting with pressure elevations to above 40 mm Hg. There is, according to Goldwyn et al., who reported a series of cases of primary open-angle glaucoma in adolescents and young adults, a 2:1 preponderance of male patients in contrast to those cases of primary open-angle glaucoma that occur after the age of 50—in which the ratio of male-to-female subjects is slightly greater than one. More than half the patients are myopic and this also contrasts with the older-age open-angle glaucoma group. Young patients with primary open-angle glaucoma therefore resemble patients classified as pigmentary glaucoma—first because they are usually myopic male patients and second because they are similar in their response to topically applied steroids. The only difference noted between the two groups is the presence of pigment dispersion in the anterior chamber. The presenile group of juvenile glaucoma resembles primary open-angle glaucoma in the older adult in that there is an absence of corneal abnormalities as to size, shape, opacities, and breaks in Descemet's membrane. Other similarities include the appearance of the anterior chamber angle, impaired outflow facility, elevated intraocular pressure, cupping and atrophy of the optic nerve head, characteristic loss of visual field, family history of primary open-angle glaucoma, response to topically applied corticosteroids, and response to antiglaucoma therapy. The disease can cause marked visual disability before it is discovered. Such cases emphasize the need for tonometry in all patients old enough to cooperate, especially in those with a family history of glaucoma.

Angle-Closure Glaucoma

The shallow anterior chamber that may result in primary angle-closure glaucoma is rare and seldom seen in young patients. The exceptions to this rule are noted with microcornea and with spherophakia. However, the depth of the anterior chamber and width of the angle are genetically determined and a history of acute glaucoma in a close relative of the patient should cause the ophthalmologist to examine the angle. Periodic visits may be advised if the angle appears unusually narrow.

The plateau iris syndrome of the young may lead to angle-closure glaucoma. The central anterior chamber is of moderate depth and the plane of the iris is not bowed forward. Gonioscopy of the peripheral anterior chamber will reveal the narrowness of the angle. (See Chap. 13.)

ANOMALIES ASSOCIATED WITH INFANTILE GLAUCOMA

There are a number of pediatric clinical manifestations which feature an elevated intraocular pressure. However, obvious developmental abnormalities are present in these cases which result in pressure rise, such as the dislocated lens displaced into the anterior chamber or the iris remnants of aniridia. These conditions are discussed in Chapter 9 as associated abnormalities.

SECONDARY GLAUCOMA IN INFANCY AND CHILDHOOD

A wide variety of conditions influence aqueous humor circulation in the infant and child and the result is therefore termed secondary infantile glaucoma. These disorders include inflammatory conditions, tumors, trauma, retrolental fibroplasia, juvenile xanthogranuloma, and others that are discussed in Chapter 11.

References

Allen, T. D., and Ackerman, W. G. Hereditary glaucoma in a pedigree of three generations. Arch. Ophthalmol., 27:139, 1942.
Arganaraz, R. Clinica del glaucoma. Dia med., 21:2673, 1949.
Aubineaux, A. Le faux glaucome. Ann. Ocul., 167:550, 1930.
Barkan, O. Glaucoma classification, causes and surgical control. Results of microgonioscopic research. Am. J. Ophthalmol., 21:1099, 1938.
Congenital glaucoma, goniotomy. Trans. Am. Acad. Ophthalmol. Otolaryng., 59:322, 1955.
Becker, B., and Shaffer, R. N. Diagnosis and Therapy of the Glaucomas. 2nd ed. Mosby, St. Louis, 1965.
Christensen, R. E., and Garai, M. H. Corneal curvature and diameter in developmental glaucoma. Am. J. Ophthalmol., 71:490, 1971.
Contino, A. Del glaucoma anteriore emorragico sua patogenesi e trapia, con particolare riguardo alla forma anteriore di Contino. Zentralbl. Ges. Ophthal., 39:580, 1937.
Das glaucoma acutum von Contino. Klin. Monatsbl. Augenheilk., 100:745, 1938.
Costenbader, F. D. Personal communication.
and Kwitko, M. L. Congenital glaucoma, an analysis of seventy-seven consecutive eyes. J. Pediat. Ophthalmol., 4:9, 1967.
Courtney, R. H., and Hill, E. Hereditary juvenile glaucoma simplex. J. A. M. A., 97:1602, 1931.
Ellis, O. H. The etiology, symptomatology and treatment of juvenile glaucoma. Am. J. Ophthalmol. 31:1589, 1948.
Gallois, J. Symptomatologie d'alerte dans quelques cas d'hypertension oculaire essentielle des jeunes sujets. Bull. Soc. Opht. France, 432, 1949.
Gerard, R. Incomplete glaucoma. Arch. Opht., 7:511, 1947.
Goldwyn, R., Waltman, S. R., and Becker, B. Primary open angle glaucoma in adolescents and young adults. Arch. Ophthalmol., 84:579, 1970.
Gorin, G. Developmental glaucoma. Am. J. Ophthalmol., 58:572, 1964.
Hitta, T. Ueber Kapselglaucoma. Zentralbl. Ges. Ophthal., 46:61, 1941.
Holm-Pederson, A. E. Glaucoma juvenile, glaucoma adultum, glaucoma juvenile i tre generationer. Nordisk Med., 39:1615, 1948.
Imachi, K., Imachi, I., and Wada, K. Angebliches gl. sympathicum und sein ausbruchmechanismus. Acta. Soc. Ophthal., Jap., 40:1916, 1937.
Lichter, P. R. Iris processes in three hundred and forty eyes. Am. J. Ophthalmol., 68:812, 1969.

Mallig, B. Einige Untersuchungen uber das sogenannte Kapselglaukom. Acta Ophthal., 16:43, 1938.

Meyer, S. J. Incomplete glaucoma. Monosymptomatic glaucomatous excavation. Eye Ear Nose Throat Monthly, 21:477, 1950.

Nemetz, U. Zur Haufung der Katarakta glaukomatosa. Wien. Klin. Wchschr., 61:606, 1949.

Obbink, I. Pseudoglaukom. Zentralbl. Ges. Ophthl., 42:455, 1938.

Perkins, E. S. Glaucoma in the younger age groups. Arch. Ophthalmol., 64:882, 1960.

Peters, A. Das Glaukom. Handb. Ges. Augenheilk, Springer, Berlin, 1930.

Pokrovsky, A. I. Difficult cases and difficult types of glaucoma. Vestnik. Oftal., 29:14, 1950.

Sampaolesi, R., Reca, R. M., and Carro, A. Pesion ocular en el nino hasta los cincos anos. Arch. Ophthal. Buenos Aires, 42:180, 1967.

Sautter, H. Eine Spatform des juvenilen Glaukoms? Ber. Deutsch. Ophthal. Ges., 63:342, 1960.

Scheie, H. G. Infantile and juvenile glaucoma. Trans. Am. Acad. Ophthalmol. Otolaryngol., 67:458, 1963.

Shaffer, R. N. Pathogenesis of congenital glaucoma: gonioscopic and microscopic anatomy. Trans. Am. Acad. Ophthalmol. Otolaryngol., 59:297, 1955.

Sorsby, A. Ophthalmic Genetics. Appleton-Century-Crofts, New York, 1970, p. 37.

Sugar, H. S. Gonioscopy and glaucoma. Arch. Ophthalmol., 25:674, 1941.

New concepts in glaucoma classification. Am. J. Ophthalmol., 32:425, 1949.

The Glaucomas. Mosby, St. Louis, 1951.

Urbanek, I. Ein Fall Von Glaukoma juvenile inversum. Z. Augenh., 71:171, 1930.

Waardenburg, P. J. Is there a genetic relationship between different clinical types of primary glaucoma? Ophthal. Lit., 3:915, 1949.

In Genetics in Ophthalmology. Ed. by P. J. Waardenburg, A. Franceschetti, and D. Klein. Blackwell, Oxford, 1961, p. 578.

Westerlund, E. On the Primary Glaucoma Diseases (Vol. 12, Opera ex Domo Biologiae Heredit. Human. Univ. Hafniensis). Munksgaard, Copenhagen, 1947.

The Pathogenesis of Symptoms in Congenital Glaucoma

Solids of an organic nature yield quite readily to tensile stress. If such a solid is stretched beyond the limit of elasticity of that tissue (i.e., the yield point) and is further subjected to the same force, a permanent deformation remains. When the force is discontinued, the material will then behave like a material with a new modulus of elasticity. When a tissue with a good elastic modulus is stressed repeatedly or continuously over a long period of time, it may fail to recover completely even though the stress is well within the elastic limits.

Distention of ocular tissues is the primary pathologic change that will occur from a continued elevation in the intraocular pressure in an infant eye. This distention may involve the cornea, the limbal area, the scleral coat, and the optic nerve in either a pure or mixed form. The classical changes seen in this disease occur because of the distinct anatomic differences that are present which distinguish the infant eyeball from that of the adult.

In this chapter the various signs and symptoms of congenital glaucoma–including photophobia, blepharospasm, hazy cornea, enlargement of the eye, and tearing–will be discussed and related to the pathologic changes known to occur in this disease.

GENERAL CONSIDERATIONS

The human eye is a thin hollow elastic sphere filled with liquid under pressure. It is made up of three main tissue components, namely, the cornea, the sclera, the optic nerve area, and their respective interfaces. The internal surface of these structures is subject to stress derived from direct pressure and from tangential forces. In the normal eye, the resultant forces produce a combination of compressive and tensile effects. The compressive force acts in a centrifugal direction while the tangential force acts in a circumferential

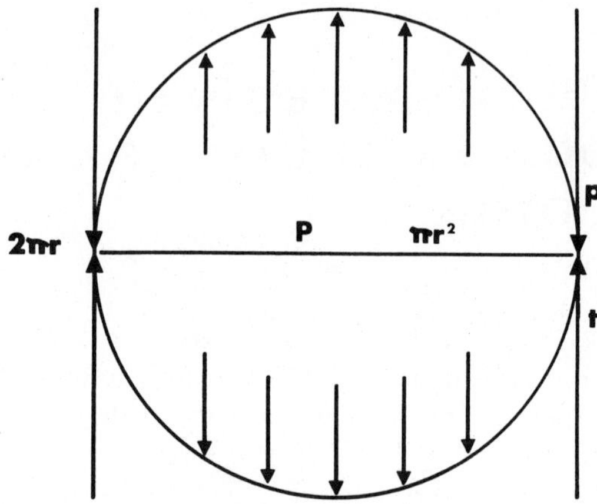

FIG. 1. Mathematical values of bursting forces in any great circle of elastic hollow sphere containing liquid under pressure. (Adapted from Friedman. Eye, Ear, Nose, Throat Monthly 45:59, 1966.)

direction. According to Friedman, these factors may be related in the form of a mathematical expression, explained as follows.

Let Fig. 1 represent a hollow sphere. The plane passing through the center will be represented by a horizontal line. The plane will generate a surface area within the sphere of πr^2.

The stresses in any great circle result from the internal forces perpendicular to the plane of that circle, which may be called the projected area of all the bursting forces. All the internal forces may be considered as applied over the area of that plane and resisted by the opposing stresses within that circumference.

The "skin" of the cross section is acted upon by a force which is the product of area (πr^2) and pressure P. Since the sphere is in equilibrium, the restraining elements are represented by the product of circumference ($2\pi r$), resistance to the internal force (tension or p), and thickness of the wall (t).

The total force $\pi r^2 \times P$ is just balanced by total resistance, $2\pi r^2 \times p \times t$. Hence $\pi r^2 \times P = 2\pi rpt$. Dividing by πr, $rP = 2pt$.

$$P = \frac{2pt}{r}$$

$$p = \frac{rP}{2t} \text{ or } p = P \times \frac{r \times 1}{2 \quad t}$$

Stress is measured as force per unit area, where
P = internal pressure
r = radius of curvature
t = thickness of wall
p = tensile stress.

It is thus shown that strains generated in the eye are the product of pressure, curvature, and thickness.

If P is kept constant and r decreases, p also decreases in the same proportion; if r increases, p also increases in a similar manner.

Tensile stress in the ocular coats is the product of intraocular pressure (P), and half the radius $\left(\frac{r}{2}\right)$ and the reciprocal of the thickness, $\left(\frac{1}{t}\right)$ of the ocular coats.

While it is not possible to measure either the stress or strain in the interior of an elastic body, when the thickness is small, the strain may be assumed to be uniform throughout the wall. For the purpose of this calculation, the eye has been treated as a sphere instead of the prolate spheroid that is its true form. For this reason, the computations which are derived from this formula are only approximations: the axial measurements were derived from the schematic eye and the values for scleral thickness are largely assumptions. Table 1 outlines the theoretical values of p in various refractive states when P is 15 mm Hg.

The radius of curvature is an important factor in determining the stress upon a specific section of the wall. The flatter the curvature the greater is the stress. If the sphere is irregular in that there are two unequally curved walls such as the cornea and sclera, each wall is under the same pressure, but not under the same stress. The cornea possesses an individual surface curvature regardless of the refractive error.

TABLE 1

THEORETICAL VALUES OF p IN VARIOUS REFRACTIVE STATES WHEN P =15 mm Hg

Refraction	P	r	t	K $\left(\frac{r}{2} \times \frac{1}{t}\right)$	p
Emmetropia	15	12	0.80	7.50	112.5
Hyperopia + 10 D	15	10	0.80	6.25	93.7
Myopia − 10 D	15	14	0.60	11.70	175.5
Myopia − 15 D	15	15	0.40	18.70	280.5
Myopia − 20 D	15	16	0.25	32.00	480.0

(P) internal pressure, (r) radius of curvature, (t) thickness of wall, (p) tensile stress
From data of Friedman. t values are assumptions due to lack of specific data.

Using the formula, the tensile strength of the inner "skin" of the cornea in an eye registering an intraocular pressure of 15 mm Hg may be calculated. Let the average corneal thickness be 0.7 mm and the radius of internal curvature be 6.8 mm.

Therefore $p = 15 \times \frac{6.8}{2} \times \frac{1}{0.7} = 73 \text{ mm Hg/mm}^2 = .99 \text{ g/mm}^2$

The sclera, which represents about 85 percent of the ocular wall surface area, exhibits a radius of curvature which varies from one eye to the other. The radius in this case is definitely related to the refractive error.

The optic nerve head provides a smooth continuation of the scleral wall. Therefore stress against the disc should vary with scleral curvature, at any given intraocular pressure.

The idealized emmetropic eye is 24 mm in length, the radius of the sclera being approximately 12 mm. A difference in axial length of 1 mm produces a change in refraction of 2.5 D. Conversely a difference of 2.5 D in refractive power corresponds to a change in axial length of 1 mm.

Applying the formula to variations in refraction and keeping P and t constant, we can calculate the effects of changes in radius:

In emmetropia $P = \frac{2pt}{12}$

The emmetropic eye must be the standard of comparison in instances of ametropia.

In axial hyperopia of + 5 D, $P = \frac{2pt}{11}$

The radius has decreased 8 percent; therefore, the stress on the ocular coats of the posterior segments of the hyperope of + 5 D should be 8 percent less than in an emmetrope with the same intraocular pressure and scleral thickness.

In the eye with congenital glaucoma, the effect of stress from the elevated intraocular pressure leads to distention of the ocular coats. In general, the distention follows one of the following patterns: (1) corneal distention; (2) limbal distention (symmetrical or asymmetrical); (3) scleral distention; (4) optic nerve cupping; and (5) mixed types. The presence of one pattern offers some protection to the other anatomical areas against stretching, i.e., when corneal distention prevails, the limbal area may remain normal. With scleral stretching, the anterior segment may remain intact. A general distention occurs in the late stages of the disease.

Shaffer and Hetherington noted the common occurrence of optic nerve cupping early in the course of the disease. According to Friedman, this condition may be due to excessive thinness of the lamina cribrosa during early life, which subjects the nerve head to multiplied stresses perhaps triple those applied against the sclera.

The influence of intraocular pressure can be calculated by using the formula. The higher the intraocular pressure the greater the influence on p in direct proportion to P. If we apply Table 1 to these calculations we find:

In emmetropia
if $P = 15, p = 15 \text{ X } 7.5 = 112.5$
if $P = 40, p = 40 \text{ X } 7.5 = 300$

In myopia
if $P = 15, p = 15 \text{ X } 32 = 480$
if $P = 40, p = 40 \text{ X } 32 = 1280$

It is obvious that in high myopia even a small increment in intraocular pressure will produce relatively large increments of stress.

According to Friedman the net result of forces derived from intraocular pressure (P) and tangential stress (p) is not obtained by simple addition, but may be derived by vectorial resolution of these forces. Since the stresses are mutually perpendicular, they can be laid out to scale as a right angle triangle and the resultant measured. In Fig. 2, the resultant will be the diagonal (D) of the stress quadrangle. Since the hypotenuse is equal to the square root of the sum of the squares of the other two sides, D can be derived as the

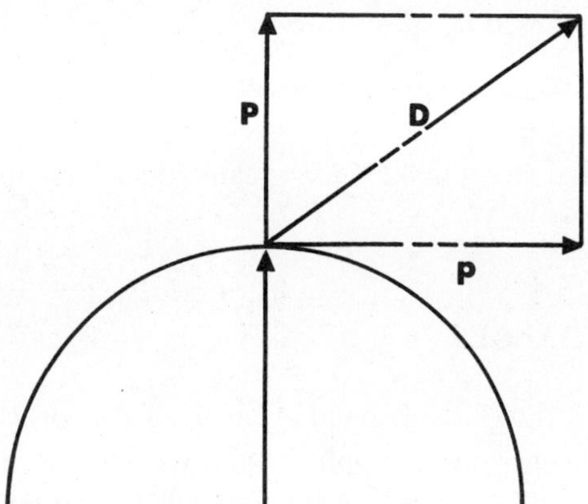

FIG. 2. Stress quadrangle to indicate vectorial resolution. *P*, internal pressure (intraocular pressure) and *p*, tangential stress. (Adapted from Friedman. **Eye, Ear, Nose, Throat Monthly** 45:59, 1966.)

geometric solution of the hypotenuse of a right angle triangle.

$$D = \sqrt{P^2 + p^2}$$

If, as in the cases with which we are dealing, one force (p) is 7.5 or more times the other, the net resultant will differ from the larger force only by a very small amount, so that the smaller force (P) may be disregarded.

Thus in emmetropia

$$D = \sqrt{15^2 + 112.5^2} = 113.5$$

and in myopia

$$D = \sqrt{15^2 = 480^2} = 480.2$$

It is essential to differentiate intraocular pressure or the compressive force (P) from tangential stress (p). Pressure is the force or weight per unit of area, such as lb/inch^2 or g/cm^2. Thus the pressure of the column of mercury 1 mm in height would be 13.6 mg/mm^2.

An intraocular pressure (P) of 15 mm Hg in an emmetropic eye would be equal to 15 X 13.6 mg = 204 mg/mm^2 or 0.204 g/mm^2 which is the compressive force.

The tangential stress would be as noted before:

$$p = 15 \text{ X } \frac{12}{2} \text{ X } \frac{1}{0.8}$$

$$p = 112.5 \text{ mm Hg} = 1.53 \text{ g/mm}^2$$

The tangential stress (1.53) is therefore 7.5 times greater than the compressive effect of direct pressure (0.204).

In a myope of –20 D

$$p = 15 \text{ X } \frac{16}{2} \text{ X } \frac{1}{.25} = 480 \text{ mm Hg} = 6.52 \text{ g/mm}^2$$

The tangential stress is 32 times greater than the compressive stress of .204.

OCULAR CHANGES

Distention of the globe with enlargement of the corneal diameters is the most obvious evidence of hydrophthalmia. An increase in the size of the orbit takes place in relation to the size of the globe. With respect to hydrophthalmia, Coronet and Aurand reported the largest globe, which measured 44 mm by 30 mm. The average dimensions of 17 specimens measured by Anderson showed that the anteroposterior diameter increased 5.6 mm, the horizontal diameter 3.2 mm, and the vertical diameter 2.5 mm.

THE CORNEA

Corneal Physiology

The normal cornea exists in a deturgesced state, that is, it contains less water than it is capable of imbibing from either distilled water or salt solutions. According to Alder the corneal stroma has a marked affinity for water because of its high collagen content and when immersed in solutions will absorb and hold water in large quantities. The anatomic peculiarities of the corneal structure, such as (1) uniformity and regularity in the arrangement of the epithelial cells, (2) the closely packed corneal lamellae of uniform size running almost parallel to each other, and (3) the absence of blood vessels are all important factors in corneal transparency. The normal state of the cornea is maintained by a variety of factors, one of which is the intraocular pressure. Should this factor reach abnormal levels, changes take place which lead first to loss of corneal transparency and later to enlargement of corneal structure.

Normal and Buphthalmic Corneas

A comparison of the findings of Gross and Merkel illustrates the striking changes that take place in the infant cornea when subjected to an increased intraocular pressure over a period of time (Table 2). The horizontal diameter may enlarge to 16 mm in the buphthalmic eye as compared with 11.6 mm in the normal. The thickness is 0.67 as opposed to 0.9 at the center and 0.47 to 1.1 in the periphery. The radius of curvature is 11.8 mm in the patient with glaucoma and 7.8 mm in the normal. Fig. 3 illustrates an

TABLE 2

COMPARISON OF THE AVERAGE CORNEAL MEASUREMENTS OF A NORMAL INFANT EYE AND A BUPHTHALMIC EYE

	Glaucoma eye (Gross) (mm)	Normal eye (Merkel) (mm)
Horizontal diameter	16.00	11.60
Thickness at center	0.67	0.90
Thickness at periphery	0.47	1.10
Radius of curvature	11.80	7.80

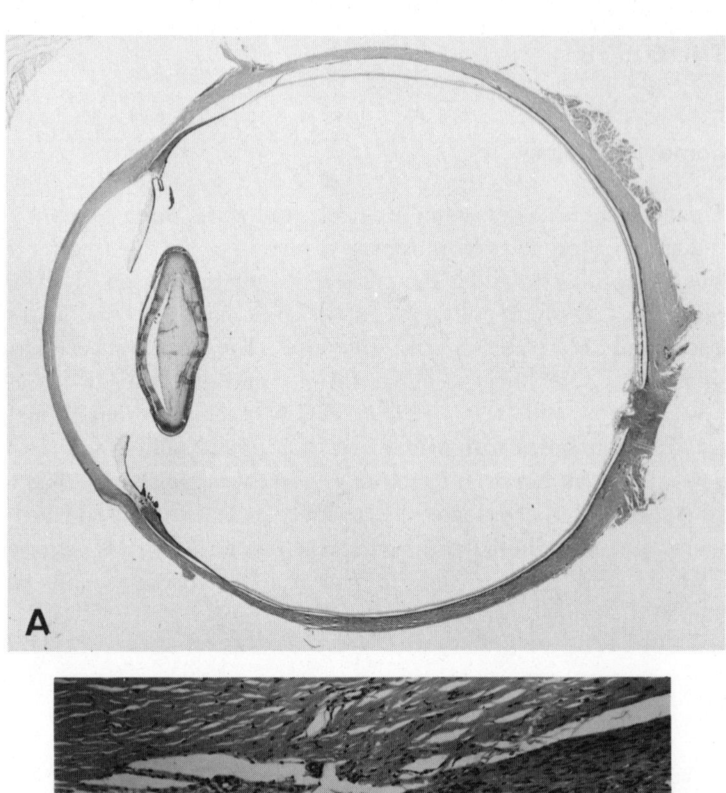

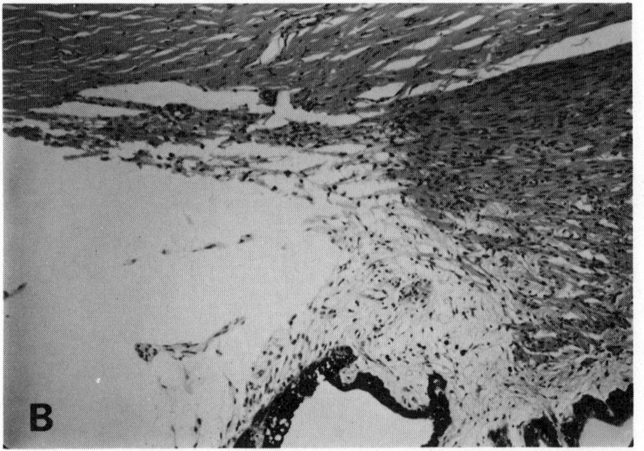

FIG. 3.A. Normal infant eye. (A. F. I. P. Neg. 939387) X 3.9. **B.** Anterior chamber angle in normal infant eye. (A. F. I. P. Neg. 939387.) (Courtesy of the Registry of Ophthalmic Pathology of the Armed Forces Institute of Pathology.) X 140.

infant eye enucleated because of a glioma of the optic nerve; it demonstrates the normal profile of the young cornea. The eye itself is otherwise unremarkable. Fig. 4 shows an advanced case of congenital glaucoma. The

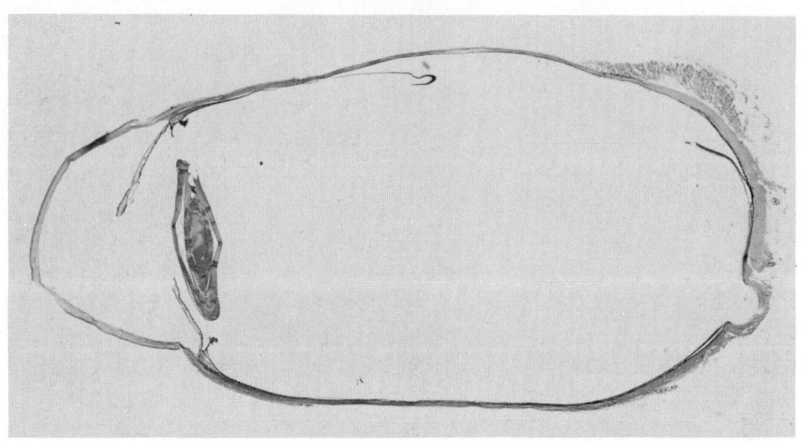

FIG. 4. Advanced buphthalmia with deep anterior chamber elongated axial length and optic nerve cupping (A. F. I. P. Neg. 935268.) (Courtesy of the Registry of Ophthalmic Pathology of the Armed Forces Institute of Pathology.) X 2.9.

cornea is enlarged, thinned at the periphery, and globular in shape. Other features include a marked increase in axial length with an associated deepening of the anterior chamber, an elongation of the corneal diameter and optic nerve cupping.

Corneal Haze

The normal cornea loses it luster and transparency as a result of an elevation of the intraocular pressure which leads to edema of the epithelium and stroma (Fig. 5). The steamy cornea of congenital glaucoma is therefore not unlike that seen in acute glaucoma of the adult. Haas reported a large series of cases which showed that the appearance of corneal haze (Fig. 6) in congenital glaucoma did not represent neglect because clouding of the cornea in infantile glaucoma was not the result of age but depended on intraocular pressure in the specific case. Opacification of the cornea to some degree is present in over 75 percent of all cases of hydrophthalmia, according to Sugar. Most of these instances result from ruptures in the endothelium together with Descemet's membrane. Damage to the endothelium removes the normal water barrier of the cornea. As the endothelium heals over the curled edges of the tears in Descemet's membrane, a new Descemet's layer is formed. The edges of the tears in Descemet's membrane always remain

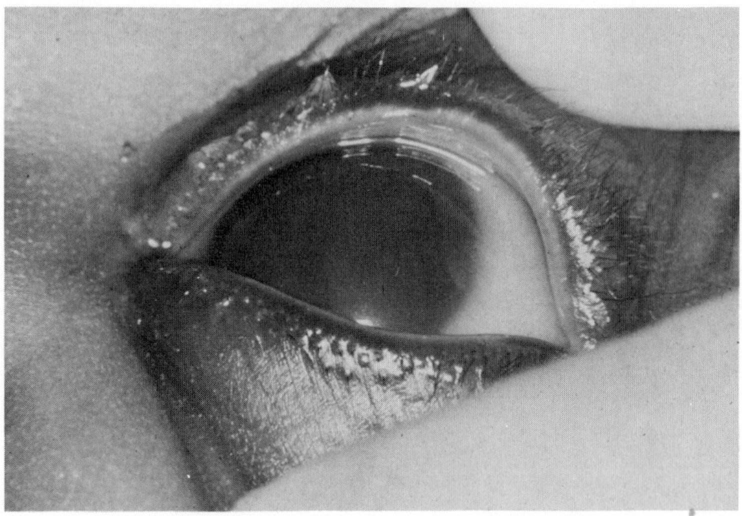

FIG. 5. Haziness of cornea in case of congenital glaucoma.

visible. Ruptures of the endothelium and Descemet's membrane are often present at birth. Their frequency varies directly with the degree of distention of the globe. Some of the ruptures are superficial and due to trauma and ulceration. Diminished corneal sensation is probably responsible for these cases. Some subepithelial colloid deposition may be found as a cause of permanent opacity in the areas overlying the tears.

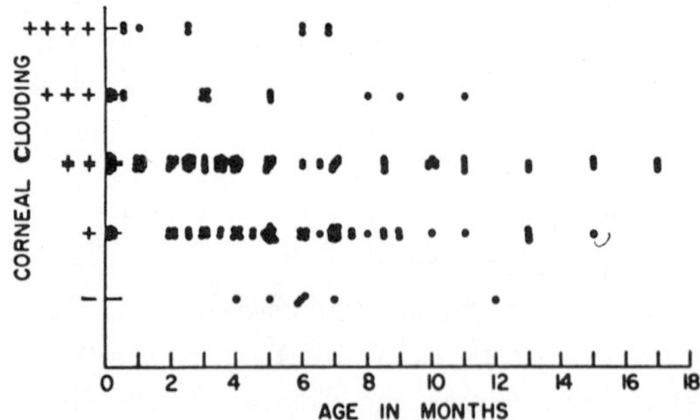

Fig. 6. Degree of corneal clouding present at time of diagnosis, revealing lack of relationship. (Adapted from Haas. **Invest. Ophthalmol.** 7:140, 1968.)

Corneal edema in congenital glaucoma takes four main forms, as outlined below.

SUPERFICIAL CORNEAL EDEMA. The generalized haziness of the cornea other than the localized areas is usually due to epithelial edema and disappears on surgical incision into the globe.

LOCAL CORNEAL EDEMA. This is caused by direct stromal absorption of aqueous humor resulting from ruptures in Descemet's membrane. This type may seriously interfere with gonioscopy. Since the haze is often localized to two or three small areas, the transparent cornea may be used to perform the goniotomy.

DIFFUSE EDEMA OF THE CORNEAL STROMA. This type of edema may interfere with detailed observation to a considerable degree, though focal retroillumination may partially remedy this. Glycerine or salt solutions are of no avail.

WHITE CICATRICIAL EDEMA. This type of edema (usually associated with bullous epithelial edema) makes contact lens visibility impossible. Prognosis in such a case is poor.

Corneal Diameter

The corneal diameter may increase to a much greater extent in proportion to the dimensions of the globe, reaching a size of 17 mm. The conjunctival vessels may become greatly dilated as the hydrophthalmic process continues. The sclera becomes thinned and may become quite ectatic near the limbus, giving a bluish-white appearance to the sclera. The thinning near the imbus leads to an enlargement and increased diameter of the cornea which is thus flattened.

Haas showed that there was no obvious relationship between increased corneal diameter and initial intraocular pressure (Fig. 7). Haab's striae, which represent tears in Descemet's membrane (Figs. 8, 9, and 10), occurred as a more localized and dense form of opacity, but did not seem to occur in corneas smaller than 12.5 mm in diameter. There appeared to be a closer relationship between corneal diameter and age of the infant at the time the diagnosis was made (Fig. 11). This would suggest that in the presence of elevated intraocular pressure, the increased corneal diameter represents a sign of elapsed time. Thus a rapidly increasing corneal diameter should arouse suspicion of glaucoma. Fig. 12 represents an advanced case of congenital glaucoma with marked asymmetric limbal distention. The increase in corneal diameter is located mainly in the limbal area so that the limbal groove is no longer present.

Costenbader and Kwitko studied a series of eyes with congenital

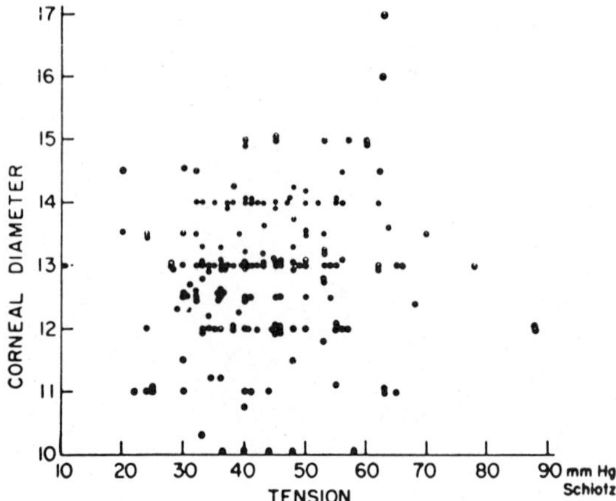

FIG. 7. Intraocular pressure of 181 eyes under miotic therapy for infantile glaucoma. Rarity of control is obvious. Corneal diameters are scattered throughout the entire range. (Adapted from Haas. **Invest. Ophthalmol.** 7:140, 1968.)

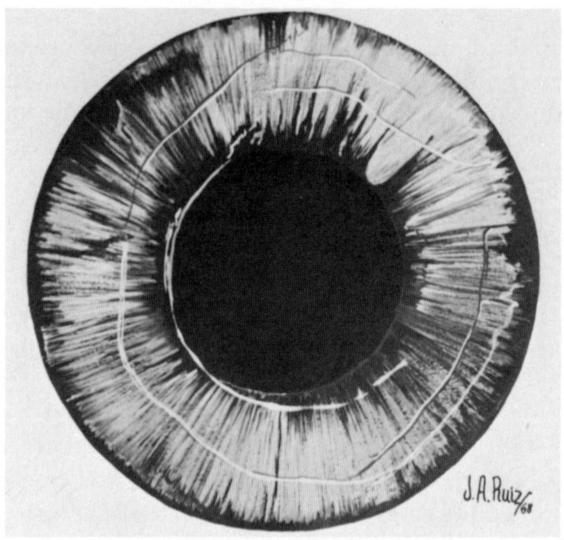

FIG. 8. Haab's striae.

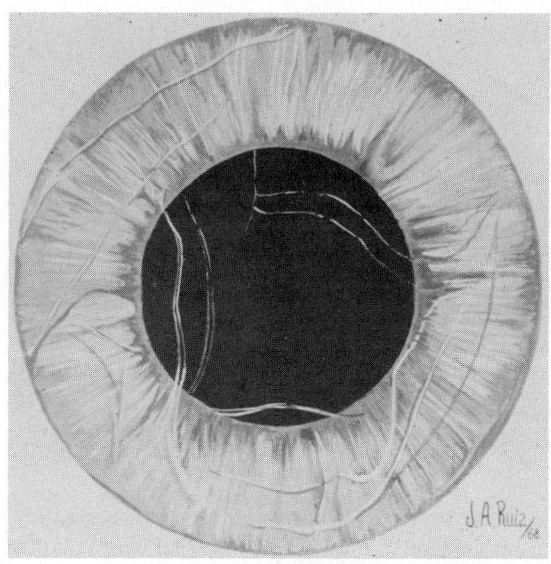

FIG. 9. Haab's striae.

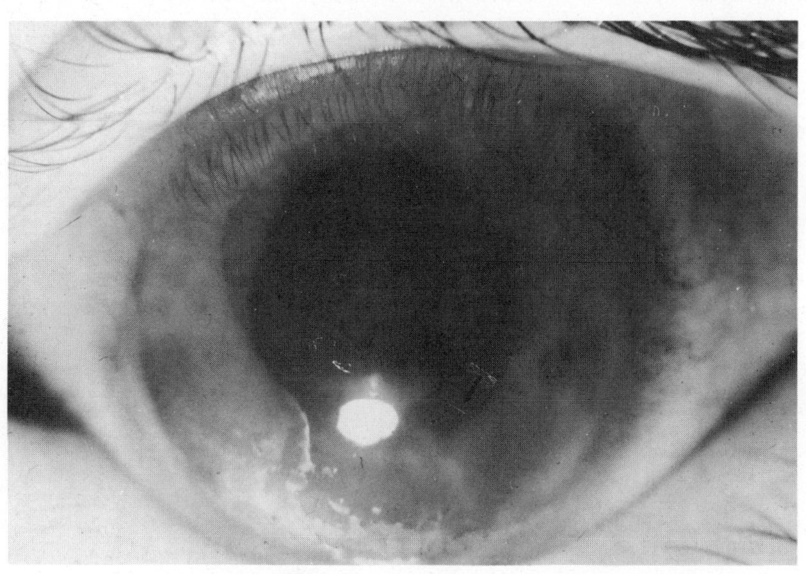

FIG. 10. Haab's striae, (*arrow*) indicates tears in Descemet's membrane.

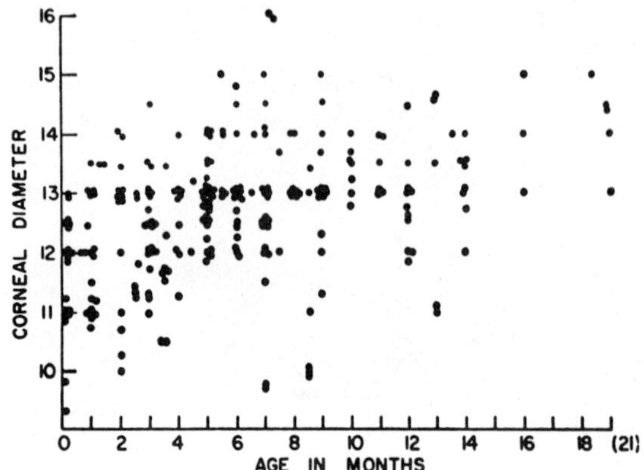

FIG. 11. Relationship of patient's age to corneal diameter at time of diagnosis. (Adapted from J. Haas. **Invest. Ophthalmol.** 7:140, 1968.)

glaucoma. The cases were arbitrarily divided into the following groups, based on age of onset: birth to five days (Table 3); five days to six months

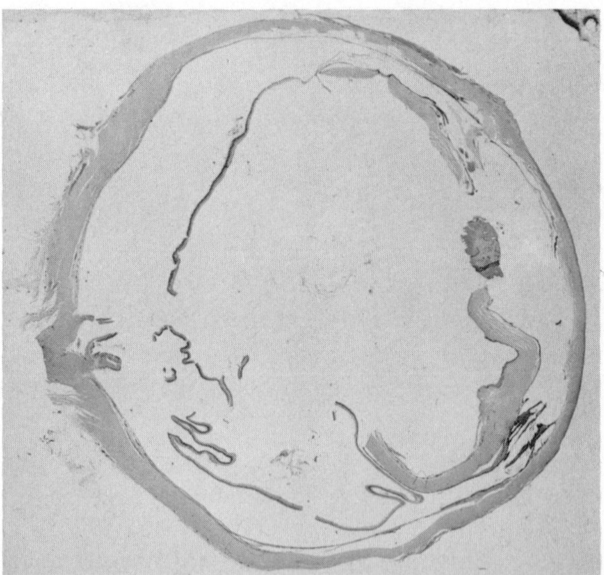

FIG. 12. Buphthalmic eye in which cornea is primarily involved. (A. F. I. P. Neg. 937392.) (Courtesy of the Registry of Ophthalmic Pathology of the Armed Froces Institute of Pathology.) X 2.9.

TABLE 3

INFANTILE GLAUCOMA–BIRTH TO FIVE DAYS: 9 PATIENTS*–16 EYES

Initial signs and symptoms	Eyes	%
Hazy cornea	14	88
Photophobia	7	44
Enlarged cornea	6	31
Enlarged eye	4	25
Epiphora	1	.06

*In one patient signs and symptoms were present at birth in one eye and began at one month in the other eye.

(Table 4); and six months to 36 months (Table 5). In the youngest group (birth to five days), a hazy cornea was noted in 88 percent of cases. Photophobia, a symptom related to corneal involvement was present in 44 percent of the eyes. The cornea was enlarged in 31 percent of cases, and the eye itself was enlarged in only 25 percent. In the older group (five days to six months), the incidence of corneal enlargement and haziness of the cornea was present in about the same proportion (76 percent and 73 percent, respectively). Photophobia was present in less than 50 percent of cases and the globe was enlarged in almost 60 percent of the eyes.

TABLE 4

INFANTILE GLAUCOMA–FIVE DAYS TO SIX MONTHS: 24 PATIENTS*–37 EYES

Initial signs and symptoms	Eyes	%
Enlarged cornea	28	76
Hazy cornea	27	73
Enlarged eye	22	59
Photophobia	15	41
Epiphora	8	22

*In one patient signs and symptoms were present at birth in one eye and began at one month in the other eye.

TABLE 5

INFANTILE GLAUCOMA–SIX MONTHS TO THIRTY-SIX MONTHS: 14 PATIENTS–20 EYES

Initial signs and symptoms	Eyes	%
Enlarged eye	17	85
Hazy cornea	14	70
Enlarged cornea	13	65
Photophobia	9	45
Epiphora	9	45

TABLE 6

COMPARISON OF THE AVERAGE ANTERIOR CHAMBER MEASUREMENTS OF A NORMAL INFANT EYE AND A BUPHTHALMIC EYE

	Glaucoma eye (Gross) (mm)	Normal eye (Merkel) (mm)
Anterior chamber depth	6.3	2.6

The study showed that the initial signs and symptoms in congenital glaucoma were those associated with the early effect of the intraocular pressure on the cornea. Hence a hazy cornea was the most common sign followed by photophobia in the newborn group of cases. The stretching of corneal tissue and corneal edema led directly to the intense sensitivity to light.

This would suggest that the cornea is more susceptible than other ocular tissues to an elevated intraocular pressure in an infant eye at an early age. When onset took place after the initial five-day period (Table 4) the signs and symptoms were those related to enlargement of the globe. The patients in the five days to six months group had enlargement of the cornea slightly more frequently than haziness of the cornea. An enlarged eye was present in 59 percent of cases. After the child reached the age of six months, an enlarged eye was the most common sign (85 percent). A hazy cornea (70 percent) and large cornea (65 percent) followed in that order.

It is possible, therefore, that prior to six months the cornea has relatively less tensile strength than the sclera and will expand more readily under the influence of a raised intraocular pressure. After six months a relative increase in tensile strength of the cornea allows it to resist elevated pressure so that the expansile effect takes place in a more uniform manner upon the scleral coat as well with a resultant enlargement of the entire globe. This is further suggested by the fact that after the five-day period photophobia, a manifestation of corneal involvement, did not appear as one of the most common symptoms.

Haab's Striae

Haab's striae represent breaks in Descemet's membrane which occur during the course of corneal stretching; they are associated with deep stromal edema. Corneal distention is almost never equally distributed but tends to be localized mainly in the horizontal meridian so that the breaks in Descemet's membrane are usually located here or concentric with the limbus peripherally. The horizontal tendency is probably due to flattening of the vertical meridian of the cornea. The corneal epithelium becomes edematous, leading to the intense photophobia and blepharospasm (Figs. 8, 9, 10).

Distention of the Limbal Area

Distention of the limbal area often occurs with corneal enlargement. In isolated cases, severe thinning-out of the limbus alone may be present. The limbal groove disappears and the limbus appears as a wide blue-colored band. If excessive limbal distention occurs, a marked enlargement of the corneal diameter results (Fig. 12). In this event Haab's striae are narrow or may be entirely absent. This type of limbal distention tends to be asymmetrical and occurs predominantly in the upper quadrant, according to Worst.

Epiphora

Tearing represents an important symptom in congenital glaucoma. The initiating cause is usually the irritation set off by an expanding cornea. In the author's series the incidence of epiphora rose from 0.06 percent in the group birth to five days (Table 3) to 22 percent in the group five days to six months (Table 4) to 45 percent in the group six months to thirty-six months (Table 5). This increase in frequency was closely associated with the increasing frequency in cornea and eyeball enlargement.

Blepharospasm

Blepharospasm is a frequent accompaniment of inflammatory diseases of the anterior segment of the globe. It forms part of the tearing-photophobia complex of congenital glaucoma initiated by the irritation induced by the expanding cornea. The reaction is probably mediated through the seventh cranial nerve, which supplies the orbicularis muscle; the muscles of the brow may also be involved.

THE ANTERIOR CHAMBER

Examination

Two important factors influence the examination of the anterior chamber. First, corneal distention leads to a rapid decrease in gonioscopic visibility and, second, the deep corneal edema which results from the elevated intraocular pressure remains even after the corneal epithelium has been removed. The anterior chamber angle, however, is temporarily exempted from ocular distention and the original angle architecture remains intact for a considerable time, according to Worst. For this reason goniotomy is still the operation of choice even with corneal distention. However, poor visibility gravely affects this procedure.

The filtration angles of congenital glaucoma, though varying in secondary changes because of stretching, have much in common amongst themselves. Some typical elements can be interpreted as having been formed from an atypical fetal angle after secondary stretching has exposed various structures. One of these exposed elements is the scalloped edge of the posterior pigment layer, which is the normal pigment layer, overstretched and in an upright position, now more visible than usual because of iris stroma atrophy (See Chap. 3, Fig. 52). Other exposed elements include the vascular loops which run upward into the depth of the angle (See Chap. 3, Figs. 45, 46).

Distention of the Limbal Area

In the early stage of limbal distention, the corneal clouding is mainly of the epithelial type and the goniotomy procedure still stands a good chance for success. In later stages secondary changes occur, resulting in a backward displacement of Schlemm's canal and associated structures with a thickening of the uveal meshwork fibers. This leads to a disappearance of the typical aspects of early congenital glaucoma toward what is considered a more normal gonioscopic image of the advanced untreated case. The characteristic feature of the anterior segment in long-standing congenital glaucoma is a fanning-out of the angle structures, which eventually become flattened out against the scleral wall (Fig. 13).

The iris is atrophic, tremulous, and in some locations adherent to the peripheral cornea. Schlemm's canal and associated networks may be entirely absent. The lens appears small in relation to surrounding distended structures

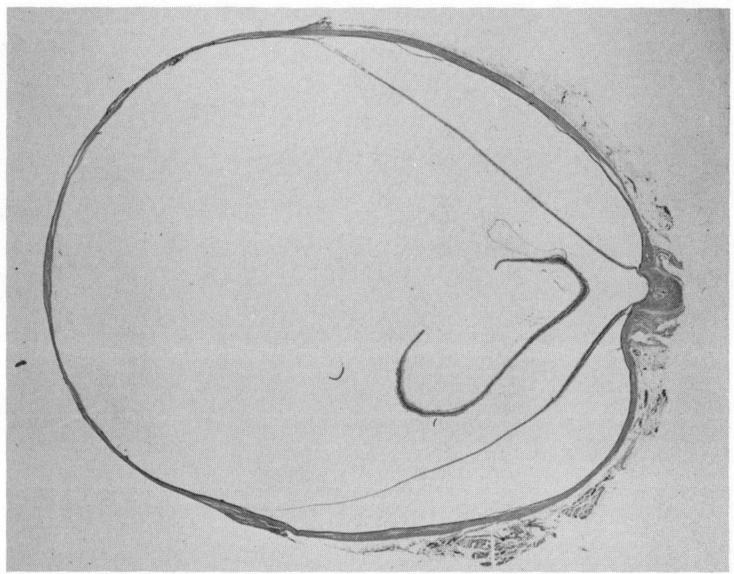

FIG. 13. Advanced buphthalmia illustrating distended limbal area and enlarged cornea. Chamber angle structures are fanned out against scleral wall. (A. F. I. P. Neg. 940482.) (Courtesy of the Registry of Ophthalmic Pathology of the Armed Forces Institute of Pathology.) X 2.9.

and is displaced posteriorly. Table 6 illustrates the marked changes that are seen in the advanced glaucoma case. The average anterior chamber depth in the buphthalmic eye exceeds the normal by 3.7 mm. The comparison is shown in Figs. 3 and 4.

TABLE 7

COMPARISON OF THE ELASTIC PROPERTIES OF AN ADULT EYE AND A THREE-DAY-OLD INFANT EYE (ACCORDING TO SQUIRE)

Thickness of scleral sack	
1. Adult av. thickness	1.09 mm
2. Infant av. thickness	0.45 mm
Adult material	2.40 times thicker
Coefficient for stretching (strip 5 mm wide by 1 mm thick)	
1. Adult	4.6 dynes/cm
2. Infant	2.7 dynes/cm
Adult material	1.70 times stronger

Adult eye has an overall strength with respect to collapse of about 4.0 times that of infant.

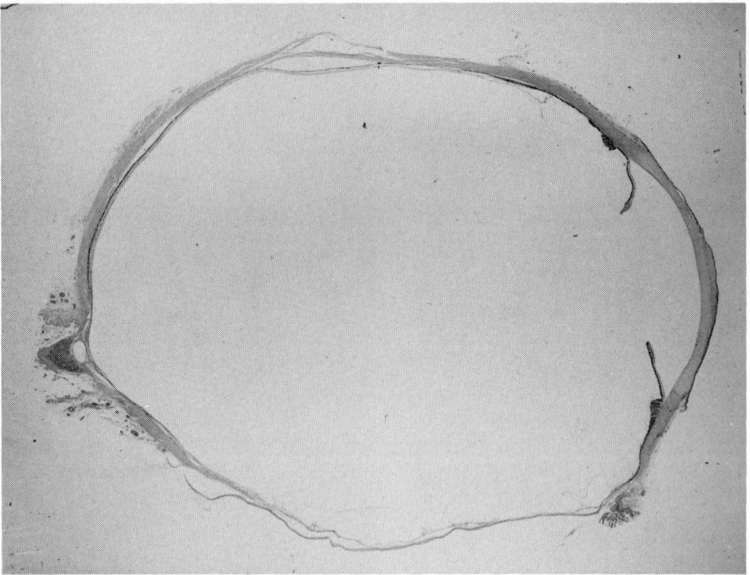

FIG. 14. Advanced buphthalmia illustrating essentially normal anterior segment including cornea, limbal area, and anterior chamber. Marked thinning is noted in sclera. (A. F. I. P. Neg. 941995.) (Courtesy of the Registry of Ophthalmic Pathology of the Armed Forces Institute of Pathology.) X 2.9.

Retention of Anterior Chamber Angle Features

The described change in the anterior chamber need not take place in every case because distention of the scleral coats may protect the anterior chamber so that it remains intact, retaining many of the typical features of congenital glaucoma. Fig. 14 illustrates an advanced case of buphthalmia in which posterior scleral distention is the prominent feature. Only moderate limbal stretching is present and the chamber angle retains many of its original characteristics. This type of distention simulates high myopia.

THE SCLERA

The expansile characteristics of the infant sclera change markedly with age (Table 7, See Chap. 4, p. 179).

It appears that there is a difference in tensile strength between the cornea and sclera which also changes with time. It is not until the child is

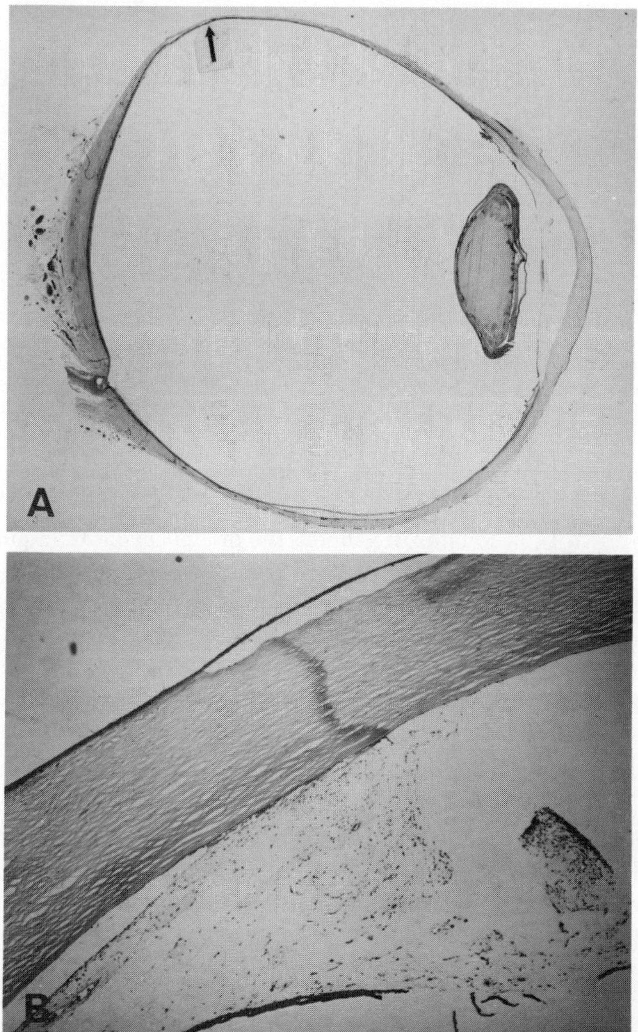

FIG. 15.A. Buphthalmic eye illustrating marked thinning of scleral coat (*arrow*). Cornea in this case shows little change. X 2.9. **B.** Anterior chamber angle illustrating broad peripheral anterior synechiae. X 22.

six months that enlargement of the eye—that is, scleral stretching—becomes the most important symptom, according to Costenbader and Kwitko.

The scleral thickness varies in different locations in the normal eye. In addition, scleral thickness seems to be related to the refractive state of the eye. Mawas measured the thickness of the ocular coats in the normal eye and

TABLE 8

SCLERAL THICKNESS ACCORDING TO LOCATION AND REFRACTION

	Normal (mm)	High Myope (mm)
Equator		
Temporally	0.80	0.30
Nasally	0.60	0.35
Posterior area (macular)		
Temporal to disc	1.10	0.25
Nasal to disc	0.80	0.10

Averaging these figures: normal thickness = 0.80 mm; Myopic eye thickness = 0.25 mm.
From data of J. Mawas. Bull. Soc. d'opht. XLVI 1:549, 1934.

in the highly myopic eye (Table 8). Although the area temporal to the disc is the thickest area in the normal eye (1.1 mm), in the highly myopic eye this area thins down to 0.25 mm. In general, the myopic eye is 0.55 mm thinner than the normal eye. A rise in intraocular pressure would probably affect the weakest areas first. Figs. 4, 14 and 15A represent cases of congenital glaucoma illustrating severe scleral stretching. The chamber angle is obstructed with broad peripheral anterior synechiae in Fig. 15B.

As the globe enlarges, the scleral coat undergoes progressive thinning, resulting in a blue-tinged appearance which is not unlike that seen in the blue sclerotic syndrome. The expanded globe may give the clinical appearance of proptosis. In other cases the steady progression of the condition may lead to a staphylomatous ectasia adjacent to the limbus.

When scleral distention takes place in congenital glaucoma the anterior segment often remains normal (Fig. 16). The chamber angle depth remains unchanged as well as the chamber angle microanatomy. When this occurs in the pure form the condition may remain undiscovered for a significant period of time as external evidence of increased intraocular pressure is not present. The axial length of the eyeball increases with an associated involvement of the optic nerve head (See Fig. 4). A diagnosis of malignant myopia may be made until tonometry reveals the true nature of the condition. It is important to note that distentional patterns that take place in congenital glaucoma differ markedly from those occurring in high myopia. In congenital glaucoma, the equatorial regions are mainly affected and little posterior pole distention occurs except for the outward bowing of the optic cup. In high myopia the pathologic changes are largely posterior. Table 9 illustrates the marked changes that are present in the scleral coat of the buphthalmic eye as compared with the normal eye. The difference between the two is 7.7 mm in the anteroposterior diameter and 2.4 mm in the vertical

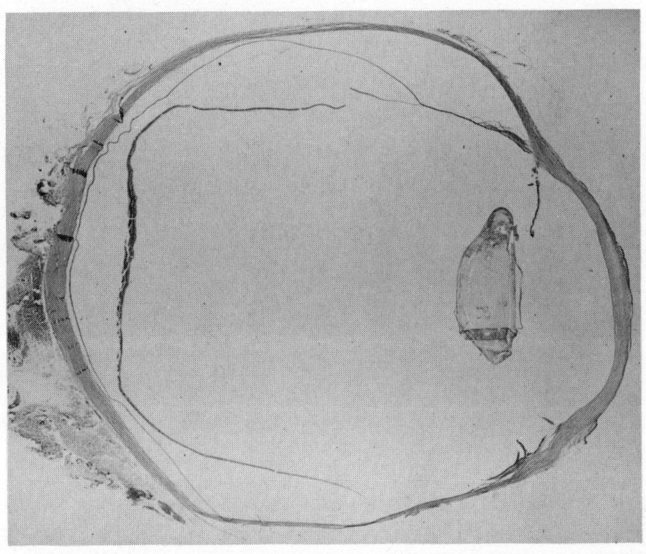

FIG. 16. Buphthalmic eye illustrating involvement of scleral sac. Cornea shows little change. (Courtesy of E. Liepa.) X 2.9.

TABLE 9

COMPARISON OF THE AVERAGE MEASUREMENTS OF A NORMAL INFANT EYE AND A BUPHTHALMIC EYE

	Glaucoma eye (Gross) (mm)	Normal eye (Merkel) (mm)
Anterior posterior diameter	32.0	24.3
Vertical diameter	26.0	23.6

diameter in this study. Fig. 16 illustrates a case of congenital glaucoma in which scleral stretching resulted in an apparent microphakia. The limbal groove is still present and the chamber angle has retained many of its original features.

THE OPTIC NERVE

Increased intraocular pressure affects the infant disc much more rapidly than the same amount of pressure in the adult (Fig. 17AB). In

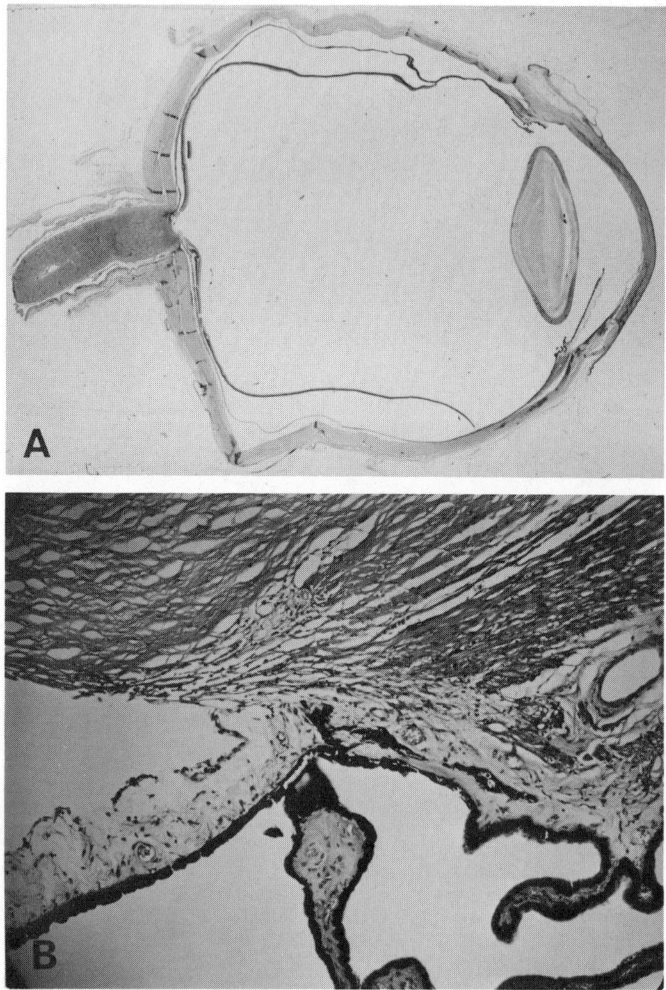

FIG. 17.A. Buphthalmic eye illustrating optic nerve cupping. Scleral coat and cornea show little change. **B.** Filtration angle in congenital glaucoma. (Courtesy of E. Liepa.) X 150.

the older patient with glaucoma, the exact relationship between elevated intraocular pressure and optic nerve excavation is still unclear for several reasons. First, despite sustained elevation of the intraocular pressure, atrophy of the optic nerve may not occur for a prolonged period; often many years are required before cupping occurs. Second, there is no definite or constant correlation between the amount of intraocular pressure and the degree of cupping of the optic nerve. This would conform with clinical experience in other fields. There is, for example, no correlation between the level of systolic blood pressure and hypertrophy of the left ventricle, the latter being dependent on many factors other than the arterial hypertension. Third, despite lowering of the intraocular pressure by adequate and timely treatment, progressive atrophic disc changes may ensue. Finally, cupping of the optic nerve may develop in a case of glaucoma even though the intraocular pressure is never greatly increased.

In the Normal Infant

In the normal infant there is general uniformity in the appearance of the optic nerve heads. Asymmetry between the two discs has been noted in only 2 to 3 percent of cases and disc cupping exceeding 0.3 disc diameter in only 3 to 10 percent of newborn infants in several large series (See Chap. 4, p. 180).

In the Glaucomatous Infant

In the glaucomatous infant an entirely different clinical picture has been noted. In infants under one year Shaffer reported that 68 percent of 126 eyes had optic nerve cupping exceeding 0.3 disc diameter. In patients in whom only one eye was involved, there was asymmetry of the discs in 88 percent of cases. Only three patients (11 percent) had cups of equal size in the two eyes and 59 percent (16 eyes) of the glaucoma eyes had disc cupping that was between three to six times the size of the cup in the normal eye. In some cases marked cupping was actually present at birth. In all eyes the disc changes had occurred in the first 12 months of life at pressures which rarely exceeded 40 mm Hg. Shaffer reported a series of 85 congenital glaucoma eyes in which 39 percent had cups which would be considered physiologic (0 to 0.3 of 1 disc diameter), 40 percent were suggestive (0.4 to 0.6 disc diameter), and 21 percent were pathologic (0.7 disc diameter or more) as judged by Snydacker's 1964 criteria. In spite of obvious cupping of the infant optic nerve there is often little functional impairment. This may be explained by the astroglial hypothesis of disc cupping described by Shaffer and Hetherington. In other instances there may be extensive damage. Prolonged pressure may cause retinal and optic nerve changes. The ganglion cells disappear. Connective tissue forms on the inner retinal surface. Sclerosis of retinal vessels and detachment of the retina may be found.

Astroglial Hypothesis of Disc Cupping

The blood pressure of infants is considerably lower than that of the adult. In the first few months of life the average blood pressure is 85/40. This gradually increases to 95/55 at the first year of life. Therefore, the effective pulse pressure passing into the infant eye is less than that of the adult. Using the ophthalmodynamometer, pallor of the whole posterior pole of the infant eye occurs as blood is forced out of either or both the choroid and Henkind's peripapillary arterial network. This is accomplished with relatively low pressures. For example at pressures of 15 to 30 g the diastolic pulse appears. The disc and peripapillary area become more and more pale until the circulation stops–usually at a pressure of 45 to 55 g. In contrast, the diastolic pulse in the adult disc is usually seen between 60 to 80 mm Hg and the systolic arrest between 100 and 120 mm Hg. Therefore, increases in intraocular pressure would be expected to shunt blood more efficiently from the infant disc than from the adult with the higher pulse pressure. Ischemia is the probable reason that cupping of the optic disc occurs so quickly in the infant, while an adult disc at the same intraocular pressure may show no cupping for many years. Once the pressure is normalized the cupping of the optic disc becomes smaller and this improvement is often permanent. If the cupping is less than 0.5 disc diameter, a field defect is usually not found.

The reason for this improvement can be explained by the astroglial hypothesis. Salzmann showed that nonmedullated nerve fibers of the optic disc located in front of the lamina cribrosa form longitudinal bundles which are surrounded by astroglial cell processes. The astroglia provide support for the bundles and separate one from the other. Some processes tend to wrap around adjacent capillaries while others form the sheath surrounding the neural bundles. The ischemia resulting from shunting blood away from the disc area when the intraocular pressure is elevated may primarily affect the astroglia. Atrophy and destruction of these cells would decrease the bulk of the optic disc, resulting in increased cupping without loss of neural elements. This would explain the lack of field defects in the presence of apparent glaucomatous atrophy such as is seen in congenital glaucoma. If the process continues the neural and ganglion cells degenerate secondarily due to loss of support and nourishment. The final result is the typical field defect of glaucoma. Since astroglial cells proliferate this would explain the decrease in cupping after normalization of tension.

The theory is based on a number of clinical observations. First, in internal hydrocephalus, the ventricles enlarge as the disease progresses.

According to Penfield and Elvidge, the cells that are primarily affected in the initial phase of the disease are the astroglial cells. The ventricles decrease in size after normalization of the intraventricular pressure has been achieved. Second, in primary optic atrophy, destruction of the neurons occurs which results in a flat pale appearance of the disc *without* cupping. This may be because the astroglial cells remain intact. Third, a small infarct involving the arterial twigs which supply the periphery of the optic disc causes an arcuate scotoma without associated cupping of the optic disc, according to Harrington.

THE LENS

The lens is affected by stretching of the zonules. Subluxation with iridodonesis and dislocation of the lens may take place. Microphakia, real or apparent, is a common feature in congenital glaucoma.

THE HYDROPHTHALMIC EYE OF A PREMATURE INFANT

Wexler and Kornzweig described the buphthalmic eye of a 6 month premature infant. Three first cousins of the mother who had normal eyes suffered from congenital glaucoma. The grandparents of the child were first cousins. The cornea of the right eye ruptured at birth for undetermined reasons but the eyeball was otherwise normal. The findings in the left eye are

TABLE 10

ENLARGED EYE OF A SIX MONTH PREMATURE INFANT WITH BUPHTHALMOS COMPARED WITH THE EYE OF A NORMAL FETUS OF THE SAME AGE

	Normal 6 month-Fetus (mm.)	6 month-Premature with Buphthalmos (mm.)
Anteroposterior diameter of globe	10.5	15
Transverse diameter of globe	10.0	14
Transverse diameter of cornea	6.0	9
Thickness of cornea at center	0.8	0.3
Thickness of cornea at limbus	0.86	0.4
Thickness of sclera at limbus	0.36	0.28
Thickness of sclera at equator	0.3	0.1
Thickness of sclera at posterior pole	0.6	0.36

From data of D. Wexler and A. Kornzweig, Arch. Ophthalmol., 37:318, 1947.

outlined in Table 1υ and compared with a normal eye of the same age. The corneoscleral sulcus was obliterated; there was practically no difference in the radius of curvature of the cornea and that of the sclera. The iris was adherent to the posterior surface of the cornea. The lens was smaller and flatter than normal but otherwise unremarkable although displaced forward. The optic disc showed glaucomatous cupping. The choroid and sclera were both reduced in thickness.

The generalized distension of the eyeball would testify to the extensive involvement of the outflow system.

References

Adler, F. H. Physiology of the Eye, Mosby, St. Louis, 1959. 3rd ed.

Anderson, J. R. Hydrophthalmia or Congenital Glaucoma: Its causes, Treatment and Outlook. Cambridge Univers., London, 1939.

Chandler, P. A. Long-term results in glaucoma therapy. Am. J. Ophthalmol., 49:221, 1960.

Coronet and Aurand. Clin. Ophthal., 18:498, 1912. Cited by Elliot, R. H. A Treatise on Glaucoma. Hodder and Staughton, London, 1922.

Costenbader, F. D., and Kwitko, M. L. Congenital glaucoma: an analysis of seventy-seven consecutive eyes. J. of Pediat. Ophthalmol., 4:9, 1967.

de Vauceleroy, M. A propos d'un cas de glaucome. Bull. Soc. Belge Ophtal., 66:13, 1933.

Ellis, O. H. The etiology symptomatology and treatment of juvenile glaucoma. Am. J. Ophthalmol., 31:1589, 1948.

Encyclopedia Britannica. Strength of materials. 15:50, 1947.

Epstein, E. Report on a case of hydrophthalmia (buphthalmos). Br. J. Ophthalmol., 30:476, 1946.

Friedman, B. Stress upon the ocular coats: effects of scleral curvature, scleral thickness and intraocular pressure. Eye Ear Nose Throat Monthly, 45:59, 1966.

Goldmann, H. Das Glaucom: Definition Allgemeines. Lehrbuck der Augenheilk, 1948, p. 372.

Gross, E. G. Betrag zur pathologischen Anatomie des Hydrophthalmus. Arch. Augenheilk., 48:340, 1903.

Haas, J. Principles and problems of therapy in congenital glaucoma. Invest. Ophthalmol., 7:140, 1968.

Harrington, D. O. The Visual Fields. Mosby, St. Louis, 1956.

Henkind, P. Microcirculation of the peripapillary retina. Trans. Am. Acad. Ophthalmol. Otolaryngol., 83:890, 1969.

Hess, L. Pathogenesis of glaucoma and glaucomatous atrophy of the optic nerve. Arch. Ophthalmol., 37:324, 1947.

Mawas, J. Introduction a l'étude de la myopie et des chorioretinites myopiques. Bull. Soc. Opht. Paris XLVI, 1:549, 1934 (Appendix I-XCIX).

Merkel, F. S. Cited by Duke Elder, W. S. System of Ophthalmology, Vol. III, Pt. 2: Congenital Deformities. Henry Kimpton, London, 1964, p. 553.

McKee, T. J. Juvenile glaucoma. Report of a case in a 19 year old soldier. Mil. Surgeon, 92:50, 1943.

Penfield, W., and Elvidge, A. R. Hydrocephalus and the atrophy of cerebral compression, pp. 1203-1217. In W. Penfield, ed., Cytology and Cellular Pathology of the Nervous System, Vol. 3. Hoeber, New York, 1932.

Phillips, C. L., and Quick, M. D. Impression tonometry and effect of eye volume variations. Br. J. Ophthalmol., 44:149, 1960.

Reis, W. Untersuchungen zur pathologischen Anatomie und zur Pathogenese des augeborenen Hydrophthalmus. Graefes Arch. Ophthal., 60:1, 1905.

Richardson, K. T., and Shaffer, R. N. Optic nerve cupping in congenital glaucoma. Am. J. Ophthalmol., 62:507, 1966.

Optic cup symmetry in normal newborn infants. Invest. Ophthalmol., 7:137, 1968.

Salzmann, M. The Anatomy and Histology of the Human Eyeball in the Normal State: Its Development and Senescence. The University of Chicago Press, Chicago, 1912.

Scheie, H. G. Infantile and juvenile glaucoma. Trans. Am. Acad. Ophthalmol. Otolaryng., 67:458, 1963.

Schmidt-Rimpler, H. Graefe Saemisch Handbuch, Vol. 6, 1908, p. 57.

Shaffer, R. N. New concepts in infantile glaucoma. Can. J. Ophthalmol., 2:243, 1967.

and Hetherington, Jr., J. The glaucomatous disc in infants, a suggested hypothesis for disc cupping. Trans. Am. Acad. Ophthalmol. Otolaryngol., 83:929, 1968.

Snydacker, D. The normal optic disc. Ophthalmoscopic and photographic studies. Am. J. Ophthalmol., 58:958, 1964.

Squire, C. Cited by Girard, L. J., Neely, W., and Sampson, W. G. The use of alpha chymotrypsin in infants and children. Am. J. Ophthalmol., 54:95, 1962.

Sugar, H. S. The congenital or infantile glaucomas. Am. J. Ophthalmol., 33:1679, 1950.

Weekers, R. Le glaucoma incomplet: contribution à l'étude du glaucome sans hypertension. Ophthalmologica, 104:316, 1942.

Nouvelle contribution à l'étude du glaucome incomplete: l'excavation glaucomateuse monosymptomatique. Ophthalmologica, 105:307, 1943.

Le glaucom incomplet. Ann. Oculist, 180:10, 1947.

Wexler, D. and Kornzweig, A. Buphthalmos in a six month premature infant. Arch. Ophthalmol. 37:318, 1947.

Worst, J. G. F. The Pathogenesis of Congenital Glaucoma. Royal Vangorcum, Ass. Netherlands, 1966, p. 31.

Congenital glaucoma: remarks on the aspect of chamber angle, ontogenetic and pathogenetic background and mode of action of goniotomy. Invest. Ophthalmol., 7:127, 1968.

7

Diagnosis and Investigation

The incidence of congenital glaucoma according to Anderson varies between 0.03 percent to 0.08 percent of ophthalmic patients. Lehrfeld and Reber noted an incidence of 0.01 percent of 250,000 patients in a study done between 1926 and 1935 at the Wills Eye Hospital. Af Ursin reported that of 1072 glaucoma cases three percent were of the infantile type. Juvenile glaucoma, taking thirty-five years of age as the upper limit, was diagnosed in 0.01 percent of out patient cases.

It has therefore been estimated that the average ophthalmologist is unlikely to see more than one new case in every five years of practice. In addition a significant number of cases arise in children after the age of three. Since glaucoma is hardly suspected at this time, such a patient might well not have his intraocular pressure measured, and a case of juvenile glaucoma would be overlooked. Other factors involved in the diagnosis of congenital glaucoma include the difficulty of examining an infant in the newborn nursery, the necessity of using a general anesthetic for each intraocular pressure measurement, and the wide variety of other conditions that may mimic the clinical appearance of congenital glaucoma (See Chap. 10). For these reasons the diagnosis and subsequent treatment remain a problem to the practicing ophthalmologist.

Congenital glaucoma is a significant cause of blindness in children. Bailliart found it to occur in 23.0 percent of children in schools for the blind while Anderson reported the incidence to vary between 2.4 and 13.5 percent. Gonin and Lamb reported a series in which from 5.0 to 13.0 percent of blind school children had hydrophthalmia; approximately two thirds were males and 70 to 74 percent were bilateral.

It is also noteworthy to remember that the characteristic feature of a congenital anomaly is that it is usually not an isolated event. That being the case it becomes necessary that the child with congenital glaucoma be investigated thoroughly apart from his eyes. To accomplish this task, several members of the medical and paramedical team must be called upon to complete this investigation so that surgical intervention may be undertaken with safety. In this chapter the role to be played by each member of the team will be outlined.

TIME OF ONSET

Gross reported that of 45 cases of hydrophthalmia, 60.0 percent were present at or very soon after birth, 13.3 percent were noted during the first year, 17.7 percent between the first and third years and 9.0 percent later. Becker and Shaffer reported that 60.0 percent of the cases of congenital glaucoma were diagnosed in the first six months of infancy and more than 80.0 percent had their onset before the first year. The author has analyzed a series of eighty-six eyes with congenital glaucoma and found that 21.0 percent were diagnosed before 5 days of life, 42.0 percent before six months, 30.0 percent before 3 years and 7.0 percent after 3 years. The studies generally indicate that congenital glaucoma is diagnosed before the sixth month of life in at least 60.0 percent of cases.

SIGNS AND SYMPTOMS

In the first instance the nursing staff in the newborn nursery must be made acutely aware of this condition. Any child exhibiting an unusually large or opaque cornea, tearing or photophobia should be brought to the attention of the pediatrician or ophthalmologist since the infant may not exhibit these symptoms at the exact time medical rounds are made.

Table 1 illustrates the initial signs and symptoms that first became evident in a series of sixteen eyes (birth to five days). A hazy appearance of the cornea (Fig. 1) was the commonest initial sign and symptom (88 percent). This was followed by photophobia (44 percent) and enlargement of the cornea (31 percent) and eyeball (25 percent, Fig. 2). Tearing was the least frequent symptom. In this series the largest cornea was 15 mm measured in the horizontal diameter.

Following discharge the child should be examined on a routine basis by the aware general practitioner or pediatrician. An enlarged eye is easily noticed and may even be interpreted by the parents as the baby's "big blue eyes." A hazy cornea will prevent a clear ophthalmoscopic observation of retinal details and this should arouse suspicion. Table 2 illustrates the signs and symptoms noted in a series of 37 eyes in an age group five days to six

TABLE 1

INFANTILE GLAUCOMA–BIRTH TO FIVE DAYS:
9 Patients*–16 Eyes

Initial signs and symptoms	Eyes	%
Hazy cornea	14	88
Photophobia	7	44
Enlarged cornea	6	31
Enlarged eye	4	25
Epiphora	1	.06
Characteristics		
Sex		
Males		78
Females		22
Bilateral		8 of 9 patients

*In one patient signs and symptoms were present at birth in one eye and began at one month in the other eye.

months. In this series an enlarged cornea (76 percent) and a hazy cornea (73 percent) were the commonest presenting signs. The largest cornea in this series was 17 mm measured in the horizontal diameter. Other less common signs and symptoms were an enlarged eye (59 percent) and photophobia (41 percent). Epiphora was the least common sign (22 percent). In the age group six months to thirty-six months (Table 3) the enlarged eye was the commonest sign (85 percent) in this series of 20 eyes. A hazy cornea (70 percent)

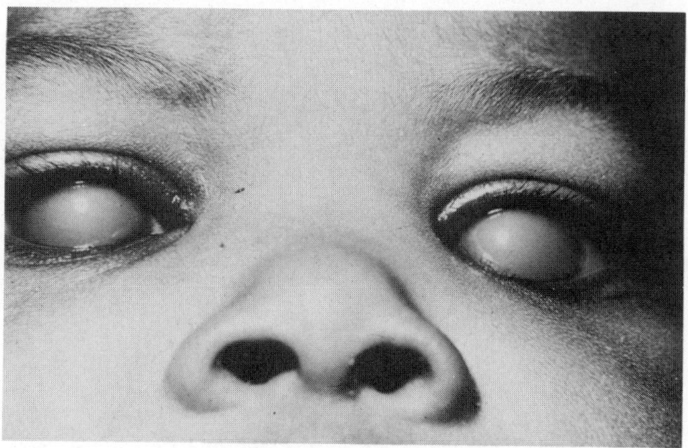

FIG. 1. Bilateral congenital glaucoma. (Courtesy of C. M. Alexander.)

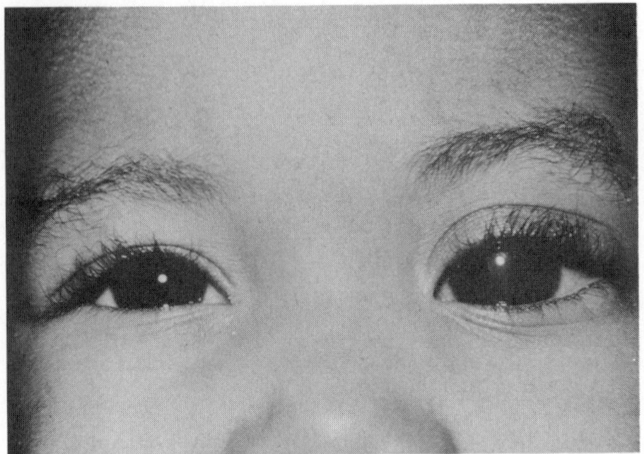

FIG. 2. Enlargement of one eye due to congenital glaucoma. (Courtesy of C. M. Alexander.)

and enlarged cornea (65 percent) followed. The largest cornea noted in this series was 16 mm measured in the horizontal diameter. The least common symptoms were photophobia and epiphora (45 percent, respectively). The typical symptom complex is illustrated in Fig. 3, which shows a photophobic child with congenital glaucoma, displaying epiphora, cloudy corneas, and blepharospasm.

TABLE 2.

INFANTILE GLAUCOMA–FIVE DAYS TO SIX MONTHS: 24 Patients*–37 Eyes

Initial signs and symptoms

	Eyes	%
Enlarged cornea	28	76
Hazy cornea	27	73
Enlarged eye	22	59
Photophobia	15	41
Epiphora	8	22

Characteristics

Sex		
Males		50
Females		50
Bilateral		14 of 24 patients

*In one patient signs and symptoms were present at birth in one eye and began at one month in the other eye.

TABLE 3

INFANTILE GLAUCOMA–SIX MONTHS TO THIRTY-SIX MONTHS:

14 Patients–20 Eyes

Initial signs and symptoms

	Eyes	%
Enlarged eye	17	85
Hazy cornea	14	70
Enlarged cornea	13	65
Photophobia	9	45
Epiphora	9	45

Characteristics

Sex		
Males		50
Females		50
Bilateral		6 of 14 patients

Whereas the newborn glaucoma cases were predominately male (78 percent) in all the other groups, males and females were equal in number although most other studies show males to outnumber females. While almost all of the newborns with glaucoma had both eyes involved, with increasing age fewer of the patients had a bilateral condition.

Fourteen of the eyes had conditions which by themselves could affect

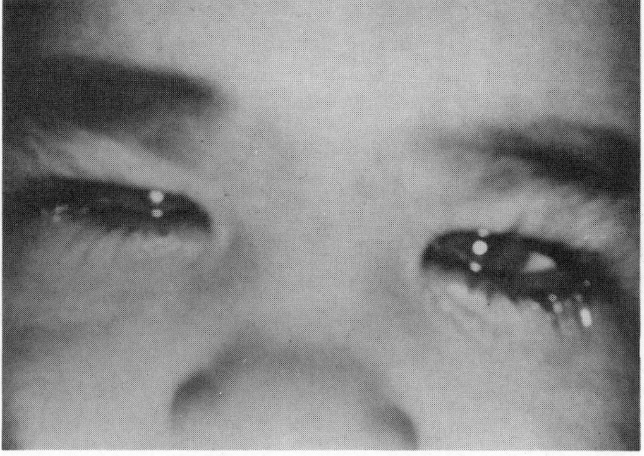

FIG. 3. Typical symptom complex of epiphora, photophobia, cloudy cornea, and blepharospasm.

visual acuity. There were seven patients with strabismus, four with nystagmus, two with congenital cataracts, and one with a corneal opacity.

Although an eye with high myopia must be differentiated from the large eye of congenital glaucoma, the two conditions may occur together. Five patients in this series had myopia in excess of 3.50 diopters. On the other hand, the eye with congenital glaucoma need not necessarily be myopic. According to Parsons, enlargement of the globe leads to a flattening of the cornea with flattening and posterior displacement of the lens. This brings about a change in the location of the cardinal points so that the eye must approach 31 mm in length for emmetropia. According to Gross the average anteroposterior diameter of the eye with congenital glaucoma is 32 mm. Therefore the eye with congenital glaucoma might well be emmetropic or have any variety of refractive error.

Blockage of the nasolacrimal system must be considered when one is examining a child with suspected congenital glaucoma. Two children in the series had to be probed. On the other hand, Scheie has noted that the nasolacrimal passages could be probed for tearing that was caused by the effects of raised intraocular pressure. In this series tearing was the least common symptom.

Any of these signs or symptoms when noted by the pediatrician or general practitioner should result in a consultation with an ophthalmologist.

OPHTHALMOLOGY OFFICE VISIT

On the initial visit to the ophthalmologist a comprehensive history should be taken from the parents. A letter from the referring physician must be noted. A careful inquiry must be made into the pregnancy, asking specifically about rubella. A good family history will reveal the presence or absence of adult glaucoma, another case of buphthalmia, or some other congenital defect. The pregnancy may have been unwanted or an abortion may have been attempted, giving rise to guilt feelings. If the child is young it will not always be possible to conduct a complete examination including tonometry, gonioscopy, and ophthalmoscopy in the office. However, a satisfactory external examination may be accomplished—especially if the mother has been wise enough to bring along a bottle or "pacifier." The infant will frequently open the eyes widely while sucking on a nipple and a presumptive diagnosis may be made. A non-dimpled Koeppe gonioscope lens (pediatric size) should be available since it is sometimes possible to insert this lens during the office examination. The eyelids are thus widely separated allowing an ophthalmoscopic examination and perhaps even gonioscopy.

Although the clinical appearance is not always characteristic even to an experienced observer (Chap. 10 outlines the various conditions which may simulate congenital glaucoma), an investigation in a hospital with the infant under general anesthesia becomes necessary when the case is highly suggestive.

It is essential that the ophthalmologist give the parents a detailed picture of their situation. They should be made aware of the protracted nature of the illness, the prognosis, the frequent necessity of repeated surgery, and the life-long necessity for continued examinations. It is often necessary to treat the anxiety of the parents as well as the physical illness of the child. Often they are young and both emotionally and economically ill-equipped to cope with the problems that have suddenly and dramatically beset them.

The ophthalmologist should familiarize the parents with the various agencies that will afford financial help if necessary. It is important to make inquiries and arrangements beforehand since it is difficult to obtain retroactive help. It is often not possible or wise to present all this information at the initial consultation. During the period of investigation in the hospital there will be ample opportunity during the frequent visits to the child's room to present the parents with the various aspects of the condition. This time and effort will reward the ophthalmologist many times over at a later date, particularly if surgical progress is not going well.

The social aspects of the disease must also be discussed. The parents must be aware of the fact that the glaucomatous condition may be arrested by means of the surgical procedure but that the vision may remain poor. They must later receive expert instruction on how to raise such a child. He may require visual aids, his cosmetic blemishes will need correction where possible, and the proper school will have to be selected.

HOSPITAL INVESTIGATION

Upon admission to the hospital, the suspected child should be thoroughly investigated to rule out possible systemic disease. Particular attention should be directed toward the cardiac status. In rubella infections for example, a well-recognized cause of congenital glaucoma, it has been shown that there is a high correlation of eye and heart involvement. The examination under anesthesia would have to be deferred if a cardiac abnormality were noted. In this event the child should be placed on acetazolamide (Diamox) by mouth in a dosage up to 15 mg/kg body weight per day. (See Chap. 13).

Acetazolamide is a diuretic and acid-base regulator of low toxicity. It is an enzyme inhibitor and acts specifically on carbonic anhydrase. The diuretic effect is due to its action on the reversible hydration of carbon dioxide and dehydration of the carbonic acid reaction in the kidney. The result is renal loss of HCO_3 ion which carries out sodium, water, and potassium. Diuresis and alkalinization of the urine thus occur. The effect of acetazolamide on the eye is due to its inhibitory effect on carbonic anhydrase in the ciliary body. The result is a decrease in aqueous humor production.

By reducing the pCO_2 the drug also has an ameliorating effect in respiratory acidosis but should be used with caution in patients depleted of sodium or potassium.

Acetazolamide is also contraindicated in Addison's disease and other types of suprarenal gland failure. Because it is a sulfonamide derivative, any of the reactions which have been reported to follow the administration of the bacteriostatic sulfonamides may occur.

The potassium level may be maintained by using Kaon elixir. This form of potassium gluconate supplies 20 mEq of elemental potassium (as potassium gluconate 4.68 g) in each 15 ml (one tablespoonful). Each 5 ml (one teaspoonful) supplies elemental potassium approximately equal to that of 0.5 g potassium chloride. In therapeutic dosage, the elixir is well tolerated without gastrointestinal disturbances. Orange juice also contains significant amounts of potassium and may be used as an alternate. Potassium should not be given when there is inadequate urinary output.

The minimal normal daily loss of potassium in a one-year-old infant is approximately 330 mg (8.5 mEq), which is equivalent to 6.3 cc of Kaon elixir. When the patient is given acetazolamide the potassium supplement should be added at the same time. Chemical analysis may be used to determine any further degree of hypokalemia.

The child should also be examined by an endocrinologist, as a variety of conditions may either be associated with hydrophthalmia or feature an ocular condition that simulates congenital glaucoma. These conditions are outlined in Chapters 9 and 10. Upon admission, in addition to the routine examinations, the following laboratory tests should be ordered. The urine should be tested for porphyrin and mucopolysaccharides, and amino-acid chromatography should be performed. The blood should also undergo amino-acid chromatography. Radiologic examination should include the hands, feet, and spinal column in addition to the routine chest x-ray. If a history of rubella exists, throat and nasal cultures should be obtained as well as determining the antibody titer of the mother.

PREMEDICATION

The pupil should be constricted with local 2% pilocarpine administered four to five times in the 2-hr period prior to surgery. The lens will thus be protected during the goniotomy procedure. If an examination is planned for diagnostic purposes only, it is best not to constrict the pupil so that an adequate examination of the fundus may be made. Atropine sulfate may be given in the premedication period because the anterior chamber is deep, the filtration angle is open, and the pupil is constricted with pilocarpine. The child may be placed on acetazolamide for several days prior to surgery in order to lower the intraocular pressure and clear the cornea. This would facilitate the examination in the nursery. However, the drug should be discontinued at least three days before the examination under anesthesia because the intraocular pressure measurement should be influenced by as few factors as possible.

Acetazolamide should not be used postoperatively since an active aqueous humor flow will help irrigate the hyphema that is usually present immediately following surgery. It would also maintain the surgical cleft in the filtration angle. Barbiturates and opiates should not be used in the preoperative medication as they tend to lower the intraocular pressure.

ANESTHESIA

Kornblueth et al. noted a lowering of the intraocular pressure in adults by an average of 6.5 mm Hg with diethyl ether, vinyl ether, cyclopropane, and sodium pentothal. The decrease was slightly less (5.7 mm Hg) with diethyl ether as compared with sodium pentothal (7.0 mm Hg). Tonography was characterized by an increase in outflow with these same agents. Using sodium pentothal, de Roetth and Schwartz reported an average fall of 19 mm Hg in intraocular pressure in cases of open-angle glaucoma, in keeping with the findings of Hallet. Morphine, Seconal, and Demerol also caused a decrease in intraocular pressure. Magora and Collins noted a decrease of from 17.3 mm Hg to 11.2 mm Hg with Fluothane, chloroform, and Trilene in normal eyes. Hetherington and Shaffer found that diethyl ether produced a decrease of 6 to 7 mm Hg in five children (10 eyes) who were undergoing follow-up examinations for congenital glaucoma.

The hypotensive effect of the anesthetic agent results from a reduction in aqueous humor production, muscle relaxation (extraocular), depression of the diencephalon and vascular changes. Muscle relaxants, which are often used during general anesthesia, may also affect intraocular tension.

Some congenital glaucoma patients may have been treated with one of the strong anticholinesterase drugs such as demecarium bromide (Humorsol), di-isopropyl-fluorophosphate (Floropryl), and echothiophate iodide (Phospholine Iodide) prior to surgery. Alfano described two patients with congenital glaucoma who developed apnea and atony following the administration of succinylcholine during the induction phase of general anesthesia. The first patient had received demecarium bromide (Humorsol, (0.25%) twice a day in the involved eye for about one year. In this case the serum pseudocholinesterase level was 80 dibucaine units but the serum cholinesterase measured 32 units (normal range 33 to 55 units). The second patient had not received anticholinesterase drugs but had a pseudocholinesterase level of 20.50 dibucaine units (normal range 71.0 to 85.0 dibucaine units). These drugs exert their effect through the inhibition of the enzyme cholinesterase, thereby preventing rapid inactivation of actetylcholine. This action occurs at the neuromuscular junctions and synapses throughout the central and peripheral nervous systems. Acetylcholine accumulates and then exerts its muscarinic action on the heart, smooth muscle, and secretory glands, and its nicotinic action on skeletal muscle and autonomic ganglia.

There are two types of human cholinesterases: (1) true acetylcholinesterase, which is present in the red bood cells, central nervous system, muscle, and motor end plate and (2) pseudocholinesterase, which is found in the plasma and various tissues. Anticholinesterase drugs may inhibit both types of enzymes. Repeated minimal exposures to anticholinesterase substances may depress the acetylcholinesterase level to a low level without producing clinical evidence of toxicity. In addition, symptoms may occur following a single large dose without significant enzyme inhibition. Leopold et al. found red blood cell and plasma cholinesterase depression in glaucomatous patients on Phospholine Iodide and on Humersol therapy for over two months. Drance described one glaucomatous patient in whom there was an immediate generalized reaction following instillation of Phospholine Iodide which consisted of abdominal pain, diarrhea, bradycardia, low blood pressure, tremors, generalized weakness, and headache. The symptoms were counteracted by the subcutaneous administration of atropine. Hiscox and McCulloch reported severe reaction in a 72-year-old glaucoma patient who had been on Phospholine Iodide for about 10 months. Both her acetylcholinesterase and pseudocholinesterase levels were markedly depressed.

When a history of the use of one of these drugs has been elicited in a patient with congenital glaucoma, succinylcholine should not be used during general anesthesia because it potentiates the anticholinesterase action. If succinylcholine must be used, serum cholinesterase levels should be determined beforehand.

INSTRUMENTATION

The operating room should be equipped with a Zeiss operating microscope which has been fitted with a Goldmann applanation tonometer (Fig. 4) as described by Leith and Chandler and Grant, as well as a slitlamp attachment. Schirmer has designed a slitlamp which may be used as an operating microscope (Fig. 5). The examination should not be undertaken until the child has reached the level of surgical anesthesia.

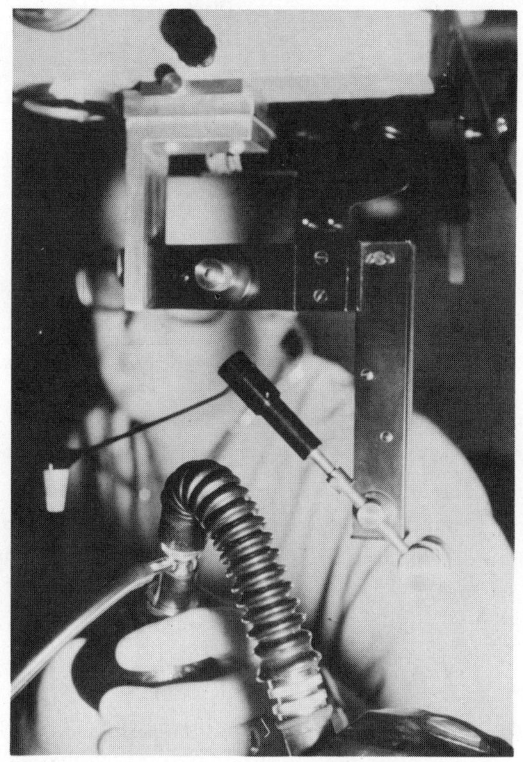

FIG. 4. Applanation tonometer fitted to a Zeiss operating microscope.

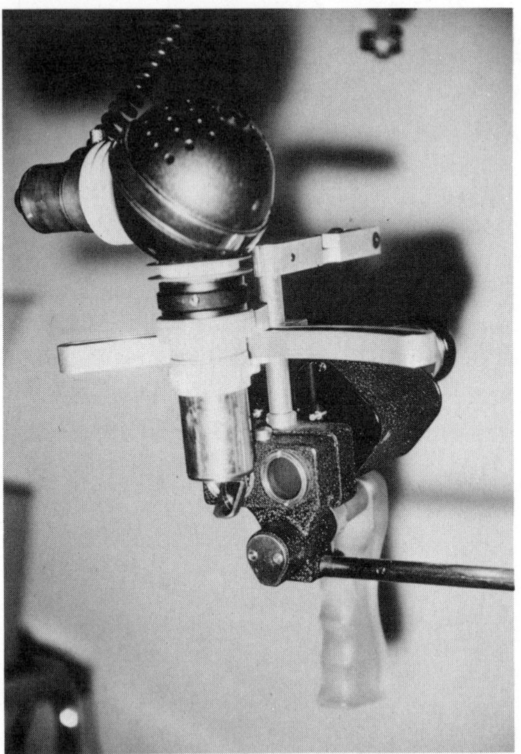

FIG. 5. Slitlamp-operating microscope. (Courtesy of K. Schirmer.)

Corneal Measurement

The corneal diameter is measured horizontally with the millimeter caliper (Fig. 6). When the horizontal end points are obscure, a vertical measurement should be included. The following figures are helpful in judging the average horizontal diameter of the cornea in infancy (Figs. in parantheses show the statistical average): at birth, 9.5 mm (9.44 mm); at 6 months, 10.5 mm (10.82 mm); and at 1 year, 11.5 mm (11.39 mm); Beyond the first year of life the corneal diameter normally increases very little. If the cornea is more than 11 mm in the newborn or more than 12 mm in diameter at any age, one should be highly suspicious. Megalocornea, an inherited corneal enlargement without associated signs of glaucoma may in some instances cause confusion in diagnosis.

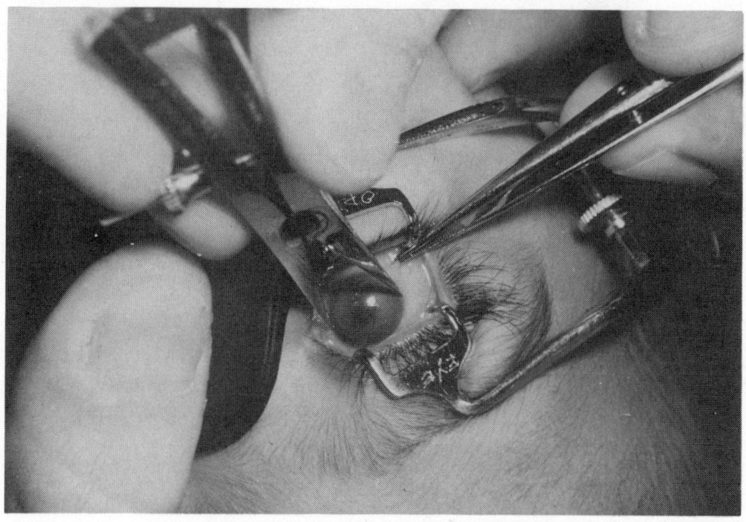

FIG. 6. Use of calipers in measuring horizontal diameter of infant cornea.

Slitlamp Examination

The cornea should be examined with the slitlamp (Fig. 7). Characteristic signs of congenital glaucoma include corneal haze (Fig. 8) and Haab's striae which represent tears in Descemet's membrane (Fig. 9A and B). Corneal clouding may occur without raised intraocular pressure in Hurler's disease by trauma, and in some dystrophic conditions. It may occur in the rubella syndrome—with or without pressure. Finally, clouding may occur not only in primary infantile glaucoma but in all of the secondary infantile glaucomas as well (Chap. 11).

Ocular Fundus Examination

An attempt should be made to examine the ocular fundus with the ophthalmoscope, with the examiner noting especially the appearance of the optic nerve head, which should be drawn, and the relative size of the optic cup recorded. The incidence of glaucomatous cupping may be as high as 50 percent on the initial examination (Fig. 10 A and B). The importance of this examination is emphasized in Chapter 11, which outlines the variety of

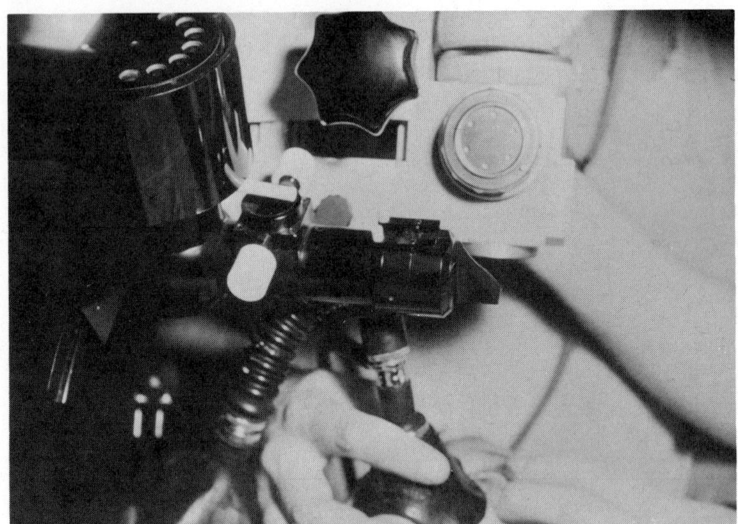

FIG. 7. Slitlamp attachment with Zeiss operating microscope.

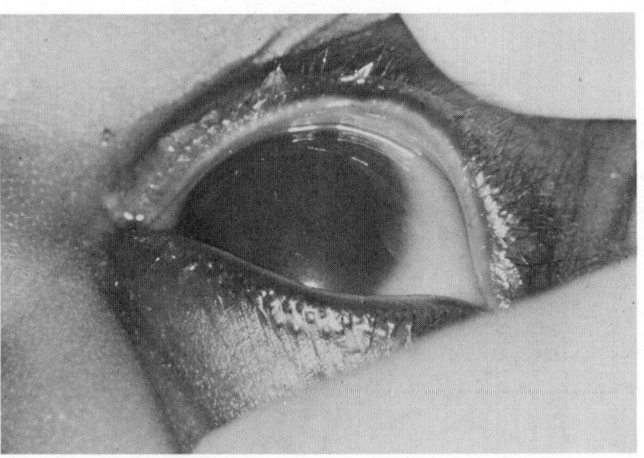

FIG. 8. Hazy cornea of congenital glaucoma.

posterior lesions that cause a rise in intraocular pressure. The miotic pupil (constricted with pilocarpine preoperatively) and hazy cornea may preclude such an examination. In this event, when a posterior lesion is suspected clinically, another examination may have to be performed at a later time with the pupil maximally dilated. When corneal irregularities obscure the

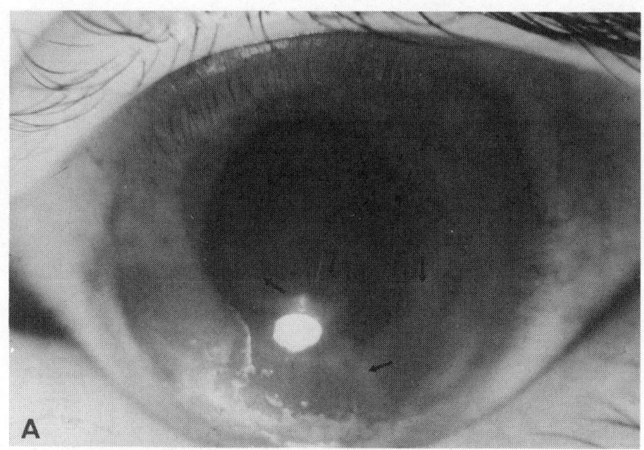

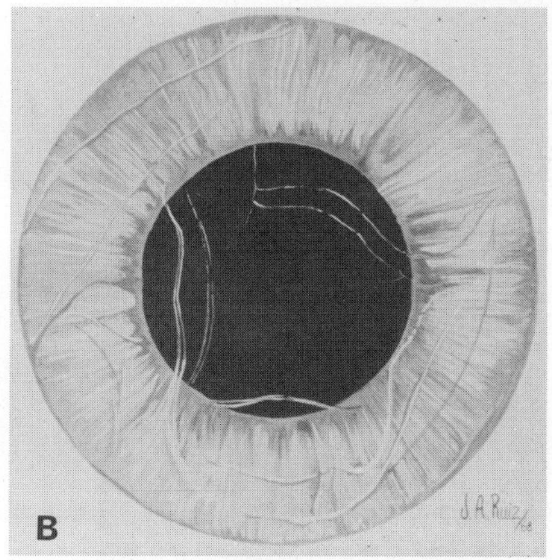

FIG. 9.A. Tears in Descemet's membrane (clinical appearance). **B.** Tears in Descemet's membrane (drawing).

fundus, the corneal epithelium may be removed with a cotton applicator, soaked in 70 percent alcohol, and the fundus viewed either directly or through the goniolens.

Intraocular Pressure Measurement

Giles reported a mean intraocular pressure of 25.8 mm Hg without the use of general anesthesia in 32 term newborns but admitted that the examination was difficult and the results possibly inaccurate. Kornblueth and co-workers found that the intraocular pressure in normal newborn infants under general anesthesia was consistently higher than in the normal eyes of adults measured under similar conditions. The average values found

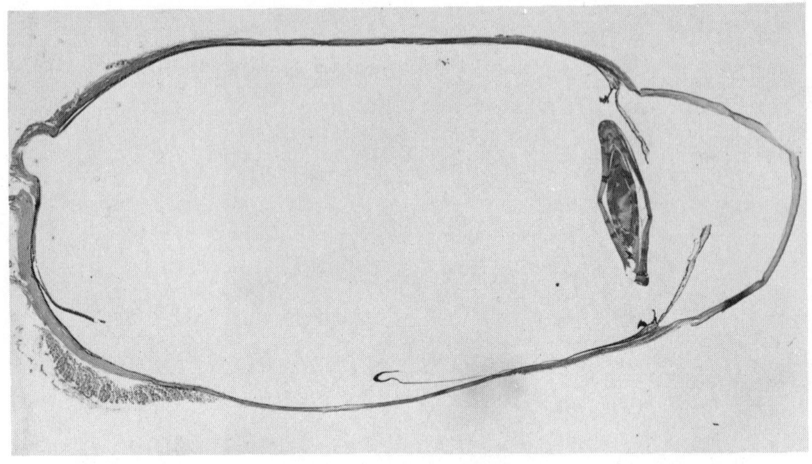

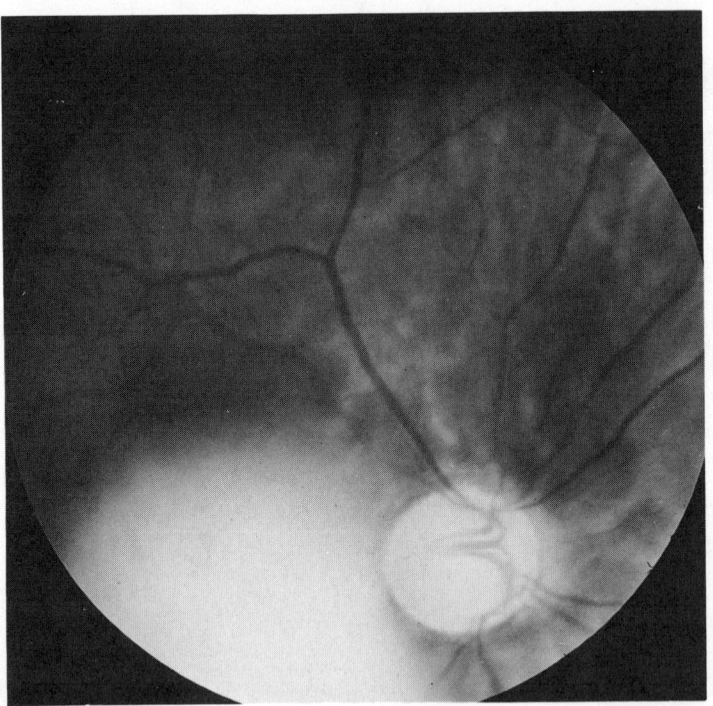

FIG. 10.A. Cupping of the optic nerve head in congenital glaucoma. (A. F. I. P. Neg. 935268.) (Courtesy of the Registry of Ophthalmic Pathology of the Armed Forces Institute of Pathology.) X 2.9. **B.** Cupping of the optic nerve in congenital glaucoma.

in this study declined gradually from 21.1 mm Hg in the youngest (birth to one year) to 15.7 mm Hg in the oldest group (eight to nine years).

With the popularity of the new anesthetic agents which were introduced over the past 20 years, initial tonometric readings found in infantile glaucoma have tended to be less constant, reducing the significance of the intraocular pressure in making the diagnosis. In general the effect of the anesthetic agent upon the intraocular pressure tends to parallel its effect on the cardiovascular status. Hence halothane (Fluothane) tends to lower the pressure. In addition succinylcholine temporarily elevates the pressure. Obviously the standardization of anesthesia for diagnosis and follow-up of congenital glaucoma is desirable and inconsistent readings should be evaluated in light of the patient's general ocular state as well as the agent in use.

Sampaolesi and co-workers found that applanation tonometry measurements in twenty-four children aged one month to five years (measurements taken under general anesthesia with methoxyflurone) varied between 7.5 and 13.5 mm Hg. Apt examined young patients under "slow induction" rectal Pentothal anesthesia and Surital anesthesia and found a normal range between 12 to 18 mm Hg.

Elevated intraocular pressure measurements with the use of the Schiötz tonometer have been recorded in normal infants during routine general anesthesia. This can occur with light anesthesia, excessive eye movements, laryngospasm, and improper positioning of the face mask or head such as would affect the endotrachial tube. Low tensions may be noted in infants with congenital glaucoma due to a relative dehydration that occurs prior to anesthesia due to food and fluid withdrawal. Moreau and Cornibert found severe hypotony associated with malnutrition. In addition the intraocular pressure varies from day to day and at different times of the same day in children as well as in adults.

Haas studied the untreated intraocular pressure in a series of 75 patients with infantile glaucoma. This study is summarized in Fig. 11A and B and shows that the intraocular pressure is independent of age and is as high in patients in whom the onset is early in life as it is with those of later onset.

Hetherington and Shaffer studied a large series of cases that included unoperated patients aged three days to one year with symptoms and signs of congenital glaucoma; patients aged three months to three years under follow-up care for congenital glaucoma; and 30 eyes of patients aged three months to seven years with no clinical evidence of glaucoma. They made the following observations. In the unoperated congenital glaucoma group at the level of surgical anesthesia, intraocular pressures were found to be below 21 mm Hg in only three eyes. The mean pressure was 32.6 mm Hg, with a

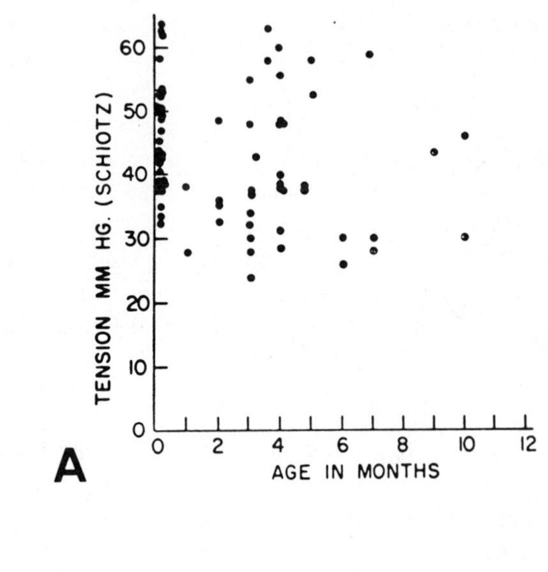

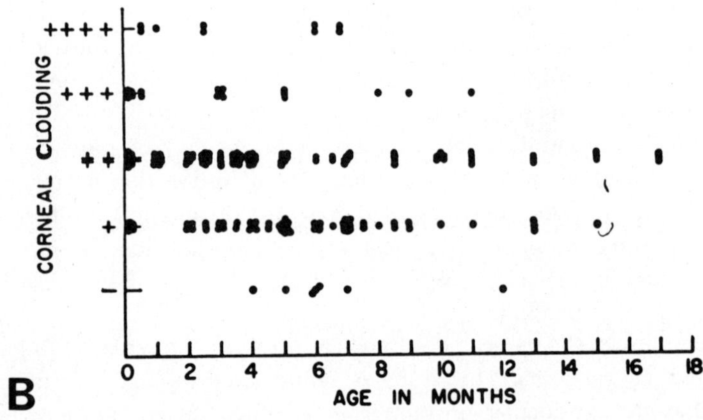

FIG. 11.A. Relationship of patient's age at time of diagnosis to intraocular pressure without treatment. Elevated pressures are similar and correspond to degree of corneal clouding. (Adapted from Haas. **Invest. Ophthalmol.** 7:140, 1968.) **B.** Degree of corneal clouding present at time of diagnosis, revealing lack of relationship as in Fig. 11A. (Adapted from Haas. **Invest. Ophthalmol.** 7:140, 1968.)

range of 17 to 59 mm Hg. In the follow-up group the mean pressure was 21.8 mm Hg with a range of 6 to 27 mm Hg under deep anesthesia. Under light anesthesia the mean pressure was 28.5 mm Hg, with a range that varied from 14 to 45 mm Hg. Therefore, with the subject under deep anesthesia the intraocular pressure decreased an average of 6.7 mm Hg. The extremes of decreases in intraocular pressure were from 0 to 28 mm Hg. Reduction in pressure occurred in 75 percent of patients and the pressure reduction during anesthesia was greater when the initial pressure was highest.

In the normal group the average pressure at the level of surgical anesthesia was 12.5 mm Hg, with a range of 7 to 22 mm Hg.

Costenbader and Kwitko examined 77 children with congenital glaucoma and made the following observations from use of the Schiötz tonometer at the level of surgical anesthesia. In the group of infants birth to five days, the average intraocular pressure recorded was 47.0 mm Hg. The highest pressure was 61.0 mm Hg (nine patients, 16 eyes). In the group aged five days to six months the average intraocular pressure was 39.9 mm Hg, with the highest recording of 60.0 mm Hg (24 patients, 37 eyes). In the group aged six months to three years the average pressure was 46.6 mm Hg, with the highest recording at 80 mm Hg (14 patients, 20 eyes). In the group over 36 months the average pressure was 43.0 mm Hg, with the highest pressure at 55 mm Hg (four patients, four eyes).

Tonography Measurements

NORMAL EYES. Graff and Dyson studied tonography values in children ranging in age from 11 to 13 years. They found that although the scleral rigidity values were higher than values attributed to adult steady-state eyes, the facility of outflow and Po/C ratio fell within limits accepted as normal for adults. Hetherington and Shaffer recorded an average coefficient of outflow of 0.15, with a range from 0 to 0.32 in infants.

Halasa studied tonography values in normal and malnourished children aged one month to one year. The mean Po value was 21 mm Hg and the mean C value was 0.33 in each group, respectively. He found a negative correlation between Po values and age and between Po values and weight.

ABNORMAL EYES. The present tonography tables are calculated for the adult cornea with glaucoma, which differs markedly in several important characteristics from the infant cornea that is affected by congenital glaucoma. Most important is the corneal edema often present in the buphthalmic eye, which results in a distinct central indentation after the foot plate of the tonometer has been applied. Since this technical aberration has not been accounted for in the present tonography tables, it should not be ignored when one is evaluating the tonography results.

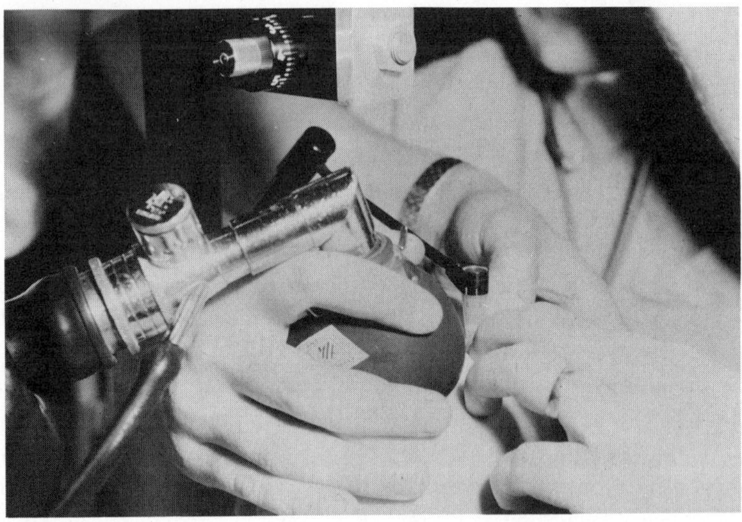

FIG. 12. Applanation tonometer in use during general anesthesia.

Hetherington and Shaffer studied tonography values in a series of patients with signs and symptoms of congenital glaucoma. In the group of

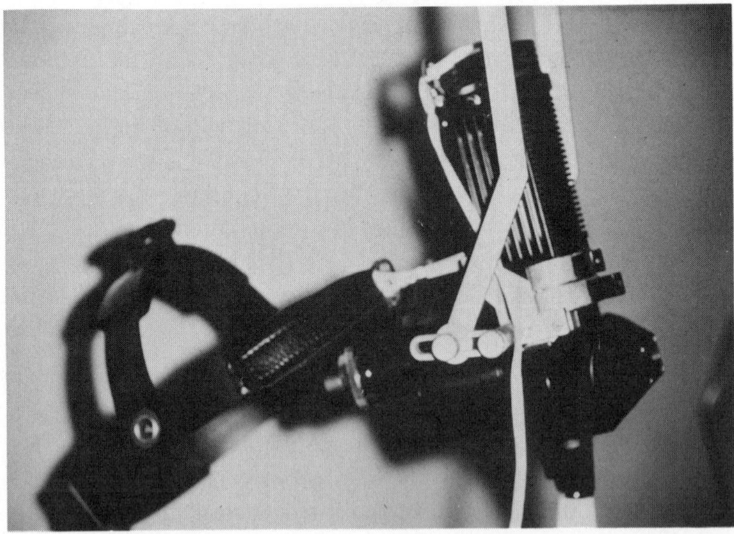

FIG. 13. Heine gonioscope, counterbalanced and fitted with headband. (Courtesy of K. Schirmer.)

patients under follow-up care tonography values varied over a wide range–from 0.02 to 0.24, with an average coefficient of outflow of 0.13. Shaffer studied the tonographic tracings of 32 goniotomized eyes. The follow-up period was from one year to 25 years. In 23 eyes (72 percent) the tonography results were technically good. An intraocular pressure of 20 mm Hg or below was noted (7 mm Hg, to 20 mm Hg, with a mean of 15 mm Hg); the facility of outflow varied between 0.19 to 0.37, with a mean of 0.25; and the Po/C ratio varied from 30 to 84, with a mean of 57. In nine eyes (28 percent) the tonography results were questionable. An intraocular pressure of 14 to 18 mm Hg was noted, with a mean of 16 mm Hg; the facility of outflow varied between 0.10 to 0.18, with a mean of 0.14; and the Po/C ratio showed a range which varied from 55 to 126, with a mean of 93.

Tonometers

Both the Schiötz tonometer and the tonography apparatus are less than ideal for measuring the intraocular pressure and analyzing the facility of outflow in young children. Scleral rigidity affects the Schiötz tonometer readings, while the 4-min interval for tonography allows the plunger to indent the edematous cornea of the hypertensive eye, yielding an unreliable tracing. Smith and co-workers compared tonometric results using the Schiötz and applanation tonometers in adults. They found that applanation values are generally higher in 84 percent of the eyes by a strikingly large spread of values. It was generally agreed that the Goldmann applanation tonometer (Fig. 12) yielded the truest measure of the intraocular pressure. This should also apply to hand-held applanation tonometers such as the Draeger instrument. The MacKay-Marg electric recording tonometer has been tested against the applanation tonometer by Hilton and Shaffer and found to compare favorably. These instruments may be used in the operating room. Intraocular pressure measurements on infants and children will of necessity be made with the patient in the supine position. It is generally agreed that in this position the intraocular pressure is higher by 1 to 2 mm Hg and lower when the patient is erect.

Gonioscopy

After the intraocular pressure has been measured and recorded, gonioscopy should be performed by using the gonioscope and Koeppe contact lens. Schirmer has modified the Heine gonioscope for use in the

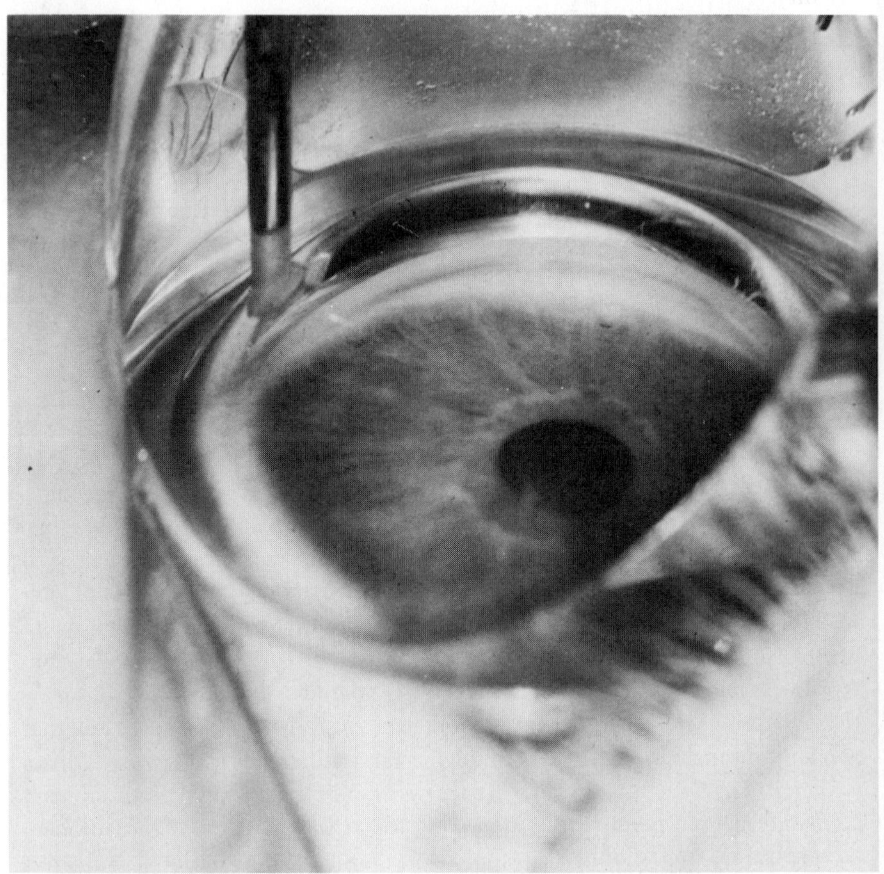

FIG. 14.A. Chamber angle of congenital glaucoma viewed with Worst lens.

operating room (Fig. 13). The Worst lens may be used with the operating microscope. If there is excessive epithelial haze this may be cleared with one or two drops of glycerine. If the haze persists the epithelium may be scraped with a scalpel (No. 15 Bard-Parker blade). Van den Heuvel uses a drop of 70 percent alcohol, which coagulates the epithelium and eases its removal with a cotton-tipped applicator. With the Koeppe contact lens in place the filtration may be observed by using the binocular microscope. A deep anterior chamber with an iris that sweeps upward toward Schwalbe's line. Fig. 14A, B, and C is characteristic of congenital glaucoma. The insertion rarely is high enough to obscure a gonioscopic view of the trabeculum,

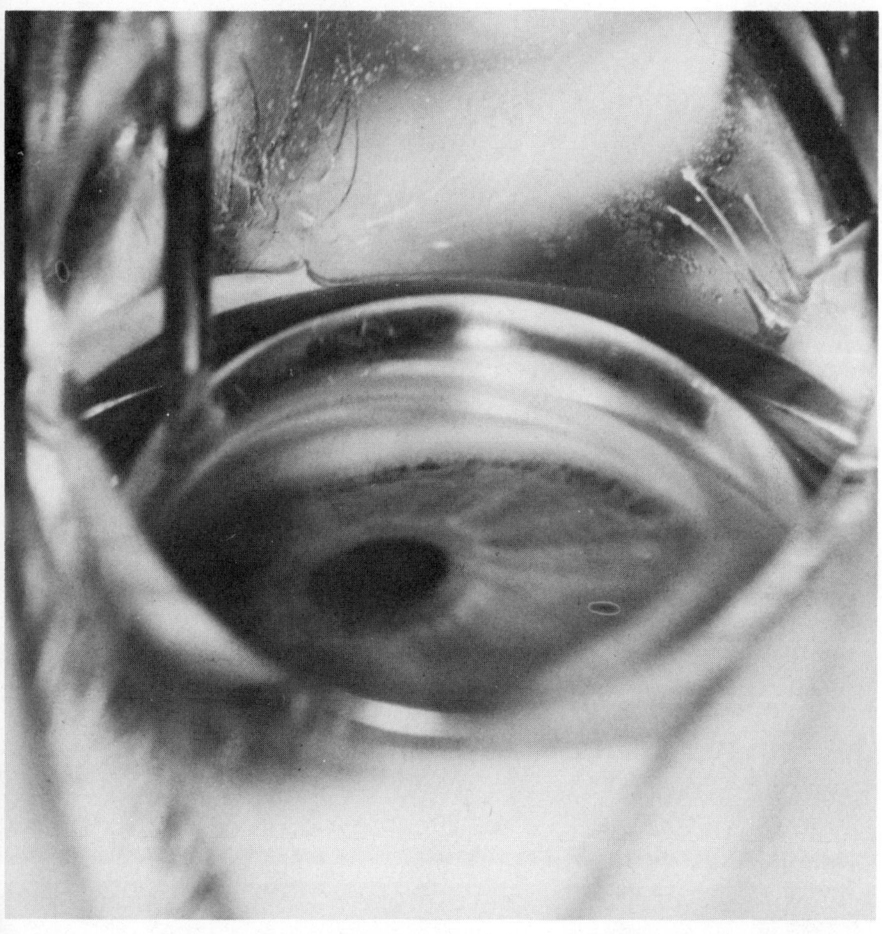

FIG. 14.B. Chamber angle of congenital glaucoma. Anterior sheet of mesoderm is partially detached from Schwalbe's line.

and frequently one can visualize a veil extending from the root of the iris along the angle wall. The iris vessels are usually hyperemic and their branches run tortuously through the angle sulcus. Pigmentary arcades may be seen through the iris stroma. When the corneal diameter is 14 mm or less the canal of Schlemm may spontaneously fill with blood or this phenomenon may be produced by compression of the jugular vein. With the canal of Schlemm filled with blood the insertion of the iris does not seem high enough to block the aqueous outflow. Thick pectinate ligaments may

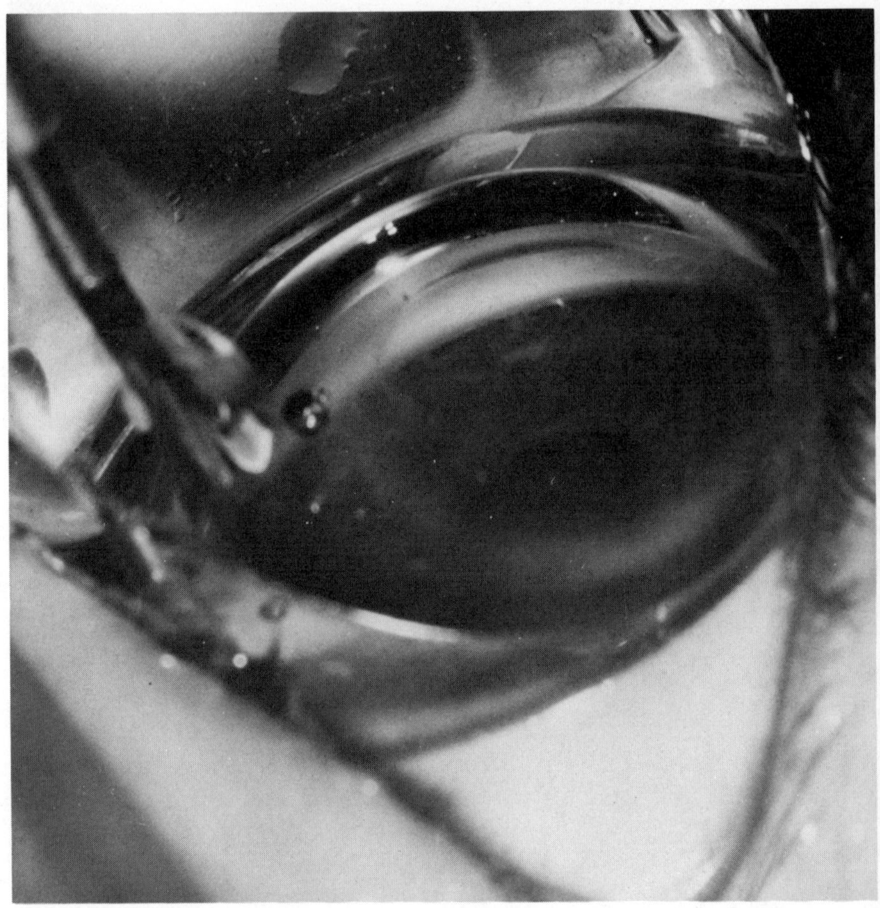

FIG. 14.C. Chamber angle of congenital glaucoma. Tears in Descemet's membrane are evident.

be present (Fig. 15), in normal as well as glaucomatous eyes. Although many patients with infantile glaucoma do not appear to have a diagnostic angle deformity, a decided difference in iris insertion may be seen in unilateral cases (Fig. 16A. and B.). Fig. 17 illustrates the normal filtration angle of a five-year-old child. The iris maintains a flatter plateau as it approaches the angle. The ciliary body may be viewed through the gonioscopic lens and blood may be seen filling Schlemm's canal. Iridocorneal adhesions and

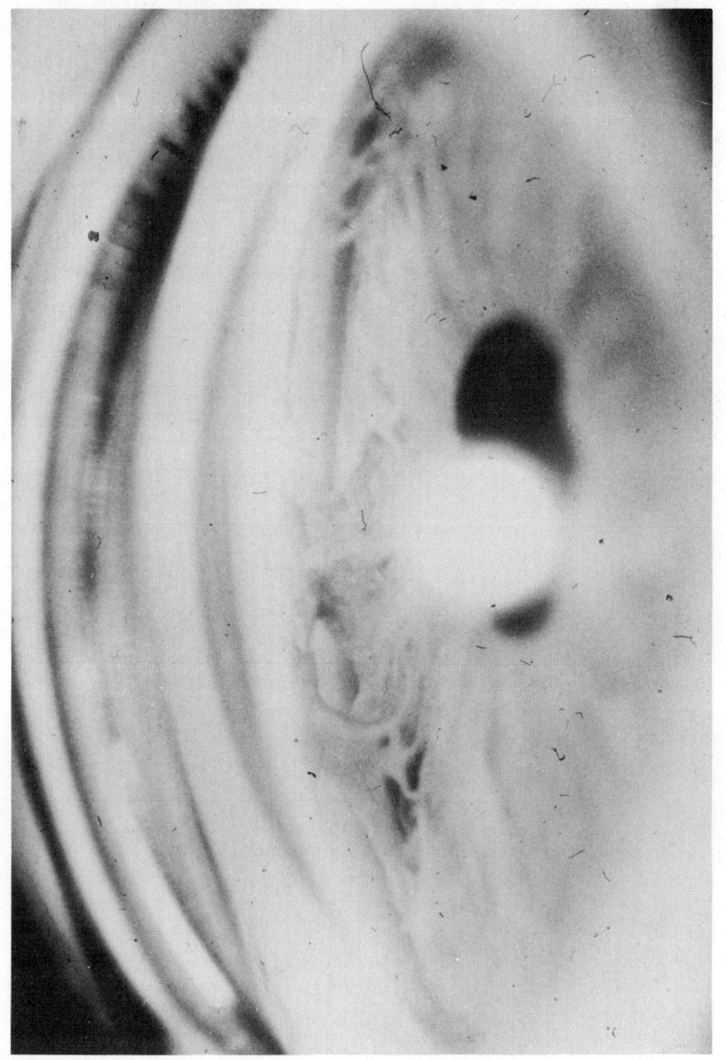

FIG. 15. Pectinate ligaments in filtration angle (Courtesy of N. Jaffe.)

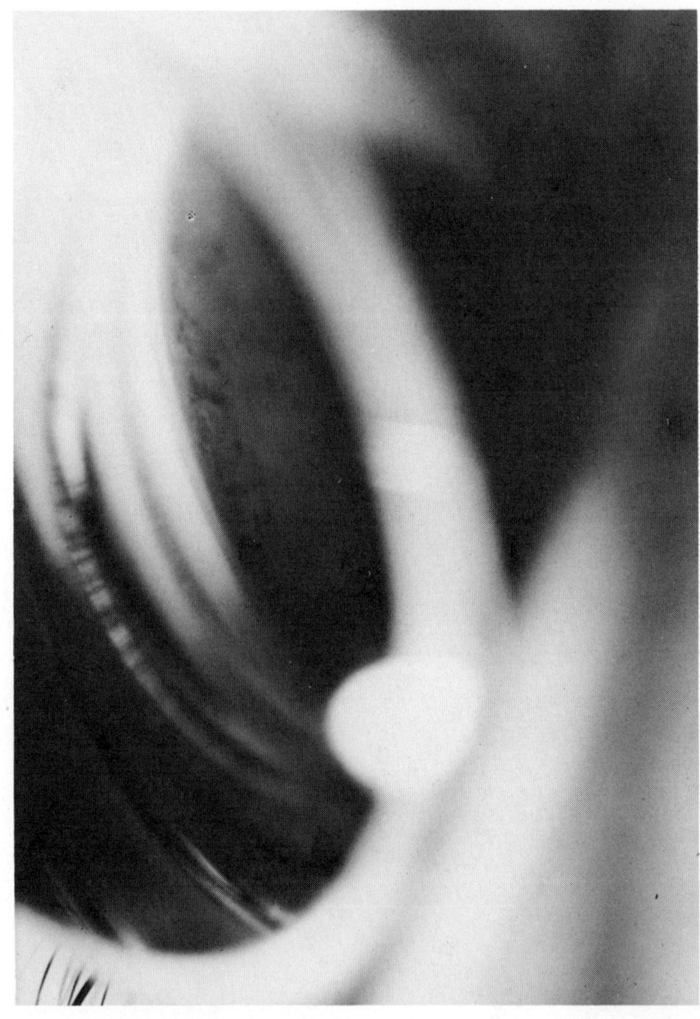

FIG. 16.A. Patient D. I. Uniocular case of congenital glaucoma, filtration angle of normal eye.

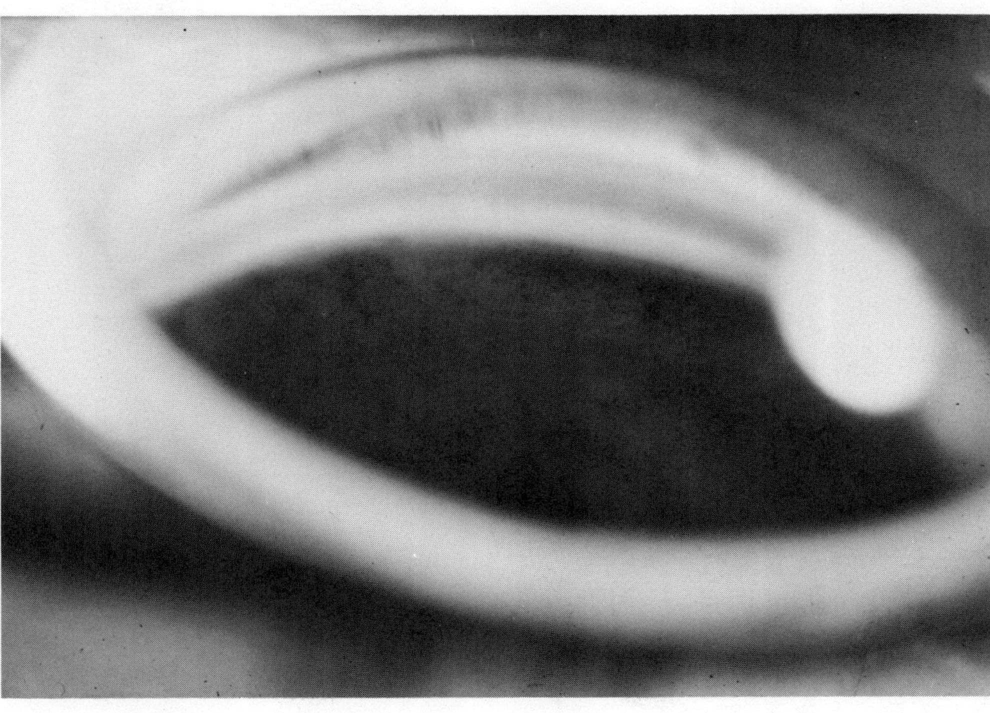

FIG. 16.B. Patient D. I. Uniocular case of congenital glaucoma, filtration angle of abnormal eye.

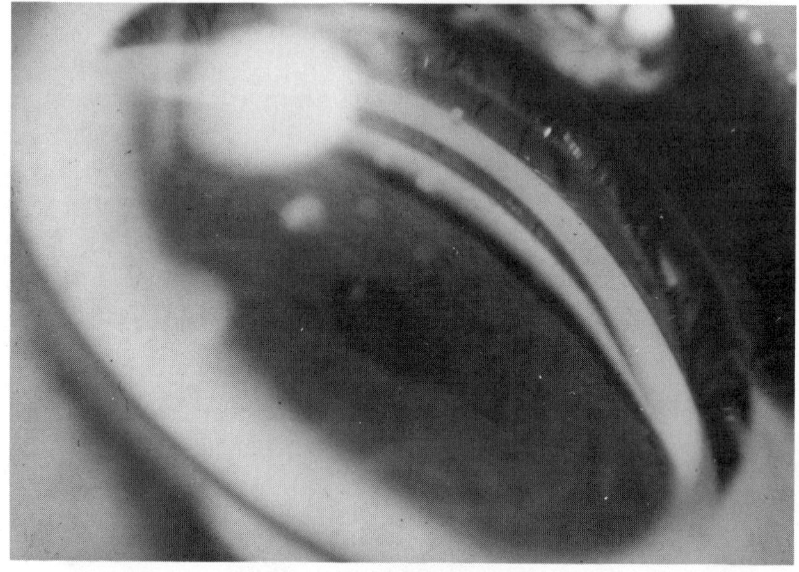

FIG. 17. Normal filtration angle of five-year-old child.

pectinate ligaments are only rarely found and when present are few in number.

After the examination is completed, a decision about the type of treatment to be undertaken is made. Since the systemic effects of the anesthesia make reliance upon the numerical values of tonometry or tonography questionable, the decision is based upon the entire clinical picture–including symptomatology, and physical findings, as well as results of tonometry. If there is any doubt as to the condition or indicated treatment, continued observation should be substituted for active therapy. The goniotomy operation produces the highest incidence of intraocular pressure normalization when the diagnosis is certain. An exception to this rule occurs when the corneal clouding precludes adequate visualization.

SUMMARY

The nature of this chapter, which describes the integrated efforts of the various members of the paramedical and medical team, makes it necessary to emphasize several points.

Congenital glaucoma may first present itself before any one of several members of the medical team—namely, the nurse in the newborn nursery, the public health nurse working in outlying areas, the pediatrician, the general practitioner, the optometrist, and the ophthalmologist. Because of the nature of the condition several other physicians may be called upon to play a valuable role, namely the cardiologist, the endocrinologist, the geneticist and the anesthesiologist. A cardiac assessment is necessary because of the frequent association of congenital glaucoma with congenital heart disease. The endocrinologist must rule out associated metabolic disturbances. The anesthesiologist must be cognizant of the various factors that would influence the intraocular pressure of the child and must therefore modify the type of anesthesia to be used.

In general the intraocular pressure will be elevated with other signs of glaucoma. However, it is important to bear in mind that as high as 75 percent of patients with congenital glaucoma will show a significant reduction in intraocular pressure when they are placed under general anesthesia.

Therefore, each patient must be evaluated individually on the basis of evidence of differences between the two eyes and abnormalities in the cornea, the optic disc, the anterior chamber, and the filtration angle.

References

af Ursin, K. V. The fate of infantile and juvenile glaucoma patients. Acta Ophthalmol., 25:345, 1947.

Alfano, J. E. Pseudocholine esterase and cholinesterase in congenital glaucoma. Am. J. Ophthalmol., 61:985, 1966.

Ocular malformations associated with congenital heart disease. Am. J. Ophthalmol., 61:1020, 1966.

Anderson, J. R. Hydrophthalmia or Congenital Glaucoma: Its Causes, Treatment and Outlook. Cambridge Univers., London, 1939.

Apt, L. Cited by Hetherington, J., Jr., and Shaffer, R. N. Tonometry and tonography in congenital glaucoma. Invest. Ophthalmol., 7:134, 1968.

Bailliart, P. Le glaucome infantile à l'Institution Nationale des Jeunes Aveugles Ann. Oculist, 180:257, 1947.

Barkan, O. Surgery of congenital glaucoma: a review of 196 eyes operated by goniotomy. Am. J. Ophthalmol., 36:1523, 1953.

Congenital glaucoma, goniotomy, Trans. Am. Acad. Ophthalmol. Otolaryngol. 59:322, 1955.

Becker, B. Diamox in glaucoma. Am. J. Ophthalmol., 37:13, 1954.

Becker, B., and Shaffer, R. N. Diagnosis and Therapy of the Glaucomas, 2nd ed. Mosby, St. Louis, 1965, pp. 218-240.

Chandler, P. A., and Grant, W. M. Lectures on Glaucoma. Lea and Febiger, Philadelphia, 1968, pp. 297-333.

Cooper, L. Z., and Krugman, S. Clinical manifestations of postnatal and congenital rubella. Arch. Ophthalmol., 77:434, 1967.

Costenbader, F. D., and Kwitko, M. L. Congenital glaucoma, a review of seventy-seven consecutive eyes. J. Ped. Ophthalmol., 4:9, 1967.

and Kwitko, M. L. Congenital glaucoma. Clin. Proc. Child. Hosp. (Wash.), 17:100, 1961.

de Roetth, A., Jr., and Schwartz, H. Aqueous humor dynamics in glaucoma: effect of ganglion blocking agents and thiopental sodium anaesthesia on aqueous humor dynamics. Arch. Ophthalmol., 55:755, 1956.

Dettbarn, W. D., Rosenberg, P., Wilensky, J. G., and Wong, A. Effect of phospholine iodide on blood cholinesterase levels of normal and glaucoma subjects. Am. J. Ophthalmol., 59:586, 1965.

Draeger, J. Simple hand applanation tonometer. Am. J. Ophthalmol., 62:1208, 1966.

Drance, S. M. Phospholine Iodide and Demecarium Bromide in the management of glaucoma. Am. J. Opthalmol., 50:270, 1960.

Galin, M. A., Melvor, J. W., and Magruder, G. B. The influence of position on intraocular pressure. Am. J. Ophthalmol., 55:720, 1963.

Geltzer, A. I., Guber, D., and Sears, M. L. Ocular manifestations of the 1964-65 rubella epidemic. Am. J. Ophthalmol., 63:221, 1967.

Giles, C. L. Tonometer tension in the newborn. Arch. Ophthalmol., 61:517, 1959.

Gonin, J. Bull et Mem. Soc. Franc. d'Opht., 38:614 1925.

Graff, E., and Dyson, C. Outflow studies in children. Arch. Ophthalmol., 74:36, 1965.

Gros, E. L. Etude sur l'hydrophtalmie au glaucome infantile. Theses Paris 1897.

Gross, E. G. Betrag zur pathologischen Anatomie des Hydrophthalmus. Arch. Augenheilk., 48:340, 1903.

Gross, B. H. Glaucome sur des June sujets Ann. d'Oculist 180:366, 1947.

Haas, J. S. Congenital glaucoma: end results of treatment. Trans. Am. Acad. Ophthalmol. Otolaryngol., 59:333, 1955.

Principles and problems of therapy in congenital glaucoma. Invest. Ophthalmol., 7:140, 1968.

Halasa, A. Tonography in normal and malnourished children. Arch. Ophthalmol., 81:328, 1969.

Hallett, E. A study of intraocular tension during general anesthesia. Trans. Ophthalmol. Soc., 24:73, 1965.

Hetherington, J., Jr., and Shaffer, R. N. Tonometry and tonography in congenital glaucoma. Invest. Ophthalmol., 7:134, 1968.

Hilton, G. F., and Shaffer, R. N. Electric applanation tonometry. Am. J. Ophthalmol., 62:838, 1966.

Hiscox, P. E. A., and McCulloch, J. C. Cardiac arrest occurring in a patient on echothiophate iodide therapy. Am. J. Ophthalmol., 60:425, 1965.

Kornblueth, W., Aladjemoff, L., Magora, F., and Gabby, A. Influence of general anaesthesia on intraocular pressure in man. Arch. Ophthalmol., 61:84, 1959.

Jampolsky, A., Tamler, E., and Marg, E. Contraction of the oculorotary muscles and intraocular pressure. Am. J. Ophthalmol., 49:1381, 1960.

Aladjemoff, L., Magora, F., and Dor, D. B. Intraocular pressure in children measured under general anaesthesia. Arch. Ophthalmol., 72:489, 1964.

Kwitko, M. L. Congenital glaucoma: a clinical study. Can. J. Ophthalmol., 2:91, 1967.

Congenital glaucoma and anterior chamber cleavage defects. Am. Acad. Ophthalmol. Otolaryngol. Course, Chicago, 1967.

Lamb, H. D. Hydrophthalmus, Am. J. Ophthalmol. 8:784, 1925.

Lederle Lab., Medical Advisory Department. Diamox. Pearl River, N. Y., 1962, p. 17.

Lehrfeld, L., and Reber, J. Glaucoma at the Wills Eye Hospital, 1935. Arch. Ophthalmol., 18:712, 1937.

Leith, A. B. Episceral venous pressure in tonography. Br. J. Ophthalmol., 47:271, 1963.

Leopold, I. H., Krishna, N., and Lehman, R. Effects of anticholinesterase agents on blood cholinesterase in normal and glaucomatous subjects. Trans. Am. Ophthalmol. Soc., 57:63, 1959.

Lowe, C. V., Terrey, M., and MacLachlan, E. A. Organic-aciduria, decreased ammonia production, hydrophthalmos and mental retardation. Am. J. Dis. Child., 83:164, 1952.

Magitot, A. Physiologic Oculaire Clinique. Masson, Paris, 1946.

Magora, F., and Collins, V. The influence of general anaesthesia on intraocular pressure in man. Arch. Ophthalmol., 66:806, 1961.

McKusick, V. A. Heritable Disorders of Connective Tissue. Mosby, St. Louis, 1966.

Meyers, S. J. Congenital glaucoma: review, summary and conclusions. Trans. Am. Acad. Ophthalmol. Otolaryngol., 59:342, 1955.

Moreau, P., and Cornibert, M. Severe hypotony and malnutrition. Bull. Soc. Franc. Ophthalmol., 63:244, 1963.

Parsons, J. H. The refraction in buphthalmia. Br. J. Ophthalmol., 4:211, 1920.

Roberts, W., and Rogers, J. W. Postural effects on pressure and ocular rigidity measurements. Am. J. Ophthalmol., 57:111, 1964.

Sampaolesi, R., Reca, R., and Carro, A. Ocular pressure in children up to five years of age. Arch. Oftal. (B. Aires), 42:180, 1967.

Scheie, H. G. Congenital glaucoma: diagnosis, clinical course and treatment other than goniotomy. Trans. Am. Acad. Ophthalmol. Otolaryngol., 59:309, 1955.

The management of infantile glaucoma. Arch. Ophthalmol., 62:35, 1959.

Infantile and juvenile glaucoma. Trans. Am. Acad. Ophthalmol. Otolaryngol., 67:458, 1963.

Schiotz, H. J. Tonometrie. Arch. Augenheilk., 62:317, 1909.

Schirmer, K. E. Personal communication.

Shaffer, R. N. Pathogenesis of congenital glaucoma: gonioscopic and microscopic anatomy. Trans. Am. Acad. Ophthalmol. Otolaryngol., 59:297, 1955.

Genetics and the congenital glaucomas. Am. J. Ophthalmol., 60:981, 1965.

New concepts in infantile glaucoma. Can. J. Ophthalmol., 2:243, 1967.

Smith, J. L., et al. The incidence of Schiötz–applanation disparity. Arch. Ophthalmol., 77:305, 1967.

Speakman, J. S., and Crawford, J. S. Congenital opacities of the corena. Br. J. Ophthalmol., 50:68, 1966.

Thomas, C. I. The Cornea. Thomas, Springfield, Ill. 1955.

Thorpe, H. Carbonic anhydrase inhibitor as a therapeutic agent in ophthalmology. Read at Meeting of the Association for Research in Ophthalmology, Eastern Section, February 18, 1953.

Van den Heuvel, Cited by Worst, J. G. F. The Pathogenesis of Congenital Glaucoma. Royal Vangorcum, Assen. Netherlands, 1966. p. 110.

Wilmer, H. A., and Scrammon, R. E. Growth of the components of the human eyeball. Arch. Ophthalmol., 43:599, 1950.

Zimmerman, L. E. The histopathologic basis for the ocular manifestations of the congenital rubella syndrome. Proc. Inst. Med. Chicago, 26:179, 1967.

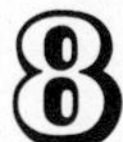

Local Malformations

Primary congenital glaucoma with the typical filtration angle configuration may occur with malformations in other parts of the eye itself in a child completely free of distant systemic conditions. The abnormality is usually present at birth, and may cloud the prognosis for good visual acuity.

The surgical procedure for ocular hypertension may indeed be completely successful but the local malformation may be such that there is only a limited visual capability. Therein lies the importance for determining the extent of these malformations. Costenbader and Kwitko reported a series of 77 eyes with congenital glaucoma and enumerated the local malformations they observed (Table 1).

Several other conditions in the immediate neighborhood of the eye are also discussed in this chapter. Here again the filtration angle displays the usual findings of congenital glaucoma.

TABLE 1

CONGENITAL GLAUCOMA: LOCAL MALFORMATIONS (77 EYES)*

Malformation	No. of eyes
Strabismus	7
Myopia	5
Nystagmus	4
Blocked tear duct	2
Cataract	2
Corneal opacities	1

*After F. D. Costenbader and M. L. Kwitko. J. Pediatr. Ophthalmol., 2:9, 1967.

CORNEAL MALFORMATION

The crucial period for corneal development occurs at the same time that the anterior chamber angle is evolving. A malformed cornea is therefore not an unlikely finding in cases of congenital glaucoma.

Corneal Opacification

Opacification of the corneal stroma is a sign of disruption of the fine architecture the cornea normally displays (Fig. 1). The disruption is on an embryological basis, which can lead to anatomical disorganization, or the opacification may be biochemical in nature related to the improper deposition of crucial elements in the corneal lamellae. Costenbader and Kwitko reported one case with corneal opacification in their series.

Macrocornea

As the intraocular pressure rises in congenital glaucoma the elasticity of

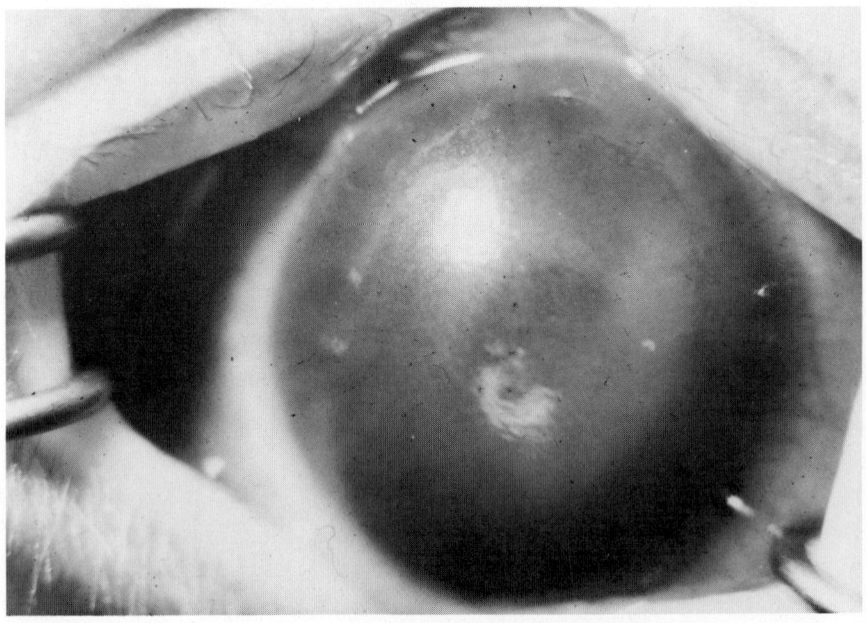

FIG. 1. Opacification of the cornea in a case of congenital glaucoma.

the infantile cornea makes it prone to enlargement. The less elastic Descemet's membrane tears to keep pace with the distending corneal lamellae. Therefore, a common finding in congenital glaucoma is a cloudy enlarged cornea with tears in Descemet's membrane and corneal edema. However, there are cases of congenital glaucoma observed where the cornea has a normal luster, the epithelium is not edematous, and Descemet's membrane is intact, yet the horizontal measurement may be up to 15 mm.

Although it is generally believed that megalocornea and congenital glaucoma are separate entities, there are families reported where some members are noted to have congenital glaucoma and other members megalocornea. In those cases where congenital glaucoma is observed in one eye and megalocornea in the opposite eye of the same patient, the megalocornea probably represents evidence of a case of arrested hydrophthalmia.

It is possible that a child could have both congenital glaucoma and macrocornea simultaneously in the same eye. The enlarged cornea, which is otherwise completely normal in a case of buphthalmia, should be an example of this occurrence. Fig. 2 illustrates a case of uniocular congenital glaucoma. The involved cornea measured 14 mm horizontally on the initial

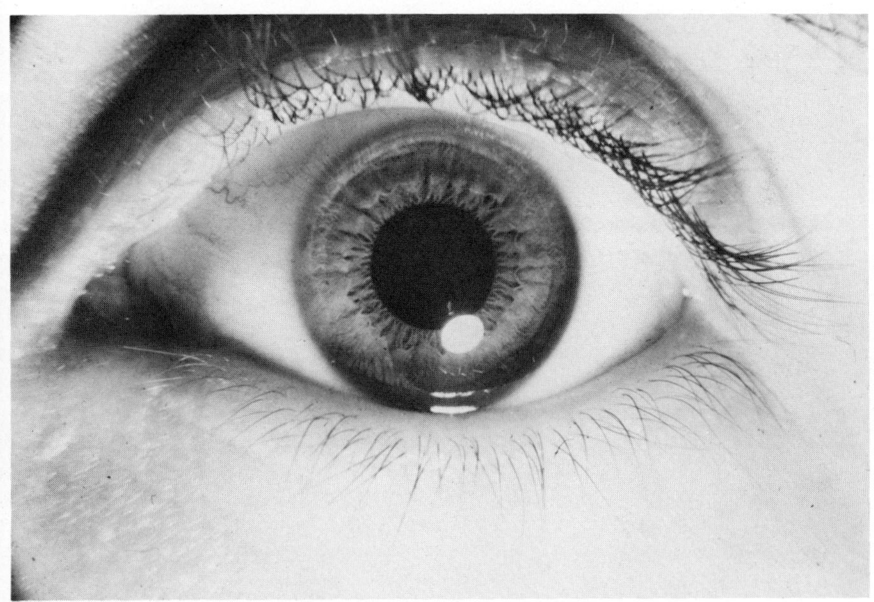

FIG. 2. Macrocornea. The intraocular pressure is elevated, yet the cornea maintains a normal luster with the epithelium, stroma and Descemet's membrane uninvolved.

examination, the intraocular pressure measured 40 mm Hg, and the visual acuity was 20/30. The corneal luster, epithelium, Descemet's membrane, and stroma were all normal. The visual field examination on this eye revealed an arcuate scotoma; the optic nerve was markedly cupped and atrophied. The arterioles at the nerve head showed pulsation, which disappeared with normalization of the intraocular pressure. The retinal blood vessels were displaced nasally and a bayonet effect was observed at the nerve head. The opposite eye was normal.

Arcus lipoidis

Faust reported the occurrence of arcus lipoidis in congenital glaucoma. Epstein reported a case of arcus juvenilis associated with buphthalmia.

LENS MALFORMATION

Microphakia

A smaller lens than normal has been observed frequently in cases of congenital glaucoma. In 1903, Gross noted that the normal lens diameter

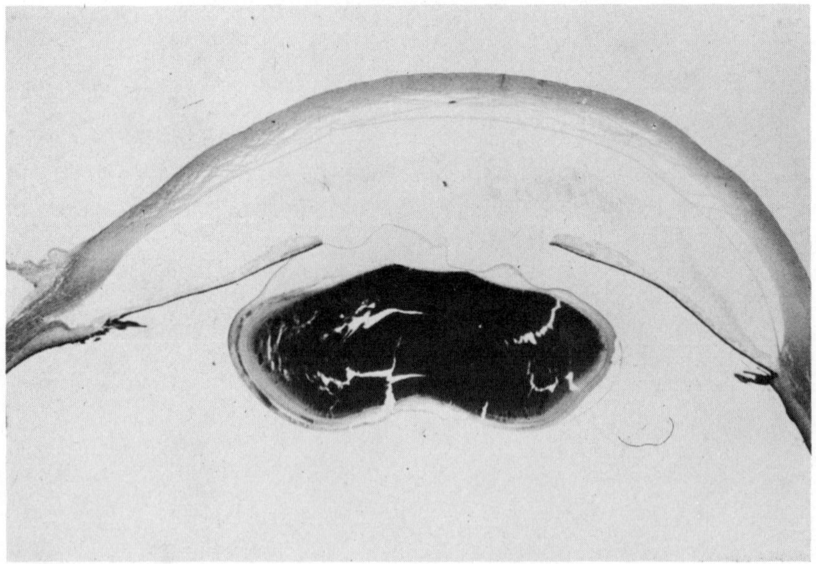

FIG. 3. Congenital glaucoma. The area occupied by the lens appears smaller than normal. (Courtesy of F. D. Costenbader.) X 30.

was 9.0 mm as opposed to a lens diameter of 6.8 mm in congenital glaucoma. These measurements have been made largely on autopsy eyes which became available because they failed to respond to treatment. A small lens has also been noted in eyes of children who suffered cardiac arrest during surgery and in whom the eye still retained its normal dimensions (Fig. 3).

Microphakia has been implicated as a factor in the etiology of congenital glaucoma. This is based on a mechanical theory that the small lens would keep the zonules on the stretch and thus hold the ciliary body in a more forward position and prevent the normal development of the filtration angle.

Congenital Cataract

A not infrequent feature of a congenital anomaly is that neighborhood structures are often similarly involved. Costenbader and Kwitko, in their series, reported two cases with congenital cataracts that were observed before the children underwent glaucoma surgery.

Dislocation of the Lens

With a normal size lens, a distending globe would put greater stress on the zonular fibers. This would be exaggerated if the lens were abnormally small. Trauma, however slight, is a likely cause of lens dislocation in congenital glaucoma. The author has noted the dislocation of the lens during a goniotomy procedure. Every case of congenital glaucoma deserves a slit lamp examination prior to surgery. In addition to the other features to be observed, signs of ectopia lentis, e.g., iridodonesis, should be looked for.

REFRACTION

The refraction of an eye is based on the anatomy of structures from the cornea anteriorly to the retina posteriorly. Any condition which changes this anatomy changes the refractive error.

Myopia

Since an enlargement of the anteroposterior diameter is a common feature in congenital glaucoma, myopia together with its associated changes should not be an unexpected finding. Costenbader and Kwitko reported 5 cases of myopia in excess of 3.50 diopters in their series. Myopia as high as -15.00 diopters has been reported.

Other Refractive Errors

In spite of the great enlargement of the eyeball in buphthalmia, the eye is often not as myopic as its abnormal axial length would suggest. The effect on refraction therefore varies since congenital glaucoma causes other optical changes besides elongation. Parsons observed that the chief factors counteracting myopia were the following.

FLATTENING OF THE CORNEA. As the cornea stretches subject to the intraocular pressure, the corneoscleral junction thins and the anterior chamber deepens. The eyeball also enlarges so that the diameter of the cornea increases, resulting in a flattening of the cornea. The curvature approaches that of the sclera.

FLATTENING OF THE LENS. The circumcorneal scleral ring (adjacent to the ciliary body) stretches and thus increases in diameter as the globe enlarges. The suspensory ligaments are thus abnormally stretched, flattening the lens and diminishing the thickness of the lens in the anteroposterior diameter. The radii of curvatures of the anterior and posterior surfaces are lengthened.

BACKWARD DISPLACEMENT OF THE LENS. As the globe enlarges (expanding the scleral ring) there is a real (although slight) displacement backward of the suspensory ligaments relative to their normal attachment to the ciliary body. In relation to the location of the anterior surface of the cornea, there is an enormous displacement backwards.

Based on these findings, Parsons calculated the location of the cardinal points of an average buphthalmic eye and showed that the eye would have to be 31.0 mm long in the anteroposterior diameter to be emmetropic. Gross found the average anteroposterior diameter in congenital glaucoma to be 32.0 mm. Emmetropia, hypermetropia and astigmatism, as well as myopia, are therefore present in congenital glaucoma.

RETINAL MALFORMATION

Retinal Dysplasia

Retinal dysplasia, although not common, may be a feature observed in congenital glaucoma (Fig. 4A and B). Figs. 5A and B illustrates two segments of involved retina. Examination of the filtration angle in this case

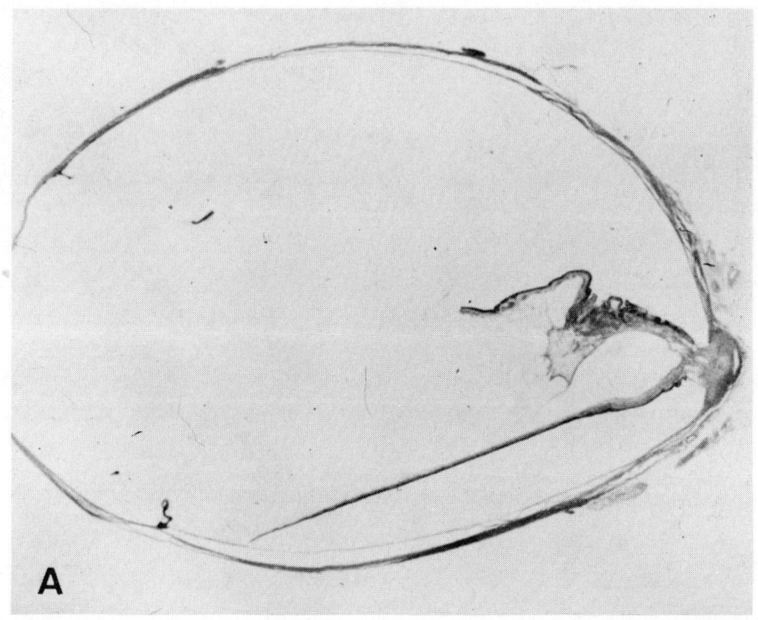

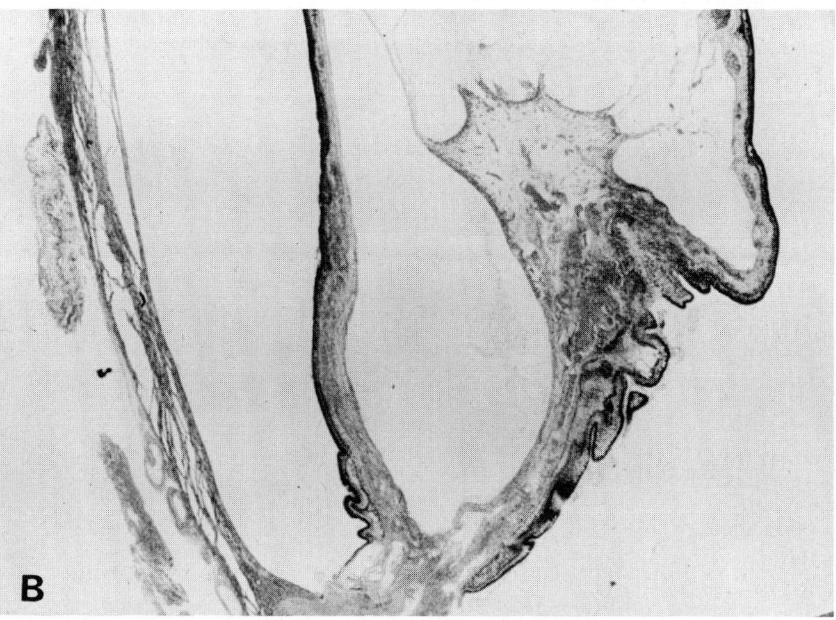

FIG. 4. Congenital glaucoma associated with retinal dysplasia. (A. F. I. P. Acc. No. 692180.) (Courtesy of the Registry of Ophthalmic Pathology of the Armed Forces Institute of Pathology.) A, X 2; B, X 7.

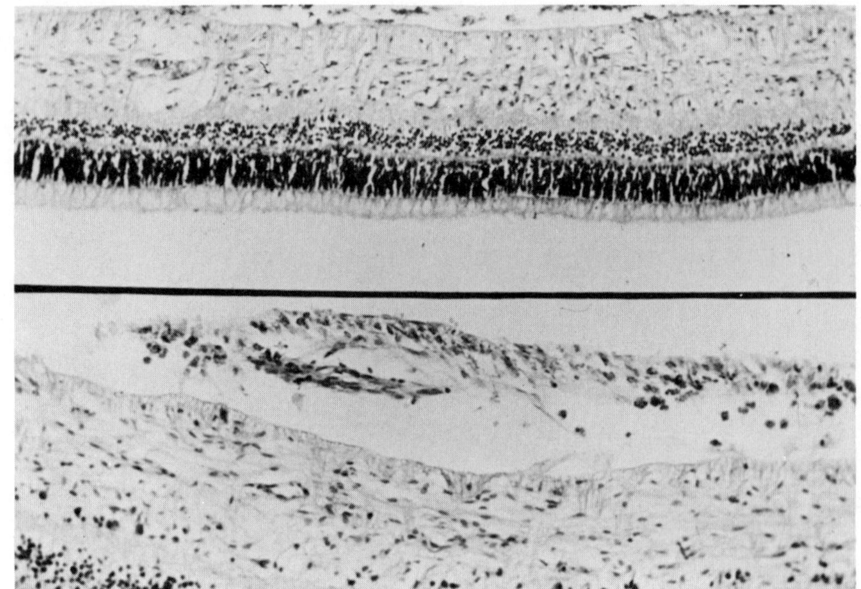

FIG. 5. Congenital glaucoma associated with retinal dysplasia. Two segments of the retina are illustrated. (A. F. I. P. Acc. No. 681622.) (Courtesy of the Registry of Ophthalmic Pathology of the Armed Forces Institute of Pathology.) Top, X 60; bottom, X 80.

shows that the longitudinal fibers of the ciliary body largely bypass the scleral spur to insert directly into the trabecular fibers (Fig. 6).

Retinal Detachment

Vos reported the occurrence of detachment of the retina in buphthalmia. Walker observed a case of congenital glaucoma that exhibited a tear in the retina which extended into the choroid.

STRABISMUS

Strabismus is a relatively common condition observed in young children. Although congenital glaucoma is relatively rare, there is no reason why these two conditions may not occur spontaneously in the same child.

Strabismus may also be found in cases of unilateral congenital glaucoma because of the anisometropia which is commonly seen in such cases. The frequent surgical procedures may result in periodic patching of the one eye,

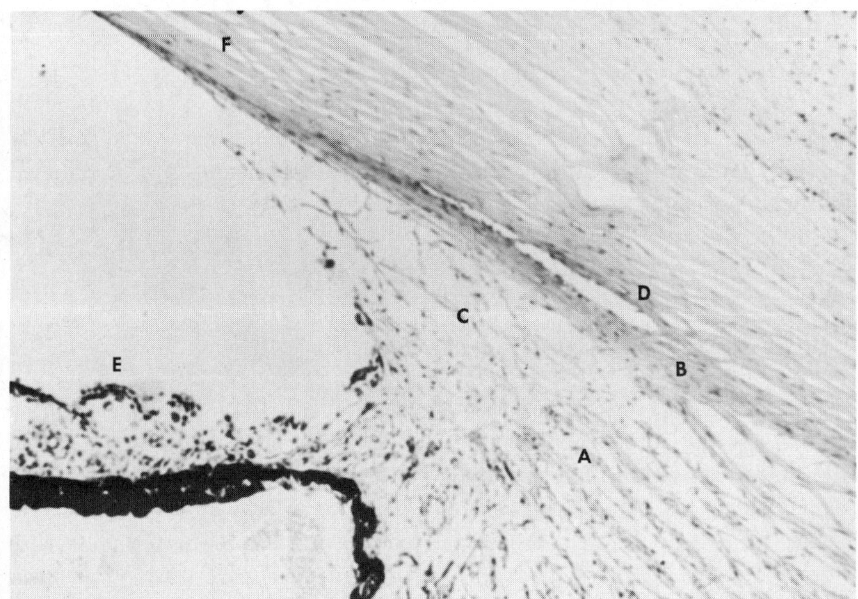

FIG. 6. Congenital glaucoma associated with retinal dysplasia. The filtration angle. The longitudinal fibers (A) of the ciliary muscle largely bypass the scleral spur (B) to insert directly into the trabecular fibers (C). (D) Schlemm's Canal; (E) iris; (F) cornea. (A. F. I. P. Acc. No. 681622.) (Courtesy of the Registry of Ophthalmic Pathology of the Armed Forces Institute of Pathology.) X 80.

which breaks up fusion. A latent case of strabismus may evolve into a frank exotropia or esotropia under these conditions.

Costenbader and Kwitko reported 7 children with strabismus that required treatment in their series of 77 eyes.

The problem of amblyopia must be energetically treated in all cases of strabismus but especially in eyes with congenital glaucoma. All the standard forms of treatment must be employed including patching, orthoptics, anticholinesterase drugs, and strabismus surgery. The child with congenital glaucoma and a normal muscle balance must also be treated for potential amblyopia, preferably by patching the normal eye and careful observation. The surgeon must not be satisfied with normalization of the intraocular pressure alone since the treated eye frequently has a lower potential for good visual acuity.

If this treatment is not instituted the normalized glaucoma eye may then become strabismic as well as amblyopic.

NYSTAGMUS

In their series, Costenbader and Kwitko found 4 patients with nystagmus. The prospects for good vision are diminished when such an abnormality is present although the nystagmoid movement is often reduced following normalization of pressure.

BLOCKED TEAR DUCT

Tearing is a common feature in congenital glaucoma. However, children at this age may also suffer from the usual causes of tearing independent of the ocular condition. Not infrequently, the lower end of the nasolacrimal duct, which normally terminates beneath the inferior turbinate, fails to open. There may be an inflammatory edema of the interior turbinate with hypertrophy and faulty positioning. As a result, excessive tearing and stasis occurs, leading to chronic conjunctivitis. The tearing may be associated with a mucopurulent secretion. Treatment is conservative with local antibiotic therapy to control the conjunctivitis and massage over the sac until the patient is 6 months of age. At this time, probing of the duct should be done if the condition persists.

In the Costenbader-Kwitko series, two patients with congenital glaucoma has blocked tear ducts and tearing which persisted after the intraocular pressure was brought under control. Probing of the tear ducts promptly caused the tearing to subside.

OTHER MALFORMATIONS

A number of other malformations immediately adjacent to the eye have been noted as findings related to congenital glaucoma. Terrien et al. reported the occurrence of facial hemihypertrophy with buphthalmia; Pesme observed a case of hydrocephalus associated with infantile glaucoma.

References

Best, F. Hydrophthalmus mit Entwicklungsstorung der Iris. Klin. Monatsbl. Augenheilkd., 82:525, 1929.

Bruckner, A. Kranheiten der Uvea. Lehr. Augenheilk., 520, 1948.

Costenbader, F. D., and Kwitko, M. L. Congenital glaucoma. An analysis of seventy-seven consecutive eyes. J. Pediatr. Ophthalmol., 2:9, 1967.
Deiter, W. Uber Aktionsstrome. Ber. Zus. Dtsch., 53:53, 1940.
Duke-Elder, W. S. System of Ophthalmology, Vol. 3, Pt. 2. Congenital Deformities. Kimpton, London, 1964, p. 554.
Eisler, P. Die Anatomie des menschlichen Auges. Kurz. Hand. Ophthalmol., 1:1, 1930.
Epstein, E. Report of a case of hydrophthalmia. Br. J. Ophthalmol., 30:476, 1946.
Faust. Arcus Lipoides bei Buphthalmus. Klin. Monatsbl. Augenheilkd., 101:287, 1938.
Franceschetti, A. Die Vererbung von Augenleiden. Kurz. Hand. Ophthalmol., 1:631, 1930.
Gross, E. G. Beitrag zur Pathologischen Anatomie des Hydrophthalmus. Arch. Augenheilkd., 48:340, 1903.
Kayser, B. Ueber die Unmoglishkeit enger genetischer Begiehungen zwishen Makrokornea resp. Megalocornea und Hydrophthalmus. Klin. Monatsbl. Augenheilkd., 102:11, 1939.
Ueber die vermiteten Beziehungen der Makrokornea zu Hydrophthalmus und uber das Fahlen ihrer Nachweisbarkiet. Klin. Monatsbl. Augenheilkd., 106:63, 1941.
Klar, R. Beitrage zur Frage der Megalokornea auf Grund von Untersuchungen eines Staroperierten Patienten und siener Sippe. Klin. Monatsbl. Augenheilkd., 104:286, 1940.
Kunz, E. Abnorme Grosse der Linse als Ursuche von jugenlichem Glaucom. Klin. Monatsbl. Augenheilkd., 87:433, 1931.
Lobek. Zur Kenntnis der Mesothoriumeinwirkung uaf das menschliche Auge. Klin. Monatsbl. Augenheilkd., 100:283, 1938.
Miklos, A. Beitrag zur Lehre der Megalokornea in Verbindung mit der sporadischen Megalokornea globosa. Klin. Monatsbl. Augenheilkd., 106:69, 1941.
Nataf, R., et Fortan, P. La megalocorneée hereditaire et familiale. Ann. Ocul. (Paris), 180:267, 1947.
Parsons, J. H. The refraction in buphthalmia. Br. J. Ophthalmol., 4:211, 1920.
Pesme, M. P. Un cas d'hydrocephalie avec glaucome infantile. Bull. Soc. Mem. Fr. Ophthalmol., 47:259, 1934.
Posthumus, R. G. Die Megalokornea in ihrem Zusammenhang mit anderen Abweichungen bei Angehorigen deiselben Familie. Klin. Monatsbl. Augenheilkd., 102:1, 1939.
Scheie, H. G., Connell, M. M., and Poley, B. J. Pediatric ophthalmology. Scope, 1:33, 1964.
Seefelder, R. Uber den anatomischen Befund in eimem Falle von Membrana pupillaris perisistens corneal adharens und angelborener Hornhauttrunbung. Arch. Augenheilkd., 69:164, 1911.
Die Entwicklung des menchiehen Auges. Kurz. Hand. Ophthalmol., 1:476, 1930.
Terrien, F., Veil, P., et Chavany, J. A. Hemihypertrophie faciale et buphthalmie. Bull. Soc. Ophtalmol., (Paris), 131, 1931.
Van Duyse. Tetratologie. Traite Ophthalmol., 1:986, 1939.
Veil, P., et Sarrazin, L. La megalocornée hereditaire et familiale. Ann. Ocul. (Paris), 176:241, 1939.
Vom Hofe, K. Weitere Untersuchungen zur Frage der Makrokornea un des Buphthalmus. Klin. Monatsbl. Augenheilkd., 104:278, 1940.
Vos, T. A. Buphthalmus en ablatio retinae. Ned. Tijdschr. Geneeskd., 82:4393, 1938.
Walker, F. O. A case of hydrophthalmos. Trans. Ophthalmol. Soc. U. K., 65:369, 1945.
Wexler, D., and Kornsweig, A. Buphthalmos in a six-month premature infant. Arch. Ophthalmol., 37:318, 1947.
Wolf-Heidegger. Entwicklungsgeschichte des Sehorgans A. Embryonalentwicklung. Lehr. Augenheilkd., 291, 1948.

9

Associated Abnormalities

Congenital anomalies of the eye result from disturbances in embryologic development. Since all 3 basic embryonic tissues contribute to the normal development of the eye, a spectrum of anomalies may arise when the normal process of development and differentiation is disturbed. These anomalies are usually present at birth; those involving the anterior segment may give rise to an elevation of the intraocular pressure, although on occasion the glaucoma does not become manifest until later childhood or early adulthood. When the intraocular pressure becomes elevated it is usually in the range of 30 to 40 mm Hg. The pressure tends to vary, however, and may not be raised on all occasions. Corneal epithelial edema develops, increasing and decreasing with changes in pressure. Epiphora, photophobia, and blepharospasm occur as in congenital glaucoma, probably related to the irritation of the edematous cornea. Ophthalmoscopy and gonioscopy may be difficult under these conditions but removal of the epithelium often permits adequate examination. Because of the degree of elasticity of the infant eye, progressive enlargment of the globe develops when the intraocular pressure remains elevated and occasionally enlargement takes place without the development of corneal edema. The corneal diameter increases, and tears develop in the less elastic Descemet's membrane. Hypotony may be noted especially shortly after a tear occurs. Cupping and atrophy of the optic discs may not be marked when the disease is first discovered, but will develop unless the intraocular pressure is controlled.

CORNEAL ABNORMALITIES

Sclerocornea

Scleralization of the cornea, or sclerocornea, is an uncommon anomaly characterized by stationary, unilateral, or bilateral opacities (Fig. 1) of the peripheral, central, or entire cornea with superficial or deep vascularization.

The cornea begins its development at the 18- to 20-mm stage and the corneal collagen appears at the 20-mm stage. Between the 25- and 28-mm stage, the corneoscleral junction becomes evident. Therefore, according to Kanai et al., sclerocornea develops at about the 20-mm stage (approximately the seventh week of gestation). The opacities are present at birth, and there is no associated interstitial keratitis, ulceration, or inflammatory disease of the cornea.

Bilateral involvement occurs in a majority of cases; males and females are similarly affected. Dominant or recessive inheritance has been described and sporadic cases also occur. Systemic abnormalities are only rarely associated with sclerocornea. They include hexadactyly of hands and feet

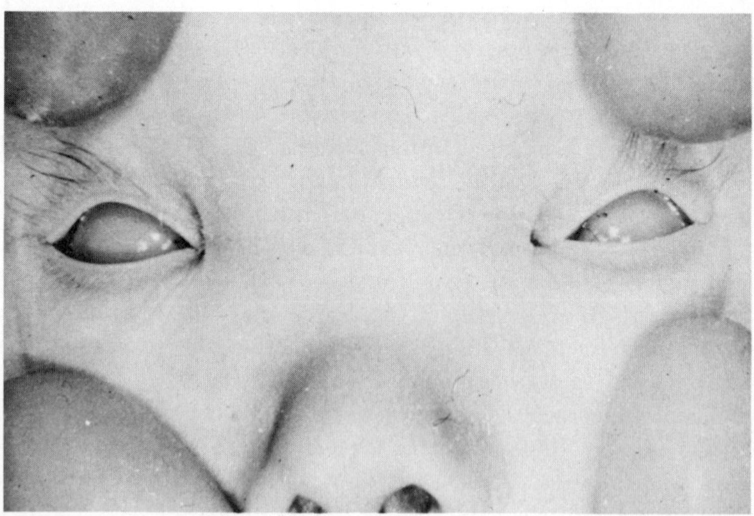

FIG. 1. Sclerocornea. The entire cornea of both eyes is involved. (Courtesy of J. S. Speakman.)

combined with lacunae of the parietal bones (possibly Biemond's syndrome); fragile bones, blue sclera, and decreased hearing (Lobstein's syndrome); features suggesting Hurler's disease; calcification of the cerebral faux, torticollis, cerebellar and psychomotor retardation, deafness, cryptorchism, and pulmonary disease; brachycephaly, facial asymmetry, including maxillary hypoplasia; dyscrania, malformed ears, occult spina bifida; prognathism with arched palate and clinical features of trisomy 18 syndrome.

Ocular examination of a patient with sclerocornea may reveal mongoloid eyelid fissures, enophthalmus and blepharoptosis with macrophthalmic, microphthalmic, and globes of normal size. Nystagmus has occurred with unilateral and bilateral cases of sclerocornea and includes intermittent, horizontal, pendular, horizontal jerk, and rotary types. Esodeviation has been reported more frequently than exodeviation. Flattening of the corneal surface (corneal plana) is frequently coexistent. The central corneal curvature has been measured to be as flat as 23 diopters, while in other patients it approaches normal values, according to Howard and Abrahams. Visual acuity has been severely diminished to as low as light perception in

TABLE 1

OCULAR ABNORMALITIES IN SCLEROCORNEA*

Anomaly	No. Patients (Total=49)
Bilateral sclerocornea	43
Enophthalmus	3
Blepharoptosis	8
Microphthalmus	4
Macrophthalmus	2
Nystagmus	9
Strabismus	12
Esotropia	7
Exotropia	4
Not described	1
Flattened cornea	38
Decreased corneal sensation	4
Transparent retrocorneal membrane	1
Shallow anterior chamber	19
Anterior synechiae	10
Posterior embryotoxin	1
Iris: Hypoplastic	8
Pupillary fibers	7
Iridoschisis	1
Pupil: Ectopic	5
Anisocoria	1
Lens: Cataractous	4
Elevated intraocular pressure	5
Fundus changes	6
Myopia	2
Coloboma	1
Glaucoma	3

*After R. O. Howard, and I. W. Abrahams, Am. J. Ophthalmol., 71:1254, 1971.

most patients. The reduced acuity is attributable to the dense corneal opacification, glaucoma, aniridia, and coloboma of the choroid and retina. The optic nerve changes of glaucoma may be observed when the fundus can be examined. The series of Howard and Abrahams (49 cases) is noted in Chapter 9, Table 1.

The electroretinogram may be normal, or diminished as in a myopic patient with a Fuch's spot. While the refractive errors in affected eyes may be minimal, both high myopia with associated changes and hyperopia have been clearly documented. Ultrasonic evaluation may provide useful information concerning the axial refractive state.

The peripheral opacified cornea is continuous with the sclera (Fig. 2) and the corneoscleral sulcus usually cannot be identified. Fine blood vessels, arising from the conjunctiva extend superficially over the peripheral cloudy cornea and terminate in arcades, leaving an ovoid, avascular area centrally, which may be opaque or clear. The corneal opacities extend through the full thickness of the stroma, and may be sufficiently dense to prevent visualization of the posterior corneal surface (Fig. 3). Corneal thickness has been estimated to be reduced, normal, or slightly increased. There is an

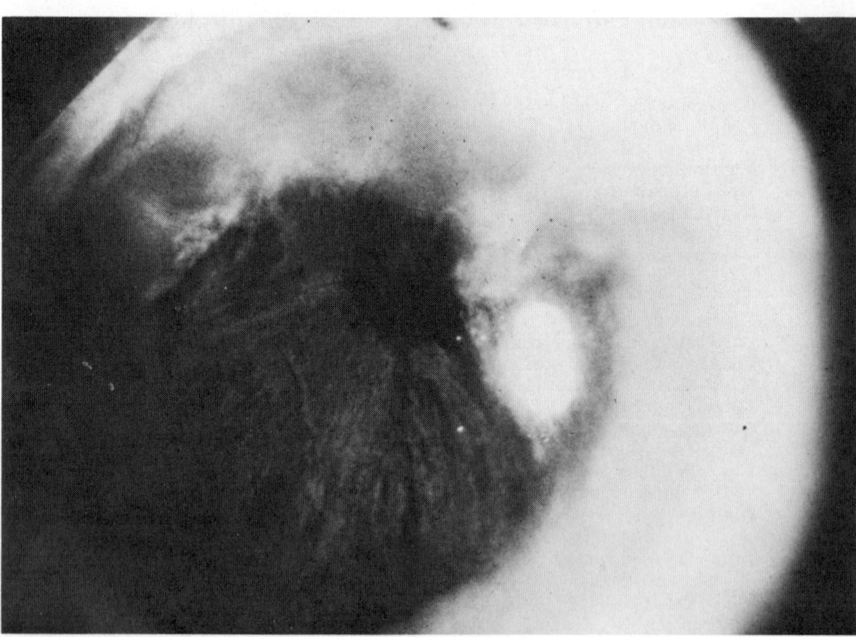

FIG. 2. Sclerocornea. Only the peripheral portion of the cornea is affected. The uninvolved cornea is clear and separated from the opaque portion by a distinct margin. A coloboma of the iris is present. (Courtesy of J. S. Speakman.)

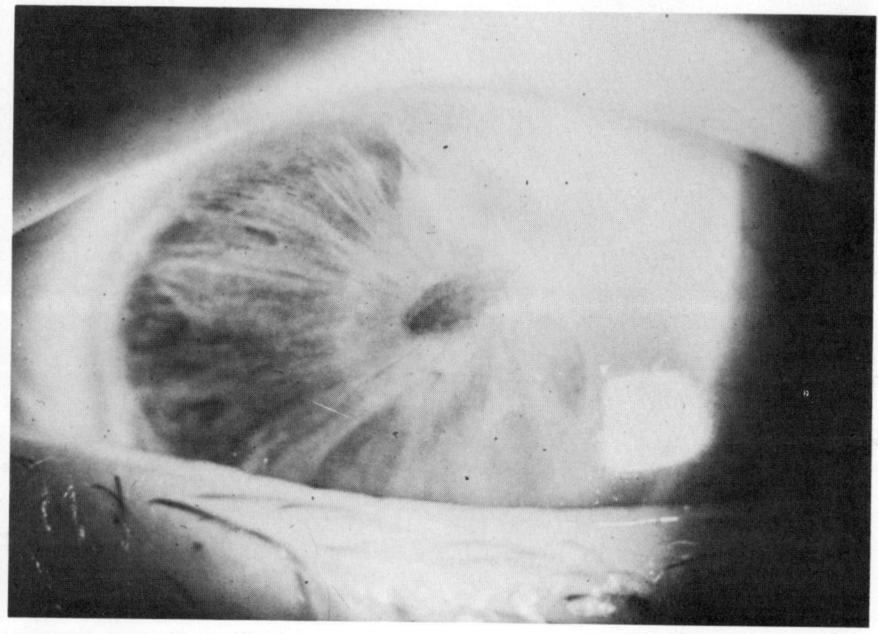

FIG. 3. Sclerocornea. The opaque portion extends to the pupil margin, which remains clearly visible.

abrupt transition from opaque to normal clear cornea when present (Fig. 4). On the basis of slit lamp and histopathologic examination, the anterior chamber is considered to be shallow. Posterior embryotoxin, and anterior synechiae extending to the center of the cornea may be present (Fig. 5). Other associated anterior ocular anomalies include hyaline membrane formation on the posterior cornea, iris coloboma, hypoplastic iris stroma, remnants of the tunica vasculosa lentis, iridoschisis and cataracts.

The intraocular pressure may only be estimated because of the abnormal cornea, but findings compatible with glaucoma have been recognized, i.e., enlarged blind spots and Bjerrum scotomas; decreased facility of outflow, enlarged cornea, and enlarged eyeball.

Goldstein and Cogan reported the pathologic findings in a case of sclerocornea. The globe was enlarged and compatible with congenital glaucoma. The cornea was of approximately normal thickness, with normal central epithelium. The peripheral epithelium, however, showed folds and underlying loose areolar tissue compatible with conjunctiva. Stromal cellularity was considered normal, and stromal blood vessels "similar to the

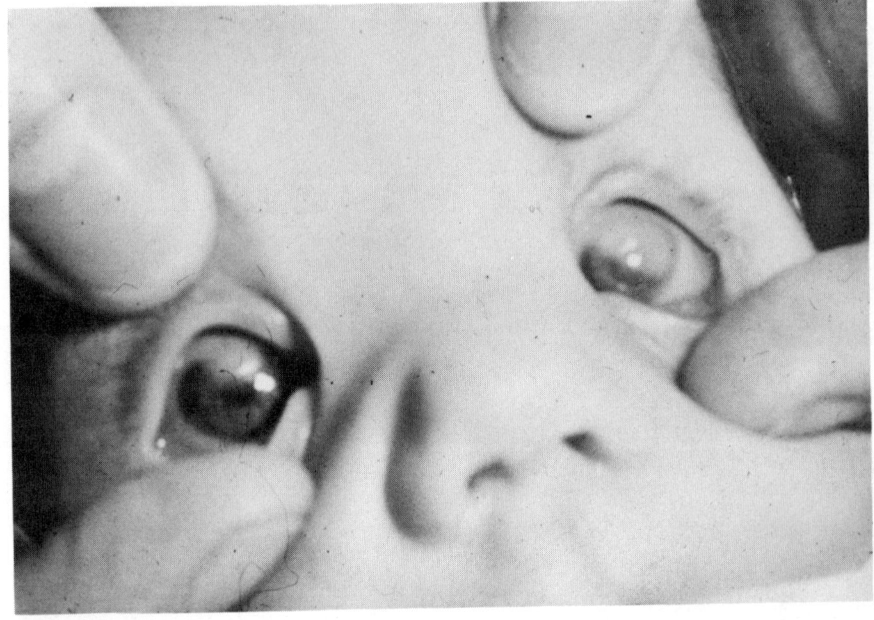

FIG. 4. Sclerocornea. Degree of involvement differs in each eye. (Courtesy of J. S. Speakman.)

sclera" were identified. Bowman's membrane was not identified, and Descemet's membrane was irregularly absent and replaced by fibroblastic proliferation. A large anterior synechiae occluded the angle. A fibroglial plaque was present on the posterior lens surface. The ciliary body was flattened and the ciliary processes atrophic. The optic nerve was cupped.

Block reported the histopathologic findings in a corneal button obtained from a penetrating keratoplasty which showed absence of Bowman's membrane, defects in Descemet's membrane, irregular stromal collagen lamellae, and anterior synechiae. Another cornea obtained at the time of penetrating keratoplasty was reported by Desvignes et al. This specimen showed absence of Bowman's membrane, diffuse stromal edema, irregular Descemet's membrane and endothelium, and a hyaline retrocorneal membrane.

Kolbert and Seelenfreund have examined two globes from an infant who died at the age of 6 weeks. One eye was microphthalmic, the other was of normal size. In both eyes, keratinization of compressed anterior corneal epithelial cells was present. Bowman's membrane was irregularly thickened or absent. The peripheral stroma was vascularized. Descemet's membrane

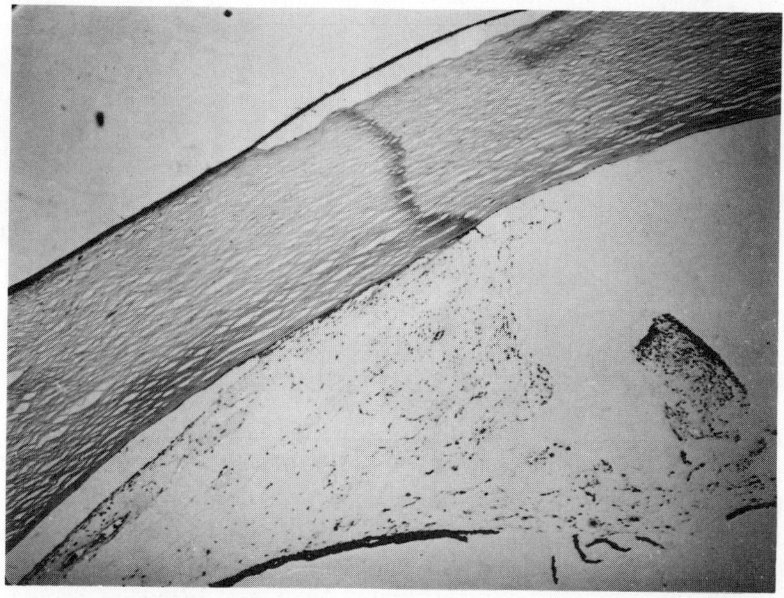

FIG. 5. Anterior synechiae. Broad iris strand extends to the central cornea. Iris stroma is atrophic. X 30.

and endothelium were irregularly absent. Anterior synechiae and a shallow anterior chamber were present. The trabecular meshwork and Schlemm's canal were present irregularly. Vacuoles were noted in the anterior subcapsular area of the normal-sized lens. These authors interpreted the findings as sclerocornea and anterior chamber cleavage syndrome.

Management of this syndrome has generally involved observation only, no specific treatment being available. Penetrating corneal grafting should be considered in patients with bilateral sclerocornea with opacifications dense enough to preclude useful vision. Surgery here should be attempted early in an effort to prevent irreversible amblyopia. The prognosis for useful vision should be guarded because of the known association of sclerocornea with other ocular abnormalities.

Microphthalmos

In 1938 Catsch found 30 cases of microphthalmos in a population of 26,735 (an incidence of 0.11 percent). Microphthalmos may be either congenital or acquired.

(1) Congenital microphthalmos may be sporadic or hereditary. Sporadic cases may be secondary to exogenous factors, such as German measles and syphilis of mother and embryo during early pregnancy. Most sporadic cases, however, are undoubtedly due to mutations and other random factors still not well understood. A family history is usually not elicited in these cases. Other cases of congenital microphthalmos, however, are inherited genetically. There are pedigrees of microphthalmos, mostly in the European literature, to illustrate all the common forms of genetic inheritance. There are some that are regularly dominant, others irregularly dominant, still others recessive, and finally, many have been described that are sex-linked, according to Zeiter.

(2) Acquired microphthalmos may be secondary to insults affecting the eyes; early in life, such as retrolental fibroplasia, pseudogliomas, arrested retinoblastomas, and infections like diphtheria and neonatal ophthalmia; or later in life, such as x-ray-induced microphthalmos and the various forms of phthisis bulbi, which only grossly can be mistaken for microphthalmos.

Complete failure of development of the optic vesicles results in anophthalmos. Once formation of the vesicles has occurred, faulty involution leads to microphthalmos and its associated local anomalies. Should the insult to the embryo be widespread deformities in many other systems will be observed.

The varieties of clinical microphthalmos may be classified as follows.

Microcornea

Microcornea may occur as an independent anomaly although it often forms an important feature of a variety of other syndromes. The anterior segment is small and the recti muscles are inserted in a more forward position. There is increased corneal curvature and an increase in the corneal refraction. Visual acuity may be unaffected only if there are no other associated ocular deformities. Microcornea arises from a defect in embryological development occurring at the fourth month of fetal life when the cornea has the same curvature as the sclera. After this time the cornea shows accelerated growth. Failure of this development to take place results in microcornea. There is a recessive characteristic with a familial tendency.

A number of ocular anomalies associated with microcornea may also be seen in sclerocornea. They include coloboma of the iris and/or retina-choroid, iridocorneal angle dysgenesis, persistent pupillary membrane, congenital cataract, glaucoma, and high refractive error. Duke-Elder has described an increased corneal curvature in some patients with microcornea, but states the curvature may also be normal, as in some patients with

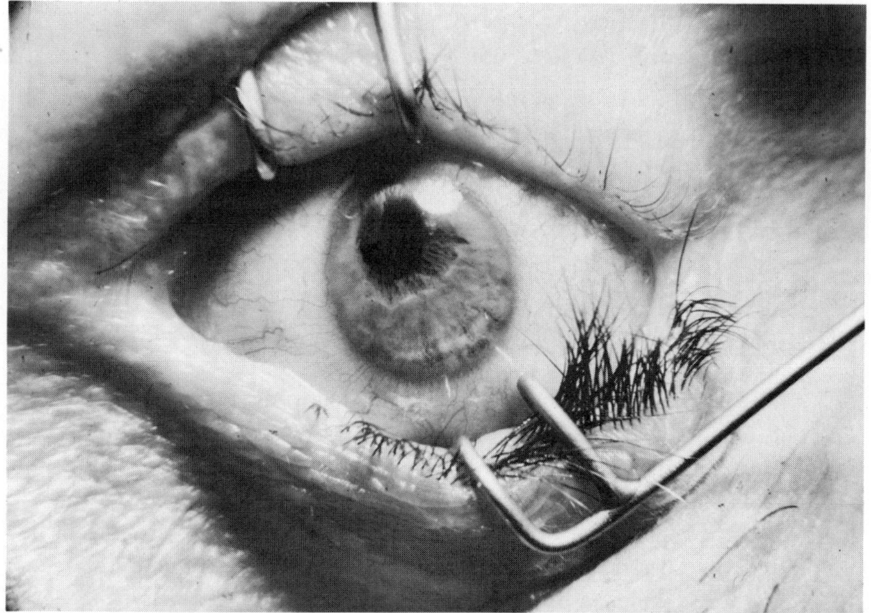

FIG. 6. Microcornea, microphthalmos, and coloboma of iris.

sclerocornea. Fig. 6 illustrates a case of microcornea and coloboma of the iris, in a patient's only eye. Fig. 7 (See colorplate, frontis.) shows a young child with unilateral microphthalmos associated with a congenital cataract which was successfully removed.

Pure Microphthalmos or Nanophthalmos

Nanophthalmos ("nanos": dwarf) is a form of congenital microphthalmos which results from an arrest in growth, caused by unknown factors sometime after closure of the fetal cleft. This produces a reduction of ocular dimensions without significant distortion of other ocular structures.

Pupillary block glaucoma may occur due to lens swelling or as a result of an anterior displacement of the lens. Glaucoma may also occur when a normal-sized lens is associated with a small anterior segment.

Visual acuity is decreased to usually less than 20/70 because of severe axial hyperopia of up to 20 diopters or because of refractive myopia. In addition there may be macular hypoplasia. Most eyes are poorly controlled with miotics or iridectomies. The large lens ultimately blocks the pupil. Cataract extraction may be necessary to control the glaucoma.

Microphthalmos with Cyst; Congenital Cystic Eyeball

When the primary optic vesicle fails to invaginate between the 2.0–mm and 7.0-mm stages of fetal development, the result is a congenital cystic eye, also called anophthalmos with cyst. Chronologically this occurs about the fourth week of gestation. Later arrest between the 7.0-mm and 14-mm stages produces the more common coloboma.

Congenital cystic eyeball, which is always present at birth, is of variable size. Typically it is a large bluish orbital mass which causes the upper lid to bulge forward. The cysts may be single or lobulated and their location in relation to the maldeveloped eye varies.

The cysts may be rudimentary and attached to the posterior wall of the microphthalmic eye or they may be located further back in the orbit, with a connecting stalk to the microphthalmic eye. Both of these types are not evident clinically and are detected only after enucleation. Other cysts are so large that they push the microphthalmic eye out of sight into the orbit, leading to the false diagnosis of orbital cyst associated with anophthalmos. However, x-ray evidence of a patient optic foramen suggests that there has been development of a rudimentary eye and that the condition is one of microphthalmos. In true anophthalmos the optic foramina would be either narrowed or completely obliterated.

Dollfus et al. reported a case of congenital cystic eyeball which affirmed the absence of a microphthalmic eye. The mass which occupied the orbit was the primary optic vesicle. The orbital cyst consisted of glial tissue arranged in layers crisscrossed by cavities. Epithelial vestiges, having the structure of the external granular layer of the retina, were present together with vestiges of the optic nerve.

Microphthalmos with Anomalous Development of Surface Ectoderm; Cryptophthalmos

The cornea, anterior chamber, and lens may be lacking and replaced by a skin appendage stretching between the eyelids, or there may be a complete absence of eye appendages, a condition known as cryptophthalmos.

Ide and Wollschlaeger reported a case of a child with bilateral cryptophthalmia (Figs. 8A and B). In addition to a number of other systemic abnormalities (Fig. 9), bilateral ankyloblepharon, small auditory meati, and syndactylia of both hands and feet were seen (Fig. 10). The eyes were small and observed only after the overlying skin was incised. The left eye demonstrated light perception with color differentiation but the right eye was blind.

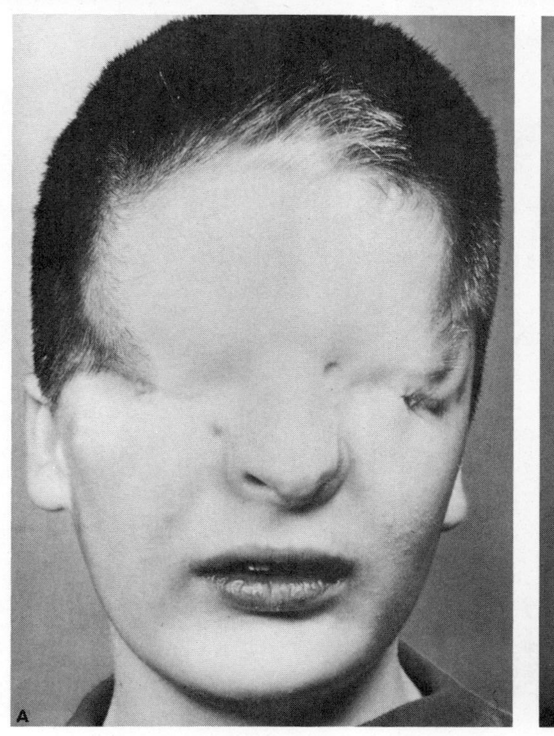

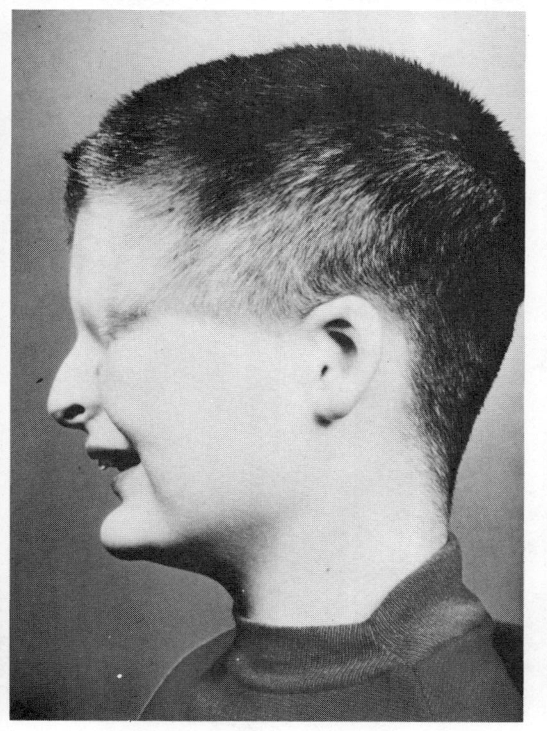

FIG. 8. Cryptophthalmia (front view and profile). Skin passes continuously from forehead to cheeks. Scars in skin overlaying eyes due to surgery performed when patient was 5 days old. (From Ide and Wollschlaeger. **Arch. Ophthalmol.** 81:638, 1969.)

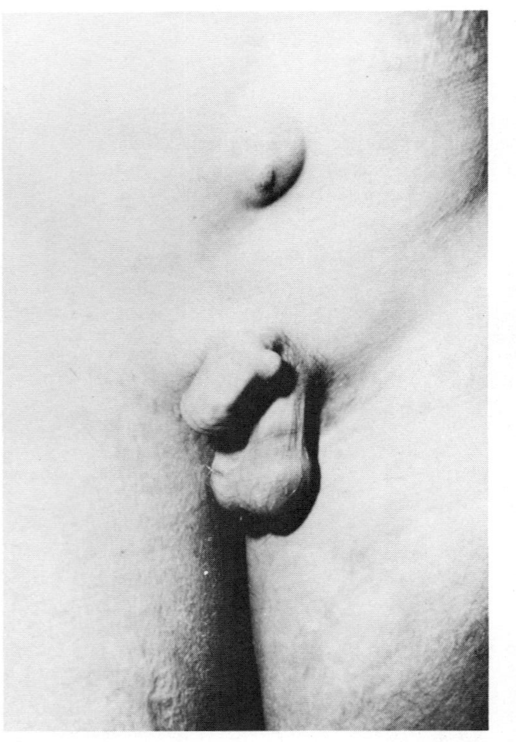

FIG. 9. Cryptophthalmia case. Umbilical hernia. Deviation of penis due to skin fold and marked chordee. Lipoma at base of penis. Healed donor sites for skin grafting on abdomen and upper thighs. (From Ide and Wollschlaeger. **Arch Ophthalmol.** 81: 638, 1969.)

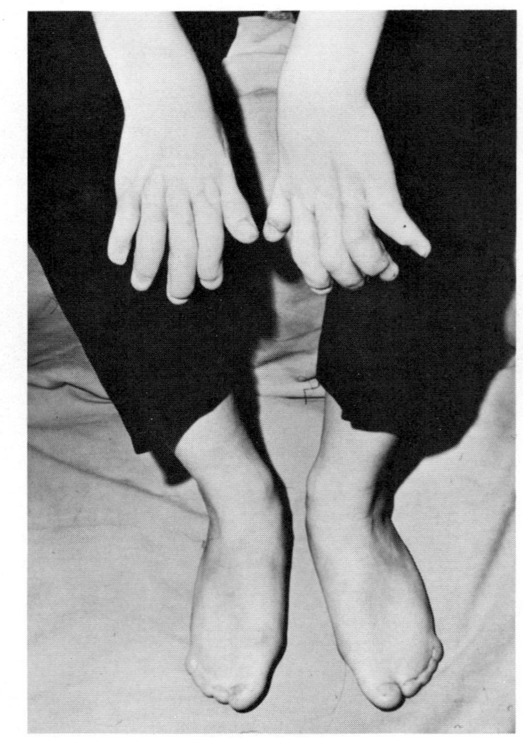

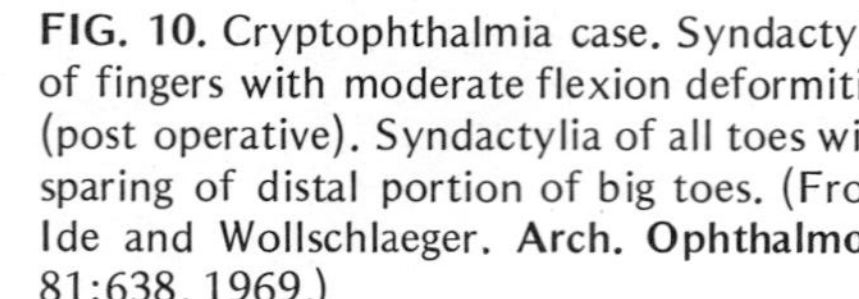

FIG. 10. Cryptophthalmia case. Syndactylia of fingers with moderate flexion deformities (post operative). Syndactylia of all toes with sparing of distal portion of big toes. (From Ide and Wollschlaeger. **Arch. Ophthalmol.** 81:638, 1969.)

Microphthalmos Associated with Multiple Ocular Defects

This is the characteristic form of microphthalmos, as evidenced by most of the 45 cases presented in Zeiter's series.

The ocular anomalies associated with microphthalmos are reviewed in Table 2. Of the 36 microphthalmic patients who survived the neonatal stage, 30 had vision no better than light perception in the affected eye. The common anomalies found included: (1) congenital cataracts and dislocated lens; (2) corneal scarring, vascular infiltration of the cornea, with indefinite limbal demarcation; (3) muscle imbalance with nystagmoid movements; (4) colobomas of the iris and choroid; (5) pupillary obstruction due to extreme miosis, pupillary membrane, or corectopia; (6) glaucoma, secondary to a combination of a large lens volume in a relatively small eye, a narrow filtration angle, and anterior synechiae; (7) retinal holes and detachment; (8) retinitis pigmentosa associated with microphthalmos and glaucoma; (9) fibrosis and shrinkage of the vitreous; (10) hypoplasia of the visual pathways up to the lateral geniculate body; and (11) hyperopia, generally, and myopia infrequently.

Systemic anomalies in the rest of the body associated with microphthalmos are even more varied. Of 44 cases 18 showed one or more of the congenital anomalies listed in Table 3. Other anomalies (each found only once) included nephrosclerosis, hydroureter, imperforate anus, fused ribs, facial hemangioma, fatty infiltration of the liver and spleen, and hemosiderosis. The cerebral and cardiovascular anomalies may be severe enough to lead to a fatal termination in the neonatal period. Of 10 microphthalmic

TABLE 2

FREQUENCY OF OCULAR ANOMALIES FOUND IN 44 CASES OF CONGENITAL MICROPHTHALMOS*

Anomaly	Frequency
Congenital cataract	14
Corneal scarring or vascularity	12
Muscle inbalance	10
Marked enopthalmos with pseudoptosis and narrowing of the palpebral fissures	11
Colobomas of iris or choroid	9
Pupillary obstruction secondary to extreme miosis or membrane	7
Narrow-angle glaucoma	4
Retinal detachments	2
Orbital cysts	2
Chorioretinitis	2
Orbital hemangioma	1

*After H. J. Zeiter, Am. J. Ophthalmol., 55:910, 1963.

TABLE 3

CONGENITAL ANOMALIES FOUND IN ASSOCIATION WITH MICROPHTHALMOS AND THEIR FREQUENCY OF OCCURRENCE*

Anomaly	Frequency
Cerebral aberation	8
Hydrocephalus	3
Microcephaly	3
Mental deficiency	5
Epilepsy	3
Congenital heart disease	5
Nonspecific	3
Tetralogy of Fallot	2
Supernumerary digits and other deformities of the extremities	8
Cleft palate and harelip	5
Cryptorchism and inguinal hernia	3
Omphalocele	2
Congenital toxoplasmosis	2

*After H. J. Zeiter, Am. J. Ophthalmol., 55:910, 1963.

newborns with associated cerebral and cardiovascular anomalies, 8 died immediately or within a few days of birth.

Zeiter reviewed the literature and classified microphthalmos as it relates to other systems of the body and syndrome complexes (Table 4). Some of these anomalies evidently appear with regular frequency, suggesting, perhaps, some special connection between them and microphthalmos. What this relation means is difficult to assess. Most of the anomalies listed in Table 4, however, appear at random and have significance only as part of a generally maldeveloped body.

Cornea Plana

Up to the fourth month of fetal life, the cornea and sclera have the same curvature, but between the fourth and fifth months an increase in corneal curvature takes place. If this process is arrested while general growth continues, cornea plana results. Flattening of the cornea may occur in varying degrees including involvement of the anterior sclera. Other features include opacification of the corneal stroma (sclerocornea), shallow anterior chamber, and astigmatism. Cornea plana may be associated with other anomalies including coloboma of the iris, congenital cataract, and ectopia lentis. Glaucoma occurs when the filtration angle is involved.

TABLE 4

CLASSIFICATION OF DEVELOPMENTAL ANOMALIES IN OTHER SYSTEMS OF THE BODY SEEN WITH MICROPHTHALMOS*

(A) Mental and neurologic malformations
- (1) Hydrocephalus
- (2) Meningocele
- (3) Encephalocele
- (4) Microcephaly
- (5) Arrhinencephaly and lack of olfactory nerves
- (6) Spina bifida
- (7) Epilepsy
- (8) Mental deficiency

(B) Congenital heart disease

(C) Deformities of the head and oral cavity
- (1) Syndrome of Jules Francois
- (2) Hallerman-Streiff syndrome
- (3) Cleft palate and harelip
- (4) Deformities of the ear
- (5) Deformities of the tongue
- (6) Dysplasia oculo-dento-digitalis
- (7) Dyscranio-pygo-phalangie
- (8) Facial hemangiomata and Lindau's disease

(D) Deformities of the extremities and fingers
- (1) Syndactylism
- (2) Polydactylism or supernumerary fingers
- (3) Talipes

(E) Other systemic anomalies
- (1) Polycystic disease of kidney, liver, pancreas, and parotid
- (2) Hemosiderosis and fatty infiltration of liver and spleen.
- (3) Genitourinary abnormalities such as nephrosclerosis, hydroureter, and cryptorchism.
- (4) Congenital toxoplasmosis
- (5) Gastrointestinal abnormalities such as omphalocele and imperforate anus

*After H. J. Zeiter, Am. J. Ophthalmol., 55:910, 1963.

Adhesions between Iris and Cornea and Associated Anomalies

Congenital ocular abnormalities involving mesodermal tissue of the anterior segment have been reported by ophthalmologists since the late 19th century. These early workers were intrigued by cases of abnormal irides and entertained the thought that the presence of such anomalous traits reflected structures normally found in the lower animals from whom man had

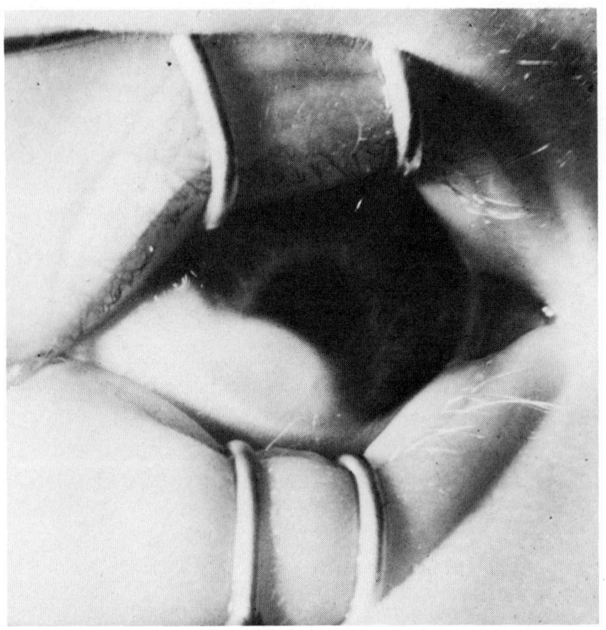

FIG. 11. Newborn. Adhesion exists between the iris and cornea with associated opacification.

supposedly evolved. Similar adhesions between the iris and cornea may also result from intrauterine corneal perforation resulting in adherent leucoma formation (Fig. 11).

Anterior Chamber Cleavage Syndrome

The anterior chamber cleavage syndrome is the current term advanced by Reese and Ellsworth for the group of congenital disorders of the anterior segment, believed to originate from faulty cleavage of the embryonic structures which eventually make up the anterior chamber of the eye. There may be a history of rubella or some other presumably viral infection during the first trimester. Abnormal iridocorneal adhesions (Fig. 12) occur either when the first and third mesodermal wave enters the anterior segment or during cleavage of the mesoderm that forms the anterior chamber. Cleavage abnormalities are divided into central and peripheral types. The corneal opacifications and adhesions may be at single or multiple focal points and the anterior chamber is irregularly shallow.

In their series of 21 patients (34 eyes), Reese and Ellsworth observed

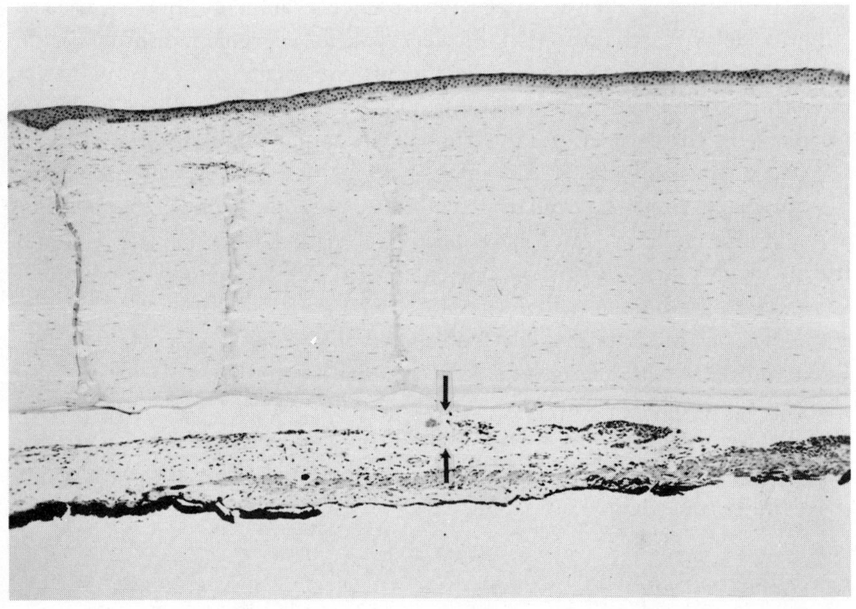

FIG. 12. Adhesion between iris and cornea. A blood vessel (arrows) passes through the adhesion. X 75.

that all cases were noted at birth or a few days later and 80 percent were bilateral. Glaucoma was present in 70 percent. Sclerocornea and cornea plana were noted in one-third of the cases. Four patients (22 percent) were mentally retarded, one had cerebral palsy, one had a cleft palate, and one had a mongolian spot.

When first seen, the dense corneal opacity may be associated with edema at the site of the adhesion. The leak may later be sealed off by the cuticular product formed by the endothelium (Descemet's membrane). Other associated systemic conditions include interventricular septal defect, anodontia partialis, myotonic dystrophy, syndactylism of both fingers and toes, oligodonty, status dysraphicus, craniofacial dysotosis, absence of intermaxillary bones and upper incisors, and malformation of the palate and lower incisors.

Peters' Anomaly, Mesodermal Dysgenesis of the Cornea

Peters' anomaly is a congenital disorder in which there is a central opacity with abnormalities of the posterior stroma and a local absence of Descemet's membrane.

The disease is believed to be a developmental anomaly that is caused by either a delayed separation of the lens vesicle, a primary disorder in the development of the endothelium of the anterior chamber, or a combination of both. Anterior synechiae extend from the pupillary zone of the iris to the periphery of the corneal opacity. Though the anomaly may be limited to the cornea, various defects in the anterior segment, including corectopia, iris hypoplasia, persistant pupillary membrane, microphthalmos, sclerocornea, and anterior polar cataract have been recorded. Glaucoma is a common feature. Eighty percent of the reported cases of Peters' anomaly are bilateral. While there are human pedigrees with combinations of Rieger's and Peters' anomalies, the latter is generally considered to involve recessive inheritance. Reese and Ellsworth have grouped this condition into their anterior chamber cleavage syndrome.

Brown reported a case with a dense bilateral central opacification in which both corneas were successfully transplanted. The author has also successfully transplanted a bilateral case.

Goniodysgenesis

Goniodysgenesis is characterized by an abnormal iridocorneal angle, iris hypoplasia, and glaucoma which develops in the first few decades of life. Inheritance is autosomal dominant.

In the large pedigree reported by Jerndal and that of Weatherill and Hart, a number of family members had "minor" dysgenesis of the angle and normal ocular pressure. Early onset of cataract was not noted in either of these pedigrees.

Henkind and Friedman reported a series of cases, with iris hypoplasia, corectopia, and filtration angle abnormalities. None of their patients suffered from glaucoma although cataracts were present. Their review of anterior segment abnormalities is summarized in Table 5.

Rieger's Disease

Rieger's disease comprises Rieger's anomaly and Rieger's syndrome. Other names designating the same condition as Rieger's anomaly have been suggested by Hagedoorn and Streiff. But Hagedoorn's "dysgenesis mesostromalis" and Streiff's "posterior marginalis dysplasia" have not proved more definitive or useful than Rieger's original classification. Rieger's anomaly includes all the primary ocular features with or without associated ocular findings. Rieger's syndrome includes all the primary ocular features with or without associated ocular findings and with one or more associated nonocular findings.

TABLE 5

COMPARISON OF THE HERITABLE ANTERIOR SEGMENT ANOMALIES*

Condition	Heredity	Ocular Abnormalities					
		Cornea	Iris	Angle	Lens	Glaucoma	Other Findings
Posterior embryotoxon	Recessive (?) Dominant (?)	Common	Occasional**	Occasional**	None	Occasional**	None
Mesodermal dysgenesis of iris and cornea	Autosomal dominant	Common	Common	Common	Occasional**	Common	May have dental or skeletal abnormalities
Peters anomaly	Recessive (?)	Common	Common	Common	Common	Common	None
Goniodysgenesis with glaucoma	Autosomal dominent	Occasional**	Common	Common	None	Common	None
Iridogoniodysgenesis and cataract	Autosomal recessive	None	Common	Common	Common	?	None

*After P. Henkind and A. H. Friedman, Am. J. Ophthalmol., 72:949, 1971.
**Involvement has been noted.

Mesodermal dysgenesis of the iris and cornea is an anomaly that was clearly delineated by Rieger in 1935. In addition to reporting two patients with anterior segment anomalies, he made a comprehensive survey of the literature on the subject. He reasoned that all the primary ocular manifestations of the disorder could be attributed to a heritable maldevelopment of the part of the mesoderm contributing to the iris and angle structures, and that the mode of familial transmission of this defect was autosomal dominant.

Since the anomaly has a dominant inheritance, one would expect, as in similarly transmitted traits, a broad range of expressivity in affected families as demonstrated by Henkind et al. There is, therefore, a great deal of difficulty in clinically separating the mild Rieger's anomaly from an eye which has markedly exaggerated "normal" structures. This dilemma frequently occurs when dominant traits are involved. Since the variability of findings in a particular pedigree would have to be assessed before the individual patient can be evaluated, ophthalmological examination of other members of the propositus' family would be necessary.

It is generally agreed that the basic malformation, be it wholly mesodermal or partially ectodermal in origin, occurs within the first two months of fetal life (12–22 mm) and that these early changes primarily affect the precursor stromal tissue of the iris, i.e., the iridopupillary lamina. Subsequent development of structures which use these defective tissues as scaffolding or support will also be affected. A great deal of developmental variation might be expected.

The primary features of Rieger's anomaly (see Table 6) are: partial or complete hypoplasia of the anterior stromal leaf of the iris; mesodermal strands, fibers, processes, or bands of a noninflammatory nature bridge the iridocorneal angle (Fig. 13) and insert into the trabecular zone or Schwalbe's line ("pectinate ligaments"), posterior embryotoxon (Fig. 14), and occasionally remnants of the pupillary membrane. The lens capsule "stars" so often seen in Rieger's anomaly (particularly in those eyes with iris colobomata) are remnants of a persistent pupillary membrane.

Gonioscopically, and in histologic sections, posterior embryotoxon appears as a thickened trabecular zone and accentuated Schwalbe's line in the presence of iris strands. It is neither embryologically nor anatomically a part of the cornea. Over 15 percent of normal eyes have been reported to have a pronounced border ring without attendant ocular abnormality (Fig. 15). Posterior embryotoxon may, however, provide the first clue to Rieger's anomaly and should be considered an important clinical finding. The great variability in its location and dimension can probably be attributed to the disturbing influence of the underlying mesodermal malformation.

TABLE 6

MESODERMAL DYSGENESIS OF THE ANTERIOR SEGMENT (RIEGER'S SYNDROME)*

Primary Features

(1) Hypoplasia of the anterior iris stroma
(2) Iris strands bridging angle (pectinate ligaments)
(3) Posterior embryotoxon

Associated Findings

Iris
- Aniridia
- Slit-like pupils
- Polycoria (true and pseudo)
- Corectopia
- Dyscoria
- Ectropion uvea (localized)
- Persistant pupillary membrane remnants
- Colobomata

Cornea
- Microcornea (real and apparent)
- Megalocornea
- Cornea plana
- Various corneal opacities (congenital)

Lens
- Colobomata
- Ectopia lentis
- Lens capsule "stars"
- Various lens opacities

Others
- Glaucoma (generally juvenile or early adult onset)
- Broad range of ametropias
- Strabismus
- Ptosis

Nonocular
- Dental anomalies—in number and shape of teeth
- Dysgnathia
- Hypertelorism
- Partial absence of facial bones
- Neurological disorders—mental retardation, hydrocephalus, cerebellar hypoplasia

*After P. Henkind, I. M. Siegel, and R. E. Carr, Arch. Ophthalmol., 73:810, 1965.

All cases demonstrate some degree of hypoplasia of the anterior stromal leaf of the iris. This can vary from a small sector defect to almost complete absence of the anterior iris leaf. The sphincter muscle usually appears prominent in these regions of hypoplasia, but the deep mesodermal and ectodermal layers are generally intact. The hypoplasia does not change with age (unless glaucoma supervenes) and can thus be distinguished from

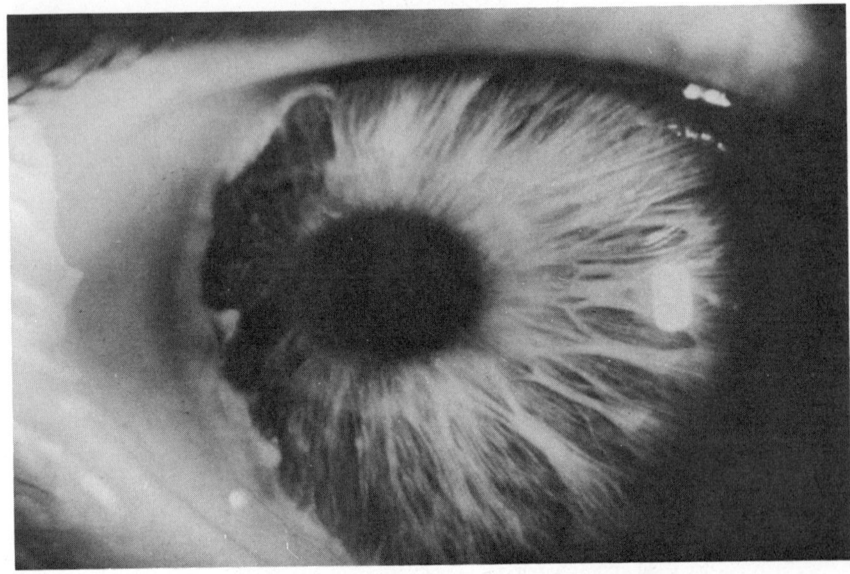

FIG. 13. Reiger's anomaly. (Courtesy of J. S. Speakman.)

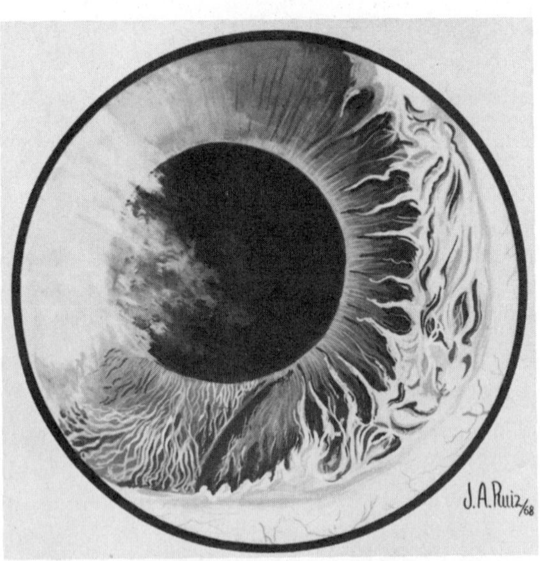

FIG. 14. Reiger's anomaly. Elevation of intraocular pressure with corneal edema.

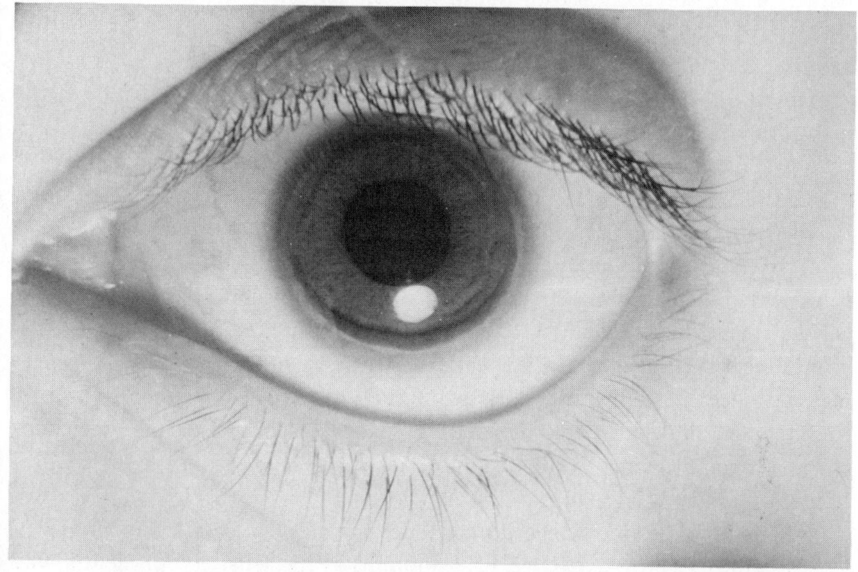

FIG. 15. Anterior border ring of Schwalbe. (Courtesy of A. H. Katz.)

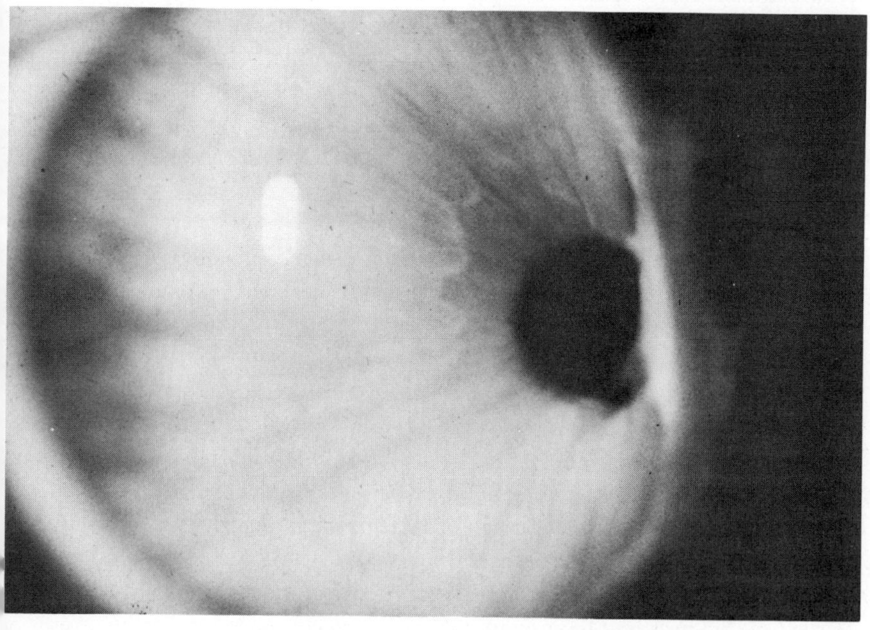

FIG. 16. Reiger's anomaly.

essential iris atrophy. Rieger felt that this maldevelopment of mesodermal tissue formed the basis for all the observable defects: "We therefore believe all cases of hypoplasia of the anterior part of the iris, regardless of whether or not irregularity and displacement of the pupil is present . . . to be a genetic entity which is initiated when the developmental disturbance of the mesoderm in the anterior segment takes place. . . ."

Iris abnormalities such as slit pupils, polycoria, and pupillary membrane remnants probably result from the disorganization of the poorly differentiated iris mesoderm. Aniridia, on the other hand, though frequently seen in cases of Rieger's anomaly, has usually been considered to be a separate, ectodermally derived malformation. Corneal abnormalities such as microcornea, megalocornea, and cornea plana are frequently seen in association with Rieger's anomaly. The appearance of microcornea in many instances may be deceiving, however, because of the presence of prominent embryotoxon or an ill-defined limbal zone. A variety of corneal lesions, including stromal opacities and hyaline membranes, have been reported in cases of Rieger's anomaly (Fig. 16).

Lens opacities have been noted, but early onset of cataract formation is not a feature. The occurrence of coloboma of the lens, ectopia lentis, and the variety of lenticular opacities are not easily explained if one accepts the notion that Rieger's anomaly is primarily a mesodermal dysgenesis. One can assume the coexistence of an independent ectodermal anomaly, but caution must be exercised in completely excluding the influence of maldevelopment in surrounding tissues.

The defects usually affect both eyes and are of themselves generally nonprogressive. On the other hand, glaucoma usually appearing in the second or third decade of life can lead to progressive ocular deterioration if uncontrolled. It is not clear whether glaucoma results from mechanical occlusion of the chamber angle by iridotrabecular adhesions or from maldevelopment of angle outflow channels. The latter explanation seems more reasonable since one frequently sees the onset of glaucoma in the face of an angle which appears largely open, gonioscopically. The glaucoma may be easily controlled or it may be unresponsive to therapy. Medical control is preferred. If surgery becomes mandatory, the external filtering operations should be employed. Goniotomy with or without goniopuncture has been reported to be effective in some younger patients (less than age 25).

Breebaart reported a case of Rieger's anomaly complicated by glaucoma, the level of which was influenced by sleep (during which time the pressure dropped). When the patient stayed awake during the night and went to sleep in the morning the pressure curves were completely reversed.

Should Rieger's anomaly be associated with dental, skeletal, or neurological defects in addition to what is considered the primary and associated ocular features, then the more comprehensive term Rieger's syndrome would apply. The skeletal changes include various dysplasias of the skull, spine, and extremities. When dental anomalies as well as lens defects are found in cases of Rieger's anomaly the reasons for advancing an independently associated ectodermal anomaly become reinforced. The existence of these associated findings results in the possibility that they represent either different aspects of a single entity or separate disorders.

Axenfeld's Syndrome

Curiously, the mesodermal anomaly so carefully delineated by Rieger is often referred to as "Axenfeld's syndrome." The preference for the latter term was probably influenced by Axenfeld's report of a patient with unusual corneal findings, which he designated as "embryotoxon corneae posterius." This patient also exhibited iris strands bridging the angle and an area of hypoplastic iris in one eye.

Although one should distinguish between mesodermal dysgenesis of the anterior segment (Rieger's anomaly) and posterior embryotoxon of the cornea (Axenfeld's syndrome) as Duke-Elder does, one should not assume that these are altogether different conditions. Indeed it is likely they are both parts of a spectrum of mesodermal abnormalities of the eye as Reese and Ellsworth have advocated.

Dominant pedigrees, particularly where there is involvement of the iris, have been reported, but autosomal recessive inheritance has also been documented. Occasional sporadic cases occur, probably representing de novo mutations.

The characteristic features include prominent Schwalbe's line (Fig. 17), the so-called posterior embryotoxon (G. embryon, embryo; G. toxon, bow) which can be seen by direct observation without gonioscopy, and prominent strands of developmental iris stroma extending from the iris root to the trabecular meshwork, Schwalbe's line, and the peripheral cornea. This attachment gives rise to a localized corneal opacity (Fig. 18). In more pronounced cases of posterior embryotoxon the iris may be hypoplastic. Such cases probably represent variants of Rieger's anomaly (Fig. 19). The anterior chamber findings vary from subtle localized involvement to extensive changes involving 360° of the angle.

The abnormal tissue may take the form of a fine delicate cellophane strand observed only on microscopic examination, or it may be seen as thick

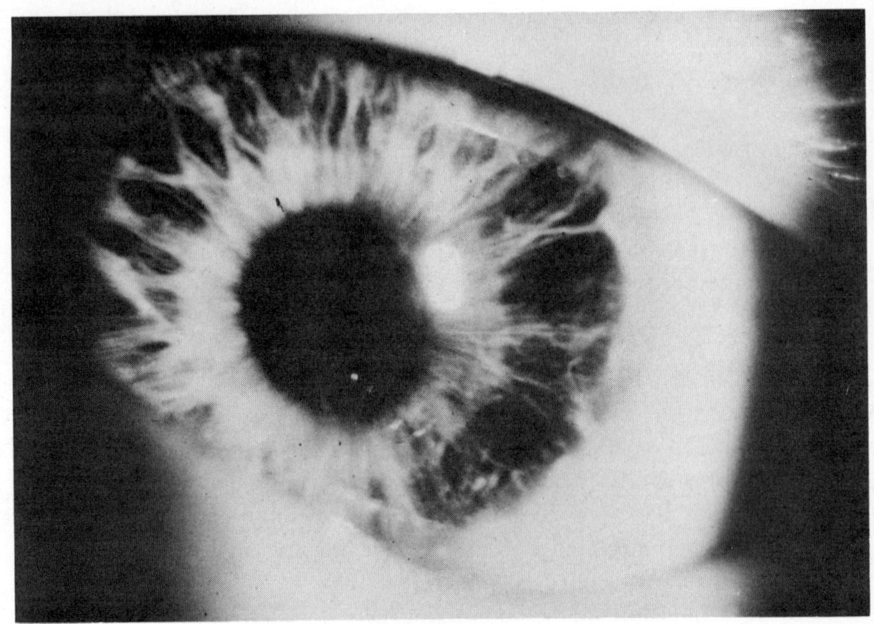

FIG. 17. Axenfeld's syndrome.

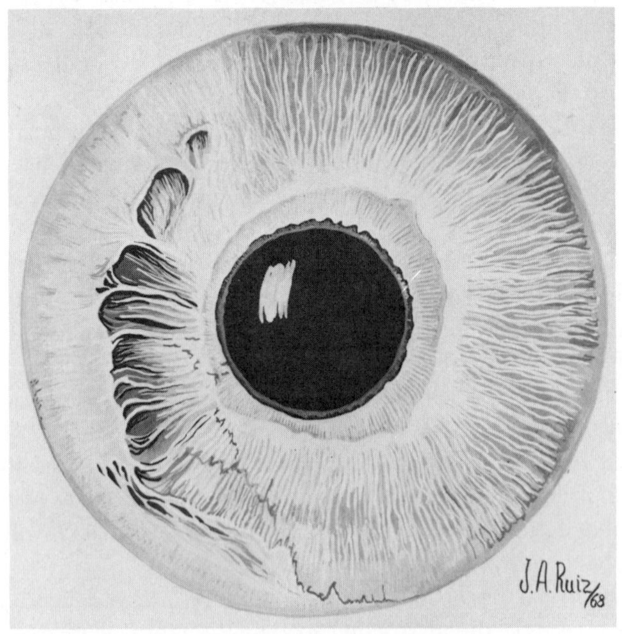

FIG. 18. Axenfeld's syndrome.

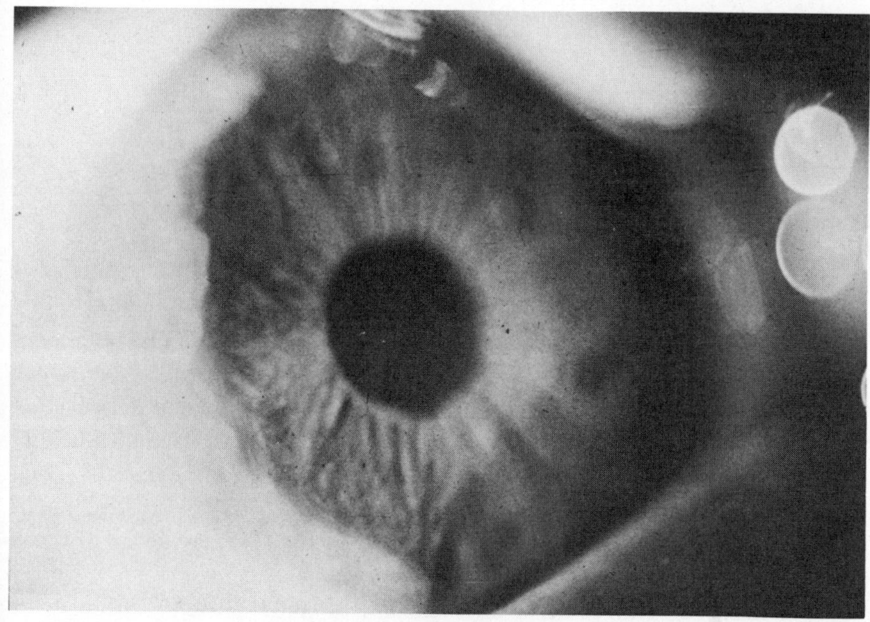

FIG. 19. Axenfeld's syndrome.

pleomorphic broad bands, often dense enough to be grossly seen, which resemble iris stroma. The trabecular zone is wide and Schwalbe's line is prominent, often displaced axially and visible on slit lamp examination as a circumferential hyaline rod which may appear to be detached from the posterior corneal surface. The eye may be microphthalmic, normal, or buphthalmic if glaucoma supervenes early in life. In this event stretching of the cornea results in the appearance of classical ruptures in Descemet's membrane. Other associated pupil and iris abnormalities include corectopia, dyscoria, various degrees of ectropion uveae, coloboma, partial aniridia and pseudopolycoria. True polycoria rarely occurs. Other anomalies are seen such as corneal opacities, lens opacities, lens coloboma, epicapsular pigment stars, ectopia lentis, strabismus, microcornea, and compound myopic astigmatism. When the condition is asymmetrical, we find anisometropia, refractive amblyopia, and strabismus.

About 50 percent of these patients have glaucoma although the severity of the hypertension may not correlate with the extent of the clinically observable angle aberrations. Onset may take place early in infancy though it usually is seen later in life, but before the age of thirty.

IRIS ANOMALIES

Aniridia

Aniridia was first described by Barratta in 1819 and Gutbier published the first pedigree in 1837. There is equal sex distribution and bilateral cases (Fig. 20, see colorplate, frontis) occur more commonly than unilateral ones in a ratio of 50:1. The term aniridia is correct only in the clinical sense since a rudimentary band of iris is always present. The apparent absence on clinical examination is due to the fact that the short stump is hidden behind the corneoscleral margin and is visible only with the gonioscope (Fig. 21). The rudimentary band of the iris root may be pulled up toward the line of Schwalbe, thus sealing the angle. The border of the lens may be grossly seen (Fig. 22).

Aniridia is said to have an incidence of 0.04 percent, although in Denmark it was estimated to be 1:100,000 by Mollenbach, and 1:50,000 in the lower Michigan Peninsula by Shaw et al.

Aniridia represents an arrest in the differentiation of the optic cup ectoderm. The defect occurs in development of the mesoderm and epidermal layers of the iris. Straub Marburg reported one family in which 114 cases were identified in 4 generations. Grove et al. reported a family study that

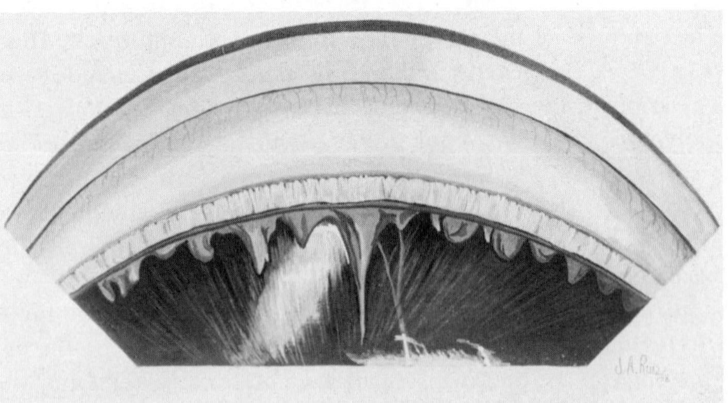

FIG. 21. Aniridia. Filtration angle showing iris stump.

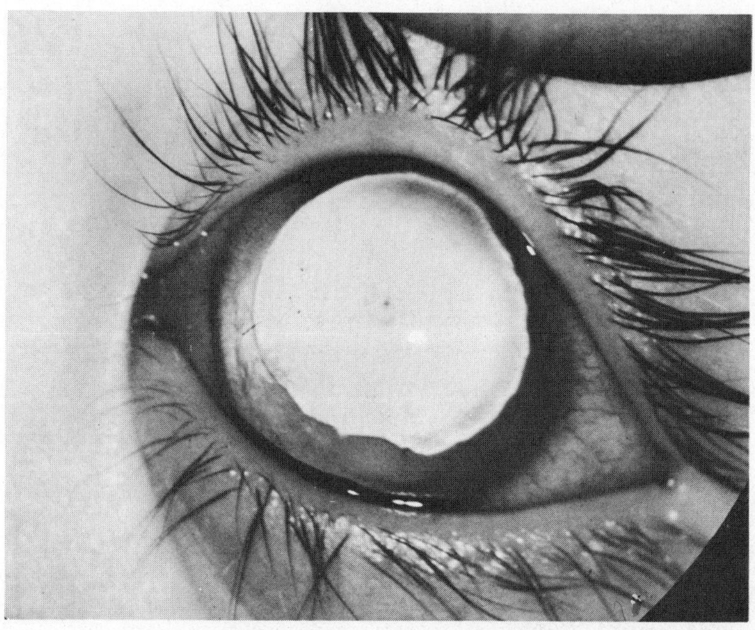

FIG. 22. Aniridia. The border of the lens is grossly visible. A coloboma of the lens is evident. (Courtesy of P. E. Milot.)

covered 5 generations in which 77 descendants of one aniridic woman, who had bilateral aniridia, were found. Ages ranged from 8 months to 68 years. Glaucoma was found in 10 individuals, and in addition, two persons had bilateral phthisis bulbi with a history of glaucoma. In this series increased intraocular pressure was not discovered under age 19. Previous findings of congenital aniridia inheritance as an autosomal dominant with relatively strong penetrance was confirmed in agreement with other authors (Franceschetti, 83.5 percent, and Reed and Falls, 92 percent). There were no cases of two parents with normal eyes having an offspring with aniridia, and there were no cases of unilateral aniridia. There are, however, some uncommon cases of recessive transmission with consanguineous parents.

Aniridia may be associated with cataract formation (Fig. 23), photophobia, strabismus, spherophakia, microphthalmos, ectopia lentis, nystagmus, corneal opacities, Bergmeister's papilla, congenital glaucoma, and aplasia of the macula (except in recessively inherited cases). Since the iris and macula develop about the same time, abnormalities may occur simultaneously. The poor visual acuity may thus be due to foveal disease. Systemic defects include polydactylia, oligophrenia, aberrent spleen, dysos-

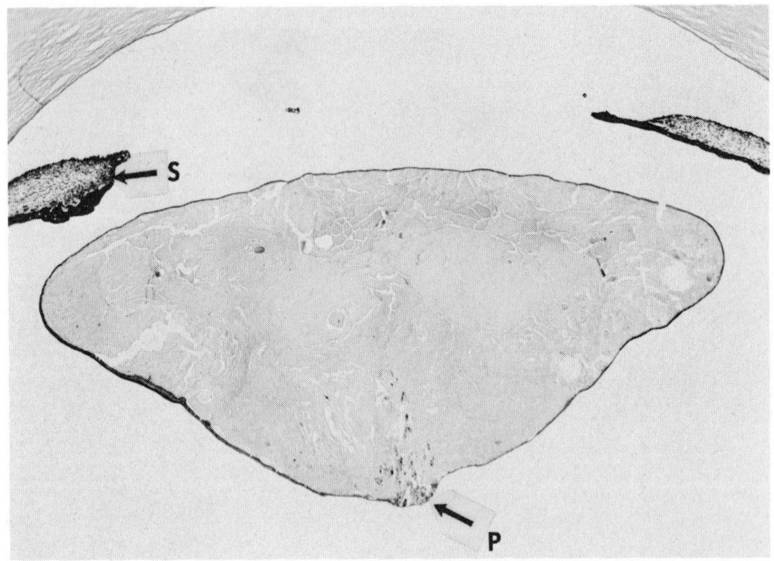

FIG. 23. Aniridia. Markedly cataractous lens with enlarged axial diameter and prominent convexity at posterior pole (arrow P), where capsule is deficient. (Dense opacity was seen in this area on gross examination.) Elsewhere capsule is of normal thickness or is irregularly thickened. In this plane of section, a small amount of sphincter is present on one side (Arrow S). (A. F. I. P. Neg. No. 65-3905.) (From Zimmerman and Font. J. A. M. A., 196:684, 1966.) (Courtesy of the authors, the American Medical Association, and the Registry of Ophthalmic Pathology of the Armed Forces Institute of Pathology.) X 22.

tosis of the skull and face, malformation of the extremities and external ears (some being low set), hydrocephalus with neurologic signs, and mental retardation.

Miller et al. first associated Wilm's tumor with aniridia in 1964. An epidemiologic study of 400 cases with Wilm's tumor indicated an incidence of aniridia of 1:59, in contrast to the usual rate of about 1:50,000. These children show some other congenital defects including hemihypertrophy, microcephaly, mental retardation, urogenital anomalies, and abnormalities of the external ears. In male patients the common urogenital anomalies are cryptorchidism, microphallus and penile hypoplasia. Lens changes (Fig. 24) and hypoplasia of the iris (Fig. 25) are both present. These may all be manifestations of the same lethal gene. The sex ratio was male: female = 9:2.

In children with aniridia, Wilms' tumor is usally diagnosed before age 3, compared to the average age of diagnosis of 3–6 years. Cases of aniridia and

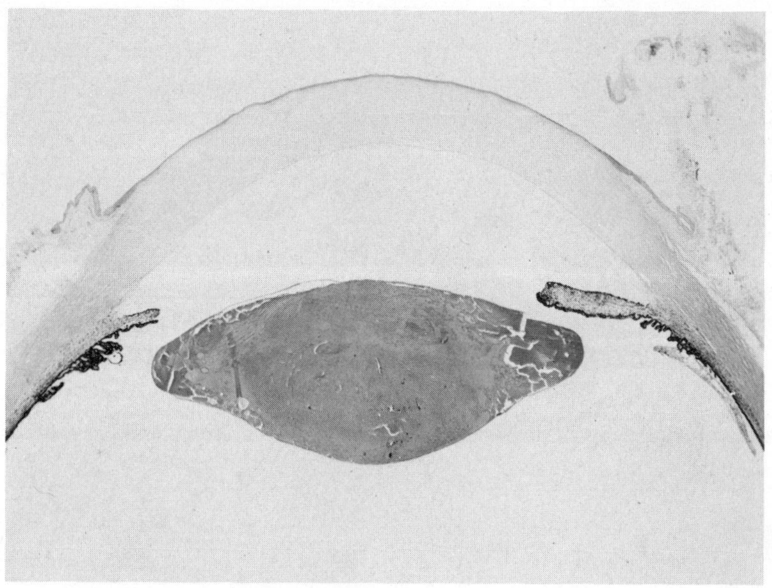

FIG. 24. Aniridia. Anterior segment of eye from mentally retarded, microcephalic 6-1/2-month-old baby who had bilateral Wilms's tumor. Degenerative changes are present throughout cortex and nucleus of lens; iris is hypoplastic. (A. F I. P. Neg. No. 65-3904.) (From Zimmerman and Font. J. A. M. A., 196:684, 1966. Courtesy of the authors, the American Medical Association, and the Registry of Ophthalmic Pathology of the Armed Forces Institute of Pathology.) X 10.

Wilms' tumor may be sporadic without family history.

The treatment of aniridia must be directed to each of the ocular symptoms. Nystagmus and photophobia may be treated with contact lenses. Enoch and Windsor reported a case of a 20-month-old child that was fitted with vented scleral contact lenses which eliminated the photophobia and caused a remission of the nystagmus. The author has treated several aniridia cases associated with macular aplasia with visual aids. One patient was able to complete undergraduate college with such a device. Lens abnormalities must undergo appropriate procedures. Blake, in 1953, reviewed the surgical treatment of glaucoma associated with congenital aniridia. He concluded that cyclodiathermy was the operation of choice in these cases. The goniotomy procedure has been used by Barkan to release the adhesions of the iris stump.

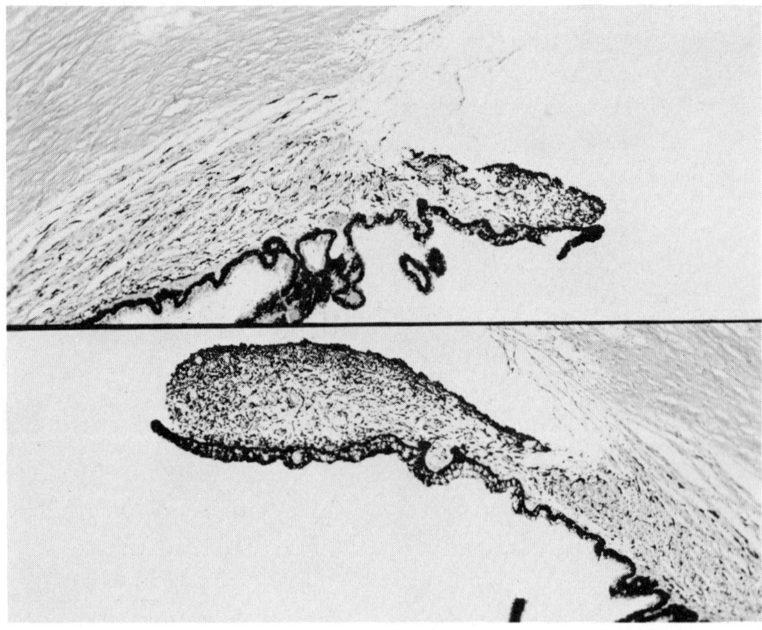

FIG. 25. Aniridia. In many planes of section the rudimentary iris contains neither sphincter nor dilator muscle. (A. F. I. P. Neg. No. 65-3910.) (From Zimmerman and Font. J. A. M. A., 196:684, 1966.) (Courtesy of the authors, the American Medical Association, and the Registry of Ophthalmic Pathology of the Armed Forces Institute of Pathology.) X 50.

Coloboma of the Iris

Coloboma of the iris occurs with faulty development of the eye during the stage of closure of the fetal fissure so that the location is downward and nasal (Fig. 26). Although a large segment may be absent the remainder of the iris is normal. Atypical colobomas of the iris result when there is an abnormal persistence of fetal blood vessels at the edge of the optic cup. Coloboma of the retina may be present as an associated condition, an example of which is shown in Fig. 27 (See colorplate, frontis.)

Coloboma of the iris may be of the total, partial, notch, or bridge type. Total coloboma of the iris (Fig. 28) displays an involvement of a whole section of the iris up to the ciliary border. In the partial coloboma only a segment is missing. A hole may be seen in the substance of the iris resulting in what is referred to clinically as pseudopolycoria. Notch colobomas may be multiple. The bridge coloboma (Fig. 29) is a rare anomaly where the defect

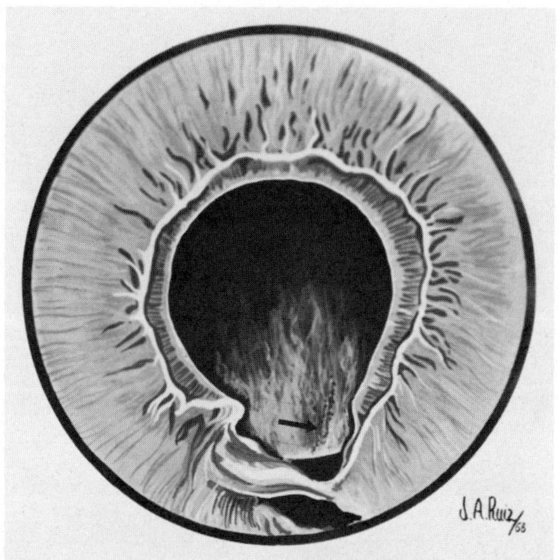

FIG. 26. Coloboma of the iris. Lens border is visible. A bridge of iris tissue spans the gap, pigment is deposited on the lens (arrow).

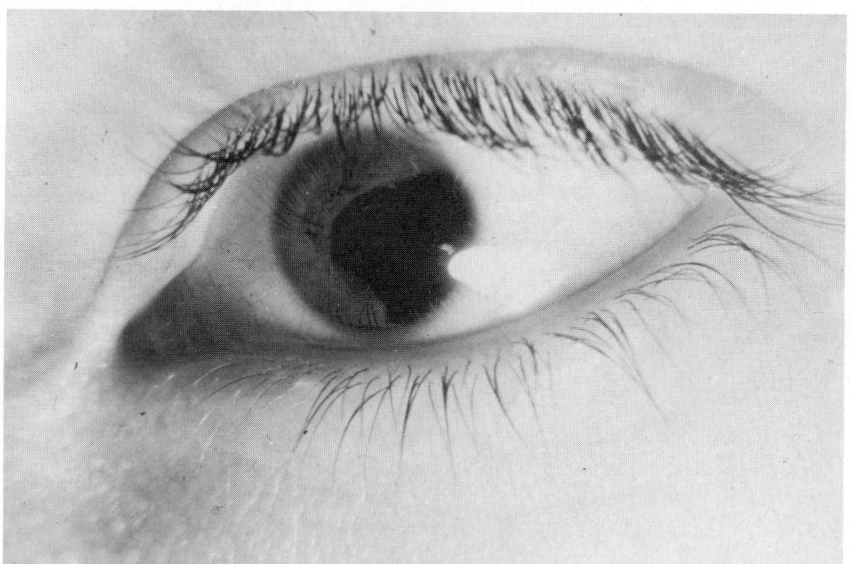

FIG. 28. Coloboma of the iris. The location is atypical. The intraocular pressure was elevated in this case.

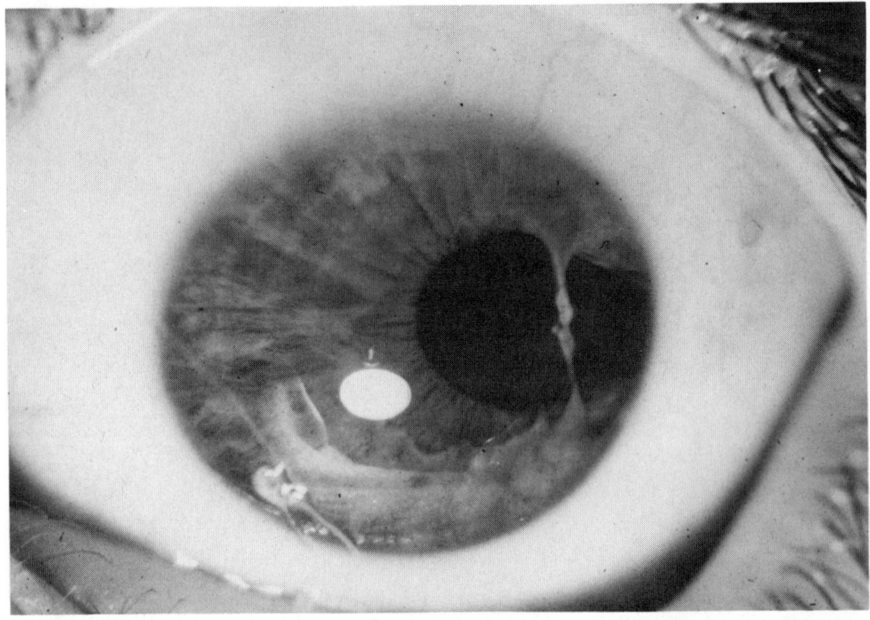

FIG. 29. Bridge coloboma of the iris. A thick strand of iris tissue crosses the defect.

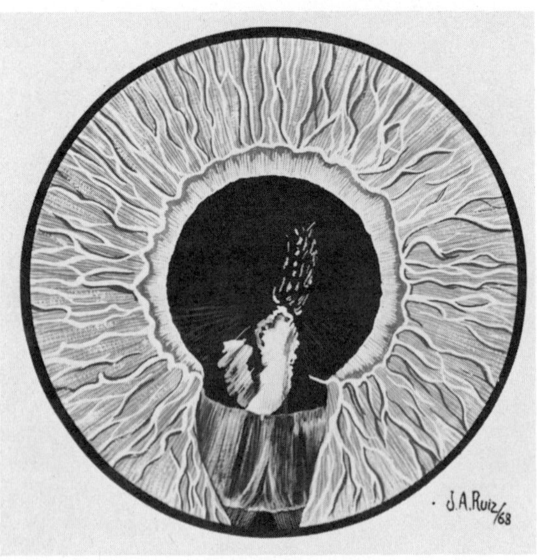

FIG. 30. Coloboma of the iris, lens, and zonules. Lens changes are illustrated.

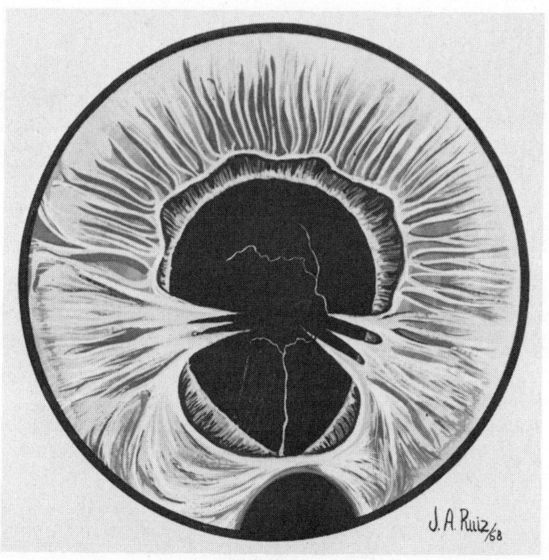

FIG. 31. Coloboma of the iris. There is persistence of the pupillary membrane. A thick band crosses the iris defect.

is spanned by mesodermal tissue derived from the anterior mesodermal layer of the iris. The bridge may be in the form of a delicate film of gossamer-like tissue bridging the gap, or it may be a stout band of tissue resembling the surrounding iris. Pits are seen in the iris surface, the floor of which is the darkly colored, pigmented epithelium.

The iris is otherwise well developed, although the sphincter muscle may be absent or poorly developed. Other abnormalities include lens changes (Fig. 30) and persistent pupillary membrane (Fig. 31).

Persistent Pupillary Membrane

Persistent pupillary membrane is a condition with a dominant transmission and consists of vascularized strands belonging to the embryonic fibrovascular capsule of the lens. There are various degrees of severity including fine filaments crossing the pupil (Fig. 32), some of which are deeply pigmented (Fig. 33). A much more severe aberration is congenital atresia of the pupil (Fig. 34).

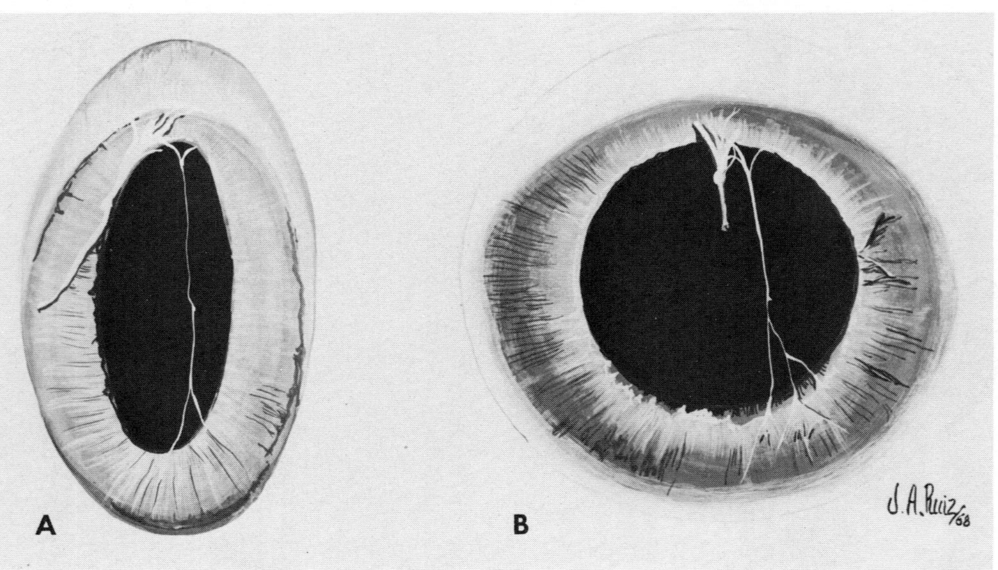

FIG. 32. Persistent pupillary membrane (front view and profile). Pupillary fibers extend across the pupil. The peripheral cornea is scleralized.

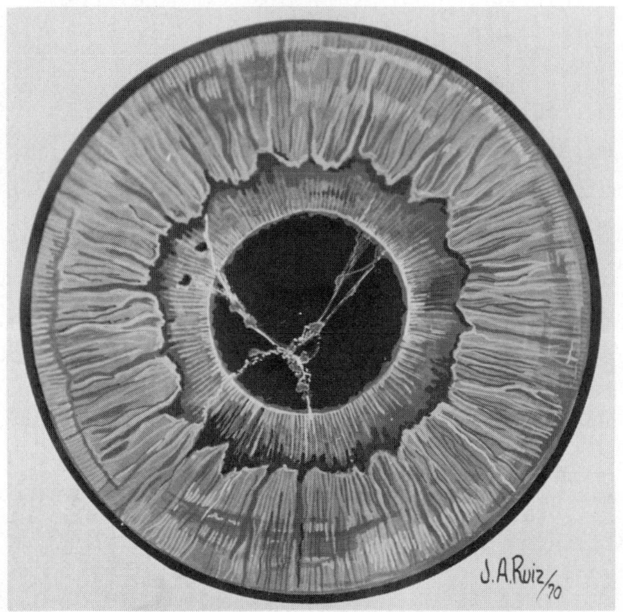

FIG. 33. Persistent pupillary membrane. Delicate pigmented filaments cross the pupil zone of an otherwise normal eye.

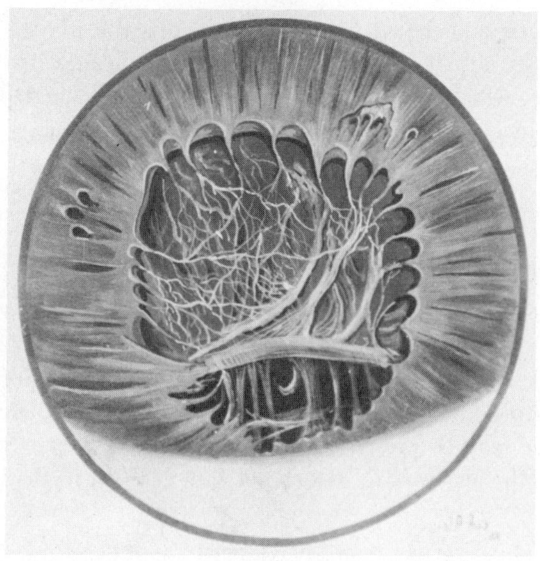

FIG. 34. Congenital atresia of the pupil with scleralization of the peripheral cornea.

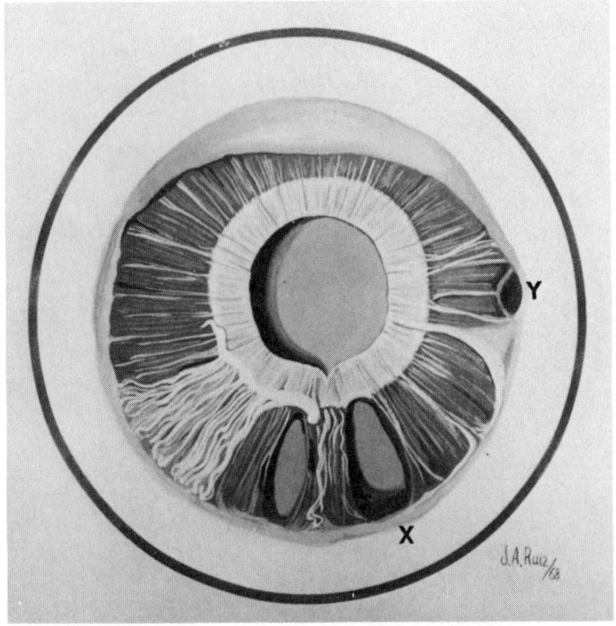

FIG. 35. Iridodehiscence (X) and iridodiastasis (Y). The peripheral cornea is opacified.

Iridodiastasis and Iridodehiscence

Iridodiastasis is a defect or separation along the iris root leaving the pupillary margin intact. There is a close resemblance to iridodialysis. Iridodehiscence, which is a splitting open of iris tissue, must be differentiated from iridodiastasis. (Fig. 35).

Hyperplasia of the Iris Layers

Anterior Layer of the Iris Stroma

The accessory iris membrane is a superficial mesodermal layer of iris which normally terminates at the lesser circle and undergoes atrophy, persisting only as a delicate tissue interspersed with pits. Sometimes it is transformed into a thick layer extending across the pupil. Irregular defects in the substance may be present, appearing as an accessory pupil. The tissue may insert into the lens capsule associated with cataract formation.

Pigment Border of Iris (Flocculi)

Darkly pigmented excrescences of the iris pigment epithelium usually present as grape-like clusters or black nodules at the upper margin of the pupil are seen. The condition is frequently bilateral. The clusters usually remain stationary but may enlarge and become cystic. They may detach and float free in the anterior chamber or retain a thin thread-like stalk.

Corectopia

Corectopia is an anomaly in the position of the pupil. Minor variations are common. The pupil may reach almost to the peripheral border of the iris. The condition is often bilateral and symmetrical. The pupil may be round, oval (Fig. 36), or irregular. Reaction to light is usually impaired or diminished. These eyes are frequently myopic and vision may be poor. The condition may be associated with ectopia lentis and lens changes.

Congenital Microcoria

The pupil is considered abnormal if, when looking at a distant object in diffuse daylight, the pupillary diameter remains less than 2 mm. Congenital microcoria is a rare, often bilateral condition which displays an absence of the dilator pupillae. Pupil reactions are minimal and patients may suffer

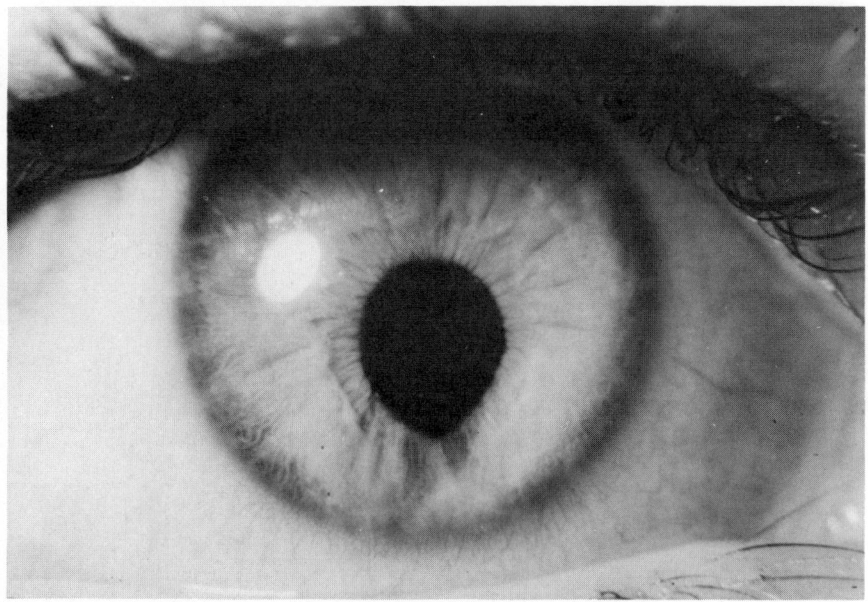

FIG. 36. Corectopia.

from twilight blindness. Circular contraction folds are usually absent with a few indications of shallow radial folds in the iris. Congenital microcoria may be treated with a surgical iridectomy.

Polycoria

In polycoria, there is actual reduplication of the pupil, each with an independent muscle supply (Fig. 37). The case reported by Jaffe and Knie demonstrated sphincter activity in each pupil. Frequently an anterior polar cataract is seen with congenital corneal opacities; glaucoma may be present. True polycoria must be differentiated from dehiscence and diastasis of the iris. False polycoria may be seen as a partial coloboma or after severe trauma to the anterior segment. Here, too, there is an associated elevated intraocular pressure.

Essential Iris Atrophy

Essential iris atrophy is a rare, progressive, usually unilateral abiotrophy of unknown origin involving the iris and trabecular meshwork. The corneal endothelium may also be involved. The iris shows progressive thinning and is

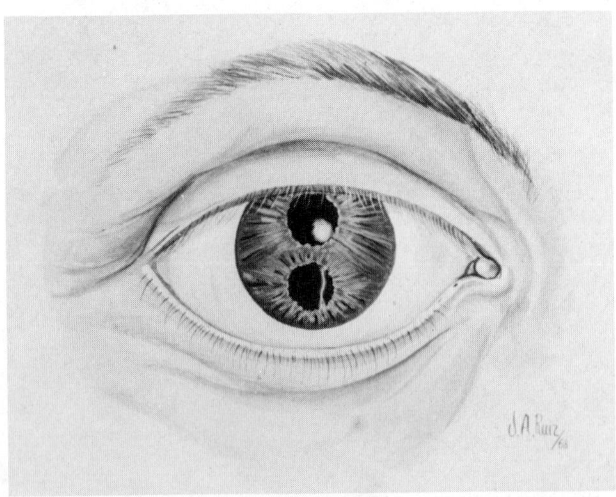

FIG. 37. Polycoria. There is reduplication of the pupillary aperture. (Redrawn from Jaffe and Knie. **Am. J. Ophthalmol.** 35:253, 1952.)

easily detected by slit lamp examination. The red reflex may be observed through the atrophied iris. Eventually a hole appears which begins in the mid-periphery. The pupil is usually displaced away from this area. Peripheral anterior synechiae form in a progressive manner leading to a gradual closure of the filtration angle.

There is no treatment for the basic abnormality. The glaucoma should be treated surgically only after all medical forms of therapy have been exhausted. A filtering operation or a cyclodialysis are the preferred procedures.

LENS AND RELATED ANOMALIES

Congenital Aphakia

Congenital aphakia may be separated into two types. In primary aphakia the condition is characterized by absence of the anterior chamber, iris, and malformation of the cornea. No lens development is recognized. An unfavorable environment causes a defect in the surface ectoderm that will form the lens vesicle. Associated ocular abnormalities are likely to be present. In secondary aphakia the lens has apparently developed to some degree. Aphakia results from a disturbance in organogenesis, possibly an abnormally thin lens capsule which perforates leading to reabsorption, or the lens may be extruded through a corneal perforation occurring during intrauterine life. According to Pratt and Richards, reabsorption is probably the commoner cause. The eye may be otherwise normal depending on the stage of ocular development during which the insult takes place.

Development of the eye as a whole is dependent upon normal development of the lens. The eyeball may be affected by any disturbance of lens metabolism either in utero or at any time before complete development of the eye takes place.

Congenital Cataract

Inflammatory

It is now clear that the rubella virus (like the causative agents of syphilis, toxoplasmosis, and cytomegalic inclusion disease) can pass through the placenta and infect the fetus. The congenital cataract is apparently the result of direct invasion of the embryonic lens. The rubella virus in these congenital infections is often widely disseminated, persisting not only throughout the gestational period but for many months after birth. It has been recovered from the throat, urine, and feces of living patients and from lymph nodes, kidneys, brain, liver, spleen, bone marrow, and ocular tissues obtained post mortem. The virus has been cultured directly from the lens in a higher titer than from several other tissues sampled at autopsy.

Gregg was the first to note that the rubella cataract was obvious at birth, as a dense, pearly white nuclear opacity occupying the entire pupillary area. The babies were characteristically small, poorly nourished, and difficult to feed. Many had congenital heart disease. Full mydriasis was difficult to obtain, and without it the cataracts seemed to occupy the entire lens. When dilatation of the pupil was possible, a much less opaque cortex that had a smoky appearance was observed surrounding the nuclear opacity (Fig. 38). The most recently formed outermost cortical layers in the periphery were often clear, and only through this portion of the lens could the normal red fundus reflex be observed. Zimmerman and Font noted how frequently the cataractous lens appeared swollen in the anteroposterior diameter (Fig. 39). This spherophakia may be important in the pathogenesis of the associated glaucoma which may be observed in the rubella syndrome. On microscopic examination, the nuclear cataract presents a distinctive picture (Fig. 40).

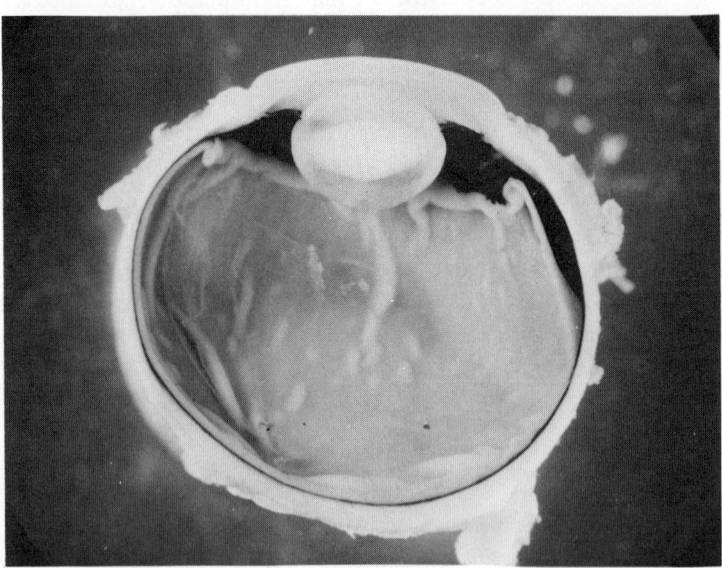

FIG. 38. Congenital rubella cataract. The dense nuclear cataract is less opaque, but degenerated and swollen cortex is characteristic. (A. F. I. P. Neg. No. 65-3166.) (From Zimmerman and Font. J. A. M. A., 196:684, 1966.) (Courtesy of the authors, the American Medical Association, and the Registry of Ophthalmic Pathology of the Armed Forces Institute of Pathology.)

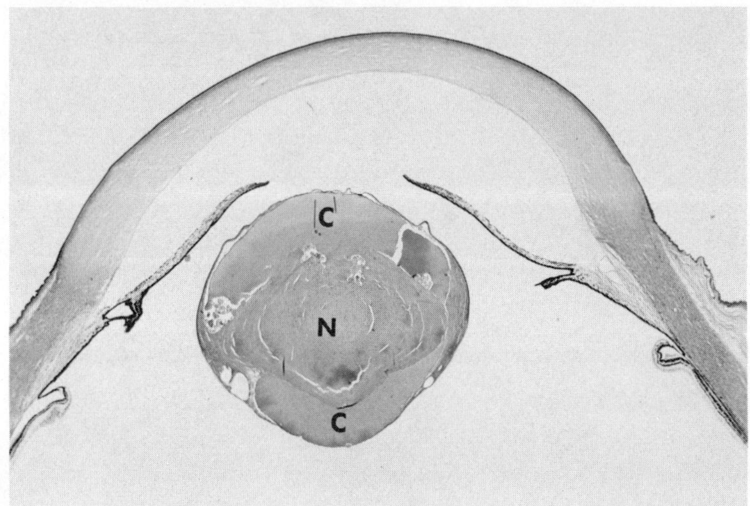

FIG. 39. Congenital rubella cataract. Spherophakia and advanced liquefaction necrosis of almost all of cortex (C) and marked sclerosis of nuclear portion (N). (A. F. I. P. Neg. No. 65-3966.) (From Zimmerman and Font. J. A. M. A., 196:684, 1966.) (Courtesy of the authors, the American Medical Association, and the Registry of Ophthalmic Pathology of the Armed Forces Institute of Pathology.) X 11.

Gregg noted that these cataracts did not correspond to any of the morphological types of congenital cataracts that had been described previously. The mysterious occurrence of unilateral cataracts could be accounted for by assuming that the virus failed to penetrate or perpetuate itself in the uninvolved lens.

The typical occurrence of dense nuclear cataracts reflects the very early entry of the virus. The variable degrees of cortical involvement could be the result of varying degrees of success the virus has in perpetuating itself.

There is no evidence that the rubella virus interferes with closure of the fetal fissure or affects retinal differentiation. Colobomas, persistence and hyperplasia of the primary vitreous, and retinal dysplasia are not observed in these cases. The rubella virus, however, does seem to have an affinity for the retinal pigment epithelium. There are focal areas of necrosis in the ciliary epithelium and a disturbance in the retinal pigment epithelium has been noted on clinical and microscopic examination.

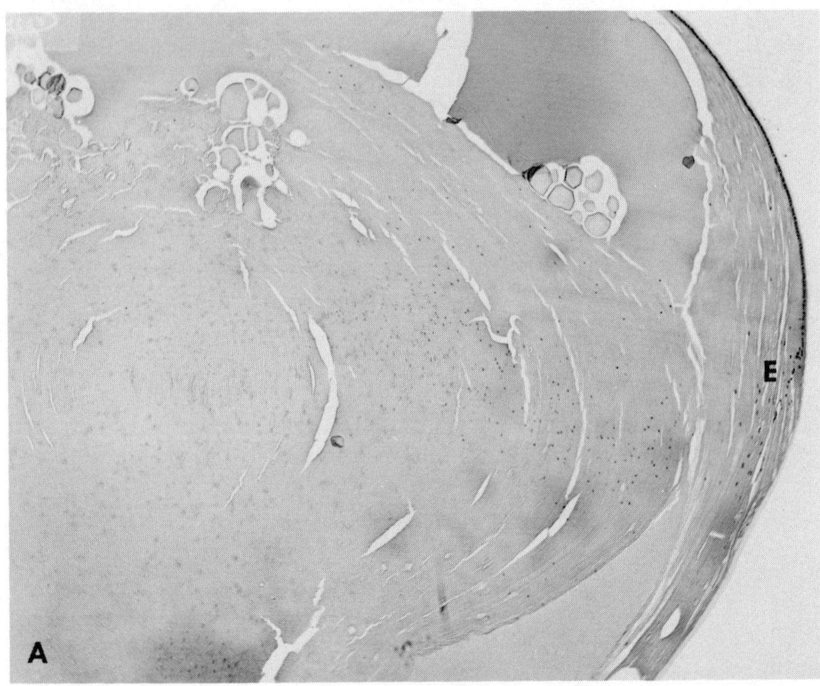

FIG. 40. A. Congenital rubella cataract. Retention of nuclei of lenticular cells in center of sclerotic nucleus is characteristic. Outer, most recently formed, cortical fibers at equator (E) appear comparatively normal. (A. F. I. P. Neg. No. 65-3972.) (From Zimmerman and Font. **J. A. M. A.**, 196:684, 1966.) (Courtesy of the authors, the American Medical Association, and the Registry of Ophthalmic Pathology of the Armed Forces Institute of Pathology.) X 50.

Impaired development of the anterior chamber angle has been observed, resulting in a picture similar to that seen in cases of congenital glaucoma. In a histopathological study of early congenital glaucoma cases, Maumenee reported that two of his 6 cases had congenital heart disease and other manifestations of congenital rubella. Two others died of cardiac arrest.

Genetic

Most hereditary cataracts are transmitted by an autosomal dominant mode of inheritance. Complete subservience of the recessive gene to its dominant partner does not always occur and minor abnormalities may be detected in the heterozygous carrier. For example, infants with galactosemia are unable to convert galactose to glucose resulting in cataract formation,

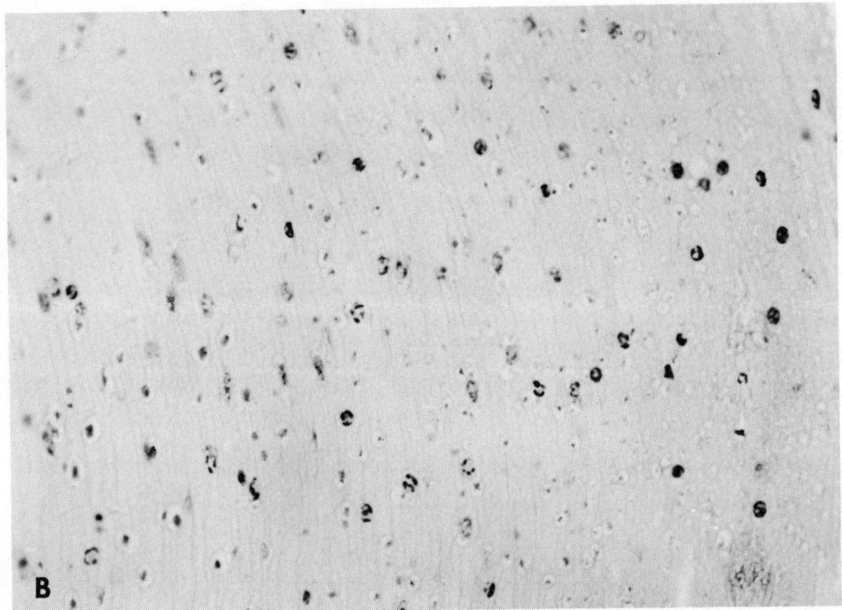

FIG. 40.B. Congenital rubella cataract. Karyorrhexis of retained nuclei produces picture stimulating infiltration by polymorphonuclear leukocytes. (A. F. I. P. Neg. No. 65-5251.) (From Zimmerman and Font. **J. A. M. A.,** 196:684, 1966.) (Courtesy of the authors, the American Medical Association, and the Registry of Ophthalmic Pathology of the Armed Forces Institute of Pathology.) X 350.

mental deficiency, and hepatosplenomegaly. This is caused by an inherited defect in the enzyme galactose-1-phosphate uridyl transferase. The heterozygous parents of such patients do not have the disease but can be shown to have a partial deficiency of transferase.

X-chromosomal linked cataracts are the least common inherited form. X-linked recessive disease is seen in a man with a defective gene on his X-chromosome or in a woman with a defective gene on each of her two X-chromosomes. However, the woman with a defective gene on only one X-chromosome (the carrier or heterozygote) may show minor manifestations of the disease. The lens may proceed to hypermaturity resulting in secondary glaucoma (Fig. 41). All daughters of an affected male inherit the defective gene and are carriers. Theoretically one-half of the sons of female carriers inherit the defective gene and are affected. The sine qua non feature of X-linked inheritance is the absence of father-to-son transmission because the man inherits his X-chromosome from his mother. The most frequently

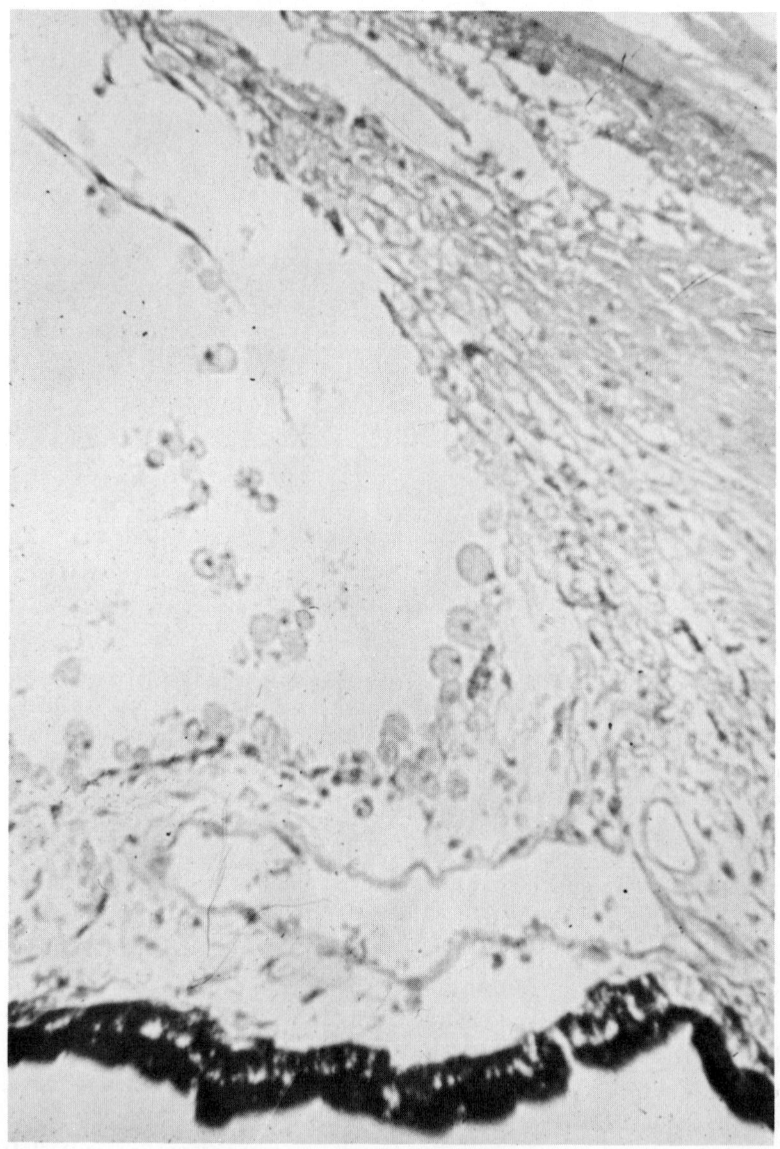

FIG. 41. Phacolytic glaucoma occurring in a hypermature cataract. The engulfed lens material is carried to the filtration angle causing a blockade to aqueous outflow. X 350.

reported X-linked inherited cataract occurs in men with the oculocerebrorenal syndrome of Lowe.

Subluxation and Dislocation of the Lens

The zonules develop from the tertiary vitreous. Duke-Elder favors an ectodermal origin for the vitreous while not excluding the possibility of a mesodermal contribution. It is generally accepted that spontaneous non-traumatic dislocation of the lens is secondary to a maldevelopment of the zonules. The lens may be displaced from its normal position in a variety of conditions. Some of these conditions are discussed elsewhere in this chapter (Marfan's syndrome, Weill-Marchesani syndrome, aniridia, homocystinuria, and sulfide-oxidase deficiency). Ehlers-Danlos syndrome and the mandibulo-facial dysostosis of Franceschetti are discussed here. Other causes of ectopia lentis include Alport's syndrome, syphilis, Crouzon's syndrome, and Kline-felter's syndrome.

Ehlers-Danlos Syndrome (EDS)

The documentation of Ehlers-Danlos syndrome dates back as far as 1682 when Job van Meekeren published a report of a 23-year-old Spaniard with unusual hyperelasticity and hyperextensibility of the skin of the right side of the body. In 1888, Kopp described the condition in a father and son. Gould and Pyle published a book in 1897 in which they made reference to an exhibitionist who was able to stretch his skin an unusual amount and also had the ability to hyperextend the joints of his hands. In 1901, Ehlers noted the association of laxity of the skin, loose-jointedness, and cutaneous fragility with subcutaneous hemorrhages. In 1907, Cohn described the coexistence of hyperelasticity and circumscribed lesions of the skin. One year later, in 1908, Danlos noted the occurrence of tumors at the site of subcutaneous hemorrhages.

EDS is a familial disorder with the basic abnormality within the connective tissue, usually transmitted as an autosomal dominant trait. The collagen bundles are defective in formation, and disorderly in structure. The collagen fibrils are thicker and more loosely connected than normal, which is believed to be responsible for the wide range of extensibility of the skin and the variability of findings in Ehlers-Danlos syndrome. The elastin fibrils have a normal structure. These patients develop a markedly hyperelastic skin which can be pulled out almost intermittently. The skin is fragile and brittle and may exhibit hemorrhages. The skin has a *velvet* feel, and when hyperextensibility of joints is a prominent feature it may be stretched some distance from the body, particularly in areas of bony prominence. When released it returns immediately to its former position. Many of these people fall into the category of "India rubbermen." These are the people who are seen as contortionists in circuses. Changes similar to those already described occur about the lids so that epicanthic folds are common.

Patients tend to develop molluscoid pseudotumors at various pressure points such as the knees, elbows, tibial surfaces, and forehead, as a result of which they have mistakenly been given the term juvenile pseudodiabetic xanthomatosis. Subcutaneous cysts which also develop are more common in the lower extremities and may calcify and present a characteristic radiologic picture. The skin of these areas may show atrophic changes, appearing shiny, thin, and alternatively hyperpigmented or depigmented with occasional fine telangiectases. The skin of the hands and soles of the feet may tend to be excessive. Wounds of the skin have a tendency to gape, and poor healing and scarring is common. The fragile skin may split spontaneously over a large hematoma or upon suddenly twisting the wrist.

Although present at birth, signs of the Ehlers-Danlos syndrome usually become manifest when the child begins to walk. Laxity of the joints causes frequent falls, and repeated dislocation of the clavicle, shoulder, radius, hip, or patella may occur. The most striking examples of joint hyperextensibility are noted in the hands, particularly in the thumbs and fingers. Some patients can extend the thumb and other fingers so that it touches the wrist. Traction on the fingers may dislocate the joints and on release the fingers snap back into place. Structural abnormalities of the feet, such as club foot or flat feet, are often noted. The frequent dislocation and strain on the joints may result in traumatic arthritis with ectopic bone formation, such as synostosis of the radius and ulna, or bony bridges between the acetabula and femur.

The basic connective tissue defect, while most striking in its cutaneous and joint manifestations, also affects other tissues of the body. Most significant, it suggests a relationship to the Marfan syndrome, because of the occurrence of dissecting aortic aneurysm, and hyperextensibility of the joints. The pathological picture, as in the Marfan syndrome, is a cystic median necrosis.

Fragility of the blood vessels is manifested by the tendency to bleed from any of the mucus membranes, especially after brushing of the teeth or other abrading procedures, the susceptibility of these patients to easy bruising, and the occasional spontaneous rupture of large arteries. Abnormal values of the Rumpel-Leede test for capillary fragility have been recorded. The hemorrhagic tendency suggests a basic defect in the clotting mechanism and such a defect has occasionally been noted. It is generally considered, however, that the main abnormality is in the supporting tissues of the blood vessel wall. Jacobs reported marked friability of the bowel at operation, and

TABLE 7

OCULAR ABNORMALITIES ASSOCIATED WITH THE EHLERS-DANLOS SYNDROME*

Lids	Hyperelasticity of the palpebral skin
	Unusually easy eversion of the upper eyelid
	Epicanthus, ptosis
Cornea	Microcornea, keratoconus
	Corneal rupture after minor trauma
	Poor wound healing with dehiscence
Angle	Filtration angle anomalies
Sclera	Blue sclera
	Posterior staphyloma
Lens	Ectopia lentis
Retina	Angiold streaks
	Macular degeneration
	Retinitis proliferans
	Rhegmatogenous retinal detachment
Vitreous	Vitreous membranes
	Vitreous hemorrhage

*After J. W. Pemberton, H. M. Freeman, and C. L. Schepens, Arch. Ophthalmol., 76:817, 1966.

McKusick mentions the unusual friability of the tissues at autopsy. The latter author cites other examples of tissue weakness, such as hiatus hernia, enteroptosis, and dilatation of portions of the bowel and respiratory tract.

The ocular manifestations of this syndrome are reviewed in Table 7 and include epicanthus, ptosis, and hypotony of the extrinsic muscles resulting in strabismus. Laxity of the palpebral tissues is evidenced by the unusual ease in everting the upper eyelid, described as Méténier's sign. Blue sclera (a common sign) and glaucoma were observed by Durham. Various corneal changes such as keratoconus and microcornea as well as corneal myopia have been described. Ectopia of the lens, postoperative dehiscence of cataract wounds, and bilateral corneal lacerations as a result of minor trauma have been observed.

Little has been reported of fundus abnormalities in the Ehlers-Danlos syndrome. Cottini and Pelbois and Rollier reported patients with angioid streaks which suggest the picture of pseudoxanthoma elasticum. Bonnet observed equatorial pigmentary changes in one patient. Bossu and Lambrechts reported a 19-year-old girl who had macular degeneration in one eye and retinitis proliferans with retinal detachment in her other eye. These changes were attributed to minute chorioretinal hemorrhages, which may be a manifestation of the basic tissue weakness. Vitreous hemorrhage has been described.

Ehlers-Danlos syndrome has been reported in association with Groenblad-Strandberg syndrome, Marfan's syndrome, mongolism, Lobstein's syndrome, Oppenheims' disease, Morquio's disease, and von Recklinghausen's disease. Ehlers-Danlos syndrome has certain features in common with Leber's congenital amaurosis including strabismus, keratoconus, retinal pigmentary changes, and occasionally variations in the size of the globe.

EDS patients can be divided into 5 distinct types: (1) gravis; (2) mitis; (3) benign hypermobile; (4) ecchymotic; and (5) an X-linked type in which all patients are males. Operative hazards are greatest in the ecchymotic patients, with vascular complications being the main problem. Patients with the gravis type of EDS also have complications at operation, but the risks are less. Few problems arise during operation in patients with the other forms of the syndrome, provided that meticulous hemostasis is achieved and suturing is done with care and accuracy.

The extreme tissue friability which may be encountered at operation can make it extremely difficult to judge the size of an incision. The tissues may tear when cutting is attempted and the wound may widen spontaneously. Closure of lacerations may be difficult since sutures tend to tear out of the wound edges. Slow healing due to wound dehiscence commonly occurs, and in some patients complete wound breakdown may require several attempts of resuturing. Stretching of scars after apparently successful primary wound healing is characteristic of the syndrome.

Mandibulofacial Dysostosis Syndrome of Franceschetti

Franceschetti and Klein proposed the term mandibulofacial dysostosis for the syndrome that consists of the following features: (1) sloping antimongoloid palpebral fissures with a notch or coloboma in the outer part of the lower eyelids, sometimes with associated anomalous cilia and atrophy of the orbicularis and tarsal tissue; (2) small and incomplete malar bones (often asymmetrical), frequently producing moderate facial asymmetry. The zygomatic process of the temporal bone may be lacking; the body and rami of the mandible are often hypoplastic as well as the maxilla. The palate is highly arched or cleft and the teeth are irregular. Malocclusion and abnormal dentition are frequently found; (3) underdeveloped small external ears, often deformed with frequent external auditory meatus atresia, sometimes associated with anomalies of the middle and inner ear with conductive deafness. Preauricular appendages and blind fistulae between the external ear and the angle of the mouth may be present; (4) macrostomia; (5) absence of nasofrontal angle; (6) hyperplasia of the frontal sinuses and absence of mastoid cells; (7) a patch of hair growing toward the cheek in front of the ear; and (8) facial clefts and skeletal deformation. Rarely seen are macroglossia, absence of parotid gland, internal hydrocephalus, lesions of the heart, great vessels, and the trachobronchial tree, cryptorchidism and mental deficiency.

The syndrome is ascribed to the effect of an incompletely penetrant dominant gene with pleiotropic manifestations. It is felt that the gene produces an inhibitory effect on the development of the facial bones derived from the first visceral arch, as well as a retarded fusion of the embryonic facial clefts.

Many incomplete forms of the syndrome have been described and patients displaying all the manifestations of the syndrome are rare. Ocular deformities include strabismus, microphthalmia and ectopia lentis.

Mandibulofacial dysostosis and ectopia lentis are inherited in a dominant manner and are probably the manifestations of a single pleiotropic gene. It seems unlikely that there are two distinct genes responsible. It is possible that the responsible gene is different from the one usually responsible for mandibulofacial dysostosis alone.

Franceschetti described incomplete and atypical forms. Incomplete forms include cases with oblique antimongoloid fissures, and malar and mandibular atrophy without auricular malformations. Abortive forms have only lid anomalies. Atypical forms show a substitution for one of the principal characteristics by another anomaly, e.g., microphthalmia for the lid deformity.

According to Sugar and Berman, the Franceschetti and Goldenhar syndromes arise at about the same period of embryonic development, the first as a genetic manifestation, the second apparently unrelated to heredity. Because of the time of origin, the two syndromes have in common certain ear deformities, and often malar and mandibular hypoplasia and palatal anomalies. They differ in the presence of epibulbar dermoids or epidermoids (only in the Goldenhar syndrome) and, usually, in the absence of vertebral anomalies in the Franceschetti syndrome. The source of much confusion in the literature is the unilateral antimongoloid slant in cases of Goldenhar's syndrome with hemifacial hypoplasia. Here the lid slant is probably the result of the facial asymmetry.

Anterior Lenticonus, Lentiglobus

Anterior lenticonus (Fig. 42) represents a congenital anomaly wherein the anterior surface of the lens protrudes to assume a conical (lenticonus) or spherical form (lentiglobus). The deformity belongs to the later intrauterine period, with the lens nucleus remaining intact although lens changes are usually present. It occurs predominantly in males and is usually bilateral.

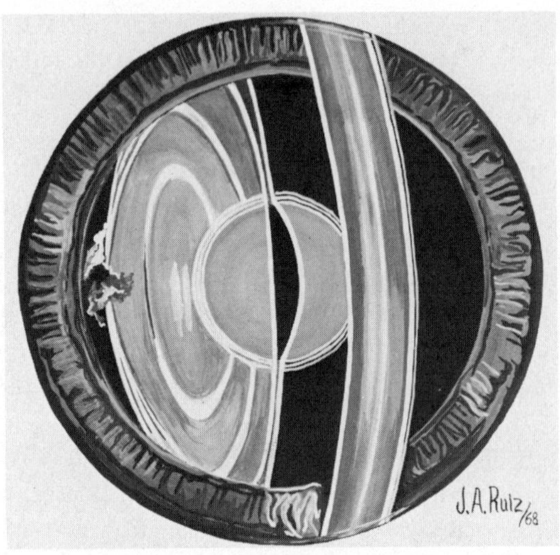

FIG. 42. Lenticonus.

The anomaly is easily detected by slit lamp examination. In the young child Purkinje images may be used as an aid to show the abnormal pattern. Anterior lenticonus is usually seen as a singular anomaly, although associated anterior segment defects may be found according to Duke-Elder.

Microspherophakia

Microspherophakia (small spherical lens) was described by Hartridge as early as 1886. In 1934, Shapira cited 11 papers from 1901 to 1931, involving 20 case reports. It has also been described in association with several systemic conditions including Marfan's syndrome, Weill-Marchesani's syndrome, Alports' syndrome, mandibulofacial dysostosis and Kleinfelter's syndrome.

Microspherophakia as an isolated anomaly is compatible with an autosomal recessive trait although Johnson et al. reported a family which appeared to be segregated in an autosomal dominant manner. Fleicher found an affected brother and sister in two families, one resulting from a first-cousin marriage. Gill described an affected brother and sister and

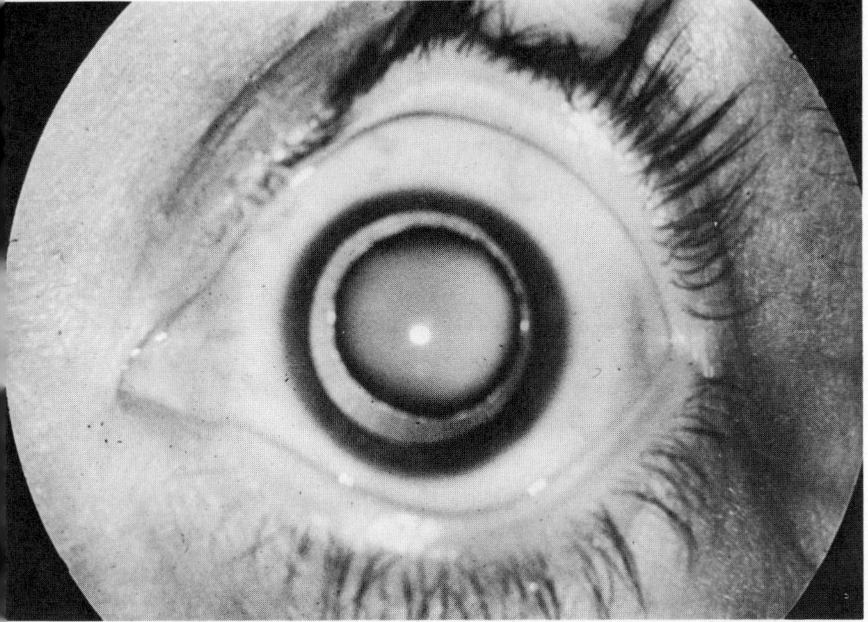

FIG. 43. Microspherophakia, pupil fully dilated. (Courtesy of D. Boyanner.)

Franceschetti reported two affected sisters, products of a first-cousin mating. Waardenberg described two affected boys and Bucklers described an affected offspring, all products of consanguineous matings.

Microspherophakia has been attributed to an arrest of development at the fifth to sixth month of embryonic life, the lens being normally spherical at this time. The cause could be a nutritional deficiency, as judged by defects in the tunica vasculosa lentis. Anomalies of the mesodermal portion of the ciliary body and of the zonules have also been implicated which could explain the association of microspherophakia with Marfan's syndrome and Weill-Marchesani's syndrome, both of these being mesodermal conditions. A zonular defect with loss of normal zonular traction on the lens would allow the lens to remain spherical instead of gradually converting to the normal biconvex shape. Glaucoma may be due to either pupillary block by the spherical and/or dislocated lens, a primary deformity of the filtration angle, or angle closure following subluxation due to an anterior displacement of the iris-lens diaphragm. Although dilation of the pupil will relieve the obstruction at the pupil (Fig. 43), in late cases peripheral anterior synechiae form so that dilation is not always effective.

Persistent Hyperplastic Primary Vitreous (PHPV)

In 1955, Reese characterized persistent hyperplastic primary vitreous as a congenital anomaly that results in an enucleation during infancy or childhood because a retinoblastoma is suspected, or because complications intrinsic to PHPV such as intraocular hemorrhage, secondary glaucoma, or corneal opacification have occurred. PHPV is present at birth as a partial (Fig. 44) or complete unilateral leukocoria (Fig. 45), often in a microphthalmic eye (Fig. 46). The basic abnormality is a persistence and overgrowth of the primary vitreous and its associated blood vessels, the hyaloid artery, vasa hyaloidea propria, and the branches contributed by the ciliary vessels. The ciliary processes are incorporated into the periphery of the membrane and are drawn centrally as the eye grows. There is an almost invariable rupture of the posterior lens capsule, which results when the lens and the remainder of the eye grow at a rate which exceeds that of the vascular retrolental membrane. Secondary cataract, which may be slow or rapid in onset, is a common sequella finally leading to intumescence.

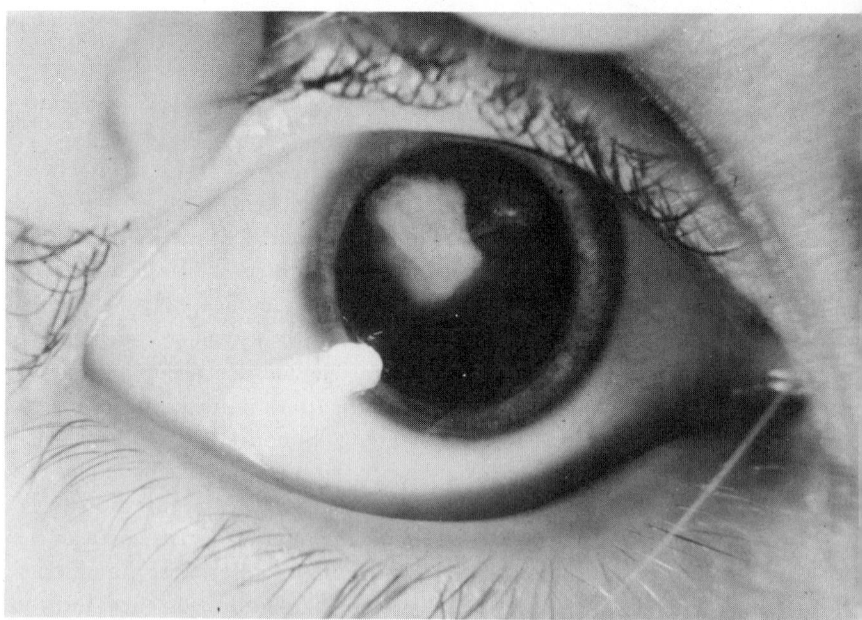

FIG. 44. Persistent hyperplastic primary vitreous, partial leucocoria.

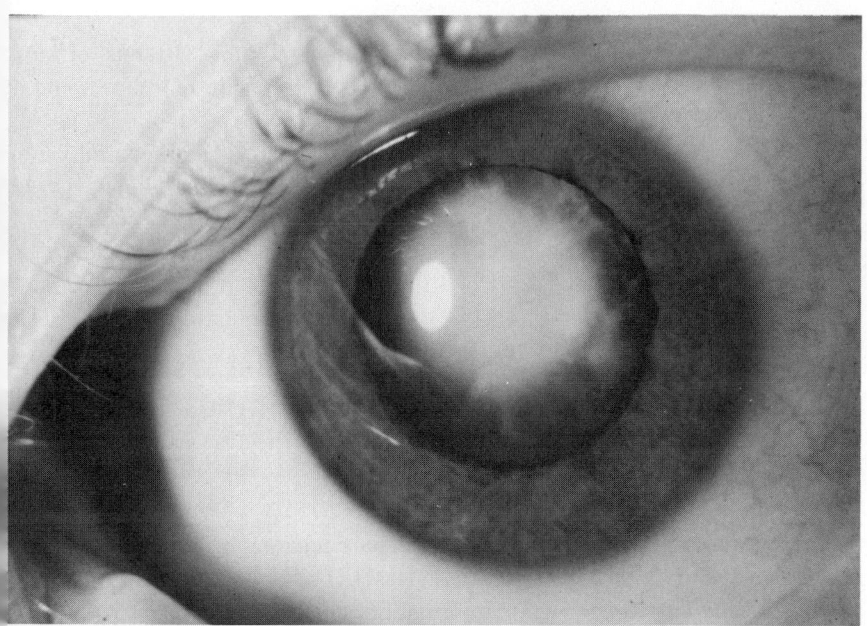

FIG. 45. Persistent hyperplastic primary vitreous, complete leucocoria.

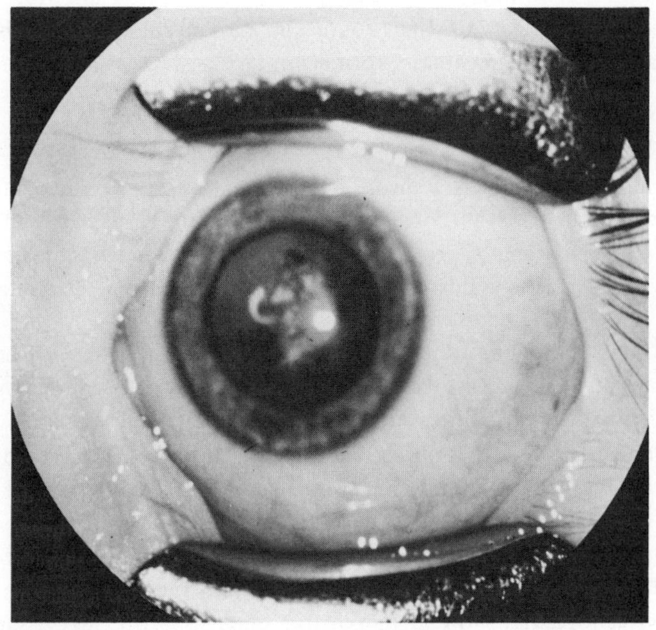

FIG. 46. Persistent hyperplastic primary vitreous, microphthalmic eye.

Spontaneous hemorrhage takes place into the membrane, vitreous, or lens, usually in early infancy. A rise in the intraocular pressure may occur and if sustained leads to buphthalmos.

Manschot and Wolter have described glial extensions originating from the retinal surface which in some instances reach the retrolental mass. Other findings include rupture of the anterior lens capsule, unusual vascularity of the iris, ectopia lentis, and coloboma of the iris, choroid, and optic nerve. Rosen and Yamashita have described the presence of a prominent circumferential ring of còllagenous connective tissue at the termination of Descemet's membrane which resembles the prominent Schwalbe's ring, described by Burian et al., in 15 percent of normal eyes.

Other Syndromes

A number of heritable conditions are characterized by the early appearance of rapidly progressive cataracts, some with filtration angle deformities or anterior segment abnormalities.

Conradi's Syndrome (Dysplasia Epiphysealis Punctata)

Conradi's syndrome has been reported to show an anterior chamber angle anomaly similar to that found in mesodermal dysgenesis. These patients also suffer from cataract formation.

Werner's Syndrome

Werner's syndrome is a disorder of premature old age associated with juvenile cataract formation, often bilateral, which develops between the ages of 20 and 35 and rapidly progress to intumescence. Glaucoma may occur in a similar manner. The syndrome is genetically transmitted, presumably as a recessive trait.

The signs and symptoms which characterize Werner's syndrome include sparse scalp and facial hair, small beaked nose, eyebrows scant at the lateral borders, and a small mouth surrounded by fine radial wrinkles. Axillary hair is scant or normal and pubic hair is scarce. Other characteristic features include bilateral arcus senilis; mild gynecomastia; small genital organs; diabetes mellitus; poor muscular development of the extremities associated with loss of subcutaneous tissues; and taut, shiny skin. The taut skin of the lower extremities impedes motion of the ankle, foot, and toes.

Roentgenograms show osteoporotic changes with soft-tissue calcification. In addition, bilateral, fairly well-demarcated patches of decreased and increased density in bones of the femoral neck may be present.

Syndrome of Francois

In 1958, Francois reported a syndrome consisting of dyscephaly with bird-like face, dental anomalies, nanism, hypotrichosis, cutaneous atrophy, congenital cataracts, and microphthalmia.

Hallerman-Streiff Syndrome (Mandibulooculofacial Dysmòrphia)

Hallerman-Strieff syndrome is characterized by dyscephaly, general brachycephaly or scaphocephaly, bird-like face, micrognathia, dwarfism, trichiasis of the lower eyelids, bilateral cataracts, microphthalmos, and congenital glaucoma. Other findings include poor hearing, microstomia, antimongolian palpebral fissure, maximally hypoplasia, anomalies of dentition, and sexual immaturity.

PHACOMATOSES

Named originally by van der Hoeve (phakoma: mother spot), these conditions occupy an intermediate place between the abiotrophies and the hereditary tumors. Involvement of the skin and possibly the central nervous system is present at birth or early infancy. The clinically distinct types have been divided into those with principally uveal tract involvement and those with principally retinal involvement. The former group includes von Recklinghausen's disease (neurofibromatosis), in addition to Sturge-Weber's syndrome (encephalooculofacial hemangiomatosis). The latter group includes von Hippel-Landau's disease (retinocerebral angiomatosis), Bourneville's disease (tuberous sclerosis) and Wyburn-Mason syndrome (arteriovenous aneurysms of retina and midbrain).

Another phacomatosis, ataxia-telangiectasis, was described by Elena Boder and Robert P. Sedgwick in 1957 and includes cerebellar ataxia and progressive oculocutaneous telangiectasia involving the bulbar conjunctiva. Oculodermal melanocytosis (blue nevus of Ota) may also be classified with the phacomatoses. Hemangioma of the choroid, a clinical entity often associated with Sturge-Weber's syndrome, may occur as an independent isolated condition associated with infantile ocular hypertension.

Neurofibromatosis; von Recklinghausen's Disease

Neurofibromatosis is considered an autosomal dominant trait with variable penetrance and a very high rate of genetic mutation. Spontaneous mutation explains why positive family histories are obtained in only 50 percent of cases. The incidence of neurofibromatosis has been documented with a frequency of one case per 2,500 to 3,300 births. Although malignancy is uncommon in most other hamartomatous syndromes there is a significant risk in neurofibromatosis where incidence has been reported from 5 percent to 16 percent. The most common malignant tumor is neurofibrosarcoma. Astrocytoma of the spinal cord and adrenal carcinoma are also found. The occurrence of uveal melanomas is distinctly increased.

Feinman and Yakovac reported a series of 46 children, all under 12 years of age, when the diagnosis was first established. Forty-three percent of 46 children manifested physical signs at birth and the remainder by one year of age. Two children had megalocornea and glaucoma.

The first clinical signs of neurofibromatosis are usually multiple café-au-lait spots and neurofibromata. The two findings may not both be found in the same patient.

The café-au-lait spots have been classically described as regularly circumscribed, macular lesions which histologically show only increased deposition of melanin in the basal cell layers of the epidermis. These lesions may be present at birth when they are considered birthmarks. They tend, however, to increase in size and number during the first and second decades. Two or less café-au-lait spots are common in childhood, and more than two spots occur in only 0.75 percent of normal children. Five spots with a diameter of at least 0.5 cm should be considered diagnostic until proven otherwise. Café-au-lait spots appeared eventually in 41 of the 46 children in the series of Feinman and Yakovac. Thirty of these children had the pathologic diagnosis of neurofibromatosis made on tissue biopsy. The 11 others had multiple café-au-lait spots but had not developed tumefactions which could be biopsied. Eight of the patients had café-au-lait spots as their only manifestation of neurofibromatosis. Included in the series were patients with such lesions as plexiform neuromas extending into the cranium from the carotid sheath and from the neck itself, neurofibroma of the sphenoid ridge and/or the orbit, and temporal lobe neurofibroma. There were no acoustic neuromas in this series although they are sometimes found in neurofibromatosis. Four cases had optic nerve gliomas associated with optic atrophy and orbital destruction.

The association of neurofibromatosis and mental retardation has been known for some time. Eleven cases in this series showed some degree of developmental or intellectual impairment. Hyperactivity and poor coordination were also prominent historical features. Six of the patients had at one time in their lives developed seizures of varying degrees of severity.

The tumors of neurofibromatosis are true hamartomas and vary in their location. Pedunculated or sessile cutaneous lesions may be quite disfiguring but are certainly less devastating than those occurring within the central neuraxis, musculoskeletal tissue, or the vascular system. Pedunculated lesions are the manifestations of long-standing or postadolescent disease and do not occur with any frequency in childhood. Instead there are subcutaneous sessile or deeper plexiform masses which are noted by the parents and result in the child's first visit to a doctor.

Bone lesions such as erosions, cysts, exostosis from cranial bones, overgrowths, pseudoarthroses, hemihypertrophy and bowing are common. Deforming scoliosis, skull, and facial bone deformities are the most frequent and serious skeletal defects.

Although the histologic appearance of central nervous system lesions may be benign, the potentially dire prognostic significance cannot be overstressed, for these tumors often involve vital structures and/or occur in closed-space locations from which they cannot be resected. Because of the intimate relationship between the axial skeleton and the central nervous system, it is often difficult to decide which is the primary determinant of the clinical findings. As an example, dumbbell-shaped neurofibromas which involve the spinal nerve roots within the intervertebral foramina can cause radicular nerve pain, lytic lesions of the vertebral column, or peripheral nerve dysfunction.

Multiple tumors of peripheral nerves, mainly in the distribution of the trigeminal and superficial cervical nerves, are found. They may, however, be met with anywhere throughout the sympathetic and peripheral cerebrospinal nervous systems.

Precocious or retarded sexual development have long been recognized as complications of neurofibromatosis. However, abnormalities of sexual maturation are usually related to neurofibromatous involvement of target organs, and include various abnormalities of menstruation and infertility. Other endocrine disorders consist of changes in height, hyperthyroidism, myxedema, Addison's disease, tetany, and diabetes.

There is a significant incidence of vascular disease in cases with neurofibromatosis including hypertension, coarctation of the aorta, renal artery stenosis, and small vessel disease.

Neurofibromatosis of the eyelid and orbit is a well recognized manifestation of von Recklinghausen's disease. The disease which often begins in early childhood may be accompanied by tumor-like masses in the subcutaneous tissue of the head and neck including the temple, and side of the face (Fig. 47). The orbital changes take place in the direction of displacement of the globe without bruit and enlargement of the optic foramen. Gliomas involving the optic nerve or optic chiasm are typically seen

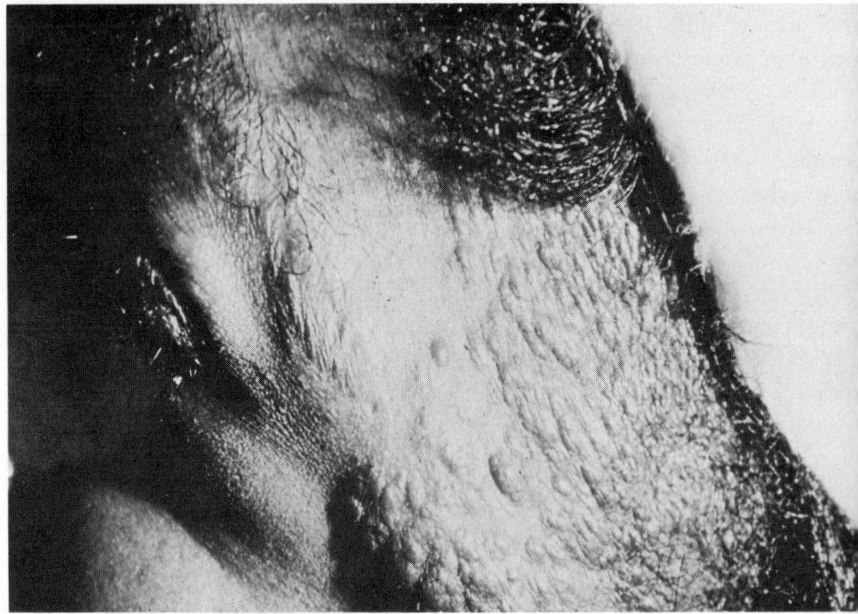

FIG. 47. Neurofibromatosis. Nodules involve the forehead and upper eyelid.

as part of neurofibromatosis. When a young child presents with monocular blindness, slight proptosis, and optic atrophy, this should be the first diagnosis considered. The eyelids may show plexiform neuroma, fibroma molluscum, Schwannoma, ptosis, and café-au-lait spots. In this event the hypertrophied nerves have a characteristic resemblance on palpation to knotted cords, a bag of worms or fiddle strings. The lids may be so extensively involved that the term "elephantiasis neuromatosa" of the lids has been used. The cornea may exhibit the so-called "lignes grises" representing large hyperplastic nerves. The iris may also be diffusely involved with small "Lisch spots"–pigmented lesions representing nevi–and, rarely, with heterochromia and ectropion uveae. The choroid and ciliary body may show diffuse thickening and hyperplasia of their neurons, Schwann cells, and melanocytes, as well as the occurrence of ovoid bodies. The retina may rarely exhibit hemangiomas.

In 1884, congenital glaucoma was first reported as one of the complications of neurofibromatosis by Schiess-Gemuseus, just two years after von Recklinghausen established the condition as a nosological entity.

As in Sturge-Weber's syndrome, involvement of the ipsilateral eyelid, with visible or palpable neurofibromata and hypertrophy of the face of the same side, is characteristically present in nearly all reported cases of congenital glaucoma complicating neurofibromatosis. When the lid is involved with multiple neurofibromata or plexiform neuroma, congenital glaucoma has an incidence of 50 percent. The glaucoma is usually associated with the presence of neurofibromatous changes involving a diffuse tumor-like hyperplasia of neuroectodermal elements in the choroid, iris, and filtration angle, seen as hypertrophied ciliary nerves and diffuse thickening of the choroid. Friedman and Ritchey described neurofibromatosis associated with congenital glaucoma in a case which also showed skeletal changes. Although the glaucoma appeared at first to be controlled with two goniotomies, the intraocular pressure began to rise and the eye was finally enucleated.

Grant and Walton have noted peculiar biomicroscopic findings in cases which had only a family history of neurofibromatosis. This was first observed by Waardenburg and consisted of the presence of neurofibromatous iris nodules. The number and prominence increase with age. Glaucoma may be present before the nodules become noticeable. The iris surface is finely irregular with numerous tiny nodules partially buried in the face of the iris and partially projecting above the surface. They are avascular and amorphous, and vary in color from light brown to colorless.

Grant and Walton noted an avascular light brown, velvety-opaque dense tissue covering and hiding the structures of the filtration angle wall in most of its circumference. This tissue extends from the periphery of the iris to the anterior portion of the corneoscleral meshwork, extending in some places as far as Schwalbe's line. The peripheral iris stroma blends with the abnormal tissue in the angle. At the juncture, the surface of the iris appears to be slightly elevated above the general plane of the iris. The periphery of the iris stroma has a coloration that is similar to that of the abnormal tissue but possesses characteristic iris structure including radial blood vessels, whereas the abnormal tissue covering the angle wall appears amorphous and avascular.

Glaucoma probably develops due to a combination of factors including: (1) infiltration of the angle by neurofibromatous tissue, obstructing the aqueous outflow pathway; (2) the neurofibromatous thickening of the ciliary body and choroid causing an anterior displacement of the iris diaphragm which narrows the filtration angle; (3) development of new fibrovascular tissue in the angle leading to synechiae formation; and (4) failure of normal tissue development of the chamber angle structures themselves.

Retinocerebral Angiomatosis; von Hippel Lindau's Disease

Arteriovenous angiomatosis may involve the abdominal viscera, retina, chamber angle, and only rarely results in vascular nevi of the face. The cerebellum is most commonly involved; the cerebrum, pons, medulla, and spinal cord are only rarely involved. Other asymptomatic undetected lesions may turn up only at autopsy.

The lesions appear as angiomas, cysts, cystic adenomas, and glial proliferations. Both the retinal and cerebellar lesions may occur independently without obvious lesions elsewhere. Transmission is autosomal dominant with varying degrees of penetrance.

The retinal lesions may be present at birth but most often manifest themselves at an average age of about 25 years, while the cerebellar symptoms are said to occur about 10 years later. However, the reverse situation has been seen. The disease has a progressive course. Typically, angiomatosis of the retina is said to be manifested by a pair of enlarged arteries and veins, coming together in the far periphery to form a large aneurysmal tumor or mass associated with glial proliferation and cystic degeneration in the surrounding retina. The lesions may be multiple; bilaterality occurs in less than 50 percent of cases. With cerebellar involvement the patient exhibits ataxia, nystagmus, headaches, nausea, vomiting, and ultimately papilledema.

Extensive hemorrhages, exudation, and retinal separation result in cataract formation and uveitis with rubeosis iridis and synechiae formation leading to iris bombe. In 1930, Ballantyne noted that eyes affected by von Hippel-Lindau's disease frequently succumb to secondary glaucoma as a complication of the progressive nature of the disease.

Oculodermalmelanocytosis; Extrasacral Mongolian Spots; Blue Nevus of Ota

Oculodermalmelanocytosis (Fig. 48) may be transmitted as a recessive trait but is more often dominant, according to Franceschetti. Most cases are, however, sporadic in nature.

The dermal manifestations may be seen at birth although they are usually noted at puberty. In female patients the pigmentation may become more intense during menses. The color varies from light brown to dark brown, gray, and blue-black (Fig. 49).

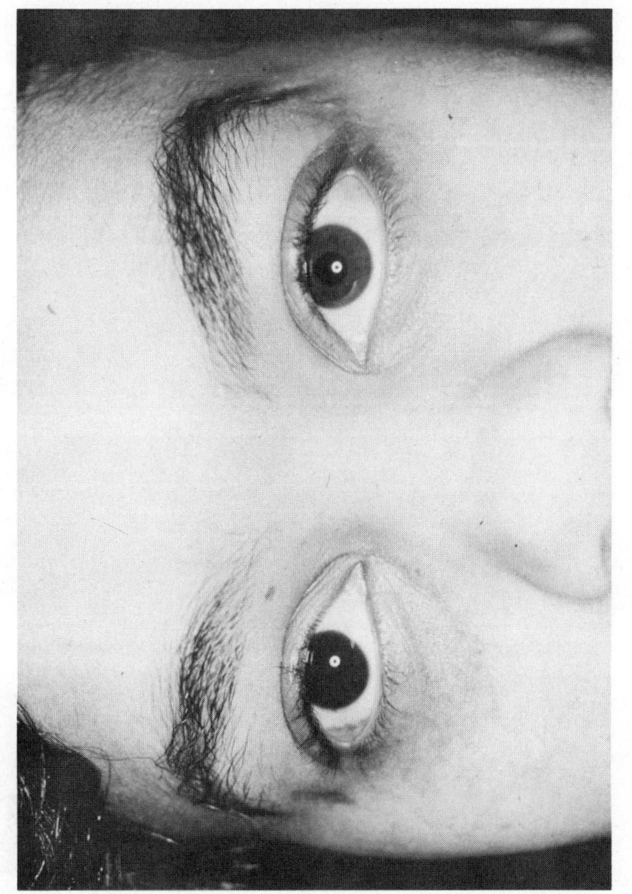

FIG. 48. Oculodermalmelanocytosis (blue nevus of Ota).

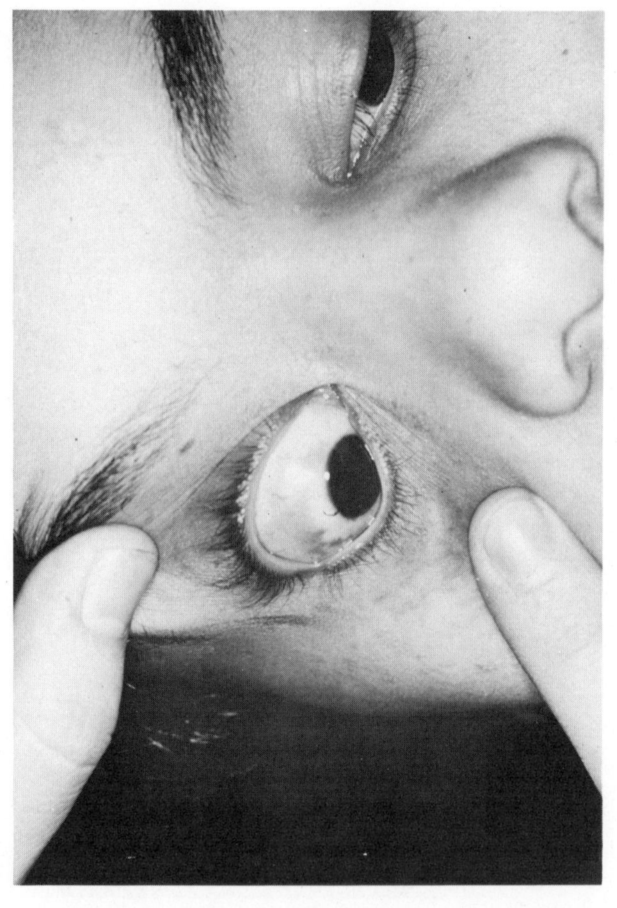

FIG. 49. Oculodermalmelanocytosis (blue nevus of Ota). Oculodermal manifestations.

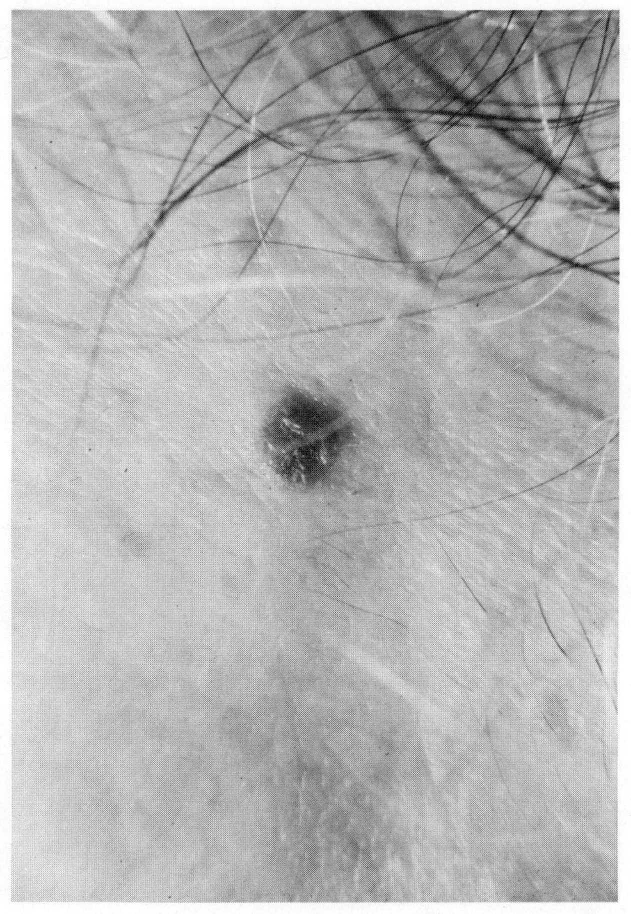

FIG. 50. Oculodermalmelanocytosis (blue nevus of Ota). Skin lesion involving the cheek.

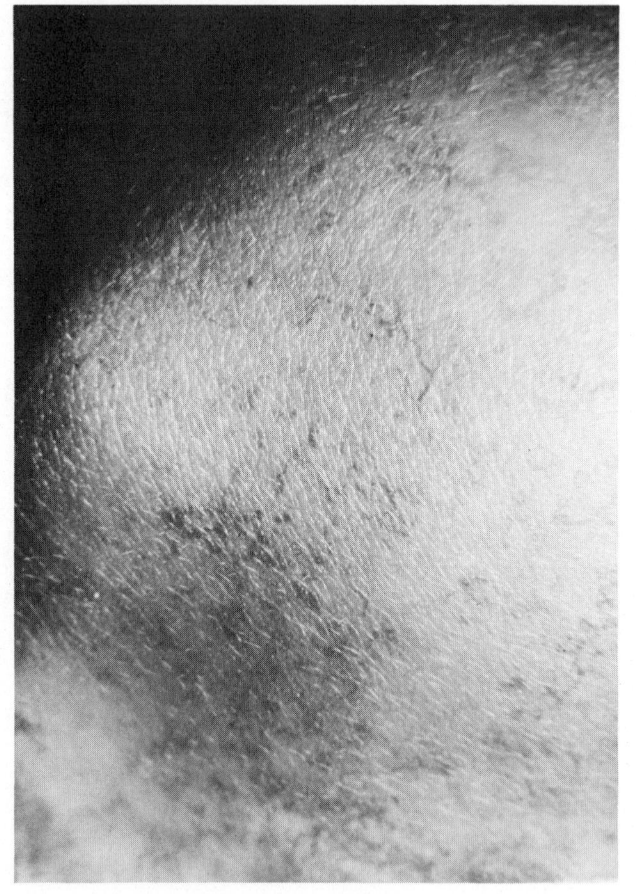

FIG. 51. Oculodermalmelanocytosis. Skin lesion involving the shoulder.

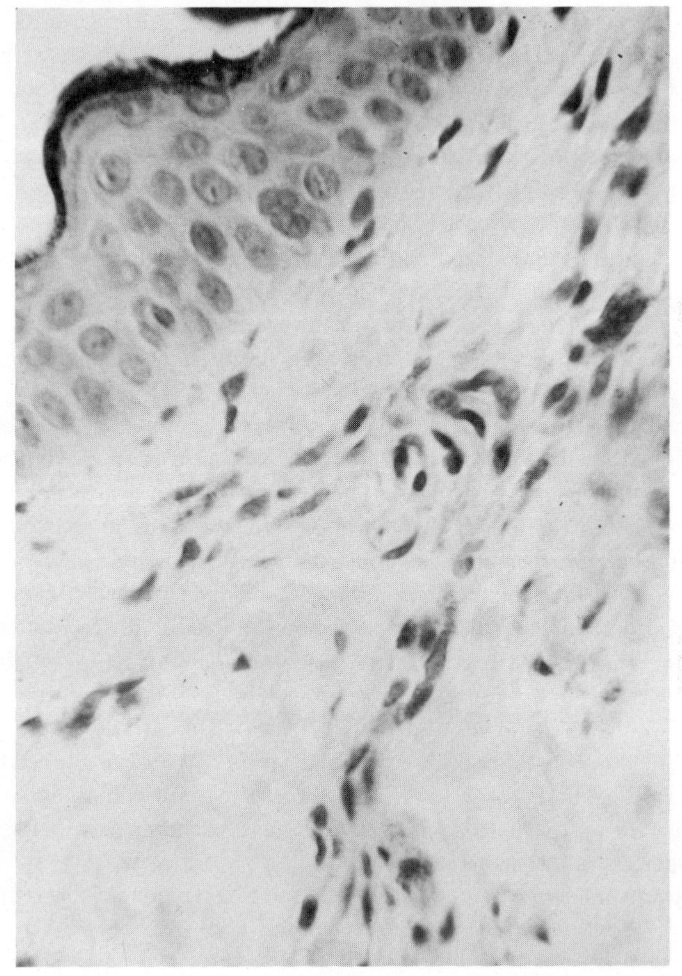

FIG. 52. Oculodermalmelanocytosis (blue nevus of Ota). Skin biopsy. (Courtesy of E. Shapiro.) X 300.

The condition has been extensively reported in Orientals and less frequently in Blacks. Swarthy Caucasians are also affected. The skin lesions usually follow the distribution of the first two branches of the trigeminal nerve on the one side with additional lesions involving other skin areas on both sides, including the upper and lower lids, frontal and temporal skin, the cheek (Fig. 50), cranial bones, orbit, the shoulders (Fig. 51), buccal mucosa, conjunctiva, sclera, optic nerve, uveal tract, palate, and gingiva. Often the most obvious sign is heterochromia of the iris.

Histological examination reveals clumps of pigment in the sclera, conjunctiva, lamina cribrosa, uveal tract, and episclera (about the emissaria). Biopsy of the skin lesion shows spindle shaped cells with long branching processes heavily laden with melanin and melanocytes located deep in the dermis (Fig. 52).

Slit lamp examination of the involved eye shows a thick, spongy, darkened appearance of the iris which has lost its normal architecture. The pupil dilates poorly and the retina on the affected side is usually darker in appearance, sometimes with an extensive accumulation of pigment about the optic nerve head.

Gonioscopic examination of the filtration angle reveals sporadic hyperpigmentation, which is thought to be the cause of elevated intraocular pressure in the instances it occurs. The uveal meshwork is heavily pigmented in some areas to the extent that normal angle structures may be completely obscured. Other areas may be only minimally involved. Such a heavily pigmented area must be differentiated from a malignant melanoma involving the filtration angle, and the condition must be differentiated from pigmentary glaucoma. In the latter case the angle structures such as the scleral spur and ciliary body band still remain definable even in the presence of excessive angle pigmentation. This helps in differentiation from pigmentary glaucoma even in the absence of the other diverse manifestations of oculodermalmelanocytosis. In the former case careful gonioscopic observation will show an increase in size of the melanoma while the benign hyperpigmentation remains the same.

There is no associated defect in vision unless glaucoma supervenes.

Encephalooculofacial Hemagiomatosis: Nevus Flammeus; Sturge-Weber's Syndrome

Encephalooculofacial hemangiomatosis or Sturge-Weber's syndrome is characterized by a port-wine facial hemangioma (Fig. 53) along the cutaneous and conjunctival distribution of the trigeminal nerve involving the

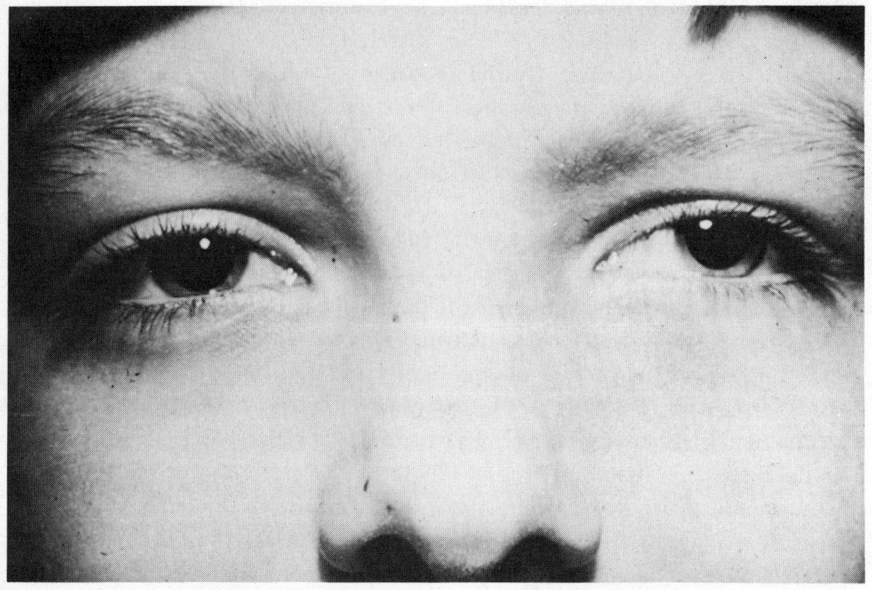

FIG. 53. Sturge-Weber's syndrome. The port-wine stain is evident on the right cheek.

lid, orbit, and scalp, ipsilateral choroidal hemangioma, ipsilateral meningeal hemangioma, epilepsy, intracranial calcification, and both congenital glaucoma and secondary glaucoma. The condition features a capillary nevus that affects the skin of the face, mucosa of the lids, mouth, and pharynx together with vascular nevi of the pia and tortuous retinal vessels. Berkow described retinitis pigmentosa associated with Sturge-Weber's syndrome. The patient also showed unilateral congenital glaucoma and buphthalmos. The limitation of the ocular, meningeal, and main facial manifestations to one and the same side is constant.

In the Sturge-Weber syndrome the defect is essentially mesodermal in origin since the anomalies involve the vessels of the pia, choroid, and skin. Though these structures are widely separated in later life, the angioma of the choroid of the eye and the common involvement of the skin in the distribution of the first and second branches of the trigeminal nerve and of the pia overlying the occipital and temporal lobes on the same side can be easily explained by the proximity of these structures during fetal development. Some conditions that are thought to be dominant fail to appear in the progeny due to poor penetrance. In Sturge-Weber's syndrome the penetrance may be as low as 10 percent.

In 1930, Ballantyne described the historical background of Sturge-Weber's syndrome as follows: "Our search takes us back to 1860 when Schirmer described a case of capillary naevus affecting the skin of the face and trunk and mucous membranes of the eye, nose, mouth, and pharynx, associated with buphthalmos of the left eye. He noted marked dilation and tortuosity of the retinal veins but no choroidal abnormality. . . . In 1879 Allan Sturge presented to the Clinical Society a patient with a congenital port-wine mark on one side of the face and affected with epileptiform convulsions on the opposite side of the body, attributed by Sturge to a naevoid condition of the vessels of the brain. The eye on the same side as the facial naevus was described as having a large cornea and very myopic refraction. The choroid was darker than that of the opposite eye and the retinal vessels were tortuous. A few years later, Horrocks showed to the Ophthalmological Society a girl, 9 years of age, with naevus of the right side of the face including the eyelids, dilatation of the anterior ciliary veins, tortuous retinal veins and enlargement of the cornea in the same eye. Clonic convulsions and spastic hemiplegia were present on the opposite side of the body. These two cases were quoted by Stephen Mackenzie in the discussion on a case described before the Ophthalmological Society by Milles, in which an angioma of the choroid demonstrated in the excised eye, had led to retinal detachment and blindness, and was accompanied by a naevus of the temporal and orbital regions on the same side. In Milles' case the tension of the eye was reported normal, but in other respects it closely resembles the case of Lawford, where, with a naevus of the left side of the face, there was a naevus of the choroid, sub-retinal haemorrhage, detachment of the retina and glaucoma, presumably secondary, in the left eye. Galezowski's case, published 38 years after Schirmer's, was a typical congenital naevus of the face, with buphthalmos of the corresponding eye, and many other examples of the same condition have been recorded by Cushing, Elschnig, Marchesani, and others. Including my own case, described above, I find records of some 31 cases which should probably be placed in this category. These cases differ widely in their characters, e.g., in Beltmann's, the naevus, though mainly in the distribution of the fifth nerve, affected both sides of the face and involved the mucous membranes of the nose, mouth and pharynx. The buphthalmos was bilateral. In Cabannes, the naevus was cavernous rather than capillary and there was marked hypertrophy of the neighbouring bones and orbit. In Kaiser's and in Marchesani's, the naevus, though predominating on the side of the buphthalmic eye, affected the neck, limbs and trunk. Rottl's case had homonymous hemianopia on the side opposite to the buphthalmos."

It is generally stated that glaucoma is associated with nevus flammeus only when it affects the lids (usually upper) or conjunctiva on the same side, and that bilateral hydrophthalmia is usually found only with bilateral nevi. This is not always the case.

Pathologic examinations have shown dilatation of the intraocular capillaries associated with angiomata of both the choroid and iris. Thus, glaucoma may be seen as a result of a secondary hemorrhagic phenomena in the posterior pole (Fig. 54) and filtration angle (Fig. 55). (See colorplate, frontis for these figs.) With angiomatous malformation of the chamber angle, neovascularization occurs which produces organized fibrous tissue, resulting in the formation of broad peripheral anterior synechiae. In other cases there may be a complete absence of uveal tract disease; examination of the filtration angle reveals a gonioscopic appearance more in keeping with that seen in congenital glaucoma.

Windsor Davies reported a case of unilateral nevus flammeus associated with glaucomatous cupping of the disc, atrophy of the optic nerve, increase in size of the cornea and eyeball, and normal intraocular pressure. This case, it would seem, could be classified as arrested hydrophthalmos.

Barkan reported that goniotomy may be effective in controlling the glaucoma. This would probably apply to a primary defect of the chamber angle. With angiomatous disease of the angle, cyclodiathermy or cyclocryothermy would be the preferred treatment.

MESODERMAL ANOMALIES

Marfan's Syndrome (Marfan-Achard)

In 1876, Williams gave an account of the symptom complex that included musculoskeletal, cardiovascular, and ocular disease. In 1896, Marfan demonstrated a condition characterized by considerable elongation of the 4 extremities in a 5 1/2-year-old girl. Other features included contractures of the fingers, poor musculature, a spur of the os calcis, a pronounced deficiency of subcutaneous fat, and a marked retardation of the development of the locomotor functions. Marfan called this syndrome dolichosténomelie and described the fingers and toes as "spider-like." The same child was followed by Méry and Babonneix and was again reported in 1902. The child could not yet walk, there was a kyphoscoliosis in the dorsolumbar spine, and the patella had not followed the growth of the femur but remained in an abnormally high position within the tendon of the quadriceps muscle. These authors proposed the name "hyperchondroplasia" because the x-rays showed an unusual degree of development of the cartilages in the epiphyses. In the same year, Achard described a girl 18 years of age in whom he emphasized the characteristic feature of comparative elongation, especially of the extremities. He chose the name "arachnodactyly" because of the spider-feet-like aspect of the fingers and toes. This name was to appear most frequently in later papers on the syndrome. Achard laid greatest stress on the gracility of the extremities, on the poor development of the soft tissues, and on the comparative length of the third phalanges of the fingers. The movements of the joints were even more free than usual, with hyperextension possible in some of the joints of the hands and feet.

According to Rados, the first paper which stressed the ocular symptoms was published by Ormond and Williams in 1924. They described a 12-year-old boy with the typical habitus, including a functional systolic murmur, slight webbing of the fingers, and a slight upward displacement of the patellas. The boy was tall, underweight, and dolichocephalic, with his hands and feet characteristically long and slender. The right eye showed a deep anterior chamber, a tremulous iris, a small but active pupil with a poor response to atropine, and postoperative aphakia. Vision was improved with a +6.00 D. sphere. Macular fixation was defective. The left anterior chamber was deep, the pupil small but active, and the iris tremulous. The lens was dislocated. The response to atropine was poor. There was a large myopic crescent and vision with a −40.00 D. sphere was 6/60.

Marfan's syndrome is a true example of systemic hypoplastic dolichomorphic mesodermal dystrophy. The condition is inherited as an autosomal dominant trait with fairly high penetrance. Skeletal abnormalities include relatively long, thin extremities, arachnodactyly, dolichocephaly, elongated narrow face, prominent chin, highly arched palate, kyphoscoliosis with shortening of the trunk, pectus excavatum, redundancy or weakness of joint capsules, ligaments, and tendons with loose-jointedness. The legs grow much faster than the trunk after birth. The skeletal proportions are more important than the patient's actual height, e.g., the fingers and toes may be too long for his particular body height. The great toes are often elongated out of proportion to the others, and the arm spread may exceed the patient's height. These patients are said to resemble the characters in El Greco paintings.

It must be remembered that the dolichostenomelic habitus can be seen in the Dinka black, in the eunuch, in Klinefelter's syndrome, delayed puberty, Rh incompatibility, intrauterine rubella infection, and in mental defectives.

Cardiovascular aberrations are caused by progressive degenerative changes in the wall of the aorta and occasionally the pulmonary artery leading to insufficiency and regurgitation from a diffuse dilatation and ectasia of the aorta. Sometimes the degeneration may result in a dissecting aortic aneurysm. Other features include striae distensae, and hypoplasia of skeletal muscle and subcutaneous fat tissue.

There are a variety of ocular findings, the most striking of which is the dislocated lens. Wachtel has noted that a constant finding in Marfan's syndrome was the direct insertion of the longitudinal muscle of the ciliary body into the trabecular fibers, almost entirely bypassing the scleral spur. The canal of Schlemm was abnormal to a variable degree, being discontinuous, hypoplastic, and atrophic in various areas. Microphakia was also observed in his report. The ciliary processes were rudimentary, asymmetrical in size and distribution, and widely spaced about the lens so that the zonules were extended over 5 to 10 times their normal span. (The attenuation and decrease in the number of zonular elements could lead to lens asymmetry and ectopia lentis. When the zonules rupture, the normal-sized and configured lens becomes smaller in the transverse diameter and greater in the anteroposterior diameter.) The iris was thin and positioned posteriorly on the ciliary body with the dilator muscle absent. (This could lead to extreme miosis and a poor response to mydriatics.)

Allen et al. reported a series of 9 cases in which the appearance of the iris and the morphology of the anterior chamber angle structure were within normal clinical limits in 4 eyes. The morphology was abnormal in 7 eyes. In one eye, the angle could not be judged because of an old injury. The abnormalities consisted of both broad and fine iris processes that extended from the iris root to the anterior surface of the ciliary body, the scleral spur, the trabecular meshwork, and less commonly to Schwalbe's line to form large, irregular spaces. Shocket reported a case of central corneal opacities with synechiae of the iris in association with Marfan's syndrome.

Von Noorden and Schultz noted peripheral mounds of iris tissue and large blood vessels located parallel to the ciliary body band. The anterior mesodermal leaf of the peripheral iris showed poor development, with a paucity of crypts and an inconspicuous cleft of Fuchs. In their study, Burian and Allan found a flatness and meager development of the ciliary body, especially in the circular fibers, which may explain the fusiform configuration of the anterior ciliary body.

The scleral spur is less prominent than normal and located at an angle more nearly parallel with the scleral collagen bundles. This may be related to the anterior insertion of the longitudinal fibers of the ciliary body. Schwalbe's line is generally somewhat inconspicuous and difficult to identify, and the anteroposterior dimension of the trabecular meshwork

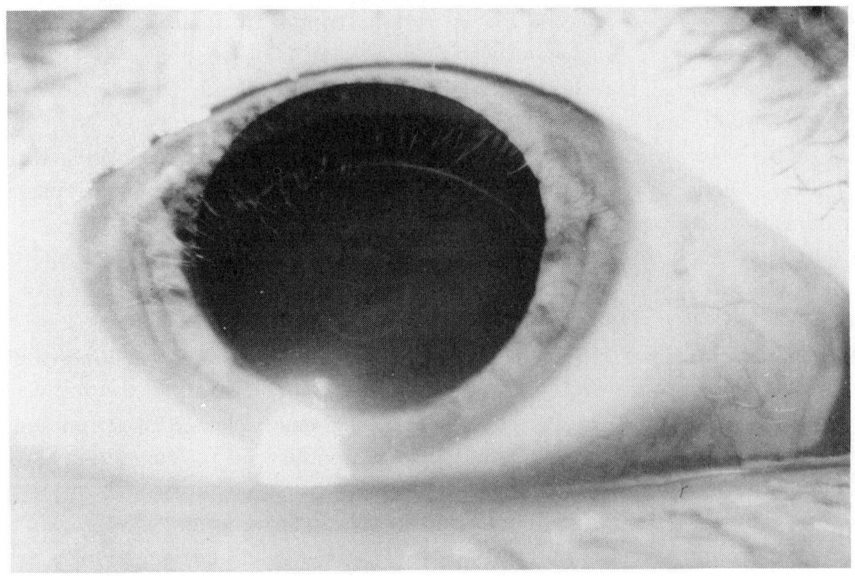

FIG. 56. Marfan's syndrome. The upper lens border is visible.

often appears greater than usual. The visible band of the anterior ciliary body is frequently wider than normal, and there is a considerable increase in the distance between Schwalbe's line and the scleral spur. The angle between the anterior iris surface and the trabecular meshwork varies widely.

Ectopia lentis is present in 60 to 80 percent of cases, usually in an upward position and often bilateral, associated with iridodonesis. The degree of displacement varies (Fig. 56) from moderate subluxation to a degree so great that the aphakic portion of the pupillary aperture is used for vision. Lens changes include microphakia, spherophakia, coloboma of the lens, minor irregularities of lens epithelium, and small cortical cataracts.

Other ocular conditions include heterochromia, a high degree of myopia (lenticular and axial); blue sclerae; tapetoretinal abiotrophy; strabismus; coloboma of the retina, macula, and optic nerve; retinal detachment; microphthalmos; megaloglobus; and keratoconus.

The chief reason for the importance of early recognition is that the ocular and systemic involvement can lead to blindness and death.

The basic defect remains unknown. There is no adequate single explanation of the Marfan syndrome for the complicated alterations which occur not only in the lens, zonule, and many other structures of the eye, but also in widely diverse body systems. However, much of the evidence points to a generalized defect of the connective tissue. The association of systemic connective tissue disorders and mesodermal chamber angle anomalies has been well established by Burian et al., who found that all patients with Marfan's syndrome as well as various idiopathic orthopedic disorders showed chamber angle changes consisting of bridging pectinate strands and iris processes, irregularity and fraying of the iris root, general thinning of the last iris roll, moundlike formations near the iris root, and abnormal vessels. These abnormalities were found in different degrees in patients with the same disease, and in different preponderance in the various systemic skeletal disorders enumerated by the authors.

Ocular enlargement is a common, if not an invariable, feature of the Marfan syndrome. The enlargement appears progressive but the degree may not be uniform. Many ocular pathologic findings appear directly related to the increased ocular size, including enlarged cornea, thinned cornea and sclera, optic nerve head deformity of the myopic type, thinned and elongated ciliary body, increased diameter of the corona ciliaris with separation of the ciliary body, disproportionate elongation of the pars plana, thinned choroid, and thinned retina with loss of specialized cells and architecture. All of these findings have been noted in patients with a normal intraocular pressure, therefore, the ocular enlargement is believed to indicate an underlying connective tissue defect of the sclera.

The feature of ectopia lentis in this disorder has been a perplexing problem, since the zonules are an ectodermal derivative and would therefore not be expected to share in a generalized connective tissue disease. The urine contains abnormal amounts of hydroxyproline suggesting a defect in the production of collagen. This could account for the weakness noted in the zonules. The generalized ocular enlargement with attendant functional and pathologic alterations may be largely a direct reflection of a fundamental collagen disorder.

The lesions in the zonule, ectopia lentis, and hypoplasia of the dilator pupillae muscle could be the polyphenic expressions of a single gene. The apparently consistent abnormalities of the anterior chamber angle structures of the iris and of the ciliary muscle appear to be developmental.

Burian postulated that the defect in Marfan's syndrome may represent an inborn error of metabolism. Indirect support of this theory is seen in the creation of defects of the connective tissue in rats fed β-amino-propionitrile, and in the recently discovered inborn error of metabolism, homocystinuria, in which arachnodactyly and ectopia lentis are commonly noted.

Glaucoma results from the angle deformity described. The dislocated lens may cause a rise in the intraocular pressure by tilting forward and narrowing the filtration angle, by blocking the pupillary aperture, and by displacing into the anterior chamber and thereby blocking the filtration angle.

Weill-Marchesani Syndrome: Spherophakia-Brachymorphia Syndrome

In 1939, Marchesani described 4 patients with short stature, brachydactyly, and spherophakia with myopia and glaucoma, and classified this syndrome as a true example of congenital systemic, hyperplastic brachymorphic mesodermal dystrophy. Genetic transmission may be dominant or recessive with partial expression in the heterozygote. The appearance of the incomplete syndromes (forme fruste), such as spherophakia with normal extremities or brachydactyly with normal eyes, suggests that mild brachydactyly represents a heterozygous intermediate while severe spherophakia (with or without brachydactyly) represent the homozygous recessive form. The occurrence of consanguinity in several of the families further favors a homozygous recessive genotype.

Weill-Marchesani and Marfan's syndromes constitute the hyperplastic (brachymorphic) and hypoplastic (dolichomorphic) forms of a systemic disorder, manifesting certain similar ocular disorders but differing in many systemic aspects. The Weill-Marchesani patient is shorter than average, heavier, and has brachycephaly. The limbs are short, the fingers are short and stubby, the hands and feet broad and spadelike with limitations at the joints and flexure deformities. The head is broad and rather square. Subcutaneous tissue is abundant and the muscles are well developed. X-ray examination reveals short fingers surrounded by a thick layer of soft tissue, with short, symmetrical, and relatively wide metacarpal bone development. Table 8 summarizes the characteristics of the important syndromes where ectopia lentis is a feature.

Ocular complications include microspherophakia, ectopia lentis (Fig. 57), and lenticular myopia. The dislocation is usually in a downward position and angle closure glaucoma may result if the lens-iris diaphragm moves forward. The lens may block the pupillary aperture and even enter the anterior chamber. Often the lens can be coaxed back into the posterior cavity with complete mydriasis and careful positioning of the patient.

Feiler-Ofry et al. described the gonioscopic appearance of the filtration angle in Weill-Marchesani syndrome. They reported the presence of numerous pigmented conical and thread-like fibers extending from the iris root to the ciliary body band and corneoscleral trabeculum, some inserting as high as Schwalbe's line and, in some places, obscuring the ciliary body

TABLE 8

COMPARISON OF SOME SYNDROMES ASSOCIATED WITH ECTOPIA LENTIS*

Features	Marfan's	Weill-Marchesani	Homocystinuria
(1) Inheritance	Autosomal dominant	Questionable	Autosomal recessive
(2) Ocular defects	Ectopia lentis, glaucoma	Spherophakia, microphakia, glaucoma	Ectopia lentis, congenital cataract, spherophakia, aniridia, retinal cyst, glaucoma
(3) Skeletal defects	Dolichomorphia, arachnodactyly loose-jointedness	Brachymorphia, reduced mobility of joints	Osteoporosis, occasional arachnodactyly
(4) Skin	Lack of subcutaneous tissue, striae distensae	Abundant subcutaneous tissue	Malar flush, livedo reticularis
(5) Cardiovascular lesions	Cystic medial necrosis, cardiac defects	No apparent increase	Vascular thromboses common
(6) Mental retardation	Absent	Frequent	Frequent

*After G. D. Presley and J. B. Sidbury, Am. J. Ophthalmol., 63:1723, 1967.

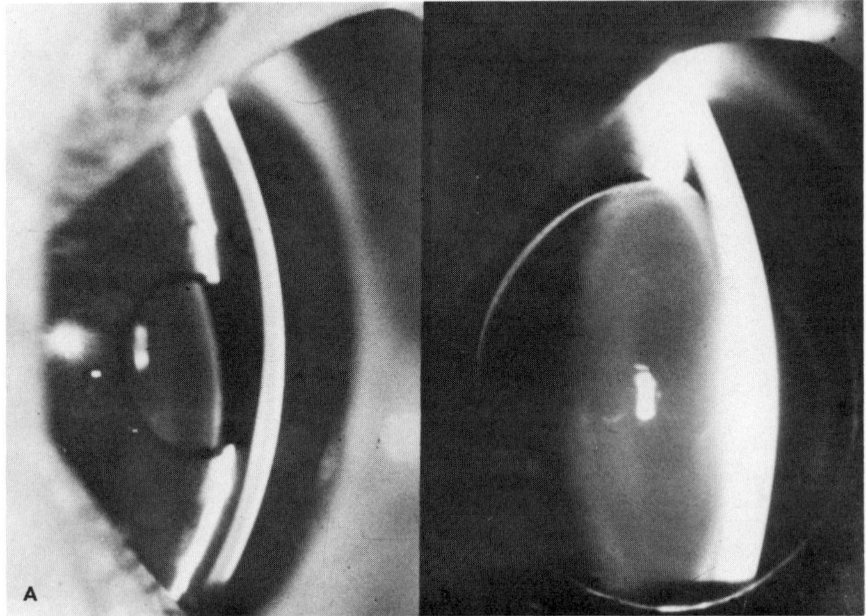

FIG. 57. Weill-Marchesani syndrome. The dislocated lens moves from the posterior cavity to the anterior chamber. (Courtesy of J. Barraquer.)

band. In addition, finer pigmented and nonpigmented fibers spread from the iris root closely adjacent to the trabeculae. The formations gave a frayed appearance to the iris root instead of the usual well defined borderline. Although the angle could be classified as medium to open, it appeared shortened in its sagittal extent.

METABOLIC DISEASE

Oculocerebrorenal Syndrome; Lowe's Syndrome

The oculocerebrorenal syndrome of Lowe, Terrey and Maclachlan was first described in 1952. Its characteristics are outlined in Table 9. The syndrome features increased organic aciduria, systemic acidosis (renal rickets), ketonuria, glycosuria, proteinuria, albuminuria, aminoaciduria, emotional irritability, skeletal changes, hypotonia, feeding problems, constipation, mental retardation, and osteomalacia. The blood shows a decreased

TABLE 9

OCULOCEREBRORENAL SYNDROME OF LOWE

Renal Symptoms
- Aminoaciduria
- Oligoammoniuria
- Albuminuria
- Intermittent glycosuria
- Renal tubular acidosis
- Low titratable acidity

Ocular Signs
- Cataract
- Glaucoma
- Corneal opacities
- Miotic pupil

Musculo-skeletal Abnormalities
- Rickets
- Osteomalacia
- Muscular hypotony
- Hyporeflexia

Retardation
- Mental
- Psychomotor
- Growth

CO_2 concentration and a decrease in serum phosphorus.

The ophthalmic findings include congenital cataracts, nystagmus, blue sclerae, bilateral corneal opacification as early as three months of age, and/or diffuse corneal edema secondary to glaucoma.

The congenital cataracts are bilateral (Fig. 58) and present in almost all reported cases. The lens capsule is irregularly thickened anteriorly and in the equatorial region where wart-like excrescences are observed (Fig. 59). In the region of the posterior pole the capsule becomes thin and defective (Figs. 60 and 61), giving rise to a prominent convexity (posterior lenticonus). Here the lens and vitreous appear to be fused. Proliferated and metaplastic cells from the migrated lens epithelium are observed among fibrils of the anterior hyaloid membrane. The filtration angle exhibits faulty development and differentiation (Fig. 62). Glaucoma is noted in about two-thirds of cases. Microphthalmia may be present even with elevated intraocular tension.

The lens is probably involved prior to the fifth week of development, whereas other ocular abnormalities occur later in embryogenesis. Female carriers frequently show scattered punctate lens opacities detected by slit lamp examination, which are not associated with visual impairment.

The essential enzyme or protein abnormality of this syndrome is

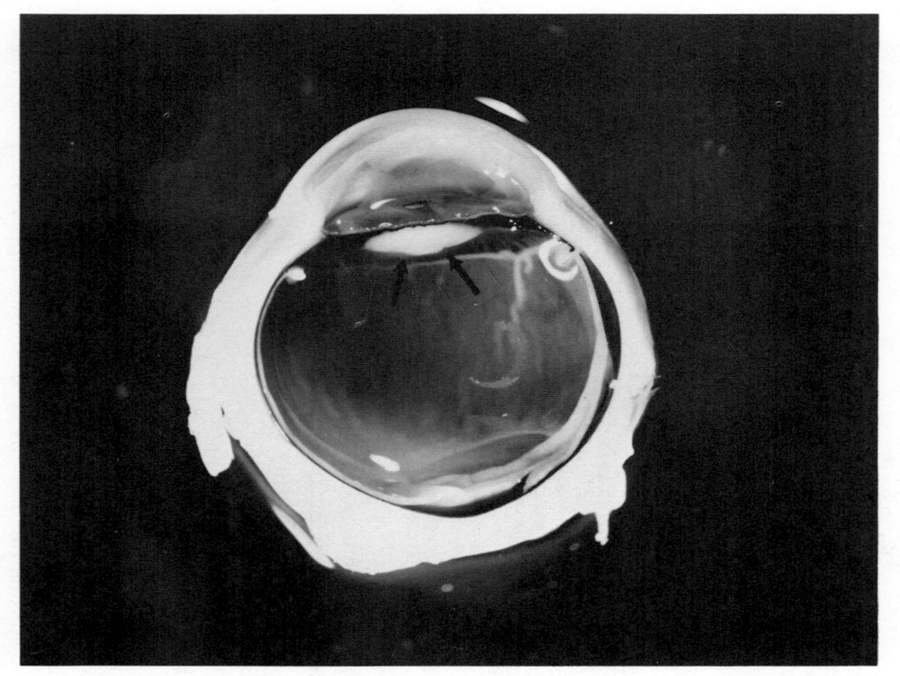

FIG. 58.A. Lowe's syndrome, 8-month-old boy, post mortem. Equatorial view. Cataractous lens is very small and disk shaped. Densely opaque subcapsular lesion with prominent convexity projects from posterior pole (arrows). Cornea and anterior chamber are larger than normal because of congenital glaucoma. (A. F. I. P. Neg. No. 63-168,1) (From Zimmerman and Font. **J. A. M. A.** 196:684, 1966.) (Courtesy of the authors, the American Medical Association, and the Registry of Ophthalmic Pathology of the Armed Forces Institute of Pathology.) X 2.

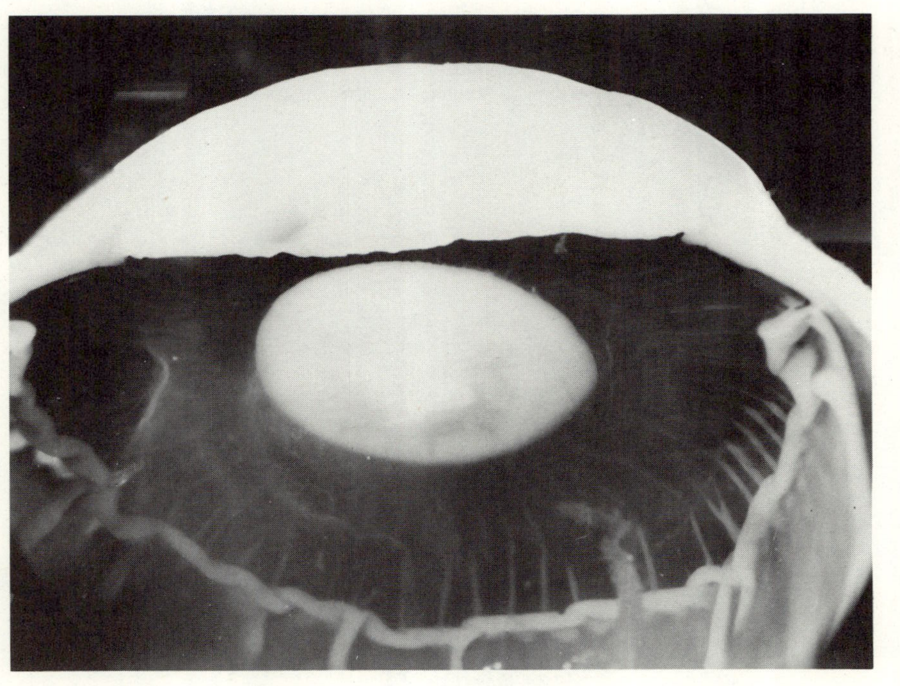

FIG. 58.B. Lowe's syndrome, 8-month-old boy, post mortem. Oblique view of posterior surface of lens. (A. F. I. P. Neg. No. 63-168,2.) (From Zimmerman and Font. **J. A. M. A.** 196:684, 1966.) (Courtesy of the authors, the American Medical Association, and the Registry of Ophthalmic Pathology of the Armed Forces Institute of Pathology.) X 6.

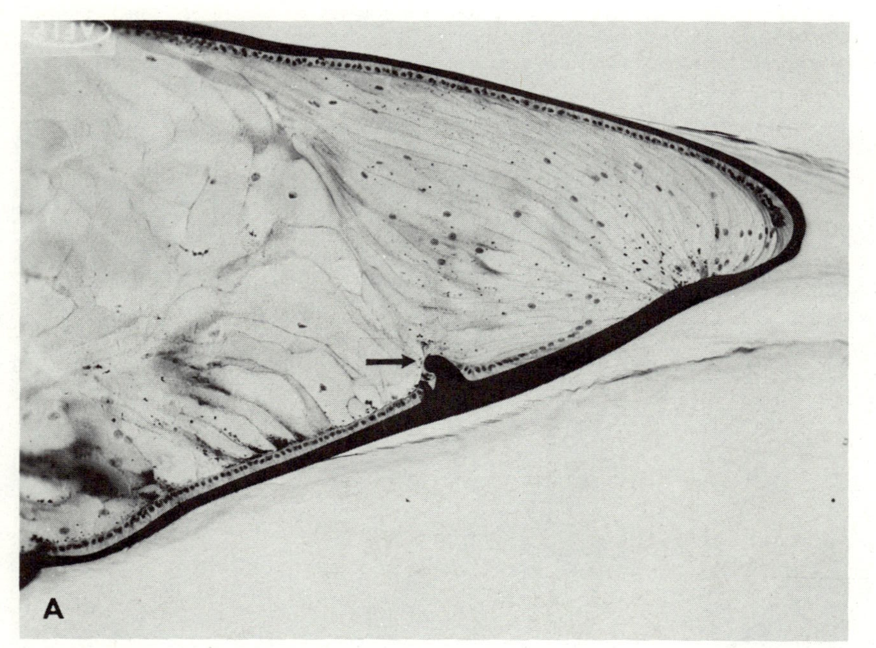

FIG. 59.A. Lowe's syndrome. Irregular thickening of lens capsule. Wart-like excrescences (arrows), posterior migration of lens epithelium and disorganization of cortical architecture are evident. (A. F. I. P. Neg. No. 63-2237.) (From Zimmerman and Font. **J. A. M. A.** 196:684, 1966.) (Courtesy of the authors, the American Medical Association, and the Registry of Ophthalmic Pathology of the Armed Forces Institute of Pathology.) X 115.

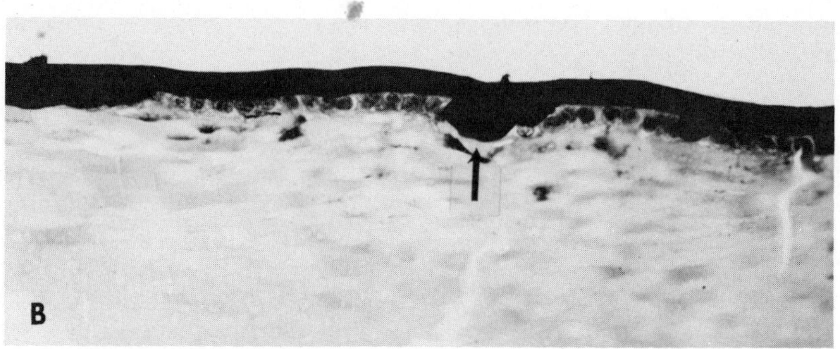

FIG. 59.B. Lowe's syndrome. Wart-like excrescence on lens capsule (arrow). (A. F. I. P. Neg. No. 63-2237.) (From Zimmerman and Font. J. A. M. A. 196:684, 1966.) (Courtesy of the authors, the American Medical Association, and the Registry of Ophthalmic Pathology of the Armed Forces Institute of Pathology.) X 305.

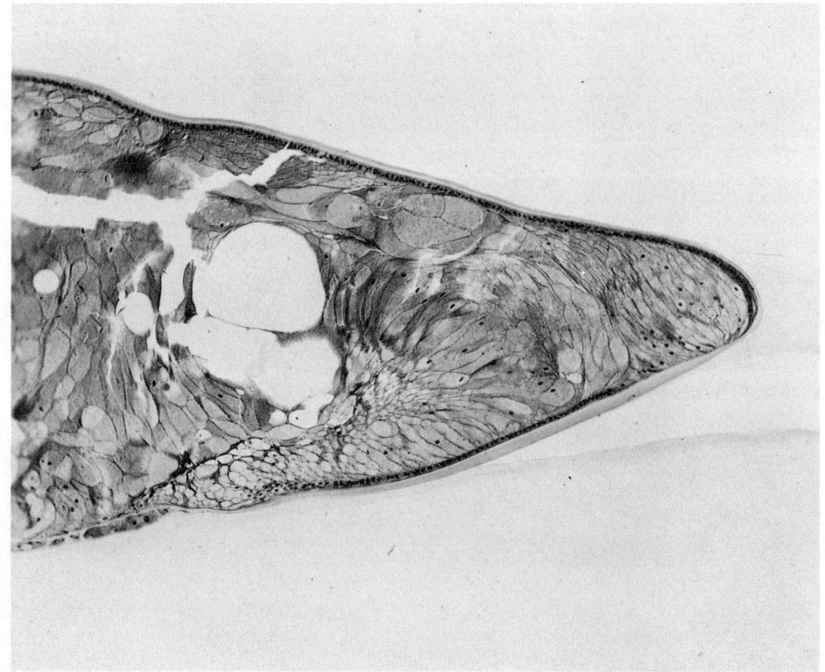

FIG. 60. Lowe's syndrome. Posterior lens capsule, while thick near equator, becomes very thin and deficient toward posterior pole (lower left side of picture). (A. F. I. P. Neg. No. 63-1636.) (From Zimmerman and Font. J. A. M. A. 196:684, 1966.) (Courtesy of the authors, the American Medical Association, and the Registry of Ophthalmic Pathology of the Armed Forces Institute of Pathology.) X 80.

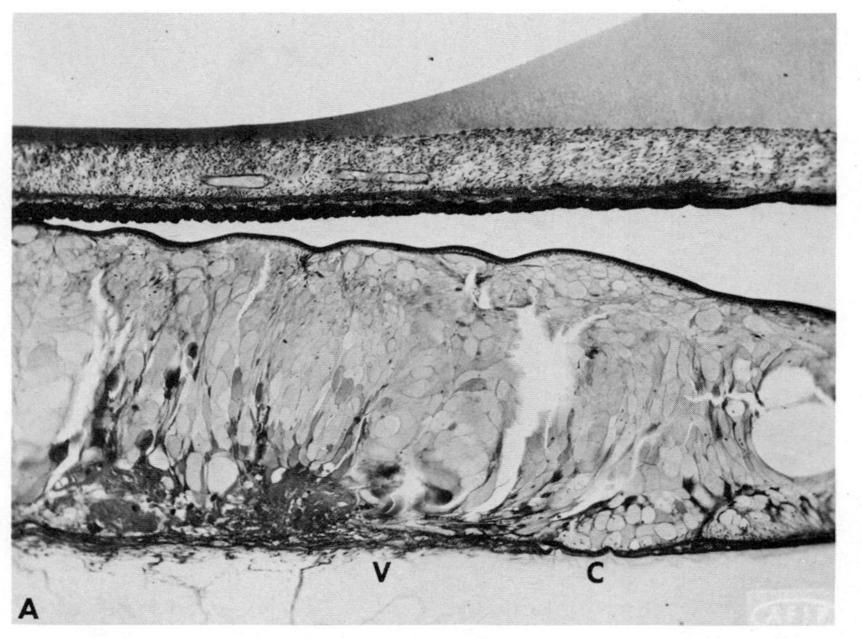

FIG. 61.A. Lowe's syndrome. In the region of posterior polar opacity, lens capsule (C) is deficient, and proliferated lenticular cells are observed among fibrils of the anterior vitreous (V). (A. F. I. P. Neg. No. 63-2233.) (From Zimmerman and Font. **J. A. M. A.** 196:684, 1966.) (Courtesy of the authors, the American Medical Association, and the Registry of Ophthalmic Pathology of the Armed Forces Institute of Pathology.) X 50.

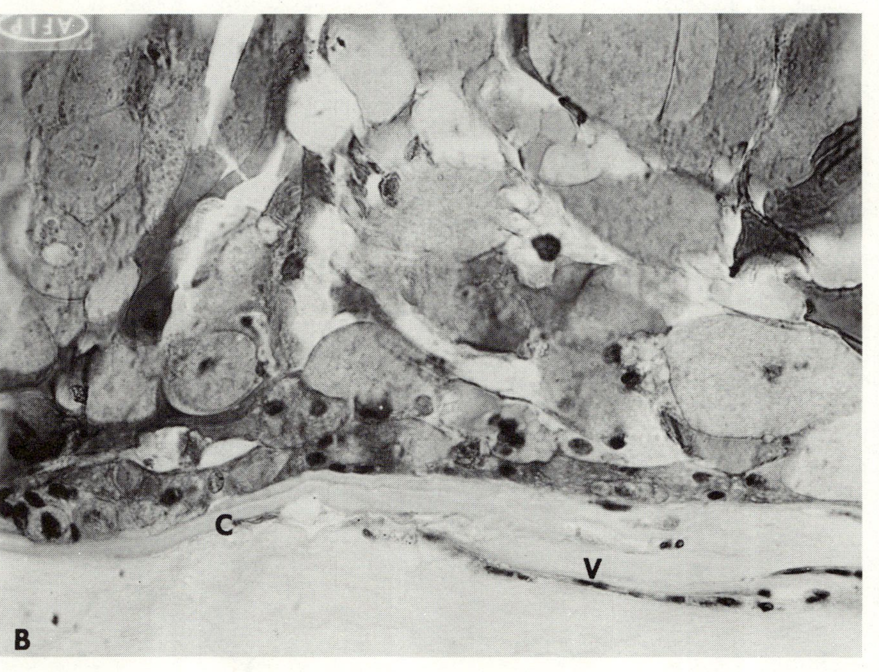

FIG. 61.B. Lowe's syndrome. Lens capsule (C). Proliferated lenticular cells are observed among fibrils of the anterior vitreous (V). (A. F. I. P. Neg. No. 63-2230.) (From Zimmerman and Font. **J. A. M. A.** 196:684, 1966.) (Courtesy of the authors, the American Medical Association, and the Registry of Ophthalmic Pathology of the Armed Forces Institute of Pathology.) X 530.

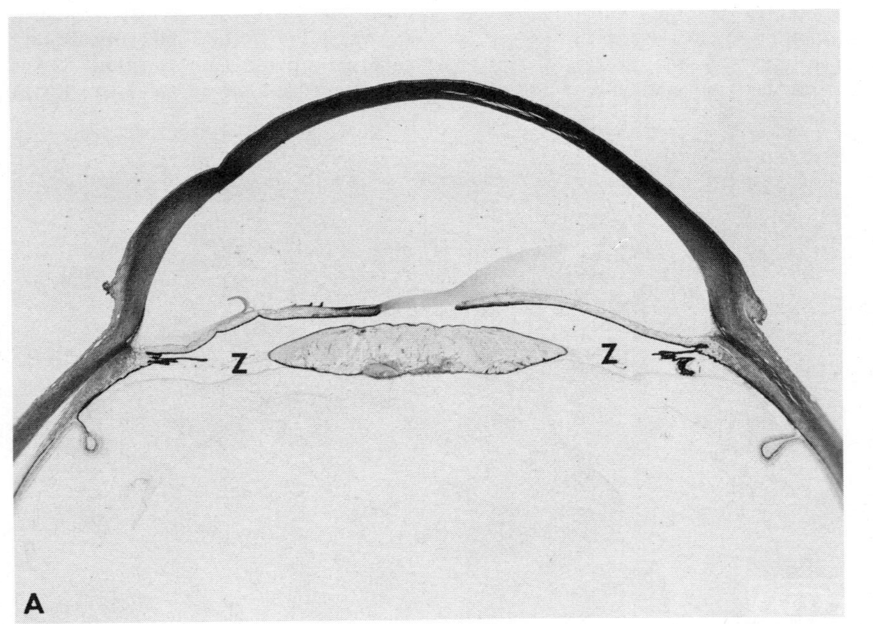

FIG. 62.A. Lowe's syndrome Anterior chamber angle is incompletely formed, and iris is incompletely separated from trabecular meshwork. Ciliary processes appear to be drawn in toward small lens by taut zonular ligament (Z) and are farther forward than normal. The ora serata is also farther forward than normal. (A. F. I. P. Neg. No. 66-2240.) (From Zimmerman and Font. J. A. M. A. 196:684, 1966.) (Courtesy of the authors, the American Medical Association and the Registry of Ophthalmic Pathology of the Armed Forces Institute of Pathology.) X 7.

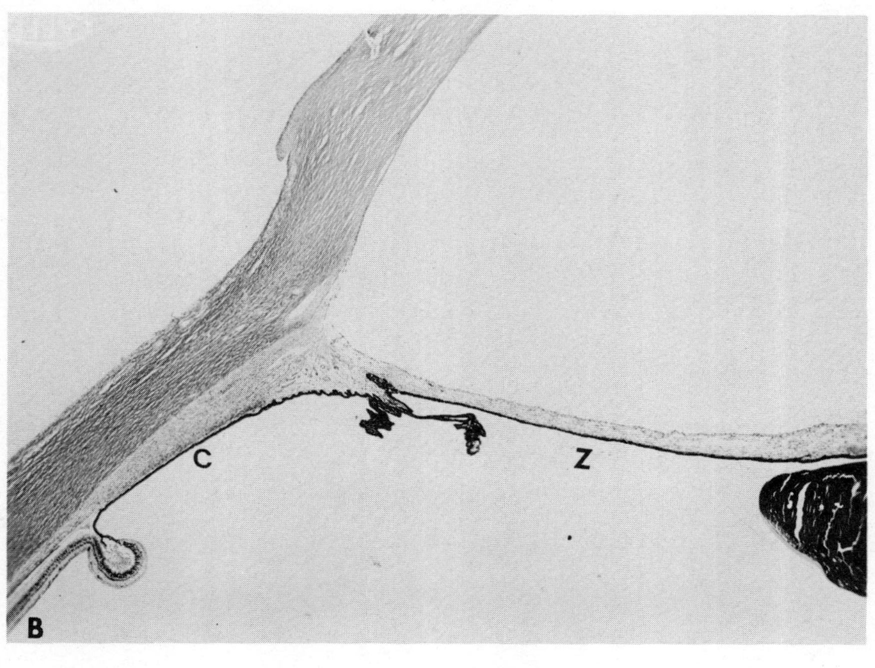

FIG. 62.B. Lowe's syndrome. Island of retinal tissue (C) is present in pars ciliaris. Zonular ligament (Z). (A. F. I. P. Neg. No. 63-1641.) (From Zimmerman and Font. **J. A. M. A.** 196:684, 1966.) (Courtesy of the authors, the American Medical Association, and the Registry of Ophthalmic Pathology of the Armed Forces Institute of Pathology.) X 18.

unknown. The condition occurs in males on the basis of a pathologic gene and is probably sex-linked. The appearance of rickets is common with this type of proximal and distal tubular disease. Generalized tubular disease is in evidence causing the systemic metabolic acidosis, alkaline urinary pH, and low specific gravity with proteinuria and glycosuria. The initial urinary problem of lack of reabsorption of phosphorus causes phosphaturia and hypophosphatemia. Bone reabsorption occurs partially under the influence of secondary hyperparathyroidism (which leads to osteomalacia in the infant) while delivering increased phosphorus from bone to plasma and then into the urine. Furthermore, the alkaline urine creates an increase in calcium loss since calcium accompanies the excretion of bicarbonate. Diminished serum calcium adds to the parathyroid stimulus and bone reabsorption. Ocular treatment consists of cataract extraction and control of the glaucoma by goniotomy.

Homocystinuria

Interest in the association of aminoacidurias and mental deficiency stimulated a survey of mentally retarded children in Ireland, which led to the discovery in 1962 of two children found to be excreting homocystine in the urine. Independently, Gerritsen et al. identified homocystine in the urine of a mentally retarded child in the United States.

Homocystinuria is a genetically transmitted enzymatic fault that represents another of Garrod's "inborn errors of metabolism" and is now well characterized clinically and biochemically. The most striking biochemical abnormalities are the presence of homocystine in urine and excess homocystine and methionine in blood. The catabolism of methionine is not completely understood, but the most important pathways appear to be those outlined by Presley and Sidbury, Spaeth and Barber. Methionine donates a methyl group (via several steps) to form homocysteine. Though this series of reactions is not reversible, homocysteine can be remethylated to methionine via a different pathway. It can also be oxidized to homocystine, which is then excreted in the urine. A major route for homocysteine is condensation with serine to form cystathionine, catalyzed by cystathionine synthetase. Mudd et al. have shown that the amino acid abnormality which results in homocystinuria is considered to be a deficiency of this enzyme. Consequently, metabolites which form prior to the metabolic block are present in increased amounts (methionine and homocystine in serum, with their increased urinary excretion) and those beyond are decreased (cystathionine is especially low in the brain, where it is normally found in relatively high concentration, and cystine is low in urine, plasma, and red blood cells). A study of cystathionine synthetase activity in the liver of a homocystinuric patient by Mudd et al. revealed no detectable enzymatic activity; in addition, parents of the patient were found to have decreased cystathionine synthetase activity in the liver but did not have homocystine in the urine.

The cyanidenitroprusside reaction for detection of cystinuria may be used for screening the urine sample. The test is done by combining 5 ml of urine with 2 ml of a 5 percent solution of sodium cyanide at room temperature. After 10 minutes, two to four drops of a 5 percent sodium nitroprusside solution are added and a beet-red color appears if cystine or homocystine is present. Cystine can then be distinguished from homocystine by high voltage electrophoresis.

One of the prominent, but by no means exclusive, signs is nontraumatic lens dislocation, and this together with other physical signs cause confusion with the Marfan syndrome. Homocystinuria exhibits a variety of signs and symptoms including homocystine in the urine; fair hair; a tall body, notably larger below the waist than above (Fig. 63, see colorplate, frontis) with long limbs and flat and turned-out feet (genu valgum and excavatum); osteoporosis and scoliosis with a tendency to vertebral fracture; a peculiar reddish skin with discoloration in the malar area of the face; dolichostenomelia; fatty livers with enlargement; epileptiform attacks; thrombotic phenomenon; hyperreflexia; cardiovascular defects; and sub-normal intelligence in about two-thirds of the cases. The general clinical findings are outlined in Table 10.

TABLE 10

GENERAL CLINICAL FINDINGS IN HOMOCYSTINURIA*

	Number	Percent
Dislocated lenses	29/31	90
Mental retardation	28/31	90
Fair skin	21/22	90
Malar flush	20/22	90
Abnormal gait	12/14	85
Light hair	20/25	80
Genu valgum	10/14	70
Thrombophlebitis	10/20	50
Convulsions	11/23	50
Marfan's syndrome	9/20	45
Premature death	13/29	40

*After G. L. Spaeth, and G. W. Barber, J. Pediatr. Ophthalmol., 3:42, 1966.

There is nothing characteristic about the mental retardation in homocystinurics, although homocystinuria may rank as the second most common metabolic disease associated with it, phenylketonuria being the first. Other causes of mental retardation associated with ocular findings include Hurler's disease, Wilson's disease, Tay Sachs' disease, and Fabry's disease. All findings may not be present in a particular individual. Spaeth and Barber described the following family. The propositus was a child with "classic" clinical and biochemical changes of homocystinuria. Her cousin excreted small amounts of homocystine but had no other clinical or biochemical abnormalities. Her parents appeared completely normal. Biochemical investigations at the National Institute of Health showed that the severity of disease was related to the degree of abnormality of the responsible enzyme, cystathionine synthetase. This variability of expression is expected, for it is known that individuals with the same genetic make-up may express their genes differently depending on environment, complement of other genes, and a multitude of other factors outlined in Chapter 1. The inconstancy of findings means that homocystinuria is frequently undiagnosed or misdiagnosed. Therefore, accurate appraisal of the incidence of the condition is difficult.

Most patients have multiple eye defects which include congenital glaucoma (Fig. 64, see colorplate, frontis), ectopic lenses, congenital cataracts, spherophakia, aniridia, optic atrophy, and retinal detachment. Other findings include microphthalmia, hyperplastic primary vitreous, myopic degeneration, colobomata, keratitis, iritis, and retinoschisis. Presley and Sidbury found that ectopia lentis occurred in 60 percent of cases, cataracts in 60 percent, optic atrophy in 30 percent, and aniridia in 10

TABLE 11

OCULAR FINDINGS IN HOMOCYSTINURIA*

	Number	Percent
Dislocated lenses	29/31	90
Myopia	6/7	90
Light irides	16/24	70
Retinal elevation	4/16	25
Cataract	5/23	20
Optic atrophy	3/21	15
Glaucoma	2/18	10
Hypotony	1/3	33
Iritis	1/18	5
Keratitis	1/18	5
Microphthalmos	1/31	3

*After G. L. Spaeth and G. W. Barber, J. Pediatr. Ophthalmol., 3:42, 1966.

percent. Table 11 outlines the incidence of these conditions as noted by Spaeth and Barber.

Carson et al. reported two autopsy eyes and noted that the zonular fibers showed degenerative changes both on light and electron microscopy. The fibers were thickened and retracted against the thickened basement membrane of the ciliary epithelium with which they were fused. Zonular material from rabbit eyes has been shown to contain cystine; thus, cystine deficiency has been offered as an explanation of the defective zonular network. Since homocystinurics are known to develop thrombosis after venous or arterial puncture due to hypercoagulation of blood, the urine of the patient with suspected Marfan's syndrome should be examined for homocystinuria before being referred for angiography.

The physician who discovers homocystinuria early in infancy must attempt to prevent the development of mental deficiency, convulsions, skeletal deformities, loss of vision, and thromboses. In the older child, stress must be laid on prevention of the vascular complications. Treatment is still not entirely satisfactory. The dislocated lens is better left alone if the eye is symptom free; glaucoma must be treated.

Sulfite Oxidase Deficiency

Sulfite oxidase deficiency is characterized by dislocation of the lens, severe neurological and mental retardation, and death in early childhood. The syndrome is due to defective activity of the enzyme that normally catalyzes the conversion of sulfite to sulfate. Sulfite oxidase deficiency joins two other causes of mental retardation, homocystinuria and cystathioninuria, as a disease of the metabolism of sulfur-containing compounds. The urine contains increased amounts of sulfite compounds and decreased amounts of inorganic sulfate. At autopsy, the patient's liver, kidney, and brain may show a virtual absence of activity of sulfite oxidase.

OTHER GENETICALLY DETERMINED DISEASES

Turner's Syndrome

Funke, in 1902, was probably the first to report a case of a female with webbed neck and sexual infantilism, but it was not until a paper by Turner in 1938 that the syndrome bearing his name was clearly defined. Turner described seven short-statured postadolescent females with sexual infantilism (underdeveloped breasts, infantile genitalia, and scanty pubic hair), loose skin folds at the back of the neck, webbing of the cervical skin (pterigium coli), and increased carrying angle of the elbow (cubitus valgus). Other conditions presently known to be associated with Turner's syndrome include coarctation of the aorta, cardiac malformations, high arched palate, multiple pigmented nevi, recurrent aural infections, low set ears, nerve deafness, diabetes, myxedema, low nuchal hairline, bilateral epicanthal folds, increased distance between nipples, shield chest, and lymphedema of the dorsum of the hands and feet during infancy. There are varying levels of ovarian function from total absence to apparent normality.

Previously this hereditary and generalized disorder was classified within the group of abnormalities known as the "Status Bonnevie-Ulrich," originally thought to be the result of endothelial dysfunction. Subsequently, females with Turner's syndrome were found to have absence of sex chromatin by buccal smear. These females usually have only 45 chromosomes, an XO karyotype, presumably from nondisjunction during maternal or paternal gametogenesis. Ford et al. reported that approximately one in every 5,000 phenotypic females possess one X chromosome instead of two and a total of 45 chromosomes instead of 46. Other sex chromosome abnormalities such as mosaicism (XO/XX) have also been demonstrated in Turner's syndrome. The female has either an absent X chromosome, a mosaic sex chromosome pattern, or a so-called isochromosome for the long arm of the X or ring chromosome of the X.

Since 1928, male patients have occasionally been reported with the classical female clinical characteristics of Turner's syndrome except for the male urogenital system. The male shows small testes with unilateral or bilateral cryptorchidism, normal scrotum, and small or moderate sized prostate. The 17-ketosteroid excretion is low-to-normal and the urinary gonadotropins are elevated. The phenotypic appearance of the male is strikingly similar to the female, e. g., short stature, webbed neck, widely spaced hypoplastic nipples, low-set ears, ptosis, high arched palate, low nuchal hairline, and abnormal configuration of the pectoralis muscle. The buccal smear and karyograph are usually normal causing some confusion as to the precise definition of male Turner's syndrome. Ocular anomalies in females include bilateral epicanthal folds, color blindness, marked myopia, hypermetropia, nystagmus, ptosis, hypertelorism, cataract, strabismus, blue sclerae, corneal nebulae, iris coloboma, and congenital glaucoma. Khodadoust and Paton reported a case of male Turner's syndrome with ocular findings that included high myopia, retinal detachment, cataract, and secondary glaucoma.

Hereditary Oculo-Dento-Osseous Dysplasia

In 1889, Brailey described a patient with microphthalmos and partial aniridia combined with the congenital absence of several teeth. In 1920, Lohmann described a syndrome of microphthalmos and camptodactyly of the fifth fingers of both hands. Ten years later Wolff described a family of 11 of whom 5 had microphthalmos, and in which one had 4 abnormally small incisors and one had supernumerary teeth. In 1938, Ciotola also reported a case with microphthalmos and syndactyly and in 1941, Berliner described two female cousins with unilateral microphthalmos and anterior synechia.

In 1957, Meyer-Schwickerath et al. described two patients with microphthalmos, dental anomalies, and a deformity of the fifth fingers

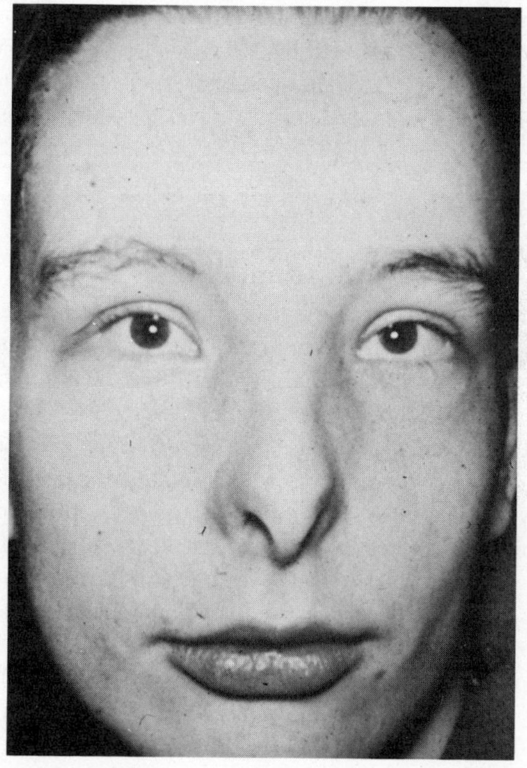

FIG. 65. Oculodentoosseous dysplasia. (From Sugar. Am. J. Ophthalmol. 61:1448, 1966.)

bilaterally consisting of a camptodactylia. The alae nasi were small with anteverted nostrils. One of the patients, a 13-year-old girl, had bilateral glaucoma. In 1964, Gillespie described a brother and a sister suffering from bilateral microphthalmos, hypotrichosis, dental anomalies (enamelogenesis imperfecta, microdontia, and missing teeth). Since these patients were siblings it was suggested that the syndrome was hereditary, being inherited as an autosomal recessive. Chromosome studies were normal.

Rajic and de Veber described 6 affected members of a family suffering from this condition. They were of normal or above normal intelligence and had normal height, weight, and growth patterns without any evidence of effects from the disturbance in the bone architecture.

Genetically, this condition was assumed by the authors to have a dominant characteristic starting as a mutant in the grandmother, since her parents were normal clinically and by x-ray. Chromosome studies on the propositus were normal as were the serum calcium, phosphorus, alkaline phosphatase, and magnesium. The bone biopsy appeared normal under the light microscope but polarized light revealed a pseudopagetoid mosaic pattern suggesting accelerated bone turnover. The children affected also showed widened ribs and clavicles. Eye findings include microphthalmos (Fig. 65) and glaucoma.

Pierre Robin Syndrome

The Pierre Robin syndrome is characterized by 3 defects: micrognathia, cleft palate, and glossoptosis. Patients are often described as having an "Andy Gump" or "bird-like" face. Other abnormalities include flattening of the base of the nose; finger, and toe anomalies; hearing loss; and hydrocephalus.

Smith and Stowe reported a history of some obstetrical mishap in about 25 percent of their cases, which included paternal influenza and maternal coryza, maternal viral infection, mild spotting to bleeding, and maternal respiratory infection. In 20 percent of cases, the mother's age averaged 36 years. A history of previous miscarriages and spontaneous abortions was not infrequent. They reported one family where the syndrome was present in 4 generations.

At the fourth month of fetal life the upper lip projects forward beyond the lower lip. Some inhibitory influence could result in failure of normal development that should take place beyond this stage. It is at about this time that the fetal filtration angle shows active development, which could be retarded by the same inhibitory influence.

Once the diagnosis is made in the newborn nursery these children must be observed with great care, since they may exhibit difficulty in swallowing, choking spells, and bouts of cyanosis due to glossoptosis (relieved by placing the child on the abdomen, which causes the tongue to fall forward) and difficulty in swallowing. Respiratory infections and failure to thrive occur at a later age. Five of the 39 cases reported by Smith and Stowe died of congenital heart disease, and 9 exhibited cardiac murmurs. The heart defects included patent ductus arteriosis and foramen ovale, auricular septal defect, and cor triloculare with coarctation of the aorta. Since these children frequently have to undergo surgery, these defects must be remembered.

The children showed a variety of ocular abnormalities including two cases of bilateral congenital glaucoma (Table 12).

TABLE 12

PIERRE ROBIN SYNDROME OCULAR ANOMALIES*

(13 major lesions in 9 patients)

Congenital glaucoma	2
Retinal detachment	1
Congenital high myopia	1
Esotropia	6
Congenital cataract	1
Moebius syndrome	1
Microphthalmos and coloboma of choroid	1

*After J. L. Smith and R. R. Stowe, Pediatrics, 27:128, 1961.

Gonioscopic examination in one case with congenital glaucoma revealed a thin, grayish, nearly translucent membrane over the trabeculum. This membrane was also observed in a case in the same series with high myopia. Early in the century Seefelter pointed out the association between congenital glaucoma and the anomaly of micrognathia and cleft palate.

With proper management, many of these children can lead nearly normal lives after age 5. However, unrecognized ocular diseases such as congenital glaucoma or retinal detachment could leave the child with a permanent disability. Therefore every infant with the Pierre Robin syndrome must have a complete ophthalmological examination prior to age 1 year.

Mongolism: Down's Syndrome

Mongolism may be associated with a variety of systemic defects and is caused by a trisomy of the 21 chromosome pair, resulting in a total of 47 chromosomes. Apparently the extra chromosome comes from a nondisjunction of a pair of chromosomes of the ovum. These children are generally born to mothers about 10 years older than the random average age.

Practically all patients with mongolism are mentally retarded with a short, wide palpebral aperture that is positioned obliquely in an upward and outward direction. Other features include a small skull; flat face; small nose, with depressed bridge; malformed ears; hypogenitalism; congenital heart disease; and a thick tongue which protrudes from the mouth. A straight line crosses the palm; the hands and feet are small. The ocular anomalies include bilateral epicanthus, nystagmus, convergent strabismus, cataract, congenital glaucoma, and keratoconus. The iris is said to show characteristic changes associated with mongolism. The first is a paucity of stromal fibers giving the appearance of iris atrophy. The other is a speckled circle of stromal condensation associated with localized atrophy, usually toward the periphery of the anterior iris surface, known as "Brushfield's spots," which are seen in 85 percent of cases. Cataractous changes are usually recognized in late childhood or early adult life. The opacities are typically dust-like or plate-like with irregularly shaped blue-white opacities that are seen in the cortex surrounding the embryonic lens nucleus. They vary in size and may be quite dense; the anterior Y suture may be opacified. Progression is slow. The keratoconus may be extreme but operation is rarely indicated, unless the visual defect is profound, because of the low IQ. Glaucoma, however, requires prompt surgical measures.

OTHER CONDITIONS

Hemangioma of the Choroid

This condition, which may occur as an independent entity, is most often associated with the Sturge-Weber syndrome. When present, the iris is darker on the affected side, the stroma appears denser than normal, and prominent vessels may be seen on the iris surface. According to Anderson the majority of choroidal hemangiomata are found near the posterior pole of the globe, particularly in the inferior temporal quadrant. This condition must be differentiated from a malignant melanoma.

Pigmentary Glaucoma

In 1940, Sugar and Barbour described pigmentary glaucoma as a clinical entity which has been observed in children as young as age 10. There is an

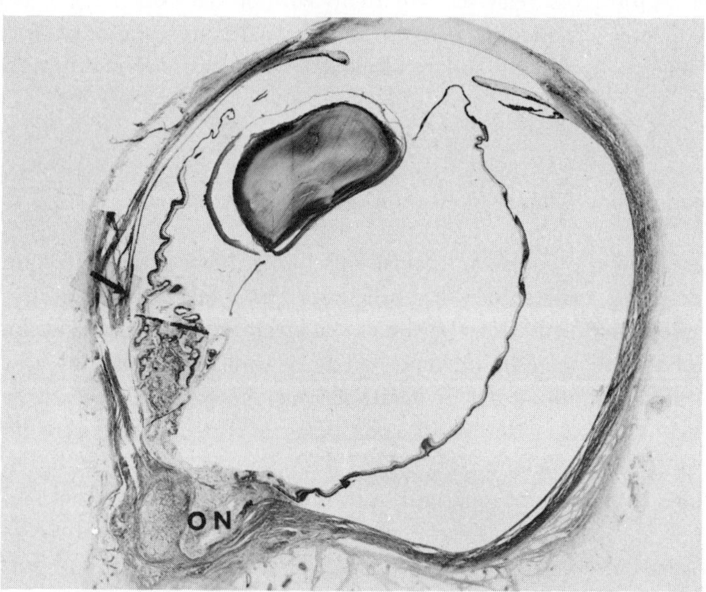

FIG. 66. Microphthalmic eye of phocomelic baby (case reported by Casanovas and Carbonnell). On left side of picture iris is very hypoplastic, and posteriorly from the arrow to the optic nerve head (ON) there is huge choroidal coloboma filled in with dysplastic retina. (A. F. I. P. Neg. No. 65-4111.) (From Zimmerman and Font. J. A. M. A. 196:684, 1966.) (Courtesy of the authors, the American Medical Association, and the Registry of Ophthalmic Pathology of the Armed Forces Institute of Pathology.) X 4.

associated concentric atrophy of the iris pigment epithelium demonstrable by transillumination. Loose pigment particles find their way, by aqueous fluid currents, around the circumference of the lens and into the filtration angle, encumbering an outflow system that may already be defective to some degree. The Krukenberg pigment spindle is present on the posterior corneal surface, and is also due to anterior chamber aqueous flow dynamics. Myopia is common.

Sampaolesi considers pigmentary glaucoma a special type of congenital glaucoma of late onset, although others suggest that it is very similar to primary open angle glaucoma, with a deep anterior chamber, decreased facility of outflow, characteristic field loss, and optic disc cupping.

Becker and Podos found that in studying a possible relationship between pigmentary glaucoma and open angle glaucoma two similarities arose. Firstly, family studies showed that both conditions occur in close relatives. Secondly, topical corticosteroid testing showed that almost an equal number of patients with normal pressure and Krukenberg's spindle responded as did close relatives of patients with primary open angle glaucoma.

Pigmentary glaucoma affects mostly males in a ratio of 5 to 6:1. Inheritance is dominant and sex-linked with occasional manifestations in women carriers.

Thalidomide (Ocular Malformations and Phocomelia)

Paresis of the ocular and facial muscles has been observed frequently in the phocomelic babies born of mothers who have taken thalidomide. All the more serious malformations of the eye associated with failure of closure of the fetal fissure may be encountered in a small percentage of cases. The defects may be unilateral or bilateral and show all degrees of severity. Involvement ranges from small colobomas of the iris to severe microphthalmia and anophthalmia.

Since thalidomide apparently produces no associated lethal malformations, few autopsies have been performed in these cases and there is almost no information concerning the pathological changes to be found in the eyes of thalidomide babies. According to Zimmerman and Font, the recent report by Casanovas and Carbonell provides the only histopathological description of a malformed eye of a phocomelic baby (Fig. 66). In this case, one eye appeared normal but the other was microphthalmic with a coloboma of the iris, choroid, and optic disk. Dysplastic retina filled the choroidal coloboma adjacent to the disk.

Rubenstein's Syndrome; Broad Thumb Syndrome

The Rubenstein syndrome exhibits unusually large thumbs and toes. Other features include hypertelorism, myopia, mental retardation, and infantile glaucoma.

References

Abbassi, V., Lowe, C. V., and Calcagno, P. L. Oculo-cerebro-renal syndrome, a review. Am. J. Dis. Child., 115:145, 1968.

Achard, M. C. Arachnodactylie. Bull. Mem. Soc. Med. Hop. Paris, 19:834, 1902.

Adams, S. T., Grant, W. M., and Smith, T. R. Congenital glaucoma (possibly Lowe's syndrome). Arch. Ophthalmol., 68:191, 1962.

Albaugh, G. H. Congenital anomalies following maternal rubella in early weeks of pregnancy: with special emphasis on congenital cataract. J. A. M. A., 129:719, 1945.

Alfano, J. E. Ocular aspects of the maternal rubella syndrome. Trans. Am. Acad. Ophthalmol., Otolaryngol., 70:235, 1966.
Experiences with congenital glaucoma. Eye, Ear, Nose, Throat Mon., 47:48, 1968.
Alford, C. A., Neva, F. A., and Weller, T. H. Virologic and serologic studies on human products of conception after maternal rubella. New Eng. J. Med., 271:1275, 1964.
Alkemade, P. P. H. Dysgenesis Mesodermalis of the Iris and the Cornea. A Study of Rieger's Syndrome and Peters' Anomaly. Van Gorcum, Assen, 1969.
Allan, R. A., Straatsma, B. R., Apt, L., and Hall, M.O. Ocular manifestations of the Marfan syndrome. Trans. Am. Acad. Ophthalmol., Otolaryngol., 71:18, 1967.
Alvis, B. Y., and Toland, V. A. Nevus flammeus associated with glaucoma. Report of a case in which cyclodiothermy was used in an attempt to control the intraocular pressure. Am. J. Ophthalmol., 26:720, 1943.
Anderson, J. R. Hydrophthalmia or Congenital Glaucoma. Its causes, Treatment and Outlook. Cambridge Univ. Press, London, 1939.
Arenberg, I. K., et al. Alport's syndrome, re-evaluation of the associated ocular abnormalities and report of a family study. J. Pediatr. Ophthalmol., 4:21, 1967.
Armaly, M. F. Ocular involvement in chondrodystrophia clacificans congenital punctata. Arch. Ophthalmol., 57:491, 1957.
Axenfeld, T. Zur Kenntnis der isolierten Dehiszenzen der Membran Descemetii. Klin. Monatsbl. Augenheilkd., 2:157, 1905.
Embryotoxon corneae posterius. Ber Dtsch. Ophthalmol. Ges. 42:301, 1920.
Aynsley, T. R. Buphthalmos and naevus. Br.J. Ophthalmol, 13:612, 1929.
Baillart, P. Le glaucome infantile a l'institution nationale des jeunes aveugles. Ann. Ocul. (Paris), 180:257, 1947.
Ballantyne, A. J. Buphthalmos with facial naevus and allied conditions. Br. J. Ophthalmol., 14:481, 1930, and 24:65, 1940.
Baratta, G. Observazioni pratiche sulle principali malatti degli orchi. Milano 1818, Tomo 2, s 349, as cited by Jungken, C. Ueber den angebornen mangel der Iris. J. Chir. Augenheilkd., 2:667, 1821.
Barkan, O. Glaucoma: classification, causes and surgical control. Results of microgonioscopic research. Am. J. Ophthalmol., 21:1099. 1938.
Pathogenesis of congenital glaucoma. Am. J. Ophthalmol., 40:1, 1955.
Becker, B., and Kolker, A. Vision and its Disorders. U. S. Dept. Health, Education, and Welfare. Bethesda, Md., 1967, p. 87.
and Podos, S. Krukenberg's spindles and primary open angle glaucoma. Arch. Ophthalmol., 76:635, 1966.
and Schaffer, R. N. Diagnosis and Therapy of the Glaucomas, 2nd ed. Mosby, St. Louis, 1965, p. 233.
Beetham, W. P. Atropic cataracts. Arch. Ophthalmol., 24:21, 1940.
Beighton, P., and Horna, F. T. Surgical aspects of the Ehlers-Danlos syndrome. Br. J. Surg., 56:255, 1969.
Bellanti, J. A., et al. Congenital rubella. clinicopathologic virologic, and immunologic studies. Am. J. Dis. Child, 110:464, 1965
Berkow, J. W. Retinitis pigmentosa associated with Sturge-Weber's syndrome. Arch. Ophthalmol., 75:72, 1966.
Berliner, M. Unilateral microphthalmia with congenital anterior synechiae and syndactyly. Arch. Ophthalmol., 26:653, 1941.
Bessiere, E., Riviere, J., and Leuret, J. P. Le rebeller, an association of Klinefelter's disease and congenital anomalies camptodactyly, microphakia. Bull. Soc. Ophtalmol., Fr., 62:197, 1962.

Bettman, J. W., and Cleasby, G. W. Congenital glaucoma. Pediatrics, 32:420, 1963.
Black, H. H., and Landay, L. H. Marfan's syndrome. Am. J. Dis. Child., 89:414, 1955.
Blake, E. M. The surgical treatment of glaucoma complicating congenital aniridia. Am. J. Ophthalmol., 36:907, 1953.
Blatt, N. Beziehungen Zwischen der intrauterinalen Resorption der Gertrubten Linse und dem Mikrophthalmus. Klin. Monatsbl. Augenheilkd., 68:761, 1922.
Bloch, N. Les differents types de sclerocornee, leurs modes d'heredite, et les malformations congenitales concomitantes. J. Genet. Hum., 14:133, 1965.
Boder, E., and Sedgewick, R. P. Ataxia-telangiectasia. Univ. S. Cal. Med. Bull., 9:15, 1957.
and Sedgewick, R. P. Ataxia-telangiectasia. A review of 101 cases. In G. Walsh (Ed.), Cerebellum, posture and cerebral palsy, Little Club Clinics in Developmental Medicine, No. 8. The National Spastics Society and Heinemann Medical Books, London, 1963, p. 110.
Boniuk, M. Ocular Manifestations of the rubella syndrome. Read before the Verhoeff Society Meeting, Washington, D.C., April 27, 1965.
Bonnet, P. Les manifestations oculaires de la maladie d'Ehlers-Danlos. Bull. Soc. Ophtalmol. Fr., 6:623, 1953.
Bornstein, M. B. Aniridie bilaterale avec polydactylie. Relations des anomalies oculaires du type colobanateux associées a des malformations squelettiques avec les formes atypiques du syndrome de Barbet-Biedl. J. Genet. Hum., 1:211, 1952.
Bossu, A., and Lambrechts, M. Manifestations oculaires du syndrome d'Ehlers-Danlos. Ann. Ocul. (Paris), 187:227, 1954.
Braendstrup, J. M. Posterior embryotoxon in three generations. Acta Ophthalmol. (Kbh.), 26:495, 1948.
Brailey, W. A. Double microphthalmus with defective development of the iris, teeth, and anus. Glaucoma at an early age. Quoted by Gillespie, F. D., Arch. Ophthalmol., 71:187 1964.
Breebaart, A. C. A case of Rieger's Anomaly with glaucoma. Influence of sleep. Arch. Ophthalmol., 76:825, 1966.
Brown, S. I. Corneal transplantation in the anterior chamber cleavage syndrome. Am. J. Ophthalmol., 70:942, 1970.
Bruno, M. S., and Narasimham, M. B. The Ehlers-Danlos syndrome. A report of four cases in two generations of a negro family. New. Eng. J. Med., 264:274, 1961.
Bucklers, M. Mikrophakie. In A. Gutte (Ed.). Hardbuck Erbkranhkeitin Erbleiden des Auges, Vol. 5. Thieme, Leipzig, p. 106.
Burian, H. M. Chamber angle studies in development glaucoma. Marfan's syndrome and high myopia. Missouri Med., 55:1088, 1958.
and Allan, L. Histologic studies of the chamber angle of patients with Marfan's syndrome. Arch. Ophthalmol., 65:323, 1961.
and Burns, C. A. Ocular changes in myotonic dystrophy. Am. J. Ophthalmol., 63:22, 1967.
von Noorden, G. K., and Ponseti, I. V. Chamber angle anomalies in systemic connective tissue disorders. Arch. Ophthalmol., 64:671, 1960.
Busacca, A., et Pinticart, E. Etude gonioscopique d'un cas de embryotoxon corneae posterius. Ophthalmologica, 115:283, 1948.
Busch, G., Weiskopf, J., et Busch, K. Dysgenesis Mesodermalis et Ectobermal is Rieger oder Rieger'sche Karnkheit. Klin. Monatsbl. Augenheilkd., 136:512, 1960.
Cabannes, C. La buphthalmie congenitale dans ses rapports avec l'hemihypertrophie de la face. Arch. Ophthalmol., 24:368, 1909.
Callender, G. R., and Tigpen, C. A. Two neurofibromas in one eye. Am. J. Ophthalmol., 13:121, 1930.

Capella, J. A., et al. Hereditary cataracts and microphthalmia. Am. J. Ophthalmol., 56:454, 1963.
Carson, N. A. J. and Carre, J. J. Treatment of homocystinuria with pyridoxine. A preliminary study. Arch. Dis. Child., 44:387, 1969.
Cusworth, D. C., et al. Homocystinuria. A new inborn error of metabolism associated with mental deficiency. Arch. Dis. Child., 38:425, 1963.
Dent, C. E., Field, C. M. B., and Gaull, G. E. Homocystinuria. Clinical and pathological review of 10 cases. J. Pediatr., 66:565, 1965.
and Neill, D. W. Metabolic abnormalities detected in a survey of mentally backward individuals in Northern Ireland. Arch. Dis. Child., 37:505, 1962.
Cassady, J. R., and Light, A. Familial persistent pupillary membranes. Arch. Ophthalmol. 58:438, 1957.
Cassanovas, J., et Carbonell, M. Malformations oculaires en la embriopatia thalidomidica. Arch. Soc. Oftalmol., Hisp. Am., 24:947, 1964.
Catsch, A. Korrelations patologiesche Utersuchungen. Arch Ophthalmol., 138:886, 1938.
Chandler, P. A., and Grant, W. M. Lectures on Glaucoma. Lea & Febieger, Philadelphia, 1965, pp. 334–335, 341.
Chu, E. H. Y., Warkany, J., and Rosenstein, R. B. Chromosome compliment in a case of the male Turner syndrome. Lancet, 1:785, 1961.
Chutorian, A., and Rowland, L. P. Lowe syndrome. Neurology (Minneap.), 16:115, 1966.
Ciotola, A. G. Microftalmo E malformazioni della dita (sindattalia; polidattilia). Boll. Ocul., 17:855, 1938.
Cogan D. G., and Kuwabara, T. The sphingolipidoses and the eye. Arch. Ophthalmol., 79:437, 1968.
and Kuwabara, T. Ocular pathology of the 13–15 trisomy syndrome. Arch. Ophthalmol., 72:246, 1964.
Cohn, P. Demonstration eines Patienten mit Gummithaut (Cutis Laxa) und eigentumlichen zirkumskrupten Hautveranderungen, braunroten eindrukabren Erhebungen Verhl. Dtsch Derm. Ges., 9:415, 1907.
Collier, M. La dysplasie marginale posterieure de la cornee dans le cabre des anomalies squelettiques et ectodermiques. Ann. Ocul. (Paris), 195:512, 1962.
Collins, E. T., and Batten, R. D. Neurofibroma of the eyeball and its appendages. Trans. Ophthalmol. Soc. U. K. 25:248, 1905.
Cooper, L. Z., et al. Rubella in contacts of infants with rubella. Associated anomalies. Morb. Mort. Wk. Rep., 14:44, 1965.
Cordes, F. C. Cataract types. Man. Am. Acad. Ophthalmol. Otolaryngol., 3rd Ed., Rochester, Minn., 1954.
Cottini, G. B. Association des syndromes de Groenblad-Stranberg et d'Ehlers-Danlos syndrome dans le meme sujet. Acta Derm. Venercol. (Stockh.), 29:544, 1949.
Crebbin, A. R. Persistent pupillary membrane and congenital ectopia lentis. Am. J. Ophthalmol., 12:87, 1929.
Curtin, V. T., Joyce, E. E., and Ballin, N. Ocular pathology in the ocular-cerebro-renal syndrome of Lowe. Am. J. Ophthalmol., 64:533, 1967.
Danlos, M. Un cas de cutis laxa avec tumers par contusion chronique des coudes et des genoux (xanthome juvenile pseudo-diabetique de M. M. Hallopeau et Mace de Lepinary). Bull. Soc. Fr. Derm. Syph., 19:70, 1908.
Davis, W. S. Nevus flammeus and arested hydrophthalmos. Am. J. Ophthalmol., 22:298, 1939.
Day H. J., and Zarafonetis, C. J. D. Coagulation studies in four patients with Ehlers-Danlos syndrome. Am. J. Med. Sci., 242:565, 1951.
Delay, J., et Pichot. P. Sur une maladie familiale caractérisée par l'association d'oligophrenie d'aniridie et de cataracte congenitale. Arch. Ophtalmol., (Paris), 8:105,

1948.

Desvignes, P., et al. Aspect iconographique d'une cornea plana dans une maladie de Lobstein. Arch. Ophthalmol. (Paris), 27:585, 1967.

Dickey, J. L. A case of congenital ectopia lentis. Am. J. Med. Sci., 89:491, 1885.

DiGeorge, A. M., and Harley, R. D. The association of aniridia, Wilm's tumor, and genital abnormalities. Trans. Am. Ophthalmol. Soc., 63:64, 1965, and Arch. Ophthalmol., 75:796, 1966.

Dollfus, M. A., et al. Congenital cystic eyeball. Am. J. Ophthalmol., 66:504, 1968.

Dorff, G. B., Appelman, D. H., and Levinson, A. Turner's syndrome in the male. Acta Pediatr. 65:555, 1948.

Duke-Elder, W. S. Text-book of Ophthalmology, Vol. 3. Mosby, St. Louis, 1941, p. 3322.

System of Ophthalmology, Vol. 2. Kimpton, London, 1969, pp. 20, 105.

System of Ophthalmology, Vol. 3, Pt. 2. Kimpton, London, 1964. pp. 127, 142, 399, 419, 451, 481, 503, 543, 550, 566, 688, 775.

System of Ophthalmology, Vol. 9. Kimpton, London, 1966, p. 823.

Dunphy E. B. Glaucoma accompanying Nevus Flammeus. Am. J. Ophthalmol., 18:709, 1935.

Durham, D. G. Cutis hyperelastica (Ehlers-Danlos syndrome) with blue scleras, microcornea, and glaucoma. Arch. Ophthalmol., 49:220, 1953.

Editorial. Genetic counselling for the family, Image, 37:2, 1970.

Efron, M. Aminoaciduria. New Eng. J. Med., 272:1058, 1107, 1965.

Ehlers, E. Curis Laxa, Neigung Zu Haemorrhagien in der Haut. Lockerung mehrerer Artikulationen. Der. Ztschr., 8:173, 1901.

Erickson, C. A. Rubella early in pregnancy causing congenital malformations of the eyes and heart. J. Pediatr., 25:281, 1944.

Falls, H. F. A gene producing various defects of the anterior segment of the eye. Am. J. Ophthalmol., 32:41, 1949.

The role of the sex chromosome in hereditary ocular pathology. Trans. Am. Ophthalmol. Soc., 50:421, 1952.

Faust, K. Arcus Lipoides Bei Buphthalmus. Klin. Monatsbl. Augenheilkd., 101:287, 1938.

Fehr, H. Gesellschaftsberichte, Sitzung vom Feb. 23, 1899, Berlin Ophthal. Ges. Abstracted, Zbl. Prak. Augenheilkd., 23:184, 1899.

Feiler-Ofry, V., Stein, R., and Godel, V. Marchesani's syndrome and chamber angle anomalies. Am. J. Ophthalmol., 65:862, 1968.

Feinman, N. L., and Yakovac, W. C. Neurofibromatosis in childhood. J. Pediatr., 26:339, 1970.

Fischer, H. La glossoptose. Le syndrome de Pierre Robin. Vigot Freres, Paris, 1932.

Fisher, N. F., Hallett, J., and Carpenter, G. Oculocerebrorenal syndrome of Lowe. Arch. Ophthalmol., 77:643, 1967.

Fleischer, B. Abnorme Kleinheit und Kugelgestalt der Linse bei Zwei Geschwisterpoaren. Arch. Augenheilkd., 80:248, 1916.

Fontana, V. J., Ferrara, A., and Perciaccante, R. Wilm's tumor and associated anomalies. Am. J. Dis. Child., 109:459, 1965.

Ford, D. E., et al. A sex chromosome anomaly in a case of gonadal dysgenesis (Turner's syndrome). Lancet, 1:711, 1959.

Ford, J. C., and Irvine, A. R. Persistent hyperplastic vitreous associated with anterior rupture of the lens capsule. Arch. Ophthalmol., 66:467, 1961.

Forsius, H., Erikson, A., and Fellman, J. Embryotoxon corneae posterius in isolated population. Acta Ophthalmol. (Kbh.) 42:42, 1964.

Fraccaro, M., Kaijser, K., and Lindsten, J. Chromosome complement in gondal dysgenesis (Turner's Syndrome). Lancet, 1:886, 1959.

Franceschetti, A. Kurzes Handbuch der Ophthalmologie. Springer, Berlin, 1930, p. 712.

Ueber Mikrophakie und deren Erbgang. Klin. Monatsbl. Augenheilkd., 85:285, 1930.
Malformations oculaires et auriculaires familiales Rev. Otoneuroophtalmol., 18:500, 1946.
Un syndrome nouveau. La dysostose mandibulo-faciale. Bull. Schwiez. Akad. Med. Wiss., 1:60, 1944.
and Klein, D. The mandibulofacial dysostosis, a new hereditary syndrome. Acta Ophthalmol. (Kbh.), 27:144, 1949.
et Klein, D. Les affections génétiques en ophtalmologie. Encyclopedie Medico-chirurgicale, Ophtalmologie, Vol. 1, 1956.
Francois, J. A new syndrome, dyscephalia with bird face and dental anomalies, nanism, hypotrichosis, cutaneous atrophy, microphthalmia, and congenital cataract. Arch. Ophthalmol., 60:842, 1958.
Heredity in Ophthalmology. Mosby, St. Louis, 1961, p. 355.
Congenital Cataracts. Thomas, Springfield, Ill., 1963, pp. 126, 265.
et Hanssons, M. Syndrome oculo-cerebro-renal de Lowe, examen histopathologique oculaire. Bull. Soc. Belge Ophtalmol., 135:412, 1963.
et Katz, C. Association homolatérale d'hydrophtalmie, de nevrome plexiforme de la paupiére supérieure et d'hémihypertrophie faciale dans la maladie de Recklinghausen. Ophthalmologica, 142:549, 1961.
Katz, C., et Lambrechts, M. Association homolatérale d'hydrophtalmie, de névrome plexiforme de la paupiére supérieure et d'hémihypertrophie faciale dans la maladie de Recklinghausen. Bull. Soc. Belge Ophtalmol., 126:1059, 1961.
Fraumeni, J. F., and Glass, A. G. Wilm's tumor and congenital aniridia, J. A. M. A., 206:825, 1968.
Freeman, D. Neurofibroma of the choroid. Arch. Ophthalmol., 11:641, 1934.
Friede, R. Uber die angeborne Entoderm-Mesoderm-Hypoplasie des Auges und deren Beziehung zur Cornea plana congenital. Klin. Monatsbl. Augenheilkd., 102:16, 1969.
Friedman, M. W. and Ritchey, C. L. Unilateral congenital glaucoma, neurofibromatosis and pseudarthrosis. Arch. Ophthalmol., 70:294, 1963.
Funke, B. Pterigium coli. Dtsch. Z. Chir., 63:162, 1902.
Gardner, H. A. Will my baby be normal? Therapeutics, 1:2, 1971.
Garrow, A., and Lowenstein, A. A case of monocular hydrophthalmia with special reference to its possible relation to Sturge Weber's syndrome. Br. J. Ophthalmol., 27:335, 1943.
Gartner, S. Malignant melanoma of the choroid and von Recklinghausen's disease. Am. J. Ophthalmol., 23:73, 1940.
Gaull, G. E. Personal communication.
Geeraetz, W. J. Ocular Syndromes. Leas & Febiger, Philadelphia, 1965, p. 139.
Gerritsen, T., Vaughn, J. G., and Waisman, H. A. The identification of homocystine in the urine. Biochem. Biophys. Res. Commun., 9:493, 1962.
and Waisman, H. A. Homocystinuria, and error in the metabolism of methionine. Pediatrics, 33:413, 1964.
and Waisman, H. A. Homocystinuria. Absence of cystathionine in the brain. Science, 145:588, 1964.
Gilkes, M. J., and Strode, M. Ocular anomalies in association with developmental limb abnormalities of drug origin. Lancet, 1:1026, 1963.
Gill, R. R. Familiare Microphakie. Klin. Monatsbl., Augenheilkd., 80:411, 1928.
Gillespie, F. D. A hereditary syndrome. Dysplasia oculodentodigitalis. Arch. Ophthalmol., 71:187, 1964.
Gitzelmann, R. Hereditary galactokinase deficiency, a newly recognized cause of juvenile cataracts. Pediatr. Res., 1:14, 1967.
Goldstein, J. E., and Cogan, D. G. Sclerocornea and associated congenital anomalies.

Arch. Ophthalmol., 67:761, 1962.
Goodman, R. M., et al. Ehlers-Danlos syndrome occurring together with Marfan's syndrome. New Eng. J. Med., 273:514, 1965.
Gould, G. M., and Pyle, W. L. Anomalies and Curiosities of Medicine. Saunders, Philadelphia, 1897, p. 217.
Grant, W. M., and Walton, D. S. Distinctive gonioscopic findings in glaucoma due to neurofibromatosis. Arch. Ophthalmol., 79:127, 1968.
Gregg, N. McA. Congenital cataract following german measles in the mother. Trans. Ophthalmol. Soc. Aust., 3:35, 1941.
Grignold, A. Su due casi di aderance congenite irido-corneali multiple associate in un paziente a deformazione de ectopia pupillare (disgenesis mesodermalis corneae et iridis de Rieger). Boll. Ocul., 28:641, 1949.
Grove, J. H., Shaw, M. W., and Bourgue, G. A. family study of aniridia. Arch. Ophthalmol., 65:81, 1961.
Guerry, D. Congenital glaucoma following maternal rubella. Am. J. Ophthalmol., 29:190, 1946.
Gutbier, S. Irideremia seu defectu iridis congenito. Dissert inaug. Wirceb. Def., Gothae 1834, p. 14, as cited by Berger, U., Beitrage Zur lehre von der irideremia von Carron du Villards, und Gutbier. Ammon's Z. Ophthalmol., 5:78, 1837.
Hagedoorn, A. Congenital anomalies of the anterior segment of the Arch. Ophthalmol., 17:223, 1937.
Haines, J. W., and Pumphrey, A., Sturge Weber's syndrome. Am. J. Dis. Child., 61:557, 1941.
Hammond, A. Dysplasia epiphysialis punctata with ocular anomaly. Br. J. Ophthalmol., 54:755, 1970.
Haut, J., et Joannides, Z. A propos de 55 cas de syndrome de Lowe. Arch. Ophtalmol. (Paris), 26:21, 1966.
Heller, H. R. The Turner phenotype in the male. J. Pediat., 66:48 1965.
Helveston, E. M., Malone, E., and Lashmet, M. H. Congenital cystic eye. Arch. Ophthalmol., 84:622, 1970.
Henkind, P., Siegel, I. M., and Carr, R. E. Mesodermal dysgenesis of the anterior segment, Reiger's anomaly. Arch. Ophthalmol., 73:810, 1965.
and Friedman, A. H. Iridogoniodysgenesis with cataract. Am. J. Ophthalmol., 72:949, 1971.
Hermann, P. Le syndrome microphtalmie-retinite pigmentaire glaucome. Arch. Ophtalmol. (Paris), 18:17, 1958.
Hertzberg, R. Twenty-five year follow up of ocular defects in congenital rubella. Am. J. Ophthalmol., 66:269, 1968.
Heuyer, G. et al., Presentation de deux Freres atteints d'oligophrenie avee cataracte aniridie et nystagmus. Arch. Fr. Pediat., 5:545, 1948.
Hindle, N. W., and Crawford, J. S. Dislocation of the lens in Marfan's syndrome. Canad. J. Ophthalmol. 4:128, 1969.
Hogan, M. J., and Zimmerman, L. Ophthalmic Pathology, an Atlas and Textbook. Saunders, Philadelphia, 1962, p. 447.
Hoog, J. Congenital luxation of the crystalline lens. Lancet, 2:583, 1876.
Hov, L. K. Bijdrage tot de Ziekte van Lignad-Fanconi of het syndrom van Debre-de Toni-Fanconi. Maandschr. Kindergeneeskd., 24:37, 1956.
Howard, R. D., and Abrahams, I. W. Schlerocornea. Am. J. Ophthalmol., 71:1254, 1971.
Hsia, D. Y. Clinical variants of galactosemia. Metabolism, 16:419, 1967.
Hung, P. T. Chromosomal aberrations following ocular irridation. Am. J. Ophthalmol., 65:866, 1968.
Ide, C. H., and Wollschlaeger, P. B. Multiple congenital abnormalities associated with

cryptophthalmia. Arch. Ophthalmol., 81:638, 1969.
Irrevere, F, et al. Sulfite oxidase deficiency, studies of a patient with mental retardation, dislocated ocular lenses, and abnormal urinary excretion of S-sulfo-L-cysteine, sulfite, and thiosulfate. Biochem. Med., 1:187, 1967.
Itin, W. Longeur axiale de l'oeil chez deux freres atteints de sclerocornee peripherique avec cornea plana, l'un presentant une haute myopie, l'autre, une forte hypermetropie. Ophthalmologica, 152:369, 1966.
Jacobs, P. H. Ehlers-Danlos syndrome. Report of a case with onset at age 29. Arch. Dermatol., 76:460, 1957.
Jaffe, N. S., and Knie, P. True polycoria. Am. J. Ophthalmol., 35:253, 1952.
Jansen, L. M. The structure of the connective tissue. An explanation of the symptoms of the Ehlers-Danlos syndrome. Dermatologica, 110:108, 1955.
Jerndal, T. Goniodysgenesis and hereditary juvenile glaucoma. Acta Ophthalmol. (Suppl.) (Kbh.), 107:1970.
Johnson, S. A. M., and Falls, J. F. Ehlers-Danlos syndrome, a clinical and genetic study. Arch. Dermatol., 60:82, 1949.
Johnson, V. P., Grayson, M., and Christian, J. C. Dominant microspherophakia. Arch. Ophthalmol., 85:535, 1971.
Jones, I. S., and Cleasby, G. W. Hemongiomia of choroid. Am. J. Ophthalmol., 48:612, 1959.
Kahlke, W. Heredopathia atactica polyneuritiformis (Refsum's Disease). In G. Schettler (Ed.), Lipids, and Lipidoses. Springer-Verlag, New York, 1967, p. 352.
Kanai, A., et al. The fine structure of sclerocornea. Invest. Ophthalmol., 10:687, 1971.
Kanof, A. Ehlers-Danlos syndrome. Report of a case with suggestion of a possible causal mechanism. Am. J. Dis. Child., 83:197, 1952.
Katz, I., and Steiner, K. Ehlers-Danlos syndrome with extopic bone formation. Radiology, 65:352, 1955.
Kayser, B. Ueber die Unmolglichkeit enger genetischer Beziehungen Zwischen Makrokornea Resp. Megalokornea und Hydrophthalmus. Klin. Monatsbl. Augenheilkd., 102:11, 1939.
Khodadoust, A., and Paton, D. Turners syndrome in a male. Report of a case with myopia, retinal detachment, cataract, and glaucoma. Arch. Ophthalmol., 77:630, 1967.
Kinoshita, J. Cataracts in glactosemia. Invest. Ophthalmol., 4:786, 1965.
Kirkham, T. H. Mandibulofacial dysostosis with ectopia lentis. Am. J. Ophthalmol., 70:947, 1970.
Klar, R. Beitrage zur Frage der Megalokornea auf Grund von Untersuchungern eines staroperierten Patienten und seiner Sippe. Klin. Monatsbl. Augenheilkd., 104:286, 1940.
Kleberger, E. Uber die Entwicklung der angeborenen zentralen Hornhauttrubung (Peterssche Defektbildung). Graefe's Arch. Ophthalmol., 175:84, 1968.
Knapp, A. A. A case of corectopia. Am. J. Ophthalmol., 13:141, 1930.
Kolbert, G. S., and Seelenfreund, M. Sclerocornea, anterior chamber cleavage syndrome and Trisomy 18. Ann. Ophthalmol., 1:26, 1970.
Kolker, A. E., and Hetherington, J. Becker and Shaffer's Diagnosis and Therapy of the Glaucomas. Mosby, St. Louis, 1971.
Kopp, A. Demonstration zweiger Falle von "Cutis Laxa." Munch. Med. Wschr., 35:259, 1888.
Krause, K. Naevus Flammeus und Glaukom. Z. Augenheilkd., 68:244, 1929.
Kreibig, W. Ueber Neurofibromatose des Auges. Klin. Monatsbl. Augenheilkd., 114:428, 1949.
Krill, A. E. Observations of the carriers of x-chromosomal linked chorioretinal degenerations. Am. J. Ophthalmol., 64:1029, 1967.

Woodbury, C., and Bowman, J. E. X-chromosomal-linked sutural cataracts. Am. J. Ophthalmol., 68:867, 1969.

Kwitko, M. L. Successful corneal transplantation in the anterior chamber cleavage syndrome. Unpublished data.

Glaucoma due to hypermature cataract. Can. Med. Assoc. J., 89:569, 1963.

Congenital glaucoma. Can. J. Ophthalmol., 2:91, 1967.

Anterior segment anomalies, a clinical pathologic report of conditions simulating congenital glaucoma. Can. J. Ophthalmol., 3:116, 1968.

Glaucoma in infants and children. Mod. Med. Can., 23:1, 1968; and Mod. Med. Aust., 3:11, 1969.

Lane, F. Persistent posterior fibrovascular sheath of the lens. A report of two clinical cases and three eyeballs examined microscopically. Arch. Ophthalmol., 48:572, 1919.

Lapayowker, M. S. Cutis hyperplastica, the Ehlers-Danlos syndrome. Am. J. Roentgenol., 84:232, 1960.

Laurent, C., Royer, J., et Noel, G. Syndrome de Turner et glaucome congenitale. Bull. Soc. Ophthalmol. Fr., 5:367 (No. 5–6), 1961.

Lehrfeld, L., and Reber, J. Glaucoma at the Wills Eye hospital. Arch. Ophthal. 18:712, 1937.

Lemmingson, W. Multiple Dysplasien in Verbindung mit der Dysgenesis Mesodermalis Corneae et Iridis, Klin. Monatsbl. Augenheilkd., 138:96, 1961.

und Riethe, P. Beobachtungen bei Dysgenesis mesordermalis Corneae et Iridis in Kombination mit Oligodontic. Klin. Monatsbl. Augenheilkd., 133:877, 1958.

Lenz, H., et al. Rundesprach uber Thalidomid und angesborne Fehlbildungen der Augen. Ber. Dtsch. Ophthalmol. Ges., 65:208, 1964.

Lepri, G. Un caso di malformazioni oculari ed extraoculari congenite (sindrome di Lohmann). Arch. Ottalmol., 53:203, 1949.

Lessel, S., and Forbes, A.P. Eye signs in Turner's syndrome. Arch. Ophthalmol., 76:211, 1966.

Leydhecker, F. Eine Familie mit Mikrophthalmia congenita. Graefe's Arch. Ophthalmol., 139:790, 1938.

Lindsten, J. The nature and origin of X-Chromosome aberrations in Turner's Syndrome. Almquist and Wiksell, Stockholm, 1963.

Lisch, A. Ueber Beteiligung der Augen, insbersondere das Vorkommen von Irisknoetschen bie der Neurofibromatose (Recklinghausen). Z. Augenheilkd., 93:137, 1937.

Lisker, R., Nogueron, A., and Sanchez-Medal, L. Plasma thromboblastin component deficiency in the Ehlers-Danlos syndrome. Ann. Intern Med., 53:388, 1960.

Lohmann, W. Beitrag Zur kenntnis des reinen mikrophthalmus Arch. Augenheilkd., 86:136, 1920.

Lowe, C. V., Terrey, M., and MacLachlan, E. A. Organic aciduria, decreased renal ammonia production, hydrophthalmos and mental retardation, a clinical entity. Am. J. Dis. Child., 83:164, 1952.

Makao, K., und Yatsutake, K. Uber die vererbung und komplikationen der kongenitalen aniridie (abstract). Zentralbl. Ophthalmol., 34:162, 1935; Acta Soc. Ophthalmol. Jap., 39:131; Deutsch Zusammenfassung, 15 (1935).

Malik, S. K. R., Sood, G. C., Gupta, D. K., and Seth, R. K. Sclero-cornea. Br. J. Ophthalmol., 49:602, 1965.

Mandelcorn, M., Merin, S., and Cardarelli, J. Goldenhar's syndrome and phocomelia, case report and etiologic consideration. Am. J. Ophthalmol., 72:618, 1971.

Mann, I. On congenital hyaline membranes on posterior surface of cornea. Br. J. Ophthalmol., 17:449, 1933.

Marfan, A. B. Un cas de déformation congenitale des quatre membres plus prononcée aux

extremites charactérisée par l'allongement des os, avec un certain degre d'amincissement. Bull. Mem. Soc. Med. Hop. (Paris), 13:220, 1896.
Margasco, A., et al. Unusual malformation association, mandibulofacial dysostosis and bilateral microspherophakia. Ann. Ottalmol., 91:489, 1965.
Manschot, W. A. Persistent hyperplastic primary vitreous. Arch. Ophthalmol., 59:188, 1958.
Marchesani, O. Brachydaktylie und angeborne Kugellinse als Systemerkrankung. Klin. Monatsbl. Augenheilkd., 103:392, 1939.
Marinesco, G., Draganesco, S., and Vasiliu, D. Nouvelle maladie familiale, caractérisée par une cataracte congénitale et un arret du dévelopment somato-neuropsychique. Encéphale, 26:97, 1931.
Mathur, S. D., Sharma, G. K., and Makhija, J. M. Spherophakia. Opthalmologica, 153:419, 1967.
McCulloch, C., and Hunter, W. S. A search for ocular anomalies in persons with abnormal number of sex chromosomes. Can. Med. Assoc. J., 86:14, 1962.
McFarland, W., and Fuller, D. E. Mortality in Ehlers-Danlos syndrome due to spontaneous rupture of large arteries. N. Engl. J. Med., 271:1309, 1964.
McGavic, J. S. Weill-Marchesani syndrome. Brachymorphism and ectopia lentis. Am. J. Ophthalmol., 62:820, 1966.
McKusick, V. A. Heritable Disorders of Connective tissue, 3rd ed. Mosby, St. Louis, 1966, pp. 41, 116, 124.
Merins, S., Crawford, J. S., and Cardaelli, J. Hyperplastic persistent pupillary membrane. Am. J. Ophthalmol., 72:717, 1971.
Méry, H., et Babonneix, L. Un cas de déformation congénitales des quatres membres. Hyperchondroplasie. Bull. Mem. Soc. Med. Hop. (Paris), 19:671, 1902.
Méténier, P. A propos d'un cas familial de maladie d'Ehlers-Danlos. These, Alger, 1930, cited by McKusick, V. A.
Meyer-Schwickerath, G., Gruterich, E., and Weyers, H. Mikrophthalmus syndrome. Klin. Monatsbl. Augenheilkd., 131:18, 1957.
Miller, R. W., Frumeni, J. F., and Manning, M.D. Association of Wilm's tumor and aniridia, hemihypertrophy and other congenital malformations. N. Engl. J. Med., 270:922, 1964.
Mills, D. W. Mesodermal dysgenesia of the anterior segment of the eye. Can. J. Ophthalmol., 2:279, 1967.
Minckler, J. Pathology of the Nervous System. Vol. 1. McGraw-Hill, New York, 1968, p. 667.
Mollenbach, C. J. Congenital defects in internal membranes of the eye. Clinical and genetic aspects. In: Opera ex Domo Biolgiae Heriditariae Humanae Universitatis Hafniensis, Vol. 15, Munkagaard, Copenhagen, 1947.
Mories, A. Ehlers-Danlos syndrome with a report of a fatal case. Scot. Med. J., 5:269, 1960.
Mudd, S. H., et al. Homocystinuria. An enzymatic defect. Science, 143:1443, 1964.
Murakami, S. Zur pathologischen Anatomie und Pathogenese des Buphthalmus bei Neurofibromatose. Klin. Monatsbl. Augenheilkd., 16:514, 1913.
Nadler, H. L. Prenatal detection of genetic defects. J. Pediatr., 74:132, 1969.
Newton, T. H., and Carpenter, M. E. Ehlers-Danlos syndrome with acroosteolysis. Br. J. Radiol., 32:739, 1959.
O'Grady, R. B. Nanophthalmos. Am. J. Ophthalmol., 71:1251, 1971.
Paganelli, V. X. L'aniridie bilaterale associée á la forme fruste de la maladie de Crouzon (dyostose cranio-faciale). These, Geneva, 1951.

Paufique, L., Etiene, R., et Moreau, P. G. Une cas de sclero cornee. Bull. Soc. Ophtalad. Fr., 2:138, 1962.
Pelbois, F., et Rollier, F. Associaton d'un syndrome d'Ehlers-Danlos et d'un syndrome de Groenblad-Strandberg. Bull. Soc. Fr. Dermatol. Syphiligr. 59:141, 1952.
Pemberton, J. W., Freeman, H. M., and Schepens, C. L. Familial retinal detachment and the Ehlers-Danlos syndrome. Arch. Ophthalmol., 76:817, 1966.
Peritz, G. Der Infantilismus. Ergen. Inn. Med. Kinderh., 7:405, 1911.
Peters, A. Ueber angeborne Defektbildung der Descemetchen Membran. Klin. Monatsbl. Augenheilkd., 44:27, 1906.
Petrohelos, M. A. Werner's syndrome, a survey of three cases with review of the literature. Am. J. Ophthalmol., 56:941, 1963.
Pfandler, U. Les consequences d'un conseil genetique qui n'a pas été suivi par les parents. J. Genet. Hum., 3:149, 1954.
Pincus, M. H. Aniridia congenita. Arch. Ophthalmol., 39:60, 1948.
Pittinos, G. E. Ehlers-Danlos syndrome with a disturbance of creatine metabolism. Report of a case. J. Pediatr., 19:85, 1941.
Polani, P. E., Hunter, W. F., and Lennox, B. Chromosomal sex in Turner's syndrome with coarctation of the aorta. Lancet, 2:120, 1954.
Ponseti, I. V., and Baird, W. A. Scoliosis and dissecting aneurysms of the aorta in rats fed with lathyrus, odoratus seeds. Am. J. Pathol., 28:1059, 1952.
Posthumus, R. G. Die megalokornea in ihrem Zusammenhang mit anderan abweichungen bei Angehorigen Derselben Familie. Klin. Monatsbl. Augenheilkd., 102:1, 1939.
Poynton, F. C. Case of atavism. Trans. Med. Soc. (Lond.), 26:338, 1903.
Pratt, J. C., and Richards, R. D. Bilateral secondary congenital aphakia. Arch. Ophtalmol., 80:420, 1968.
Presley, G. D., and Sidbury, J. B. Homocystinuria and ocular defects. Am. J. Ophthalmol., 63:1723, 1967.
Prunty, F. T. G., McSwiney, R. R., and Clayton, B. E. Primary gonadal insufficiency in a girl and a boy. Metabolic effect of estrogen and testosterone. J. Clin. Endocr., 13:1480, 1953.
Rados, A. Marfan's syndrome, arachnodactyly coupled with dislocation of the lens. Arch. Ophthl. 27:477, 1942.
Raeder, J. G. Einige Falle von Invertierung, der Intraoculare Druckschwankung bei netzhautablosung mit Sekundarglaukom. Klin. Monatsbl. Augenheilkd., 74:424, 1925.
Rahn, E. K., et al. Lever's congenital amaurosis with an Ehlers-Danlos like syndrome. Arch. Ophthalmol., 79:135, 1968.
Rajic, D. C., and de Veber, L. L. Hereditary oculo-dento-osseous dysplasia. Ann. Radiol. (Paris), 9:1, 1966.
Rasmussen, D. H., and Ellis, P. P. Congenital glaucoma in identical twins. Arch. Ophthalmol., 84:827, 1970.
Reed, T. E., and Falls, H. F. A pedigree of aniridia with a discussion of germinal mosacism in man. Am. J. Hum. Genet., 7:28, 1955.
Reeh, M. J., and Lehman, W. L. Marfan's syndrome (arachnodoctyly) with ectopia lentis. Trans. Am. Acad. Ophthalmol. Otolaryngol., 58:212, 1954.
Reese, A. B. Congenital cataract and other anomalies following German measles in the mother. Am. J. Ophthalmol., 27:483, 1944.
Persistent hyperplastic primary vitreous. Am. J. Ophthalmol., 40:317, 1955.
Tumors of the Eye. Hoeber, Harper & Row, New York, 1963, p. 198.
and Ellsworth, R. M. The anterior chamber cleavage syndrome. Arch. Ophthalmol., 75:307, 1966.
and Payne, F. Persistence and hyperplasia of the primary vitreous. Am. J. Ophthalmol., 29:1, 1946.

Reforzo-Mebreves, J., Trabusco, A., and Escardo, F. A case of rudimentary testes, delayed growth and congenital malformations. Turner's syndrome in a male. J. Clin. Endocr., 9:1333, 1949.

Rieger, H. Verlagerung und shlitzform der Pupille mit hypoplasie des Irisverderblattes. Z. Augenheilkd., 84:98, 1934.

Beitrage zur kenntnis seltener missbildungen der Iris. I. Membrana Iridopupillaris persistens. Graefe's Arch. Ophthalmol., 131:523, 1934.

Beitrage zur kenntnis seltener Missbildungen der Iris. II. Uber Hypoplasie des Irisvorderblattes mit Verlagerung und Entrundung der Pupille. Graefe's Arch. Ophthalmol., 133:602, 1935.

Erbfragen in der Augenheilkunde. Graefe's Arch. Ophthalmol., 143:277, 1941.

Robin, P. La glossoptose, un grave danger pour nos enfants. Paris Gaston. Doin., 1929.

Glossoptosis due to atresia and hypotrophy of the mandible. Am. J. Dis. Child., 48:541, 1934.

Sabata, J. Marphanuv syndrom-dystrophia mesodermalis congenitadysmorpho dystrophia mesodermalis congenita. Lek. Listv., 3:477, 1947.

Scheie, H. G. Infantile and juvenile glaucoma. Trans. Am. Acad. Ophthalmol. Otolarygol., 67:458, 1963.

Schiess-Gemuseus, U. Vier Falle angeborner Anomalie des Auges. III. Hydrophthalmos mit keratoglobus. Arch. Ophthalmol., 30:195, 1884.

Schimke, R. N., et al. Homocystinuria. Studies of 20 families with 38 affected members. J. A. M. A., 193:711, 1965.

Schirmer, R. Ein Fall von Telangiektasie. Arch. Ophthalmol., 7:119, 1860.

Schlaegel, T. F. Uveitis in childhood. J. Pediatr. Ophthalmol., 6:66, 1969.

Schmid, A. E. Dysmorpho-dystrophia mesodermalis congenita. Ophthalmologica, 111:28, 1946.

Schocket, S. S. Anterior cleavage syndrome in a patient with Marfan's syndrome. 66:272, Am. J. Ophthalmol. 1968.

Sever, J. L., et al. Rubella virus. J. A. M. A., 182:663, 1962.

Shaffer, R. N. New concepts in infantile glacoma. Can. J. Ophthalmol., 2:243 1967.

Shapira, T. M. Microphakia and spherophakia with glaucoma. Am. J. Ophthalmol., 17:726, 1934.

Shaw, M. W., Falls, H. G., and Neel, J. V. Congenital aniridia. Am. J. Hum. Genet., 12:389, 1960.

Shirley, S. T. Congenital glaucoma without megalocornea. Trans. Can. Ophthalmol. Soc., 10:51, 1958.

Sjogren, T. Klinische und vererbungsmedizinische Untersuchungen uber ologophrenie mit kongenitaler Katarakt. Z. Ges. Neurol. Psychiat., 152:263, 1935.

Smith, J. L., Cavanaugh, J. J. A., and Stone, F. C. Ocular manifestations of the Pierre Robin syndrome. Arch. Ophthalmol., 63:984, 1960.

and Stowe, F. R. The Pierre Robin syndrome (glossoptosis, micrognathia cleft palate). Pediatrics, 27:128, 1961.

Smith, M. E., Sander, T. E., and Bresnick, G. H. Juvenile xanthogranuloma of the ciliary body in an adult. Arch. Ophthalmol., 81:813, 1969.

Snell, S., and Collins, E. T. Plexiform neuroma (elephantiasis neuromatosis) of temporal region, orbit, eyelid, and eyeball. Trans. Ophthalmol. Soc. U. K., 23:157, 1903.

Sohar, E. Renal disease, inner ear deafness and ocular changes, a new heredofamilial syndrome. Arch. Intern. Med., 96:627, 1956.

Spaeth, G. L., and Barber, G. W. Homocystinuria, in a mentally retarded child and her normal cousin. Trans. Am. Acad. Ophthalmol. Otolaryngol., 69:912, 1965.

and Barber, G. W. Homocystinuria, its ocular manifestations. J. Pediatr. Ophthalmol., 3:42, 1966.

Spaulding, A. G., and Naumann, G. Persistent hyperplastic primary vitreous in an adult. Arch. Ophthalmol., 77:666, 1967.
Speakman, J. S., and Crawford, J. S. Congenital opacities at the cornea. Br. J. Ophthalmol., 50:68, 1966.
Stanbury, J. B., Wyngaarden, J. B., and Fredrickson, D. S. The Metabolic Basis of Inherited Disease. McGraw-Hill, New York, 1966.
Stephenson, W. V. Anterior megalophthalmos and arachnodoctyly, a case report. Am. J. Ophthalmol., 28:315, 1945.
Stoermer, J., und Anton, H. U. Beitragzur problematik des sog. mannlichen Turner's syndrome. Med. Welt., 7:362, 1960.
Straub, W. Beitrag zur angeborenen Total-trubung der Hornhaut. Ophthalmologica, 120:401, 1950.
Beitrag zur Klinik der persistierenden Glaskorpearterie. Ophthalmologica, 121:194, 1951.
Streiff, E. B. Dysplasie marginale posterieure de la cornee (embryotoxon posterius Axenfeld) dans le cadre des malformations irido-corneennes. Ophthalmologica, 118:815, 1949.
Straub, W., and Golay, L. The ocular manifestations of the Lowe syndrome. Ophthalmologica, 135:632, 1958.
Strelling, M. K. Ehlers-Danlos syndrome. Br. J. Dermatol., 72:164, 1960.
Sugar, H. S. The Glaucomas. Hoeber, New York, 1952.
Juvenile glaucoma with Axenfeld's syndrome. Am. J. Ophthalmol., 59:1012, 1965.
and Barbour, F. A. Pigmentary glaucoma. Am. J. Ophthalmol., 32:90, 1949.
and Berman, M. Relationship between the mandibulofacial dysostosis syndrome of Franceschetti and the oculo-auriculo-vertebral dysplasia syndrome of Goldenhar. Am. J. Ophthalmol., 66:510, 1968.
Summer, G. K. The Ehler-Danlos syndrome. A review of the literature and report of a case with a subgaleal hematoma and Bell's palsy. Am. J. Dis. Child., 91:419, 1956.
Swan, C. Study of three infants dying from congenital defects following maternal rubella in early stages of pregnancy. J. Pathol. Bact., 56:289, 1944.
et al. Congenital defects in infants following infectious diseases during pregnancy. Med. J. Aust., 2:201, 1943.
Symposium of Surgical and Medical Management of Congenital Anomalies of the Eye. Transactions of the New Orleans Academy of Ophthalmology. Mosby, St. Louis, 1968.
Tallan, H. H., Moore, S., and Stein, W. H. L-cystathionine in human brain. J. Biol. Chem., 230:707, 1958.
Terslev, E. Two cases of aminoaciduria, ocular changes and retarded mental and somatic development (Lowe's syndrome). Acta Pediat., 49:635, 1960.
Theobold, G. D. Neurogenic origin of choroidal sarcoma. Arch. Ophthalmol. 18:971, 1937.
Histologic eye findings in arachnodactyly. Am. J. Ophthalmol., 24:1132, 1941.
Theodore, F. H. Congenital opacities of cornea, Arch. Ophthalmol., 31:138, 1944.
Thomas, C., Cordier, J., et Algan, B. Les alterations oculaires de la maladie d'Ehlers-Danlos. Arch. Ophtalmol., 14:691, 1954.
Cordier, J., et Algan, B. Une etiologie nouvelle du syndrome de luxation spontanée des cristallins; la maladie d'Ehlers-Danlos. Bull. Soc. Belge Ophtalmol., 100:375, 1952.
Tikhomirov, P. E. Arachnodactyly and ectopia lentis. Vesnik Oftalmol., 7:591, 1935.
Tolman, M. M. Ehlers-Danlos syndrome. Arch. Dermatol., 82:447, 1960.
Toselli, C., e Volpi, U. Gigantismi parziah e facomatos l'ipertrofia emifacciale neurofibromatosa con buftalmo omolaterale. Ann. Ottalmol. Clin. Ocul., 89:791, 1963.

Turner, H. H. A syndrome of infantilism, congenital webbed neck and cubitus valgus. Endocrinology, 23:566, 1938.
Turner, L. Marchesani syndrome. Proc. Staff Meet. Div. Ophthalmol. School, Med. Univ. North Carolina, 1963.
Vail, D. Primary glaucoma. Etiology and general considerations. Am. J. Ophthalmol., 41:207, 1956.
Van Der Hoeve, J. Trans. Ophthalmol. Soc. U. K., 52:391, 1932.
Van Meekeren, cited by McKusick, Va. Heritable Disorders of Connective Tissue, 3rd ed. Mosby, St. Louis, 1966, pp. 179–229.
Velicky, J., and Vrabec, F. Cornea plana congenita. Ann. Ocul. (Paris), 184:707, 1951.
Von Grolman, W. Ueber Mikrophthalmus und cataracta congenital Vasculosa. Graefe Arch. Ophthalmol., 35:187, (No. 3) 1889.
Von Hess, C. Pathologie und Therapie des Linsensystems. In A. Graefe, and E. T. Saemisch, Handbuch der Gesamten Augenheilkunde, Vol. 6, 3rd ed. Springer, Berlin, 1911.
Von Hofe, K. Wietere Untersuchungen zur Frage der Makrokornea und des Buphthalmus. Klin. Monatsbl. Augenheilkd., 104:278, 1940.
Von Noorden, G. K., and Shultz, R. O. A gonioscopic study of the chamber angle in Marfan's syndrome. Arch. Ophthalmol., 64:929, 1960.
and Baller, R. S. Chamber angle in split-pupil. Arch. Ophthalmol., 70:598, 1963.
Vos, T. A. Embryonal Synechiebildurg zwischen Augenbecherrand und Linse. Klin. Monatsbl. Augenheilkd., 96:452, 1936.
Vrabec, F. Leucogoria-pseudoglioma. Eye, Ear, Nose, Throat Mon., 48:78, 1969.
Waardenburg, P. J. Gross remnants of the pupillary membrane, anterior polar cataract and microcornea in a mother and her children. Ophthalmologica, 118:828, 1949.
Vereeiginsverslagen. Nederlandsch Oogheelkundig Gezelschap. 87, ste Vergadering op 16 en 17 December, 1933, in het Nederlandsch Gasthuis voor Ooglijders te Utrecht. Ned. Geneeskd., 78:1695, 1934.
Genetics and Ophthalmology Vol. 2. Van Gorcum, Assen, Netherlands, 1963, pp. 1340-1356.
Sperophakie, in Das menschliche Auge und seine Erbanlogen. Nijhoft, Der Haag, Netherlands, 1932.
Franceschetti, A., and Klein, D. Genetics and Ophthalalmology, Vol. 1. Van Gorcum, Assen, Netherlands, 1961, pp. 570, 572, 851, 960, 965, 967.
Wachtel, J. G. The ocular pathology of Marfan's syndrome. Arch. Ophthalmol., 76:512, 1966.
Walsh, F. B., and Murray, R. G. Ocular manifestations of disturbances in calcium metabolism. Am. J. Ophthalmol., 36:1657, 1953.
Weatherill, J. E., and Hart, C. T. Familial hypoplasia of the iris stroma associated with glaucoma. Br. J. Ophthalmol., 53:433, 1969.
Weill, G. Ectopie dus cristallin et malformations generales. Ann. Ocul. (Paris), 169:21, 1932.
Weller, T. H., and Neva, F. A. Propagation in tissue culture of cytopathic agents from patients with rubella-like illnesses. Proc. Soc. Exp. Biol. Med., 11:215, 1962.
Weiss, D. I. Congenital mesodermal anomalies and glaucoma. Invest. Ophthalmol., 7:123, 1968.
Weve H. Uber Arachnodaktylie (Dystrophia mesodermalis congenita typus Marfan). Arch. Augenheilkd., 104:1, 1931.
Wiedemann, H. R. Einiges zum Syndrom von Ehlers und Danlos. Monatsschr. Kinderkeilkd., 100:252, 1952.

Wiegmann, E. Membrana pupillairis persistens bei einen Z. Willingspaar. Klin. Monatsbl. Augenheilkd., 47:592, 1909.

Wiessenberg, S. Eine eigentumleche hautafaetensiedung am halse. Anthr. Anz., 5:141, 1928.

Wilkins, L., Grumback, M. M., and Van Wyk, J. J. Chromosomal sex in "ovarian agenesis." J. Clin. Endocr., 14:1270, 1954.

Williams, E. Rare case with practical remarks. Trans. Am. Ophthalmol. Soc., 2:291, 1873–1879.

Wilson, W. Congenital cataracts. Arch. Ophthalmol., 67:143, 1962.

Richard, W., and Donnell, G. Oculocerebralrenal syndrome of Lowe. Arch. Ophthalmol., 70:5, 1963.

Wolff, E. A microphthalmic family. Proc. Roy Soc. Med. Sect. Ophthalmol., 23:623, 1930.

Wolter, J. R. Nerve fibrils in ovoid bodies. Arch. Ophthalmol., 73:696, 1965.

Corneal involvement in choroidal neurofibromatosis. J. Pediatr. Ophthalmol., 3:19, 1966.

and Butler, R. G. Pigment spots of iris and ectropion uveae with glaucoma in neurofibromatosis. Am. J. Ophthalmol., 56:964, 1963.

and Flaherty, M. W. Persistent hyperplastic vitreous. Am. J. Ophthalmol., 47:491, 1959.

and Gonzales-Sirit, R. Neurofibromatosis of the choroid. Am. J. Ophthalmol., 54:217, 1962.

Zabriskie, J. and Reisman, M. Marchasani syndrome. J. Pediatr., 52:158, 1958.

Zamorani, G. Microftalmia e Glaucoma. Boll. Ocul., 39:746, 1960.

Zeiter, J. H. Congenital microphthalmos, a pedigree of four affected siblings and an additional report of forty-four sporadic cases. Am. J. Ophthalmol., 55:910, 1963.

Zimmerman, L. E. Histopathologic basis for ocular manifestations of congenital rubella syndrome. Am. J. Ophthalmol., 65:837, 1968.

and Font, R. L. Congenital malformations of the eye, some recent advances in knowledge of the pathogenesis and histopathological characteristics. J. A. M. A., 196:684, 1966.

10

Differential Diagnosis

An astute diagnosis is based upon a carefully taken history, a thorough physical examination, and a judicial analysis of laboratory data. In addition, it is essential to be aware of those illnesses which simulate the condition under question. There are a large number of diseases and syndromes which present with many of the cardinal signs of congenital glaucoma (Table 1). Specialists in this field are acquainted with the case of megalocornea which "responded" to a goniotomy, or worse perhaps, a fistulizing operation. They might also be aware of a case of congenital corneal dystrophy which, for no reason other than the corneal appearance, was subjected to glaucoma surgery.

The diagnosis in congenital glaucoma is, therefore, not based upon a single clinical observation or a solitary laboratory reading. In most cases a variety of positive clinical tests are needed to make the diagnosis, as shown in Chapter 7. In this chapter we will discuss conditions which bear many semblances to, and may therefore mimic, the clinical appearance of congenital glaucoma. Under the correct set of circumstances, each one could cause the observer certain doubts as to whether he is indeed observing a case of buphthalmia. As in the problem with many classifications it is not possible to sharply define each condition into a single group. The reader will quickly observe that some of these conditions, e.g., onchocerciasis, corneal staphyloma, and congenital corneal leucoma, may in fact have a rise in the intraocular pressure as part of the disease and are therefore also discussed in Chapter 11. In addition, other conditions such as gargoylism generally do not present the diagnostician with a problem when the other components of the syndrome are obvious. However, this is not always the case.

TABLE 1

DIFFERENTIAL DIAGNOSIS

Inflammation

- Intrauterine corneal inflammation
  - congenital syphilis, interstitial keratitis
  - nonluetic interstitial keratitis
  - rubella keratitis
- Infantile corneal inflammation
  - Chemical keratitis
  - Tuberculosis
  - Common wart keratitis
  - Herpes simplex
  - Varicella herpes zoster
  - Variola and vaccinia
  - Trachoma
  - Molluscum contagiosum
  - Onchocerciasis
  - Mumps keratitis
  - Staphylococcal blepharokeratoconjunctivitis
  - Acute bacterial conjunctivitis
  - Inclusion conjunctivitis
  - Adenovirus
  - Measles keratoconjunctivitis

Corneal Disorders Associated with Inflammation

- Keratectasia
- Anterior corneal staphyloma

Systemic Disease

- Corneal lipoidosis
- Hyperlipemia
- Hypercholesterolemia
- Arcus lipoides juvenilis
- Hereditary dystopic lipidosis; Fabry's disease
- Lignac-Fanconi syndrome (cystinosis)
- Disorders of calcium metabolism
- Mucopolysaccharidosis (MPS)
- Congenital porphyria
- von Gierke's glycogen storage disease
- Hand-Schüller-Christian disease
- Morquio Ullrich's syndrome
- Osteogenesis imperfecta (blue sclerotic syndrome)
- Riley-Day syndrome; Familial dysautonomia
- Cogan's syndrome
- Acrodermatitis enteropathica
- Block-Sulzberger's syndrome
- Wilson's disease
- Other systemic disorders
  - Psoriasis
  - Benign mucus membrane pemphigus
  - Erythema multiforme
  - Rosacea
  - Sjögren's keratoconjunctivitis sicca
  - Leprosy
  - Drug eruptions

Trauma

- Rupture of Descemet's membrane
- Post natal trauma

Skin Diseases

- Congenital icthyosis
- Congenital dyskeratosis

Corneal Dystrophy

- Congenital hereditary corneal dystrophy
- Congenital idiopathic corneal edema
- Granular dystrophy (Groenouw's I, Bückler's I)
- Macular dystrophy (Groenouw's II, Bückler's II)
- Lattice dystrophy (Biber-Haab-Dimmer, Bückler's III)
- Crystalline corneal dystrophy of Schnyder
- Hereditary epithelial corneal dystrophy
- Hereditary nonprogressive deep corneal dystrophy (hereditary polymorphous deep degeneration of the cornea)

Genetic Disorders

- Down's syndrome (Mongolism)
- 13—15 Trisomy syndrome

Birth Anomalies

- Congenital corneal leucoma
- Persistent hyperplastic primary vitreous
- Large cornea of high myopia
- Megalocornea

Corneal Deformation

- Keratoconus
- Keratotorus
- Keratoglobus

Orbital Hemangioma

Keratomalacia

INFLAMMATION

Bacteria such as syphilis and gonorrhea and viruses such as smallpox and chicken pox may affect the cornea during pregnancy. Blepharitis, keratoconjunctivitis, and keratitis may be seen in the newborn on a chemical, allergic, bacterial, or viral basis.

Intrauterine Corneal Inflammation

Congenital syphilis

Luetic interstitial keratitis usually manifests itself between 5 and 15 years of age. The child suffers from photophobia and lacrimation and the cornea is hazy and vascularized, usually in both eyes (Fig. 1). Folds are present in Descemet's membrane. Penicillin should be given to untreated patients for the general systemic effects. Topical steroid drops applied hourly to the affected eye relieve symptoms promptly and resolve corneal infiltration and vascularization in early cases, but must be continued for lengthy periods. Atropine drops should also be used. The condition runs its course of 3 to 8 weeks and then clears from the periphery toward the center. Some corneal haze often remains (Fig. 2). Congenital syphilitics are known for the Hutchinsonian Triad which includes pegged upper central incisors

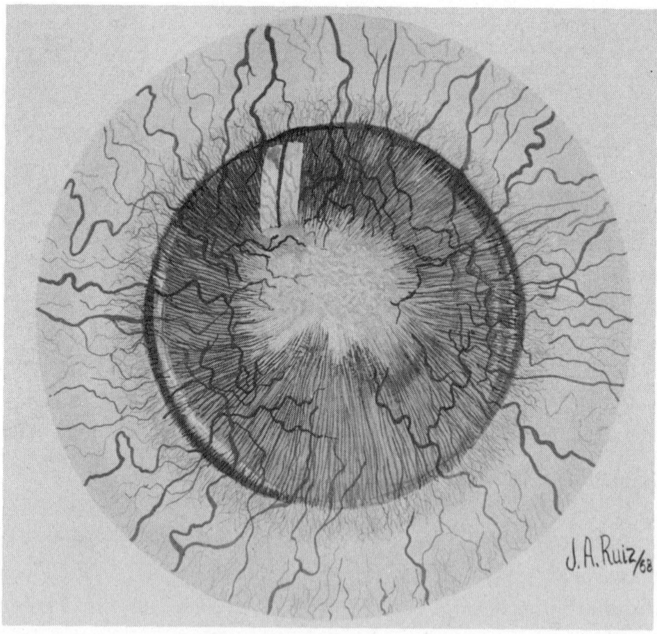

FIG. 1. Interstitial keratitis in congenital lues. Advanced stage. The entire cornea is involved.

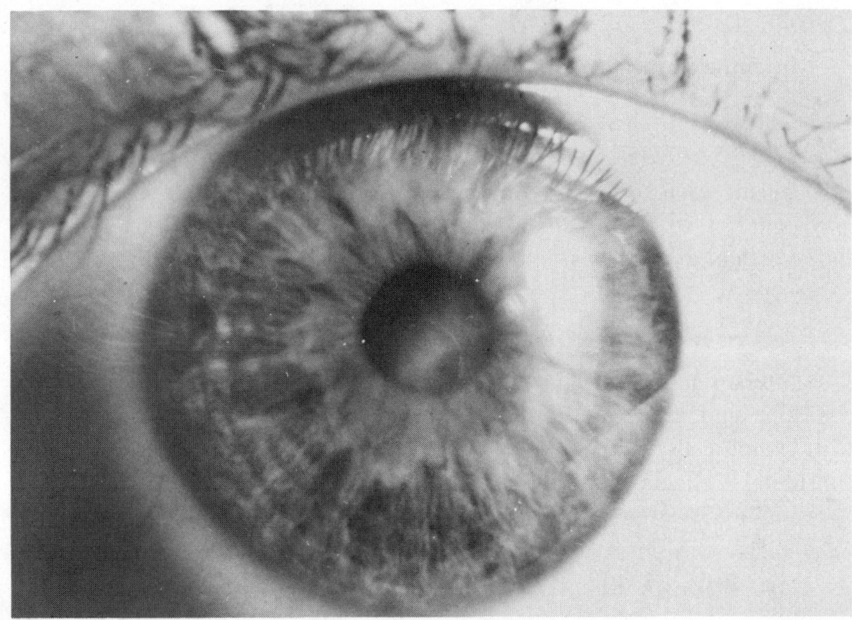

FIG. 2. Interstitial keratitis in congenital lues. Quiescent stage. A marked haze is present in the central cornea.

and deafness, in addition to interstitial keratitis. Other associated findings are gummata, saddle nose, saber shins, rhagades, frontal bossing, palatal scars, and chorioretinitis. Elevation of the intraocular pressure may also be observed (Chap. 11).

Nonluetic Interstitial Keratitis

Interstitial keratitis, which is often bilateral, may be seen at birth, in the absence of syphilis both on clinical grounds and by laboratory testing in the mother and the child. Fig. 3 (See colorplate, frontis.) illustrates an infant's eye that displayed intense photophobia and tearing at birth which responded to local atropine and steroids. Tonometry with the Goldmann applanation tonometer was necessary to differentiate this case from congenital glaucoma. Tests for lues were all negative.

Rubella Keratitis

Rubella keratitis has been described as a cause of corneal cloudiness even when not associated with infantile glaucoma.

Infantile Corneal Inflammation

Chemical Keratitis

Agents used to prevent ophthalmia neonatorum, such as silver nitrate, may give rise to an inflammed cornea and conjunctiva as well as inhibiting the growth of gonococcus, resulting in a cloudy appearance of the cornea.

Tuberculosis

Interstitial keratitis due to tuberculosis may show central scarring on clinical examination, and on histological section we see a panus infiltration with lymph cells, epithelioid cells, and Langhan's giant cells. There may be considerable edema of the corneal stroma.

Common Wart Keratitis

The common wart carries a specific scientific interest since it, like molluscum contagiosum, represents two of the few tumors induced in man by viruses. The association of verruca vulgaris of the lid margins with keratitis and conjunctivitis has been known for many years. Warts of the lid margin are a common occurrence but the cornea and conjunctiva are only involved infrequently. In this event the typical corneal picture is seen as multiple punctate epithelial erosions, together with conjunctival infiltration. The keratitis is usually a chronic epithelial disease that responds to removal of the lid margin nodules, indicating that there is no true localization of the virus on either the cornea or conjunctiva.

Herpes Simplex

According to Thygeson, herpetic keratitis is the most important specific type of keratitis occurring in the United States. The clinical types of herpetic keratitis are noted in Table 2.

Herpes simplex is caused by a small virus and results in small papular crusting lesions on the skin and mucus membranes. Occasionally the primary manifestation of the disease is an acute keratoconjunctivitis with preauricular adenopathy, follicular hypertrophy, and in some cases conjunctival pseudomembrane formation. The characteristic fluorescein-stained dendritic branching figure, which has a knob at the terminus of each branch, usually appears and provides the basis for the clinical diagnosis, even in the absence

TABLE 2

HERPES SIMPLEX KERATITIS*

Superficial Types

(1) Dendritic keratitis
(2) Geographic ulcer
(3) Chronic herpetic epithelial keratitis
(4) Herpetic neuroparalytic keratitis
(5) Rare transitory types
  (a) Herpetic punctate and striate keratitis
  (b) Herpetic filamentary keratitis
  (c) Herpetic vesicular keratitis

Deep Types

(1) Disciform keratitis
(2) Diffuse interstitial keratitis
(3) Deep ulcerative keratitis with hypopion (often complicated by secondary bacterial or mycotic infection)
(4) Keratouveitis (with or without secondary glaucoma)

*After P. Thygeson. Tr. Am. Acad. Ophthalmol. Otolaryngol. 62:411, 1958.

of a slit lamp. In infants and young children it is sometimes difficult to detect dendritic figures. However, a common experience is to find one or the other of the parents with a history of fever blisters 2 or 3 days prior to the onset of herpetic keratitis in the child. There are frequent recurrences of the corneal lesion which may finally result in a permanent corneal haze (Fig. 4A).

Laboratory identification of the virus may be made by experimental infection of the rabbit cornea, inoculation of the chorioallantois membrane, or in tissue culture by transfer of scrapings. There is a rise in the antibody titer in the first week of infection. Multinucleated giant epithelial cells may be noted in the scrapings of the cornea, lid margins, and skin lesions.

Herpes Zoster

Herpes zoster not uncommonly affects the ophthalmic division of the fifth cranial nerve. The frontal branch is almost always affected but the lacrimal and nasociliary branches frequently escape infection. When the latter is involved the cornea usually becomes involved as a by-condition.

Herpes zoster is seen as a hemifacial skin lesion which begins with erythematous papules, proceeds to crusting, and tends to stop abruptly in the midline. It may be accompanied by extraocular muscle palsies and severe persistent nerve-type pain that involves even the hair. The pain may persist a

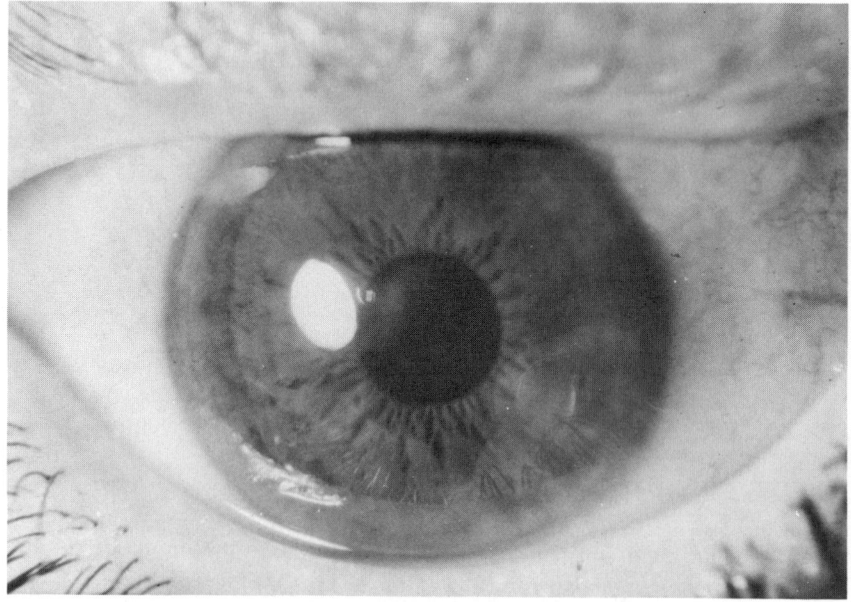

FIG. 4. A. Corneal haze resulting from recurrent dendritic ulcers.

year or more after the skin lesions have disappeared. The disease is due to a large virus which resembles the virus of chicken pox.

A coarse punctate subepithelial keratitis is seen. Opacities 1 to 2 mm in size, ragged and irregular in shape and outline, are present, leading to spontaneous desquamation and healing. The denuded area may be quite large, requiring ocular occlusion to facilitate healing. Disciform lesions may also occur and, if peripherally located, vascularization may be seen depending upon the severity of the condition. Severe cases often leave a corneal scar. The author has treated several cases which resisted standard medical treatment of ocular ointments and patching and healed only after tarsorrhaphies were performed.

An elevation in the intraocular pressure may appear anywhere from a month to a year after the onset of the disease, or it may be seen almost immediately when it is impossible to do tonometry in the presence of an inflammed cornea. Scrapings of lid lesions may be made for multinucleated giant cells. Complement fixation and precipitin tests may be performed. The virus may also be grown in fibroblast cultures. Kielar et al. have postulated that an IgA deficiency and absent delayed hypersensitivity may have

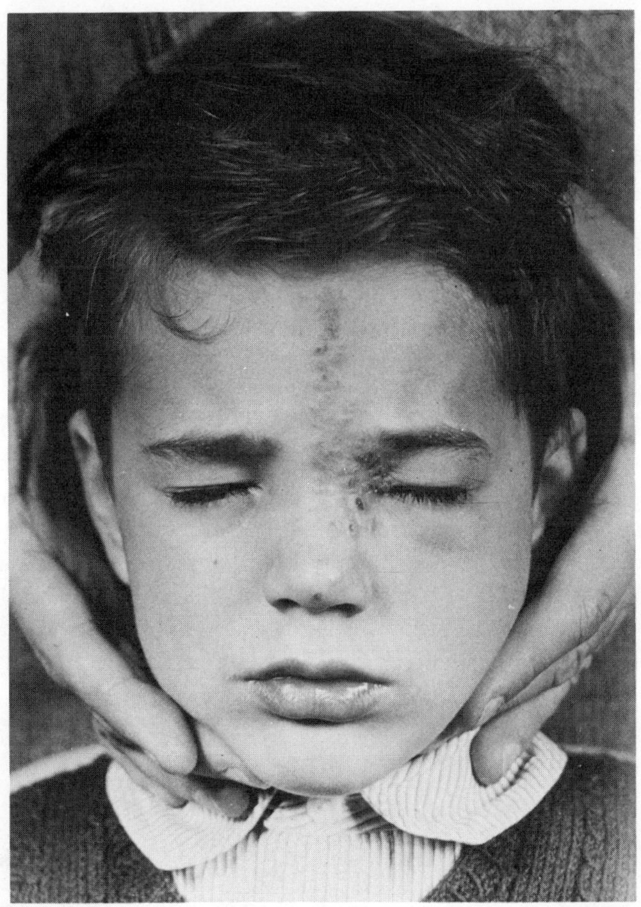

FIG. 4.B. Herpes zoster, 5-year-old child exhibiting hemifacial skin lesion. (Courtesy of M. I. H. Kaufmann.)

increased the susceptibility to, and prolonged the clinical course of this disease in a child they reported. Kaufmann has also observed herpes zoster ophthalmicus in a 5-year-old child (Fig. 4B).

Varicella

This common exanthematous disease of childhood only rarely develops ocular lesions. Vesicles of the eyelids are most common. Vesicles may also appear on the cornea, usually late in the course of the disease, associated with an injected bulbar conjunctiva. The vesicles may progress to small ulcers which heal spontaneously. Usually the visual acuity remains unaffected. Diagnosis is based on the clinical picture, but elementary bodies and intranuclear inclusions may be seen in scrapings from varicella vesicles. On slit lamp examination the cornea appears swollen, usually to full thickness, in the region of the opacity. There may be evidence of generalized varicella.

Variola and Vaccinia

Smallpox (variola) has become so rare in the United States that many a physician will never see a case during his lifetime. However, it is important to remember that the disease was at one time a major cause of corneal scarring from pox formation.

Accidental vaccinal infection of the eyelids' (Fig. 5) conjunctiva and cornea, on the other hand, is not uncommon. The infection occurs by autotransfer from a recent vaccination. Ulcers are noted in the corneal epithelium, ranging in size from pinhead to lesions which involve the peripheral, the central, or the entire cornea. Vascularization, both superficial and deep, occurs in severe cases. The small lesions evolve into a grayish punctate subepithelial keratitis which is usually disciform, and may lead to extensive scarring. Conjunctival exudate contains both poly- and mononu-

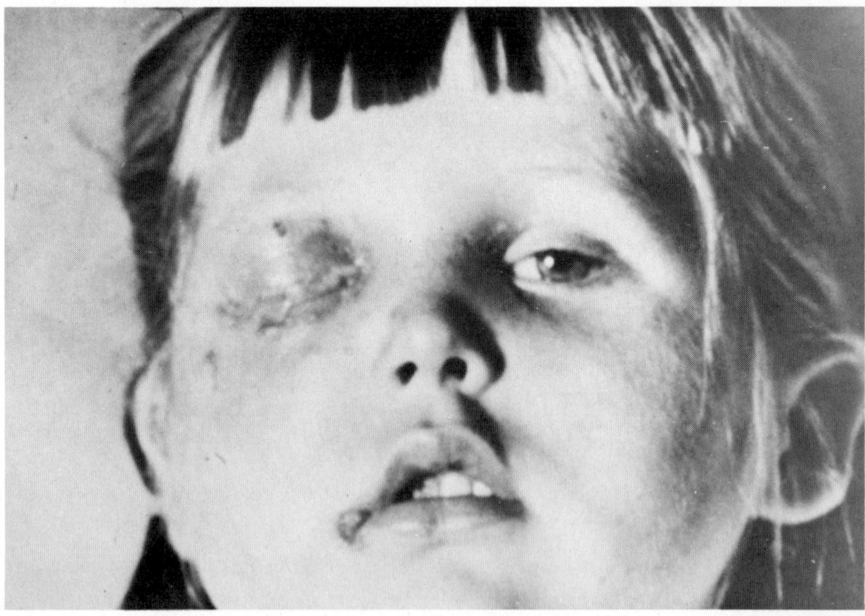

FIG. 5. A. Accidental vaccinal infection of eyelids, mouth.

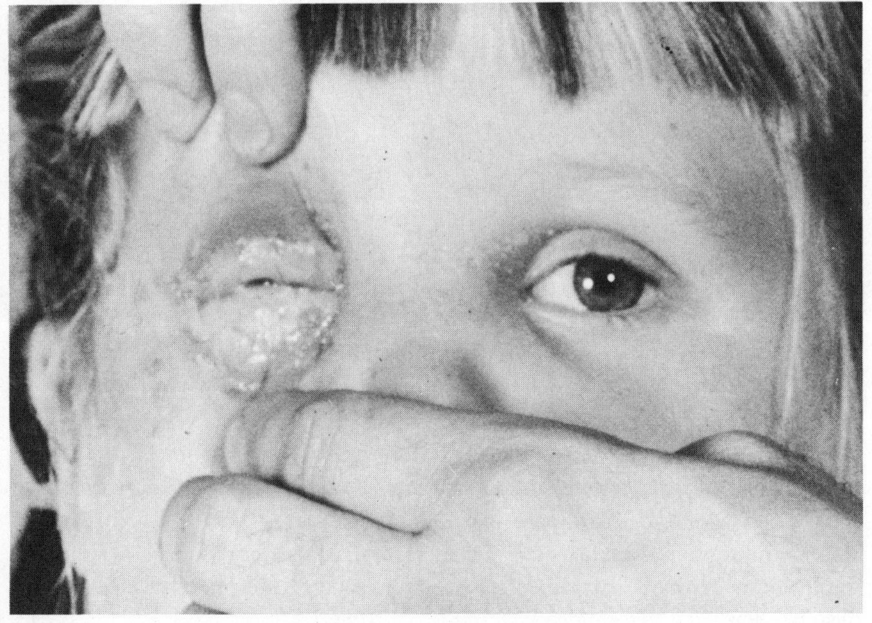

FIG. 5.B. Accidental vaccinal infection, eyelids separated.

clear cells; the virus may be isolated on chorioallantois.

Trachoma

The diagnostic clinical picture of trachoma consists of conjunctival follicles selectively affecting the upper tarsal plate, combined with upper limbal changes consisting of extension of limbal vessels, punctate epithelial keratitis, and subepithelial infiltrates. The later upper limbal changes include limbal follicles and thereafter their cicatricial remains—Herbert's peripheral pits.

There is a diffuse epithelial opacification. The stromal component appears dirty yellow when the process is active but becomes gray with time. Maximal changes occur in the upper half of the cornea, which are accompanied by the extension of superficial capillaries into the cornea to form a pannus. Halberstaedter-Prowazek inclusions in conjunctival scrapings are obtained by iodine or Giemsa stain. Polymorphonuclear leukocytes and mononuclear cells appear in the exudate. Isolation of the virus in yolk sac culture may also be successful.

Molluscum Contagiosum

Molluscum contagiosum is a benign disease of considerable ocular interest because of the virus nodules which form on the lid margins and the associated chronic follicular conjunctivitis that supervenes. The lid nodule represents one of the few tumors induced in man by viruses. The conjunctivitis and the keratitis which accompany it are entirely dependent on desquamation of the lid margin nodules, indicating that there is no true viral invasion of the conjunctiva and corneal cells but only a toxic reaction from the desquamated necrotic material. When the nodule is excised, the keratoconjunctivitis subsides. A fine punctate epithelial keratitis is present, scattered or confluent, and is more common in the upper part of the cornea. Subepithelial punctate erosions with small gray spots may be seen. As a result of its rarity and the severe reaction which results from a single small nodule on the lid margin the disease may be misdiagnosed, and cases have been seen which had progressed to pannus formation and corneal scarring. The conjunctivial exudate is usually mononuclear. Typical lesions of molluscum contagiosum may be seen elsewhere and material from such lesions identified histologically.

Onchocerciasis

Onchocerciasis is found in various areas of Africa as well as in parts of North and South America. The disease is known in Mexico, Guatemala, Venezuela, Colombia, and elsewhere.

The etiologic organism is a nematode parasite of the Filariodea family, Onchocerca volvulus. It is carried by flies of the Simulidae family as well as certain others. These act as vectors for the disease of which man is the definitive host. The adult worms are found in nodules which are generally subcutaneous. The microfilariae travel in the skin and other tissues and frequently enter the eyes, producing corneal changes, iritis, uveitis, cataracts, choroidoretinal degeneration, and optic atrophy. Sometimes the organisms can be seen with the slit lamp as they travel through the cornea and anterior chamber.

In addition to the subcutaneous nodules which contain the adult parasites, there are inflammatory skin lesions which may be either acute or chronic. If the disease has not been previously treated, the organism involved may be found in skin snips. Other ocular lesions are found in the orbit, conjunctiva, lids, iris, ciliary body, vitreous, retina, and choroid.

Showers of subepithelial corneal lesions are noted particularly at the periphery, at intervals of weeks to months. Superficial stromal lesions can also occur. Secondary glaucoma is another feature of this condition (Chap. 11).

Mumps Keratitis

A drop in visual acuity may occur during the illness but spontaneous recovery is the rule. The change is related to a transient interstitial keratitis, that is, edema without necrosis (according to Thygeson). On rare occasions mumps has been known to cause a true disciform keratitis with subsequent scar formation. The isolation of the virus on monkey kidney cells may be accomplished in as short a time as three days. The virus has been isolated from the urine as late as thirteen days after onset of the disease.

Staphylococcal Blepharokeratoconjunctivitis

Usually the lower half of the cornea is affected by fine punctate epithelial erosions in this disease. Marginal infiltrates and peripheral vascularization may occur. The diagnosis may be confirmed by smear and gram stain for the organism. Culture of the lid margin is also helpful.

Acute Bacterial Conjunctivitis

Punctate corneal epithelial erosions may complicate simple conjunctivitis. Those caused by Neisseria may produce large, punctate, yellowish, superficial stromal lesions which may enlarge and coalesce, progressing to perforation. Diagnosis is made by direct examination of gram-stained smears and cultures.

Inclusion Conjunctivitis

The occurrence of this mild venereal disease is dependent upon the presence of inclusion virus cirvicitis and inclusion virus urethritis. The lower half of the conjunctiva is usually maximally involved, but there is no conjunctival scarring and no pannus formation found. The cornea is often not affected, but occasionally severe keratitis with epithelial and subepithelial involvement does occur. The lesions vary in size from about 0.25 to 1.5 mm and are chiefly centrally located. Stromal elements may become gray in color. The incidence of this type of nonbacterial ophthalmia neonatorum appears to be steadily decreasing.

Adenovirus

Pharyngoconjunctival fever is an acute infection characterized typically by fever, pharyngitis, and acute follicularconjunctivitis. These manifestations may occur singly or together, with a wide range in degree of severity. Conjunctivitis in some degree or other occurs in almost all cases, and is severe enough in about 70 percent to be recognized as an acute conjunctivitis with follicular hypertrophy and mild preauricular adenopathy. In some cases the ocular condition is the presenting symptom and the fever and sore throat are found only if specifically sought. The conjunctivitis is clinically indistinguishable, according to Thygeson, from the disease described years ago as "Beals' acute follicular conjunctivitis."

The condition may occur sporadically but is usually epidemic in nature. Children are most often affected and there is a frequent association with swimming pools. A mild transient keratitis, usually epithelial but occasionally subepithelial, may develop.

In the adenoviruses Types 3 and 4, small and medium-sized epithelial lesions are noted. The stromal opacity is less than 1.0 mm in size and not visible to the naked eye. The lesion clears within several weeks to months. In adenovirus Type 7, a similar reaction to Types 3 and 4 is seen but larger stromal opacities may occur and take up to a year to disappear. In adenovirus Type 8 (epidemic keratoconjunctivitis), round subepithelial opacities, 1.0 to 1.5 mm in diameter, are visible to the naked eye, appearing from 7 to 10 days after onset of the disease and may persist for one year or more after the disappearance of the conjunctival inflammation. Epithelial keratitis may break down to form tiny staining ulcers. About one-third of the cases have pseudomembranes during the initial phase of the conjunctival disease. Epidemic keratoconjunctivitis is an important cause of temporarily reduced marked visual loss which often occurs during the early stages when the infiltrates involve the pupillary area, as opposed to pharyngoconjunctival fever in which visual symptoms are minimal. Unlike pharyngoconjunctival fever, which is known to have occurred in epidemic form for many years, epidemic keratoconjunctivitis was unknown in the United States before World War II. It was introduced in 1941 from Hawaii, where an epidemic of more than 25,000 cases occurred. Unlike pharyngoconjunctival fever, epidemic keratoconjunctivitis affects adults predominantly and has not been transmitted characteristically in swimming pools. Diagnosis is made by the isolation of the virus in HeLa cells, plus a rising complement fixation and precipitin antibody titer for the group (not reliable for a specific virus).

Measles Keratoconjunctivitis

The conjunctivitis of measles is typically nonpurulent and nonfollicular. Koplik spots may be noted, particularly on the semilunar fold. The keratitis is mild and entirely epithelial, consisting characteristically of multiple punctate epithelial foci which probably account for the photophobia. These cases are susceptible to secondary bacterial infection which would result in pseudomembrane and corneal ulcer formation.

CORNEAL DISORDERS ASSOCIATED WITH INFLAMMATION

Keratectasia

When the cornea is weakened by inflammation, e.g., interstitial keratitis or ulceration, even the normal intraocular pressure may cause a thinning and subsequent ectasia with scarring and vascularization. Perforation does not occur and the iris remains free of the cornea, as opposed to the corneal staphyloma where the iris forms much of the protuberant scar. If the protrusion is extensive Descemet's membrane may rupture, yielding a picture not unlike that seen in congenital glaucoma. The infection may be of viral or bacterial origin and can begin in utero. Often there is a history of viral, bacterial, or other infectious illnesses of pregnancy, with obvious signs of sepsis in the mother and/or child. The condition may be bilateral.

Anterior Corneal Staphyloma

Corneal perforation from injury, inflammation, or ulceration at birth or often in utero, causes a protrusion and scarring of the corneal stroma with incarceration of the iris within the opacified thin and bulging cornea (Fig. 6). The condition may also develop as a congenital anomaly. The presence of uveal pigment lining the posterior corneal surface gives the cornea a blue color as the dark uveal pigment shines through the bands of scar tissue. This severe inflammatory process may be of bacterial or viral origin and the condition may be bilateral. Bowman's and Descemet's membrane are usually absent to some degree; the corneal lamellae are replaced by irregular cellular stromal tissue. There is a gradual conversion of the iris stroma to fibrous tissue by the activity of its fibroblasts and those of the adjacent corneal lamellae. Eventually, the entire area becomes covered with endothelium (Fig. 7). The filtration angle is often involved and the resultant secondary glaucoma causes the weak corneal scar to bulge, exaggerating the staphy-

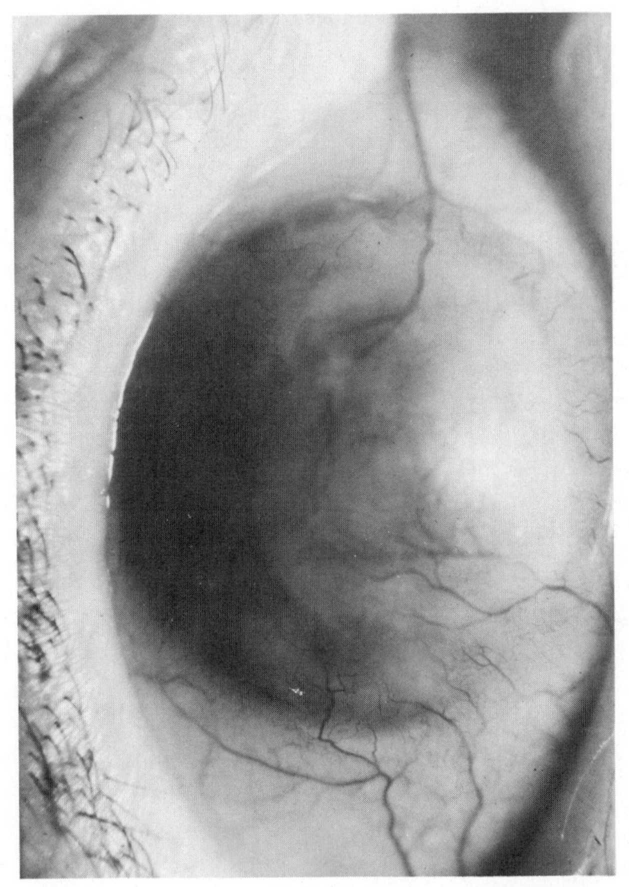

FIG. 6. Anterior corneal staphyloma.

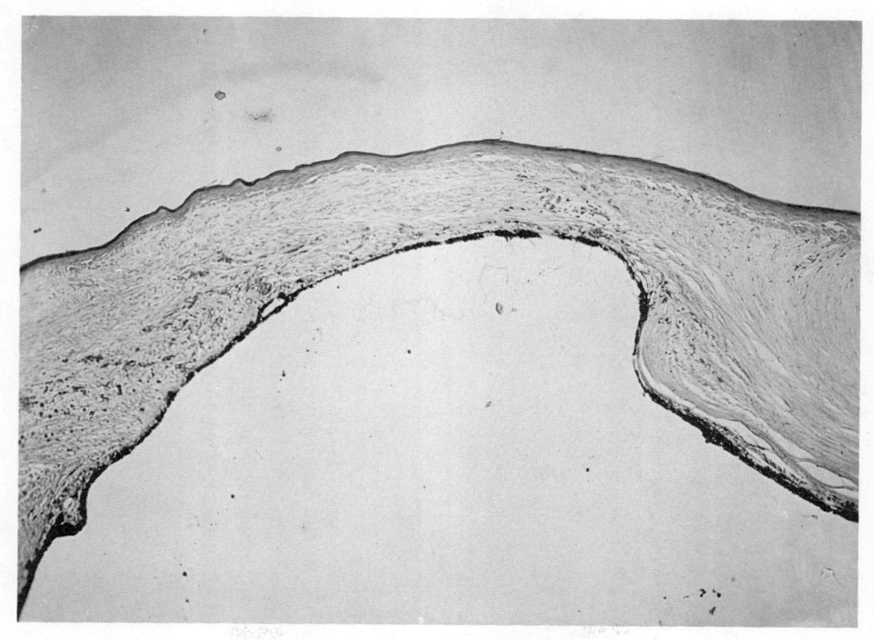

FIG. 7. Anterior corneal staphyloma. (A. F. I. P. Acc. No. 940867.) (Courtesy of the Registry of Ophthalmic Pathology of the Armed Forces Institute of Pathology.)

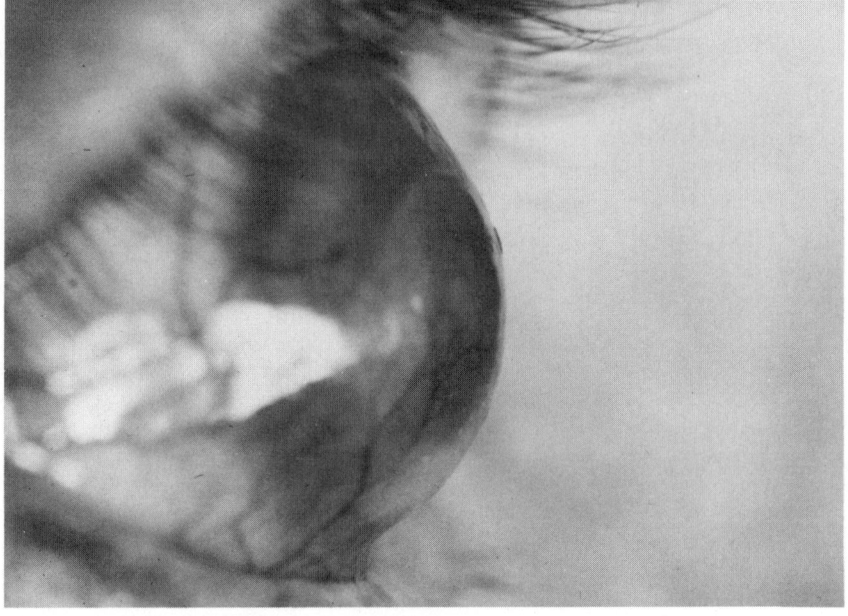

Fig. 8. Anterior corneal staphyloma (profile view).

loma. Whereas the buphthalmic eye develops a uniform enlargement of the cornea, the staphyloma may be irregular and conical, bulging prominently through the eyelids (Fig. 8). Even when the staphyloma is extensive, a peripheral zone of normal cornea is usually present. Vision is almost always poor and the cornea may ulcerate and even perforate. The lens may be absent, shrunken, or cataractous.

SYSTEMIC DISEASES

Corneal Lipoidosis

Familial lipoidosis may be associated with a cloudy appearance of the cornea. A general lipoid storage in the eye (lipoidosis bulbi) can be produced experimentally by feeding experimental animals a cholesterin-rich diet which results in the production of an arcus lipid infiltration of the cornea and nodules of cholesterol in the iris (Figs. 9-11). Kwitko and co-workers, using New Zealand albino rabbits, were able to limit this deposition of lipid material to some degree by adding magnesium to the feed.

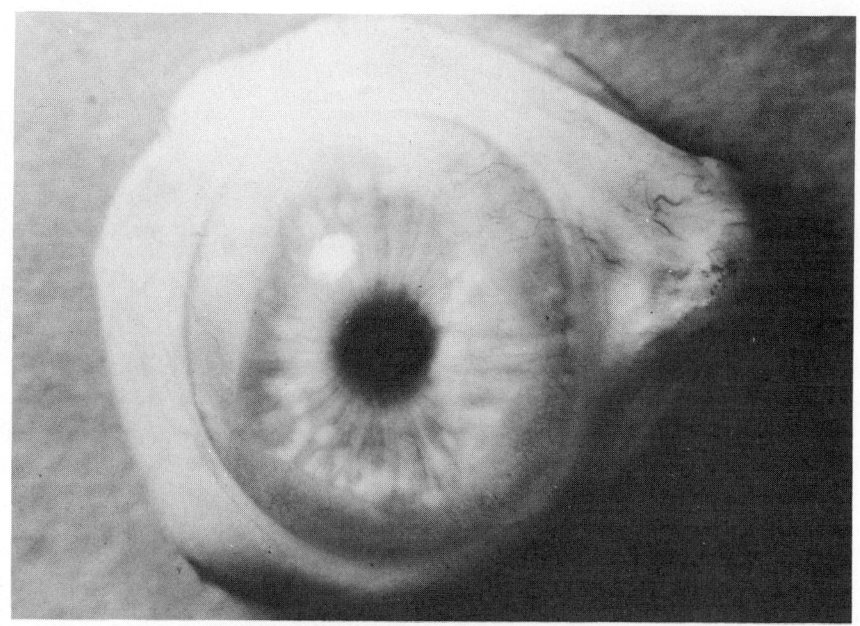

FIG. 9. Lipoidosis bulbi in a New Zealand albino rabbit (gross specimen). Both the cornea and iris are involved.

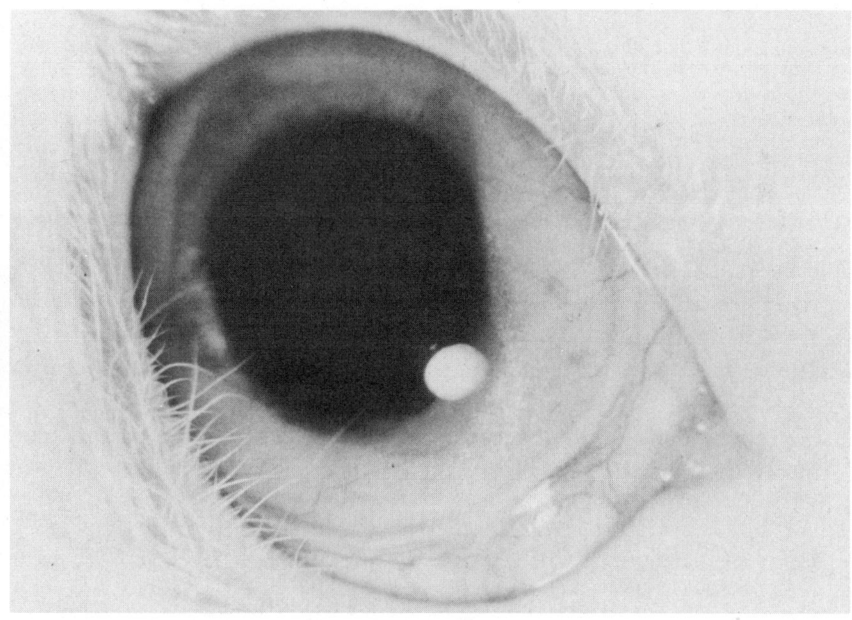

FIG. 10. Lipoidosis bulbi in a New Zealand albino rabbit. The cornea is primarily involved.

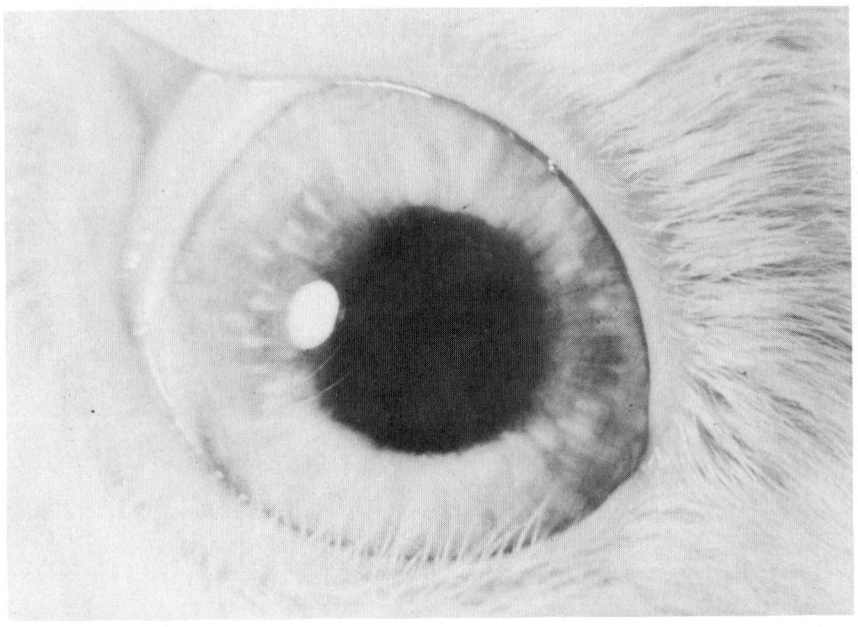

FIG. 11. Lipoidosis bulbi in a New Zealand albino rabbit. The iris is primarily involved.

Hyperlipemia and Hypercholesterolemia

Xanthomas of eyelids (Fig. 12) and tendons may be present. Bilateral lipid interstitial keratitis has been described, with wedges of closely packed fat granules arranged in bands radiating from the periphery toward the center of the cornea. Unaffected corneal sections remain clear. Neutral fats may be as high as 4,000 to 5,000 mg per 100 ml. The condition can occur in diabetes mellitus, extreme starvation, and lipoid nephrosis. An increase in cholesterol and phospholipids may be found. Vision may be impaired due to involvement of the retinal arterioles. A dominant hereditary pattern is noted.

Arcus Lipoides Juvenilis

Peripheral corneal deposits of lipid substances are most commonly seen in the annular form (Fig. 13). When they appear in an apparently normal cornea they may be the result of a systemic fat disorder. Vision is not

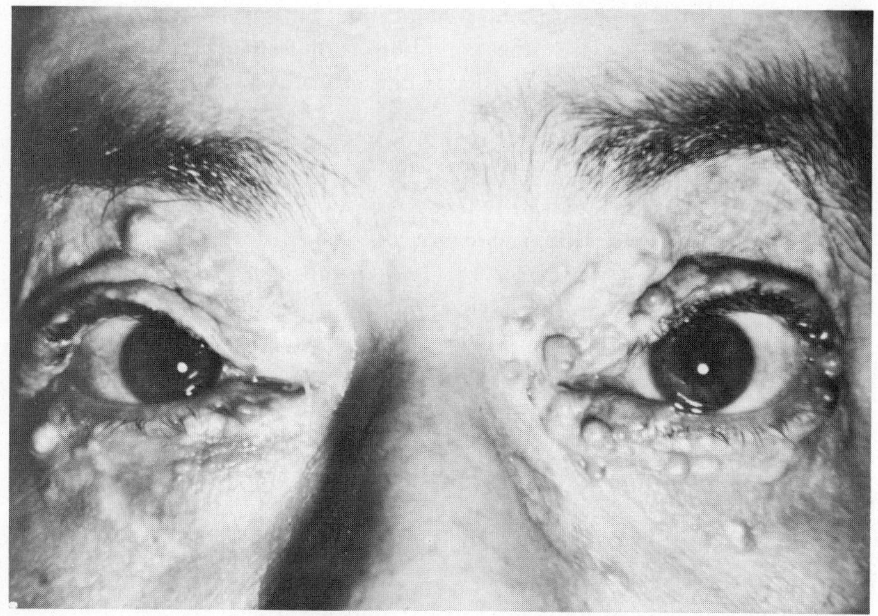

FIG. 12. Xanthomas of eyelids.

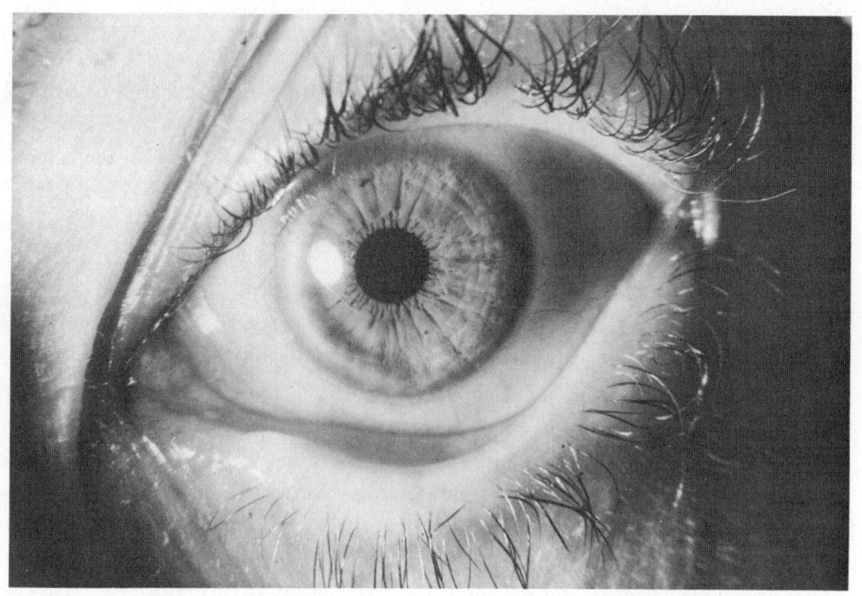

FIG. 13. Arcus juvenilis. (Courtesy of J. Decarie.)

affected unless the opacity is central in location. Signs of associated systemic disease should be sought. The condition may also occur secondary to calcification from a primary disorder of the cornea.

Hereditary Dystopic Lipidosis (Fabry's Disease)

This rare disease, transmitted as a sex linked recessive trait, was first described by Fabry in 1898 as a dermatological entity. However, it is now known to be an inborn error of lipid metabolism with a generalized glycolipid deposition in the myocardium, the smooth muscle of blood vessels, the epithelium of the kidney, and the central nervous system. The disease begins early in life with macular and papular skin eruptions, and primarily affects males.

Ocular involvement includes typical ampulliform dilatations similar to those which cause the dermal eruptions and a characteristic type of corneal opacity which affects the deeper layers of the epithelium. The main retinal feature is a corkscrew tortuosity of the vessels, mainly in the veins near the posterior pole, sometimes associated with retinal hemorrhages and a perimacular edema. Spaeth and Frost found that retinal vascular evidences were not as frequent as the corneal (90 percent) and conjunctival (60 percent) manifestations of the disease.

Lignac-Fanconi Syndrome; Cystinosis

The hallmark of childhood cystinosis is the generalized deposition of cystine crystals in various organs. Ophthalmologically, corneal and conjunctival birefringent crystals afford a convenient means of diagnosis by slit lamp biomicroscopy (Fig. 14). Cystinosis or cystine storage disease is a generalized disturbance of the amino acids appearing as an aminoaciduria with the accumulation of cystine in the liver, spleen, lymph nodes, kidneys, bone marrow, and ocular tissues including the cornea, conjunctiva, choroid, iris, ciliary body, and sclera. The birefringent iridescent crystals are concentrated anteriorly in the corneal stroma and located intra- and extracellularly in the stroma, leaving the uninvolved stroma clear (Fig. 15). Other features include dwarfism, wasting, osteoporosis, vomiting, renal rickets, polydypsia, polyuria, dehydration, acidosis, and sometimes tetany. Urinalysis reveals glycosuria, albuminuria, ketonuria, and aminoaciduria. Hematological analysis reveals acidosis, hypopotassemia, and sometimes hypocalcemia. According to Cogan, the corneal crystals are not present at birth but begin between the third and sixth month of life. They increase progressively and may give rise

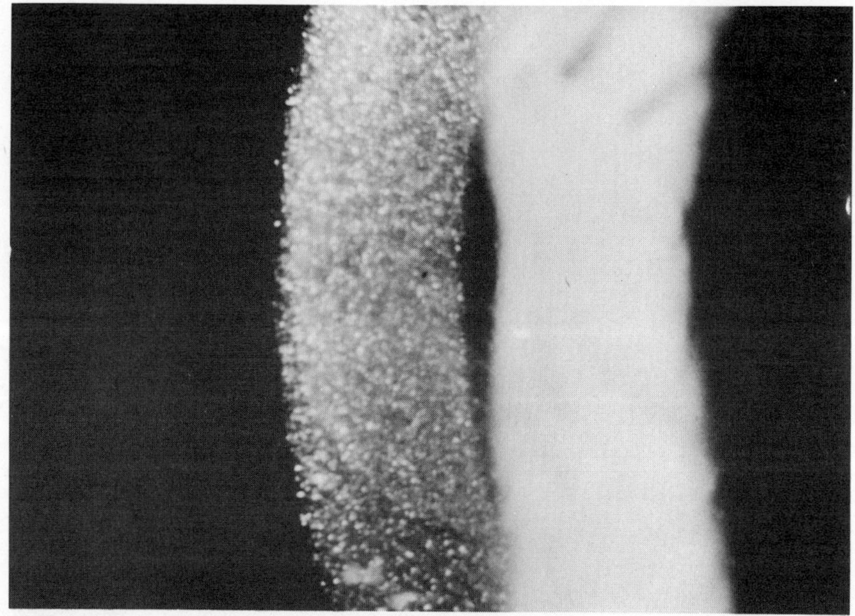

FIG. 14. Cystinosis. Corneal crystals noted on slit lamp examination. (Courtesy of B. Streiff.)

to a "glare" type of photophobia. Band-shaped keratopathy has been described.

Disorders of Calcium Metabolism

According to Gardner and Bergstrom, idiopathic hypercalcemia and failure to thrive are features of a syndrome which includes mental retardation, elfin facies, pallor, vomiting, constipation, polyuria, and osteosclerosis. The wide-eyed look of the child may suggest an ocular enlargement (Fig. 16).

A band-shaped opacity is seen in hyperparathyroidism, vitamin D intoxication, sarcoidosis, and uremia. Deposits of calcium are noted in the conjunctiva, corneal epithelium, and subjacent stroma. Lesions may be diffuse and involve the entire surface as a band-shaped opacity. In less severe cases there may be white flecks or glass-like crystals aggregated toward the limbus. The condition may be associated with essential (familial) hypercholesteremia. On slit lamp examination, highly refractile fatty droplets are

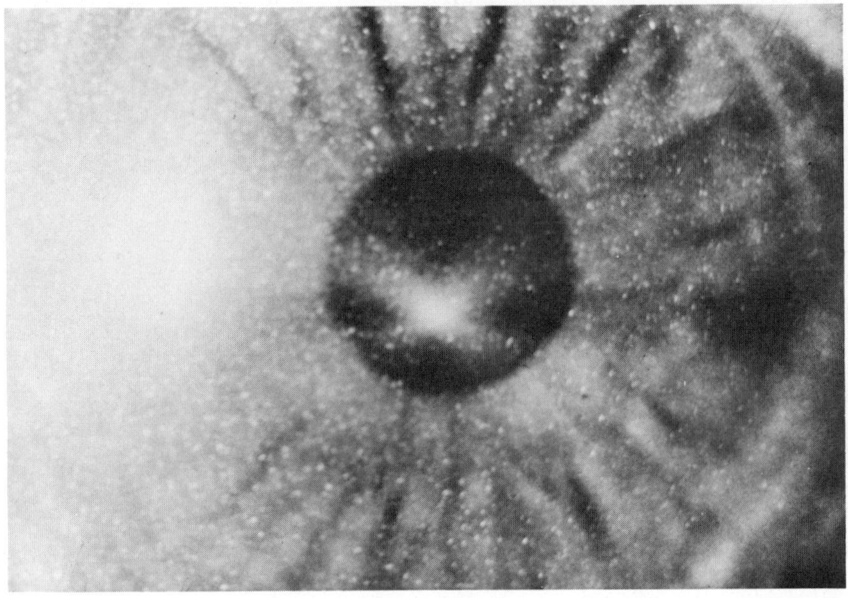

FIG. 15. Cystinosis. Birefringent crystals are separated by clear corneal stroma. (Courtesy of B. Streiff.)

noted at the level of Bowman's membrane which then spread through the stroma. A clear zone is present between the deposits.

Mucopolysaccharidosis (MPS)

Hunter's syndrome (systemic mucopolysaccharidosis, type II) is one of several genetic disorders of mucopolysaccharide metabolism which have been included under the term "gargoylism." It resembles Hurler's syndrome (mucopolysaccharidosis type I) in that dwarfing, stiff joints, hepatosplenomegaly, and gargoyle-like facies are commonly observed. However, it is clinically less severe. Features differentiating it from Hurler's syndrome are the mode of inheritance which is X-linked recessive rather than autosomal recessive, absence of lumbar gibbus, the occurrence of a perceptive type of deafness, and most important, the absence of corneal clouding.

Dysostosis multiplex, lipochondrodystrophy, or Hurler's syndrome results in a lymphoid infiltration of many body tissues including the cornea, giving it a ground glass appearance (Fig. 17) which must be differentiated from the cloudy cornea of congenital glaucoma. The orbit is usually

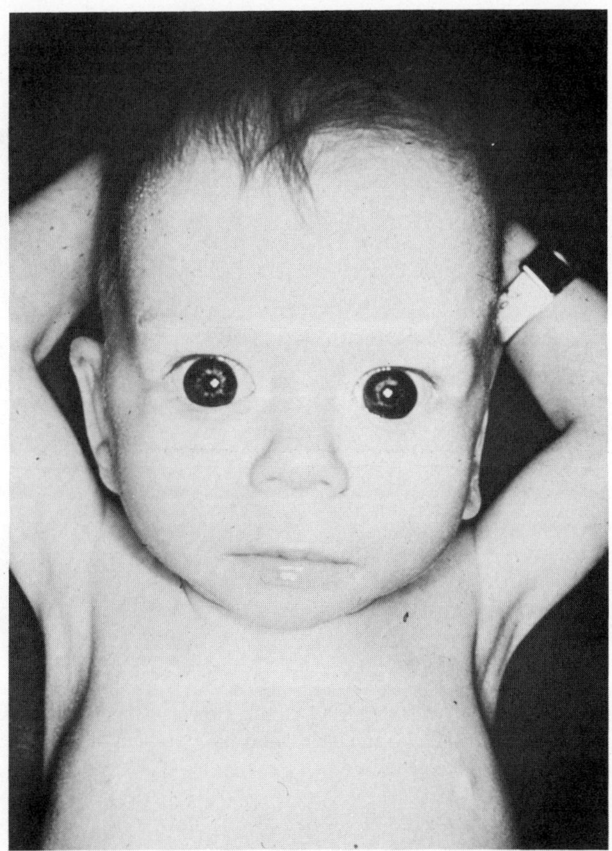

FIG. 16. Idiopathic hypercalcemia.

involved. Chondrodystrophic skeletal changes, dwarfism, kyphosis, large head, grotesque facies, mental deficiency, deafness, hepatosplenomegaly, and short claw fingers make up the syndrome. Corneal opacities may be bilateral and present soon after birth. They may become progressively dense with increasing age. On slit lamp examination, small whitish gray spots or filaments involving the central portion of the corneal stroma, especially anteriorly, are seen. Opacities are not found in the sex-linked recessive form.

Brante, in 1952, showed that Hurler's disease is a mucopolysaccharidosis. While chondroitin sulfate B is usually the predominant acid mucopolysaccharide stored, heparitin sulfate is also abnormally deposited. Carlisle and Good were the first to point out that the application of the Rebuck skin

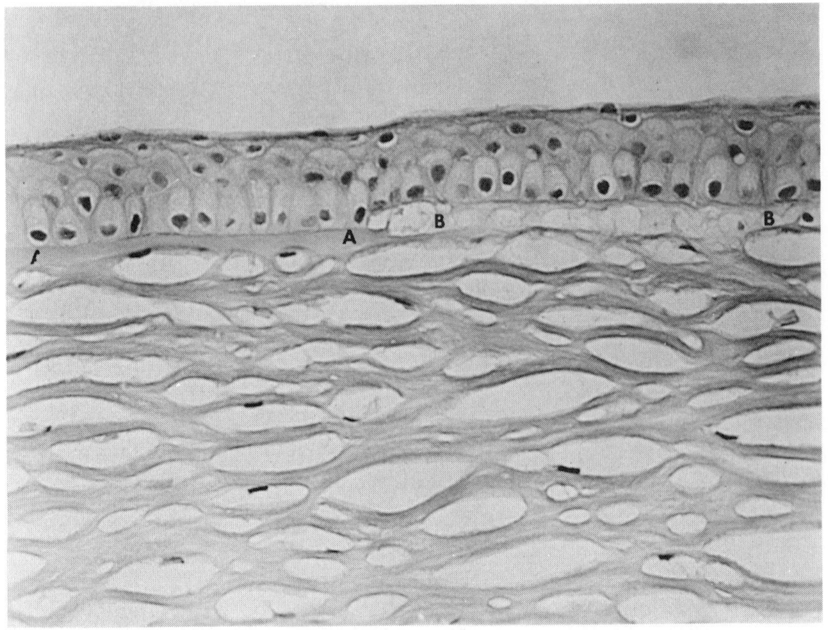

FIG. 17. The cornea of a case of Hurler's syndrome. Bowman's membrane (A) is replaced with cells containing glycoprotein and acid mucopolysaccharide (B). The result is a ground-glass appearance of the cornea.

window inflammatory lesion to suspected individual yielded the most rapid and certain production of diagnostic mononuclears presenting the abnormal metachromatic inclusions. Such diagnostic mononuclear phagocytes have been designated as "Hurler's" cells.

Scheie utilized the characteristic skin window findings of this disease to expand our concepts of mucopolysaccharidosis. In a newly recognized forme fruste of Hurler's disease (mucopolysaccharidosis type V), typical Hurler's cells were found in the skin windows of adult patients who presented with corneal clouding as the chief finding and lacked the extensive systemic involvement of the classical cases of Hunter and Hurler. Recently, Rebuck and Schiller were able to produce typical Hurler cells in the skin windows of normal controls merely by the application of chondroitin sulfate B to the test lesions. None of the other known purified acid mucopolysaccharides, similarly applied, were capable of eliciting such Hurler cells. Normal lymphocytes, monocytes, and histiocytes ingested and stored the chondroitin sulfate B to form classical Hurler cells within a 14 to 24 hr period after the initiation of the inflammation. Blood analysis reveals Reilly bodies in white cells, while the bone marrow shows Bühot cells. Urinalysis reveals increased chondroitin sulfate B and heparin monosulfuric acid. Radiological examination reveals an enlarged sella turcica, hook-shaped vertebrae, long bones, and enlarged diaphyses tapering toward the metaphyses. Ribs are spatula shaped and there is delayed maturation of ossification centers. Glaucoma and buphthalmos have been reported in cases of Hurler's Syndrome.

Congenital Porphyria

Congenital porphyria is a rare metabolic disorder resulting in porphyrinuria, which is inherited as a recessive character and is commoner in males (ratio 2:1). It may be present at birth and has been described in the fetus, according to Nelson. The classical clinical manifestations of this disorder are the excretion of a Burgundy red urine, discoloration of the bones and teeth, extreme sensitivity of the skin to light, and hirsutism. Hepatic and splenic enlargement is common. Not all these symptoms may be evidenced at one time and in one patient.

Conditions other than porphyrinuria may cause a reddish urine so that hemoglobinuria, myoglobinuria, and hematuria must be differentiated. Like many other fluorescent compounds, the porphyrins are sensitized by light and become powerful proteolytic agents. There is also a frequent accumulation of refractile droplets in the conjunctiva and cornea. The ocular involvement may be severe enough to cause blindness.

Von Gierke's Glycogen Storage Disease (Hepatonephromegalia: Glycoginica)

The genetic nature of this disease, first described by von Gierke in 1929, is strongly supported by the familial occurrence in a number of instances, and the history of consanguinity in others. The inefficiency or failure in forming glucose from hepatic glycogen results in great instability of the blood sugar content, and in hypoglycemia during periods of stress and fasting. The consequent excessive utilization of fat and protein leads to retardation of growth and finally to wasting. Other features include (1) an enlarged liver containing 12 to 16 percent glycogen (normal range 3.2 to 7.6 percent): (2) hyperglycemia after meals of high glucose content because the liver, choked with stored glycogen, no longer serves as a depot for excess glucose; (3) severe acidosis owing to the accumulated ketones from excessive fat combustion and to the increased lactic acid content of the body fluids which accompanies hypoglycemia; and (4) fat accumulation which gives many of these dwarfed children a doll-like appearance. Von Gierke's glycogen storage disease displays cloudiness at the margin of the cornea owing to the accumulation of glycogen.

Hand-Schüller-Christian Disease

Hand-Schüller-Christian syndrome consists of exophthalmos, diabetes insipidus and multiple defects in membranous bones, especially the cranium. This triad is relatively uncommon, according to Gellis, but the manifestations may occur singly or in combination with other characteristic lesions such as xanthoma disseminatum, mild hepatomegaly, seborrhea of the scalp, pulmonary infiltration, and stomatitis. The onset of the disease is insidious and usually occurs before the age of 6 years. At an early stage, a roentgenogram of the skull usually discloses sharply defined defects or areas of bone rarefaction. A biopsy will show the histologic picture of a granuloma with a few scattered foam cells. Future growth and sexual development may be retarded and diabetes insipidus may develop. Exophthalmos results from the accumulation of xanthomatous tissue in the retroorbital region. The course of the disease is chronic but spontaneous remissions may occur. Lipid infiltration of the cornea, which may be diffuse on rare occasions, results in corneal opacities. Corneal biopsy reveals squamous cells containing birefringent lipids associated with an inflammatory reaction.

Morquio Ullrich's Syndrome

A homogeneous cloudiness of the entire corneal stroma is noted in Morquio Ullrich's syndrome, owing to the presence of fine yellowish gray refractile particles distributed throughout the stroma both peripherally and centrally. The endothelium is normal. Deafness, flaring rib cage, hypotonia, kyphosis, genu valgum, pes planus, increased anteroposterior diameter of the chest, dwarfism, short neck and trunk, and long extremities are features of the syndrome together with hypoplastic enamel. Cardiac defects and hepatosplenomegaly may also be present. Hematological analysis reveals Reilly granulations in the polymorphonuclear leukocytes. Urinalysis shows increased mucopolysaccharides, occasional keratosulfate, and a small amount of chondroitin sulfate B. Radiological examination demonstrates coarse trabeculation of the humerus, ulna, and radius. Many epiphyses are irregularly shaped and poorly ossified. Short metacarpals and phalanges are noted together with narrow anterior portions of the vertebrae. Ribs are wide and spatulous. A related condition is Morquio syndrome (mucopolysaccharidosis type IV) or hereditary chondro-osteodystrophy. The cornea is not involved in this disease.

Osteogenesis Imperfecta (Blue Sclerotic Syndrome)

The osteogenesis imperfecta syndrome is genetically transmitted as an autosomal dominant and occasionally recessive condition, characterized by widespread defective mesodermal germinal tissue including bones, ligaments, and sclera. The blue sclera is the most common feature. Other features include otosclerotic deafness in which 50 percent of the occurrences are noted in the second and third decade, occasional congenital heart disease, lacerability of blood vessels leading to gastrointestinal hemorrhage, megalocornea, myopia, keratoconus, and corneal infiltrates. Fragile bones (fragilitas ossium) and lax joint capsules are the cardinal features of the disease, leading to multiple fractures and dislocations. The parathyroid glands may be involved and hyperthyroidism may be present.

A bluish tint to the sclera is normal among very young children. This is caused by an infantile translucency of the sclera which allows the color of the choroid to show through. However, the blue coloration fades in later months. In the blue sclerotic syndrome, a reduction of collagenous fibers with thinning and diminution of the opaqueness of the sclera allows the uveal pigment to be seen more readily, giving the sclera the blue color. Buphthalmia also leads to thinning of the scleral coat, but only as a secondary phenomenon. Blue sclerotic syndrome must be differentiated from (1) Van der Hoeve's syndrome, a mesodermal disease which features a blue sclera; (2) Ehlers-Danlos syndrome, blue sclera; (3) Marfan's syndrome, blue sclera; (4) Block Sulzberger's syndrome; and (5) Lobstein's disease, which consists of optic atrophy, strabismus, synostosis of the major and minor alae of the sphenoid bone, blue sclera, deafness, and osteoporosis causing spontaneous fractures.

Riley-Day Syndrome (Familial Dysautonomia)

In 1949, Riley et al. described a series of patients with a new syndrome inherited in a recessive manner, consisting of deficient lacrimation; excess sweating and salivation; abnormal reaction to minimal emotional stress characterized by transient, extreme elevation of blood pressure; development of bilateral, symmetric, sharply demarcated erythematous blotches of the skin which tended to recur in similar configurations; motor incoordination with awkwardness of the hands; peculiar shuffling gait; thickened speech; hyporeflexia; and a relative indifference to pain (Fig. 18).

Other symptoms frequently found include cyclic vomiting, pulmonary infection, unexplained high fever, breath holding spells in infancy, urinary

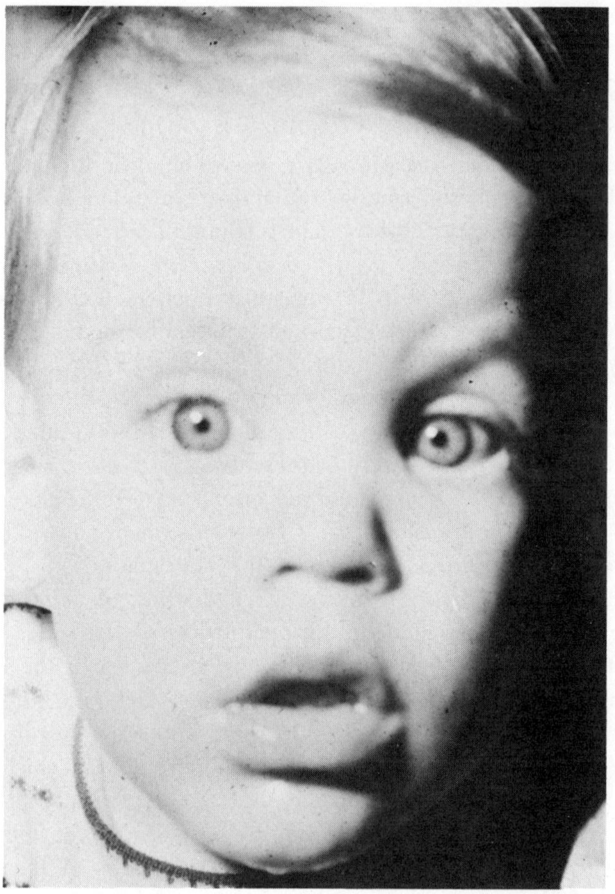

FIG. 18. Riley-Day syndrome. Excess salivation is evident.

frequency related to nervous tension (not to a neurogenic disturbance of the bladder), mental retardation, and convulsions.

Dunnington describes only two constant ocular findings in this disease: defective lacrimation and corneal hypesthesia. Lacrimation cannot be induced by external irritation or stellate ganglion block; no more than a drop or two of tears is secreted during crying, although the eyes may appear normal. Corneal sensitivity is either completely absent or greatly diminished. Retinal vascular tortuosity of a mild to moderate degree may also be noted.

Liebman has divided the corneal lesions into three types. (1) Severe central ulcerative lesions resembling neuroparalytic keratitis, and keratomalacia with extensive opacification of the central cornea. These lesions respond only to tarsorrhaphy. (2) Mild superficial lesions in the lower third of the corneal epithelium without active ulceration but with considerable turbidity of the corneal stroma. These lesions resemble exposure keratitis and respond to bland ointments and eyedrops. (3) This type consists of faint scarred areas of the lower cornea just inside the limbus which resemble etched glass, without any history of ocular symptoms. The precise cause of the ocular manifestations of this disease is yet to be defined although there are some interesting avenues being pursued.

Kroop has found that when β-methyl choline (mecholyl) is injected subcutaneously, tear formation is observed. This is interpreted as a normal end organ response to stimulation by a parasympathomimetic drug. The defect in lacrimation could therefore depend on an abnormality of nerve pathways. In addition, Smith and Dancis showed that three-fourths of their patients had pupillary constriction when 2.5 percent mecholyl was instilled, a result similar to its action in Adie's syndrome. This effect is interpreted as evidence of cholinergic insufficiency.

Kritchman et al. have reported severe hypotension and instances of cardiac arrest during general anesthesia, so that the consideration of any type of surgery must be undertaken with great caution. Confirmation of diagnostic suspicions is obtained by finding an absence of fungiform papillae in the tongue together with an abnormal histamine reaction in the skin.

Cogan's Syndrome

Cogan's syndrome features interstitial keratitis, vertigo, tinnitus, profound nerve deafness, nystagmus, blurred vision, photophobia, pain, and conjunctival injection. Nodular yellow white opacities of the cornea may be associated with polyarteritis or may occur following vaccination. The intraocular tension is normal. Examination using the slit lamp shows opacities through the deep portion of the cornea with endothelial pitting. Blood analysis reveals leukocytosis and eosinophilia. Hearing loss is shown by audiometry and the Wassermann test is negative.

Acrodermatitis Enteropathica

Acrodermatitis enteropathica is characterized by the symmetrical distribution of a rash over the face, ears, back of scalp, buttocks, elbows, hands, and feet. Lesions are at first bullous, erythematous, and later, squamous. There is evidence of paronychia and dystrophy of the nails. Other features include blepharitis, conjunctivitis, photophobia, decreased visual acuity, intermittent diarrhea, and alopecia with loss of eyelashes and eyebrows. There is also a low growth rate and death usually occurs before 10 years of age. Slit lamp examination reveals radial fanlike stripes in the cornea with both intraepithelial and subepithelial opacities in the central portion. Fluorescein stain is negative. Cases have been reported with corneal opacities which regressed on chloroquin therapy. The disease has a familial characteristic.

Block-Sulzberger's Syndrome (Incontinentia Pigmenti)

The Block-Sulzberger's syndrome, or incontinentia pigmenti, was first described in 1926 in a patient with striking skin changes and an intraocular pseudoglioma. Since that time more than 200 cases have been reported in the dermatology literature and countless others are known to practitioners of that specialty. More than a curious skin disorder, the disease is a generalized ectodermal dysplasia with involvement of the eyes, hair, teeth, and central nervous system. There are two types: (1) patchy pigmentary dermatosis, which occurs at birth; and (2) a reticular form which begins after age two. In two-thirds of the patients, the pigmentation is preceded by an acute inflammation of the skin which resembles herpetiform dermatitis. The skin manifestations are pigmented macules arranged in flecks, whorls, spiders, or linear patches; they do not follow the lines of cleavage or distribution of nerves (Fig. 19). This pigmented stage is characterized histologically by loss of pigment from the basal cells of the epidermis and the presence of pigment, free or in macrophages, in the dermis. This appearance suggested to early observers that the basal cells simply had become incontinent of pigment and led to the name of the syndrome. Dental anomalies are common and include delayed eruption, malformation, and absence of teeth. Osseous abnormalities are frequent and there may be an associated baldness. Neurologic disorders including mental retardation, seizures, and spastic paralysis have been seen. Most of the cases occur in young females (20:1). In 1959, Wollensack described anomalies of the eye in 26 percent of cases which included corneal opacities, congenital cataract, strabismus, nystagmus, blue scleras, myopia, iris malformations, persistent hyperplastic primary vitreous, pseudoglioma, prenatal and postnatal uveitis, papillitis, and retinal detachment (Fig. 20).

Wilson's Disease

Wilson's disease, or hepatolenticular degeneration, characteristically involves the basal ganglia. This degeneration is associated with cirrhosis of the liver, and the presence of a brownish or yellow green pigment in Descemet's membrane on the posterior surface of the outer margin of the

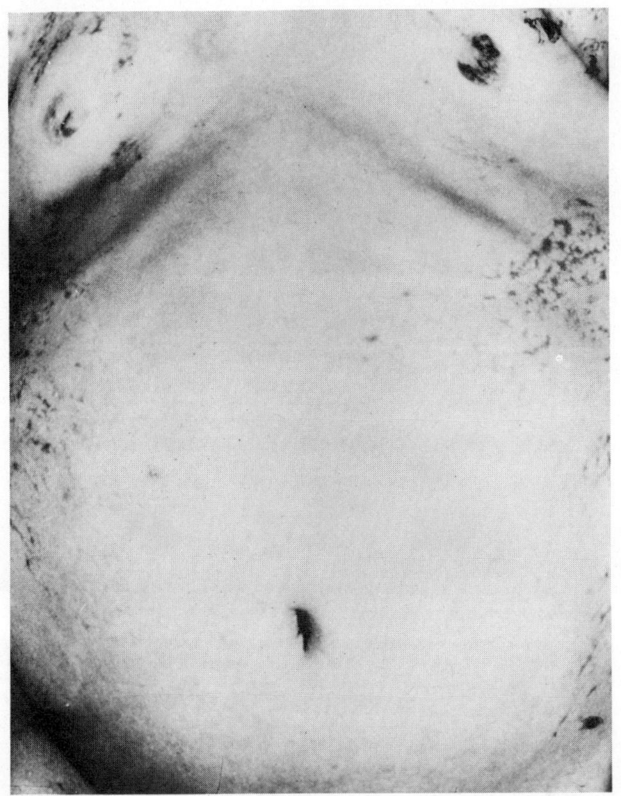

FIG. 19. Block-Sulzberger's syndrome. Distribution of pigment on the trunk. (From Zweifach. **Am. J. Ophthalmol.** 62:716, 1966.)

cornea (Kayser-Fleischer ring). The onset is usually in the latter part of childhood. Clinically, the condition is characterized by a rigidity of the skeletal musculature and involuntary movements. The facial appearance is usually one of constant smiling. Speech is jerky and irregular.

Other Systemic Disorders

In addition to the diseases listed above, corneal opacities have also been described in psoriasis, benign mucous membrane pemphigus, erythema multiforme, rosacea, Sjögren's keratoconjunctivitis sicca, and leprosy. Corneal deposits, which are often transient, are seen in association with drug eruptions, occurring with the use of antimalarials and arsenicals.

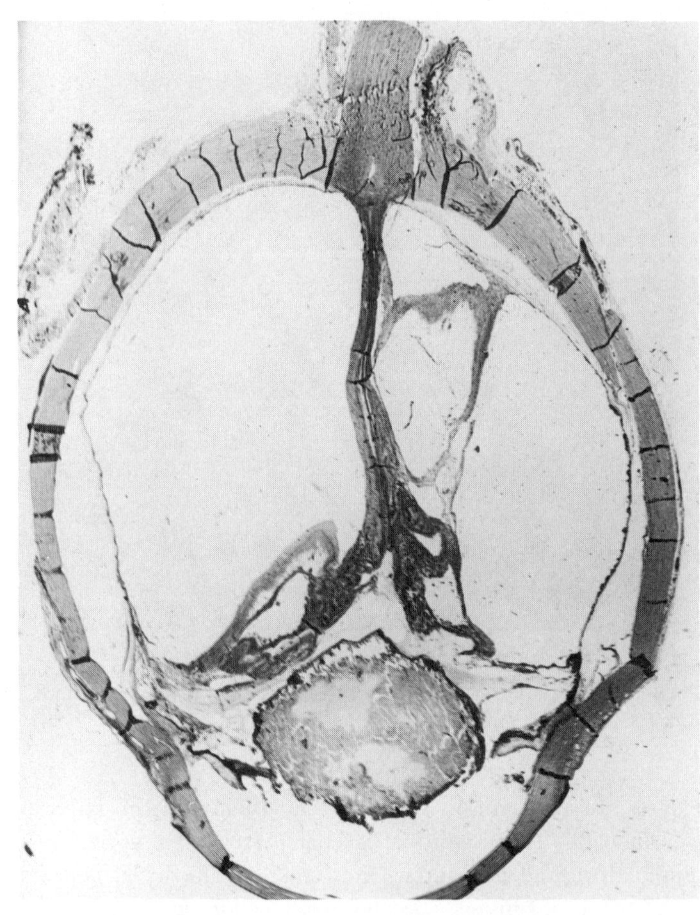

FIG. 20. Block-Sulzberger's syndrome. The retina eminates from the nerve in the form of a pipelike stalk. (From Zweifach. **Am. J. Ophthalmol.** 62:716, 1966.)

TRAUMA

Rupture of Descemet's Membrane

Breaks in Descemet's membrane owing to trauma, as seen with a difficult forceps delivery, may simulate the breaks in Descemet's membrane observed in congenital glaucoma (Fig. 21). If damage to the endothelium is extensive, the cornea may become edematous and take on a ground glass or steamy appearance in the first days of life. A hyphema may be present. Clearing usually takes place within 3 weeks, when the aqueous leak is sealed off by a new Descemet's membrane formed by the endothelium. A patchy appearance may then be seen, with bands crossing the cornea representing

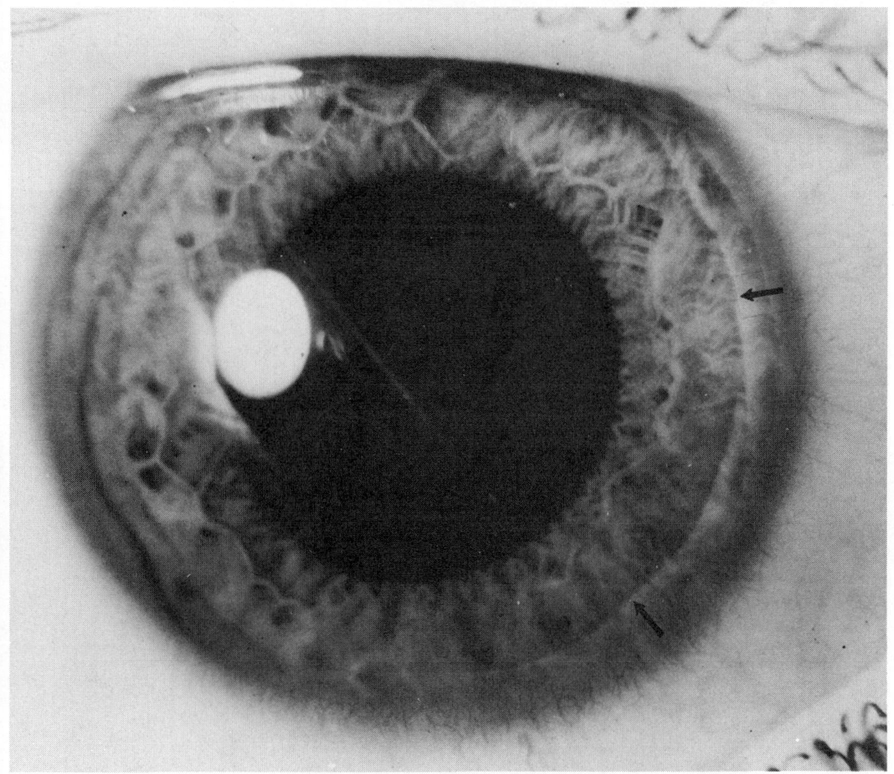

FIG. 21. Rupture of Descemet's membrane following difficult forceps delivery. Note the presence of the anterior border ring of Schwalbe nasally (arrow).

the edges of the ruptured membrane. Photophobia and tearing may be present and the clinical picture may present a problem in differentiation from congenital glaucoma. There is no elevation of the intraocular pressure and the corneal diameter is normal. Involvement may be bilateral. Spencer et al. observed 4 patients with unilateral corneal injuries produced by obstetrical forceps at birth, who developed corneal edema and bullous keratopathy 25 to 44 years later. The patients were asymptomatic in childhood but eventually developed intermittent episodes of severe foreign body sensation, tearing, and inflammation in the injured eye. The corneal edema and bulla formation tended to remain localized to the area of the breaks in Descemet's membrane. Successful keratoplasties were performed in each case. Presumably, the irregular thickened Descemet's membrane laid down by the corneal endothelium eventually permits the accumulation of fluid in the cornea as the individual ages, and the subsequent development of bullous keratopathy. Corneal vascularization did not develop.

Postnatal Trauma

The corneal lesion in postnatal trauma is characterized by punctate epithelial erosions which are usually discrete. There is often a history of

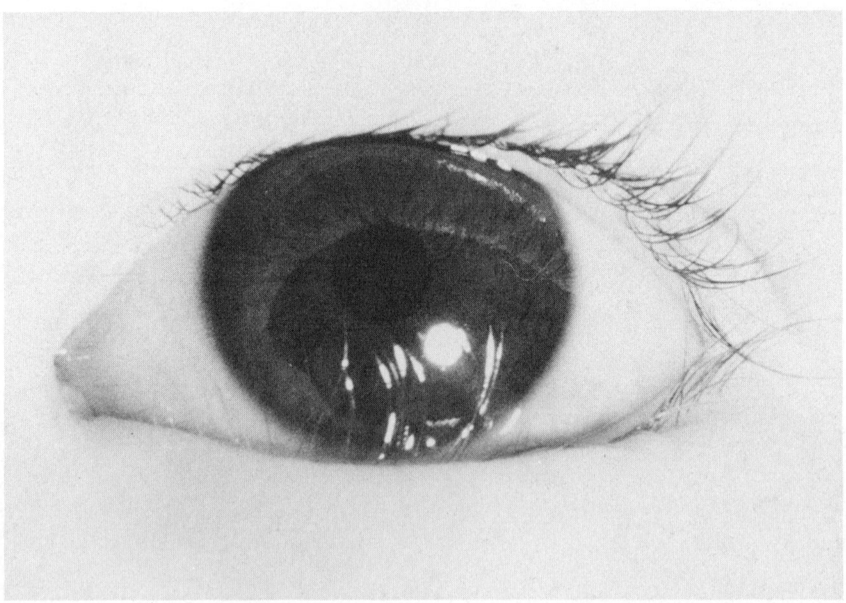

FIG. 22. Congenital entropion resulting in corneal involvement.

trauma, presence of a foreign body, or the occurrence of congenital entropion (Fig. 22).

SKIN DISEASES

Congenital Icthyosis

Congenital ichthyosis is a cutaneous disease of unknown etiology which is characterized by hyperkeratosis of the horny layers of the skin. This leads to a dry, harsh, scaly appearance due to the absence of the secretion of the sweat and sebaceous glands. Features of the disease include pseudosclerodermal facies, furrowing of the extremities with fissures and rhagades interrupting the continuity of the parchmentlike skin, erythroderma, dermal edema, and ectropion of mucous membranes. Corneal involvement may be seen as a multitude of fine punctate and linear opacities in the superficial stroma, or present in the form of a band-shaped degeneration associated with a dystrophy of the deeper corneal layers together with retinal atrophy, retinitis pigmentosa, microphthalmos, and arachnodactyly.

Congenital Dyskeratosis

Congenital dyskeratosis, as noted by Duke-Elder, was described by Spanlang, in 1927, in a patient with palmer and plantar dyskeratosis. Corneal involvement was in the form of a symmetrical, tongue-shaped, vascularized opacity extending horizontally almost completely across the cornea, affecting the epithelium and the superficial layers of the substantia propria.

CORNEAL DYSTROPHY

Congenital Hereditary Corneal Dystrophy

The opacities of congenital hereditary corneal dystrophy are frequently present at birth. They are usually stationary and may improve with passing years. There is no photophobia or inflammation. Corneal sensitivity is normal. The condition is usually bilateral and may respond to the application of 3 percent saline or 50 percent glucose to the surface of the cornea. The corneas are diffusely edematous and avascular, and exhibit a ground-glass appearance which varies from a slight haze to dense white, involving the entire thickness of the stroma. Intraocular pressure measurements are within normal limits (Fig. 23, see colorplate, frontis). Visual acuity varies from normal to bare light perception. Slit lamp examination reveals a ground-glass bluish white opacity of the entire thickness of stroma. Biopsy shows hydropic swelling of the basal layer of the epithelial cells, together with thinning of Descemet's membrane and degeneration of Bowman's membrane in some areas. The primary degeneration occurs in the corneal endothelium, initially affecting the central portion after the fifth month of gestation, and subsequently progresses peripherally, according to Kenyon and Artine. A secondary development is the diffuse stromal and epithelial edema which produces the clinically apparent clouding of the affected cornea. The clinical appearance of this condition bears many features common to congenital glaucoma. Feigin and Caplan described the following case.

"She was readmitted to the hospital at 3 months of age for a repeat tonometry. Diffuse bilateral corneal opacifications were still present and unchanged, but wandering nystagmus had developed. The ability of the child to perceive light was questioned. The corneas measured 11.0 mm, O.D., and 11.5 mm, O.S. A normal tension was recorded in both eyes by Schiötz tonometry performed under anesthesia. Bilateral goniotomy was performed. Following this procedure, no change was noted in the pressures and the opacities failed to clear."

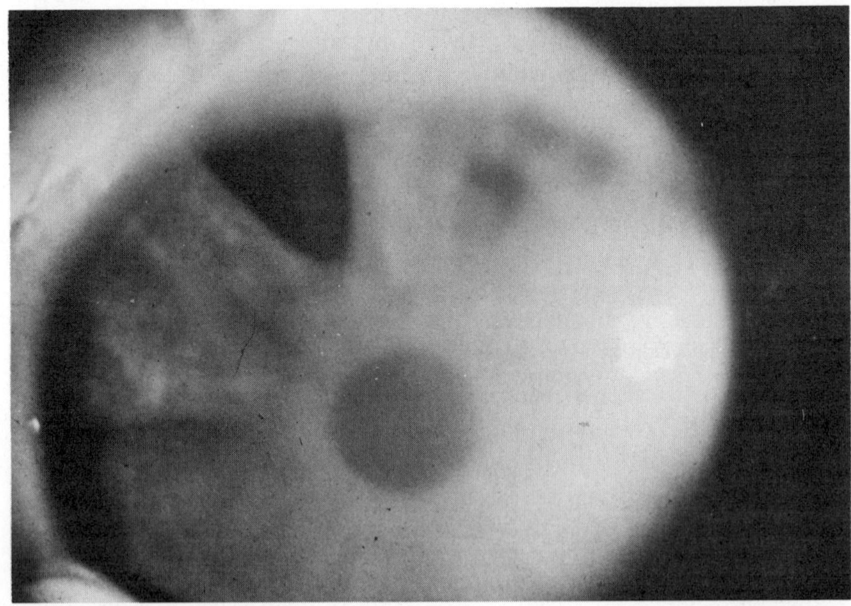

FIG. 24. Glaucoma operation performed in a case of congenital corneal dystrophy.

The author has also seen several cases which were operated under the supposition that the surgeon was indeed treating a case of congenital glaucoma. Fig. 24 illustrates such a case where glaucoma surgery was performed. The cornea failed to clear as expected. Great emphasis must be placed on the fact that the diagnosis of congenital glaucoma is not made by the observation of one striking feature, e.g., a cloudy cornea. On the contrary, the absence of other symptoms itself should cause the surgeon to lay aside the goniotomy knife and ponder the advantages of watchful waiting.

Congenital Idiopathic Corneal Edema

Edema of the cornea in a young infant may be on the basis of a metabolic disorder or may be a well advanced form of corneal dystrophy commencing during fetal life (Fig. 25, see colorplate, frontis). It may take the form of essential (Aubineau) corneal edema where the condition is recurrent and worse in the morning. Visual acuity may be affected. The endothelium remains intact. Corneal sensitivity and the intraocular pressure are normal. The attacks are often self-limited and may respond to local steroids. Fuch's epithelial-endothelial dystrophy has been observed in young children. In this case the endothelium has lost its integrity, the epithelium becomes edematous, and bedewing occurs followed by bullae formation. Corneal edema in the infant is summarized in Table 3A and B.

The healthy endothelium, because of its metabolic activity, is a prime factor in maintaining the proper fluid balance of the cornea. These cells are derived from para-axial mesoderm. In man the cells appear just before the 12-mm stage, and consist of a sheet of approximately 500,000 cells which are hexagonal in shape with oval nuclei. These cells exhibit great metabolic activity and contain mitochondria, endoplasmic reticulum, and Golgi apparatus. The abundant endoplasmic reticulum in these cells is related to the manufacture and maintenance of Descemet's membrane.

The endothelium of the infant is packed with nuclei with a high cell density per unit area. As the individual ages, fewer cells per unit area are seen, and the cells appear to spread out to cover the growing area since there is little or no mitotic activity. The cytoplasm becomes more prominent, helping to cover the area. The variation in cell concentration and cell quality of the endothelium may have two effects. It may (1) determine or influence the onset, duration, and severity of corneal edema in different patients having diseases of similar nature and severity; and (2) it might dictate the levels of intraocular pressure that govern the onset of corneal edema.

TABLE 3A

CLASSIFICATION OF PRIMARY CORNEAL EDEMA*

(1) Aubineau or essential corneal edema
(2) Fuch's epithelial-endothelial dystrophy
(3) Congenital hereditary corneal dystrophy
(4) Congenital idiopathic corneal edema

*Modified after M. Grayson. Eye, Ear, Nose, Throat Mon. 47:441, 1968.

TABLE 3B

CLASSIFICATION OF SECONDARY CORNEAL EDEMA*

Epithelial Edema

(1) Superficial bacterial infection
(2) Herpes simplex
(3) Ectodermal dysplasia
(4) Corneal erosion
(5) Allergy

Stromal Edema

Edema results when the epithelium (less severe) or endothelium (more severe) are affected. Persistent edema leads to scarring.

Endothelial Edema

(1) Severe cornea guttata
(2) Disciform keratitis or deep corneal ulcer
(3) Iritis
Inflammatory products and/or iris synechiae may cause glaucoma, which endangers that part of the normal cornea having the lesser concentration of endothelial cells.
(4) Keratoconus
Development of acute hydrops
(5) Iatrogenic injury to endothelium during surgery
Drug installation into anterior chamber, mechanical trauma during corneal, glaucoma, and cataract surgery, e.g., inadvertent corneal penetration with goniotomy knife while approaching filtration angle
(6) Delayed edema
Injury to Descemet's membrane, e.g., birth injury
(7) Constant vitreous touch
(8) Hyphema
Free blood in anterior chamber may affect endothelium.
(9) Intraocular infection
(10) Toxic material
Penetration of toxic material by exogenous or endogenous routes causes corneal edema.

*Modified after M. Grayson. Eye, Ear, Nose, Throat Mon. 47:441, 1968.

Granular Dystrophy (Groenouw's I; Bückler's I)

Granular dystrophy is characterized by discrete, grayish white opaque granules or rings with sharp borders, mainly in a disc-shaped area in the central region of the cornea. The periphery of the cornea is always entirely free of granules and corneal stroma between the opacities remains clear. In some cases only the superficial stroma appears to be involved, while in others the lesions may be found at all levels of the stroma. The disease may begin during the first 10 years of life. Visual acuity is usually good during childhood. Slit lamp examination reveals findings similar to those of gross inspection. Microscopically, the opacities consist of focal areas of hyaline degeneration in which the stromal fibers appear finely granulated. They are less PAS-positive and less birefringent than the uninvolved stroma. These latter two features, together with the fine granularity of the lesions, serve to differentiate granular from lattice dystrophy. Granular dystrophy is inherited as a dominant characteristic.

Macular Dystrophy (Groenouw's II; Bückler's II)

Macular dystrophy is characterized by irregular, grayish opaque opacities with borders not sharply demarcated. They are scattered throughout the cornea, but are especially dense in the central zone and involve all levels of the stroma. Some opacities extend to the limbus. The cornea between the spots is diffusely cloudy. The condition may manifest itself in the first decade of life. Visual acuity in childhood may be normal but usually there is severe impairment early in life. Slit lamp examination reveals the site of involvement to be in the stromal lamellae, corneal corpuscles, and endothelial cells. Corneal biopsy shows a mucoid degeneration of stromal lamellae, accumulation of pools of mucoid material within the endothelial cells and corneal corpuscles, and the disappearance of stromal cells. This mucoid material stains with Alcian blue or colloidal iron, and is not sensitive to hyaluronidase. Macular dystrophy is inherited as a recessive characteristic.

Lattice Dystrophy (Biber-Haab-Dimmer; Bückler's III)

Lattice dystrophy is characterized by branching, grayish, linear lesions, translucent by retroillumination and limited mainly to a zone between the center of the cornea and the periphery, usually not extending to the limbus (Fig. 26). The lesions are located in the stroma but the deeper layers may be spared. The cornea between the opacities, including the periphery, is relatively clear. Visual acuity may be reduced. Slit lamp examination reveals

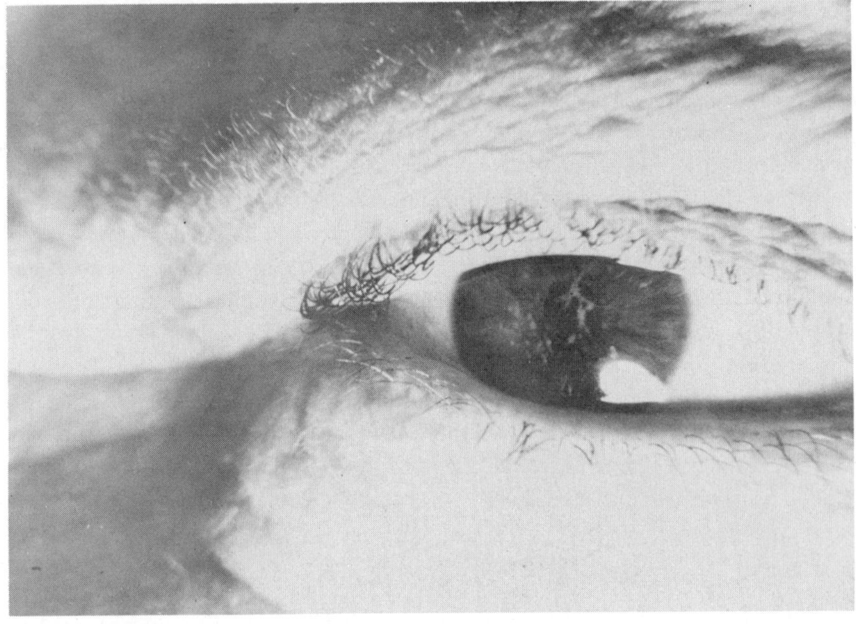

FIG. 26. Lattice dystrophy.

nonspecific epithelial and subepithelial changes which may be severe enough to obscure the typical linear lesions in the stroma. Microscopically, the characteristic stromal lesions are fusiform areas of hyaline degeneration lacking the granular character of lesions seen in granular dystrophy. They are PAS-positive. Dense accumulations of hyaline are usually observed between the irregular epithelium and Bowman's membrane, according to Hogan and Zimmerman. While these are of no significance in the differential diagnosis, they are of paramount importance clinically because of their effect on visual acuity. Lattice dystrophy has a dominant hereditary pattern.

Crystalline Corneal Dystrophy of Schnyder

Crystalline corneal dystrophy of Schnyder begins early in life, often associated with arcus juvenilis. It is usually not progressive. An oval or annular cloudy opacification is present mainly in the central portion of the cornea. The periphery of the opacity gradually extends outward but leaves a narrow, clear area between its margin and the limbus. Occasionally the entire cornea is involved. Visual acuity is moderately decreased. Corneal sensitivity is normal. Slit lamp examination reveals an opacified area which contains many small iridescent needle-shaped crystals. The opacity is located in the anterior portion of the stroma just deep to Bowman's membrane. The epithelium is normal. There is a dominant inheritance.

Hereditary Epithelial Corneal Dystrophy

Hereditary epithelial corneal dystrophy may be seen as early as 7 months of age. Fine gray punctate opacities are present, more numerous in the center of the cornea, but also involving the remainder of the cornea to within 1 to 2 mm of the limbus. Fluorescein reveals fine punctate staining of the entire corneal surface. Slit lamp examination shows opacities just beneath the epithelium, which are finely irregular and anterior to Bowman's membrane. The opacities take the form of minute, almost transparent droplets with smooth, well defined borders of varying size. Bowman's membrane, the corneal stroma, Descemet's membrane, and the endothelium are all uninvolved. There is a dominant inheritance pattern.

Hereditary Nonprogressive Deep Corneal Dystrophy (Hereditary Polymorphous Deep Degeneration of the Cornea)

This condition is generally nonprogressive but an extremely slow progression may occur. A faint haze is seen clinically in both corneas. Slit lamp examination shows the epithelium, Bowman's membrane, and most of corneal stroma to be unaffected. The entire posterior surface of the stroma is studded with multiple small nodular and larger vesicle-like excrescences which are equally distributed over the entire cornea. The nodular lesions are small, with increased translucency. The vesicle-like lesions are less common, larger, irregular, and of varying clarity, with margins outlined by areas of increased infiltration and translucency. Some appear to protrude into the anterior chamber.

GENETIC DISORDERS

Down's Syndrome (Mongolism)

Ocular findings in mongolism include the mongoloid slant of the palpebral apertures, epicanthal folds, convergent strabismus, keratoconus, nystagmus, ectropion, and high myopia. Brushfield's spots are noted during infancy but tend to disappear with advancing age. Cataracts in Down's

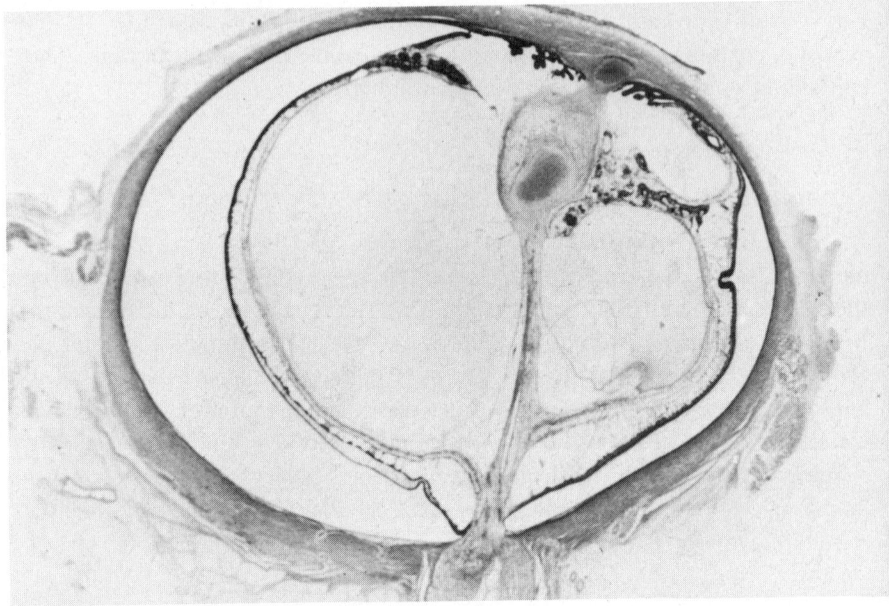

FIG. 27. Trisomy 13–15 syndrome. (Courtesy of D. Barsky.)

syndrome are similar to metabolic cataracts of other etiology. When associated with thyrotoxicosis, symptoms include lid-lag, stare, lid retraction, exophthalmos and corneal opacities. The abnormality exists in chromosome 21.

The Trisomy 13-15 Syndrome

The Trisomy 13-15 syndrome results from the presence of an extra autosomal chromosome of the 13-15 or D group. The following abnormalities reviewed by Yanoff et al. have been noted: mental retardation, deafness, heart defects, hemangiomata, cleft lip, cleft palate, motor seizures, low-set ears, polydactyly, and horizontal palmar creases. The ocular findings include microphthalmia (Fig. 27), iris coloboma, persistent pupillary membrane, congenital cataract, retinal dysplasia, corneal opacities, and hyperplastic primary vitreous. Cogan and Kuwabara have noted the apparent characteristic of a cartilage mass, extending from the retrolental region to the sclera in the region of the coloboma (Fig. 28).

Ginsberg and Perrin reported a transcleral herniation of dysplastic retina into the orbit and optic meninges, arterial endothelial proliferation in

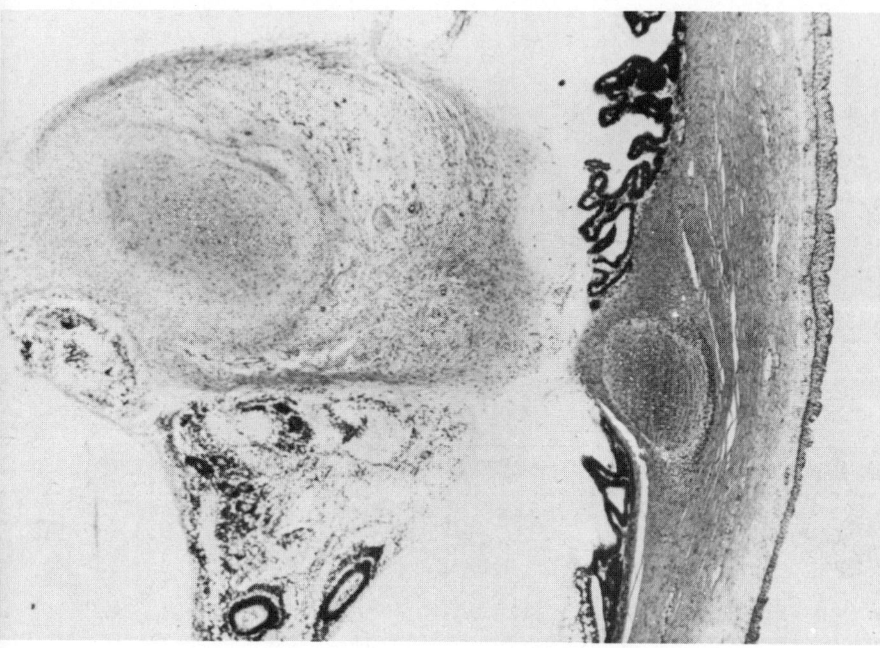

FIG. 28. Trisomy 13–15 syndrome. The characteristic cartilage mass extends from the retrolental region to the sclera in the region of the coloboma. (Courtesy of D. Barsky.)

the choroid and orbit, partial absence of ciliary nerves, and hypertrophy of optic nerve meninges.

BIRTH ANOMALIES

Congenital Corneal Leucoma

Congenital corneal opacities present in a variety of forms. They may be localized (Fig. 29) or diffuse (Fig. 30); they may involve the deep and/or superficial cornea and they may occur in association with a number of other conditions, including microphthalmos, coloboma of the iris or choroid, persistent pupillary membrane, and iris adhesions.

The dense leucomas are located deep in the central cornea, often attached to the iris. Descemet's membrane is usually absent in the region of the opacity. The lesion may result from (1) a defect in the separation process of the embryonal lens from the surface ectoderm; (2) birth injury; or

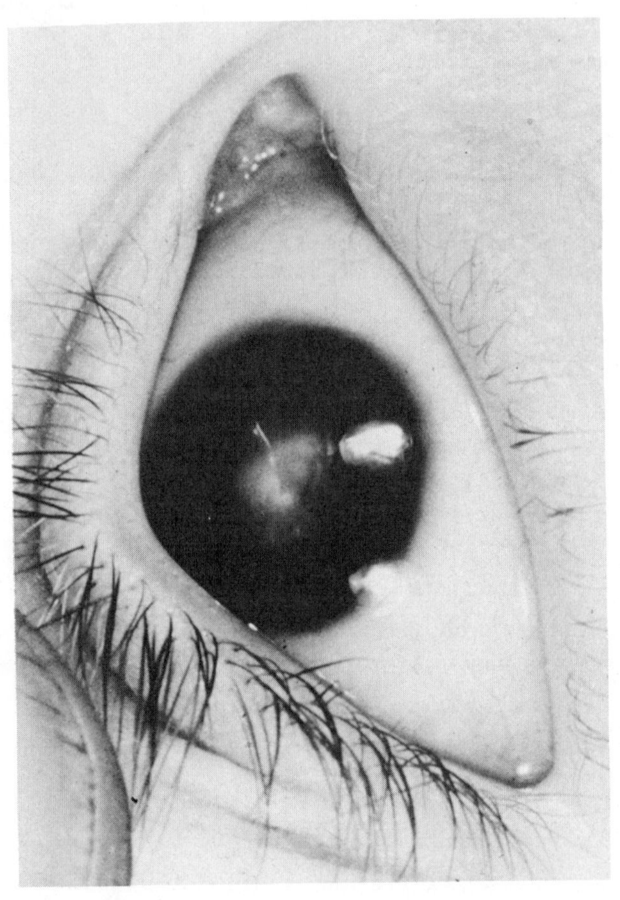

FIG. 29. Congenital corneal leucoma, localized.

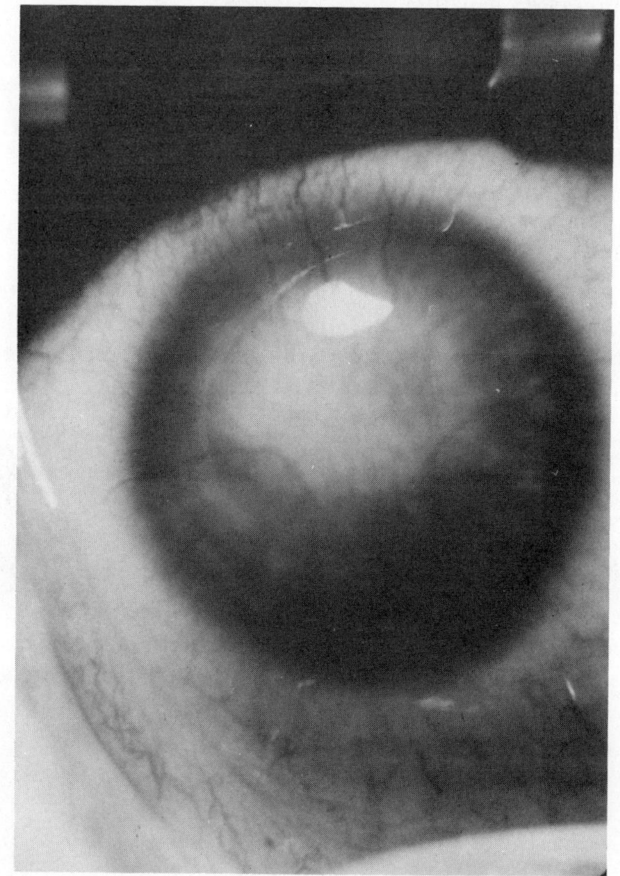

FIG. 30. Congenital corneal leucoma, diffuse.

(3) intrauterine inflammation. The leucoma may become ecstatic and perforation may occur. A familial tendency is noted.

Peters anomaly, according to Nakanishi and Brown, is a congenital central corneal stromal opacity usually associated with a defect in the posterior stroma and Descemet's membrane, together with anterior synechiae which extend from the pupillary zone of the iris to the periphery of the corneal opacification. Glaucoma is a common feature of this condition (see Chap. 9).

Persistent Hyperplastic Primary Vitreous (PHPV) (Persistent tunica vasculosa lentis; Persistent fetal fibrovascular sheath of the lens.)

Persistence of hyperplastic primary vitreous is seen as a fibrovascular tunic of the lens and part of the hyaloid vascular system, resulting in the presence of a dense fibrovascular retrolental mass (Fig. 31) often extending laterally to the equator, occupying the circumlental space to which ciliary processes extend. Elements of the peripheral retina are continuous with the mass. Spontaneous intraocular hemorrhage may occur at the periphery of the tissue. A defect in the posterior lens capsule may be present to which

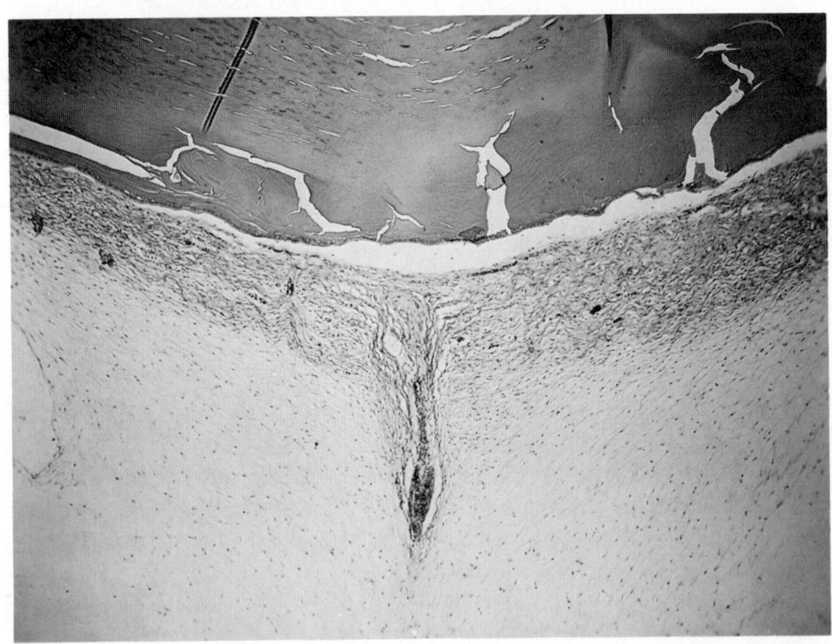

FIG. 31. Persistent hyperplastic primary vitreous. (A.F.I.P. Acc. No. 943372.) (Courtesy of the Registry of Ophthalmic Pathology of the Armed Forces Institute of Pathology.)

fibrous tissue and blood vessels extend, thus involving the lens cortex and leading to liquefaction of cortical fibers. Other lens changes occur in the form of intumescence which may produce angle closure or pupillary block. The cataractous process progresses while the liquefied elements may undergo absorption. Clinically, PHPV is manifested by a uniocular white reflex behind the pupil so that the condition is often confused with retinoblastoma. The anterior chamber is shallow and the iridocorneal angle may show retarded development. When this occurs, glaucoma is a common complication. (Chap. 9).

Large Cornea of High Myopia

Although high myopia and congenital glaucoma may both appear clinically as an enlarged eye, they differ in that the postequatorial region is first affected in myopia, while in congenital glaucoma many of the early changes take place in the anterior part of the globe (Fig. 32, see colorplate, frontis).

A buphthalmic eye need not necessarily be myopic. According to Parson, enlargement of the globe leads to a flattening of the cornea with flattening and posterior displacement of the lens. This would bring about a change in the location of the cardinal points, so that the anteroposterior diameter of the eye must approach 31 mm in length for emmetropia. According to Gross, the average anteroposterior diameter of the eye with congenital glaucoma is 32 mm. In unilateral myopia the patient is asymptomatic and the eye is not congested. There are none of the characteristic signs of congenital glaucoma evident, e.g., corneal haze or tears in Descemet's membrane. A fundus picture characteristic of high myopia is present, and the intraocular pressure is normal.

Anterior Megalophthalmos (Megalocornea; Keratomeglia)

The condition once referred to as hydrophthalmos sanatus bears no relationship with congenital glaucoma although intermediate states are found which can cause confusion. According to Anderson, Horner's original title, "megalocornea globosa," is most appropriate. The ciliary ring circumference is enlarged; the corneal curvature and diameters are increased, even reaching 18 mm (Fig. 33, see colorplate, frontis). There is often a high astigmatic error present but visual acuity may be normal. On gonioscopy, the anterior segment usually exhibits a deep anterior chamber and a broad ciliary body band with an unusually prominent scleral spur (Fig. 34). Pigment is deposited heavily in the trabeculum and may be seen on the posterior surface of the cornea (Krukenberg's spindle). The iris may be stretched,

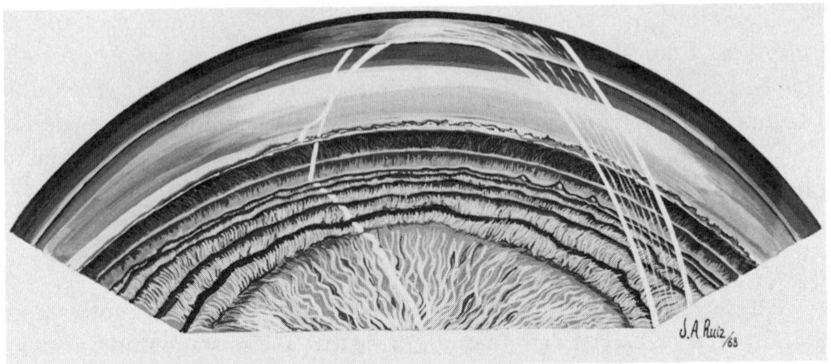

FIG. 34. Lower quadrant of chamber angle in megalocornea. Deep anterior chamber. Broad ciliary body band. Unusually prominent scleral spur. Heavily pigmented corneoscleral trabeculum. Ring of Schwalbe protruding prominently into anterior chamber in several places. Pigment on posterior corneal surface. (Modified from L. Allan.)

showing atrophy of the stroma and dilator pupillae resulting in miosis. Partial dislocation of the lens is an infrequent finding, associated with iridodonesis. Remnants of the pupillary membrane are often seen. Ectopia pupillae, cataract changes, and embryotoxon may also be found. The posterior portion of the eye is not overly enlarged. Megalocornea and congenital glaucoma have been found in members of the same family (Figs. 35 and 36 A and B), while congenital glaucoma has been noted in one eye and megalocornea in the opposite eye of the same patient. In megalocornea there are no signs of ocular congestion, the cornea is clear, and there are no tears present in Descemet's membrane. Some cases of megalocornea, however, do develop an elevated intraocular pressure, although this is unusual and some are associated with arachnodactyly. This bilateral nonprogressive condition is transmitted as a sex-linked trait and occurs almost exclusively in males (92 percent) except in cases of consanguinity.

CORNEAL DEFORMATION

Keratoconus

This congenital anomaly which shows a hereditary tendency rarely causes symptoms before adolescence. While the cornea and neighboring

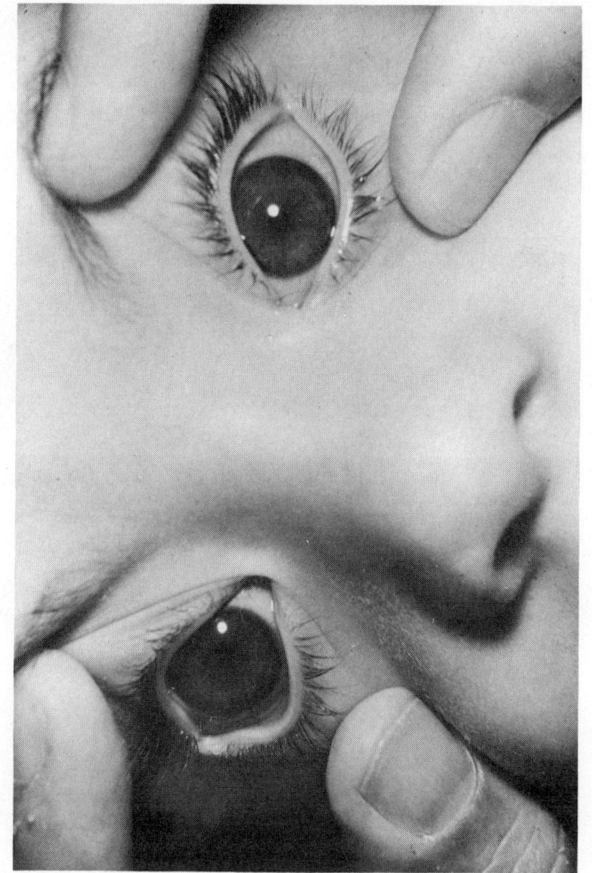

FIG. 35. Megalocornea, bilateral, one-year-old child.

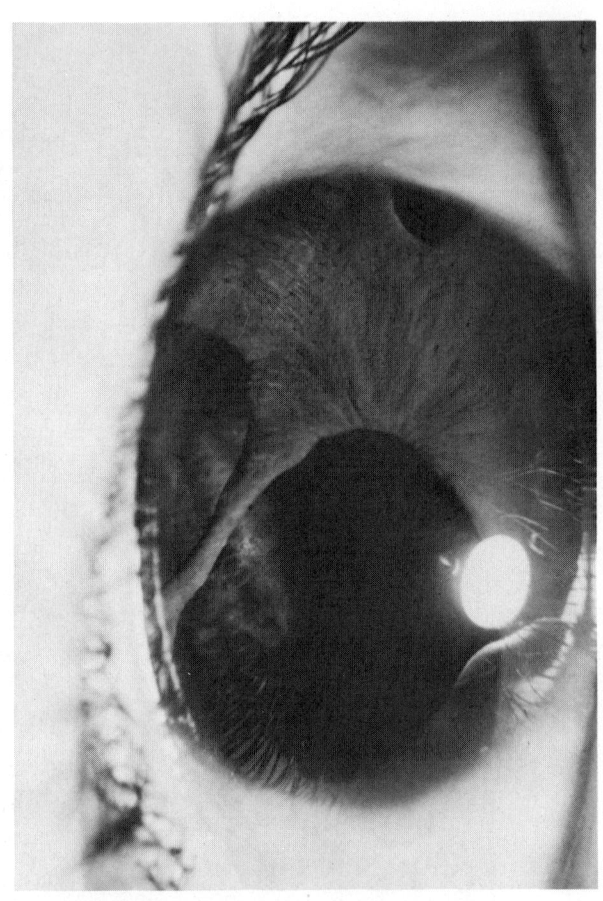

FIG. 36.A. Congential glaucoma in father of case in Fig. 35. Right eye. This eye has undergone several operations.

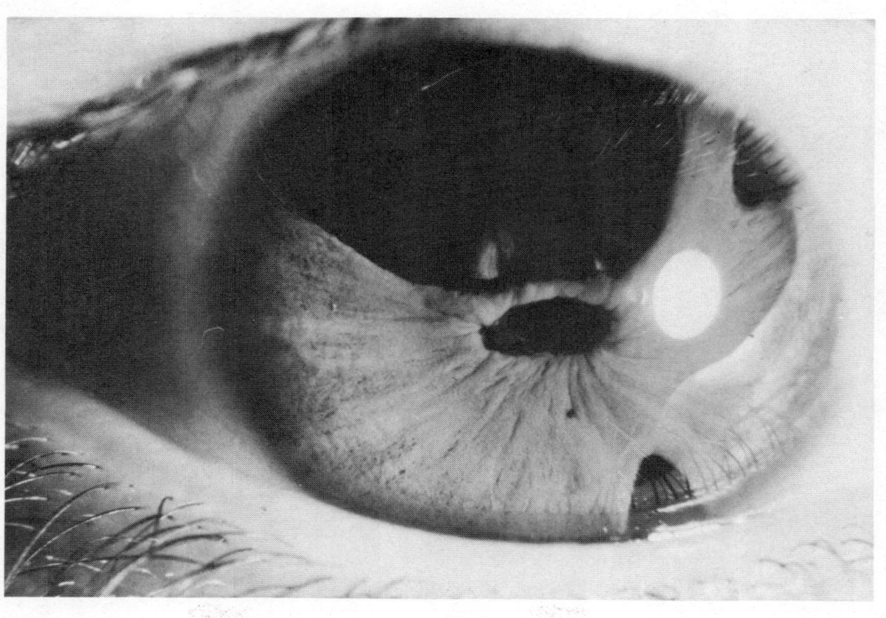

FIG. 36.B. Congenital glaucoma in father of case in Fig. 35. Left eye. This eye has undergone several operations.

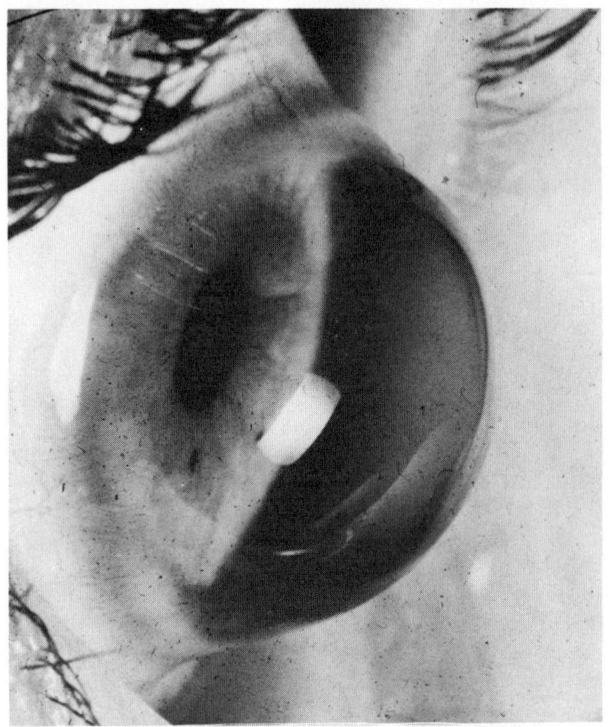

FIG. 38. Keratoglobus. (Courtesy of J. Buxton.)

sclera are greatly enlarged and the cornea flattened with ocular hypertension, keratoconus represents a form of keratectasia in which only the central cornea bulges forward, becoming thin and prominent, often surrounded by a pigmented ring (Fig. 37, see colorplate, frontis). The characteristic appearance distinguishes this condition from congenital glaucoma, even though tears in Descemet's membrane appear frequently. A marked astigmatism is present. Keratoconus may occur at birth and may be associated with congenital cataract, aniridia, and ectopia lentis.

Keratotorus

Keratotorus, according to Duke-Elder, is characterized by a toric or vault-like ectasia of the cornea with thinning of the central area. Other features include a pigmented line of hemosiderin and high myopic astigmatism.

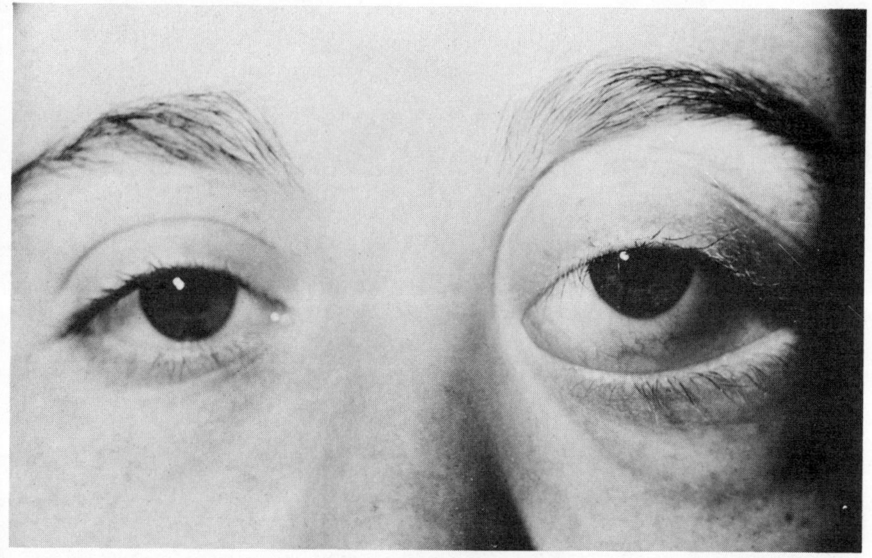

FIG. 39. Orbital hemangioma.

Keratoglobus

In keratoglobus the cornea is enlarged in a globular fashion and protrudes in the form of a pendulant breast with a thinned peripheral corneal stroma. The condition is usually stationary, (according to Duke-Elder) and symptomless (Fig. 38). Keratoglobus may be a sign of arrested buphthalmos. The author has treated advancing keratoglobus with a thick lamellar doner graft implanted eccentrically in a shallow recipient bed that involved the weakened cornea.

ORBITAL HEMANGIOMA

Orbital hemangiomas are the most common of all orbital tumors and usually become evident in early childhood. Their size varies greatly and, when large, they may be seen as a unilateral exophthalmos. This in turn may give the appearance of an enlarged globe (Fig. 39). On microscopic examination the younger the infant, the more cellular and invasive the tumor appears, according to Hogan and Zimmerman. Malignant in appearance, they almost always behave in a benign fashion.

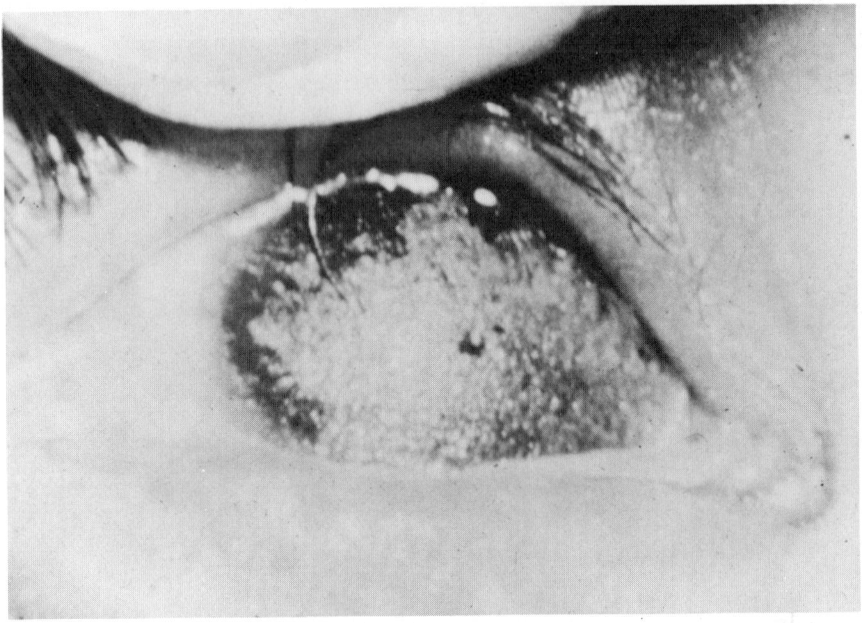

FIG. 40. Xerosis of the cornea in a 19-month-old child. (Courtesy of A. Ferry.)

KERATOMALACIA

Keratomalacia causes blindness in approximately 20,000 children each year. Xerophthalmia and nyctalopia (night blindness) are the two chief ocular signs of vitamin A deficiency. The former term includes both xerosis (Gr.dry) and keratomalacia. Xerosis (Fig. 40), a dry, lackluster cast of the cornea, is an ominous finding usually related to vitamin A deficiency, unless there is a condition of the lids or of lacrimation to account for it. Keratomalacia, a sudden whitening and softening of the cornea, is the final stage of corneal xerosis, and does not occur in the absence of vitamin A deficiency. This has been shown both on experimental and clinical grounds. Acquired night blindness is another reliable indication of vitamin A deficiency, but many children with xerophthalmia are too young to be tested for this reversible retinal dysfunction.

Bitot spots, characteristic triangular, foam-like lesions, usually located within the palpebral fissure at the temporal limbus, were first described in children with night blindness. The spots were once thought to be pathognomic of vitamin A deficiency but this is no longer considered to be

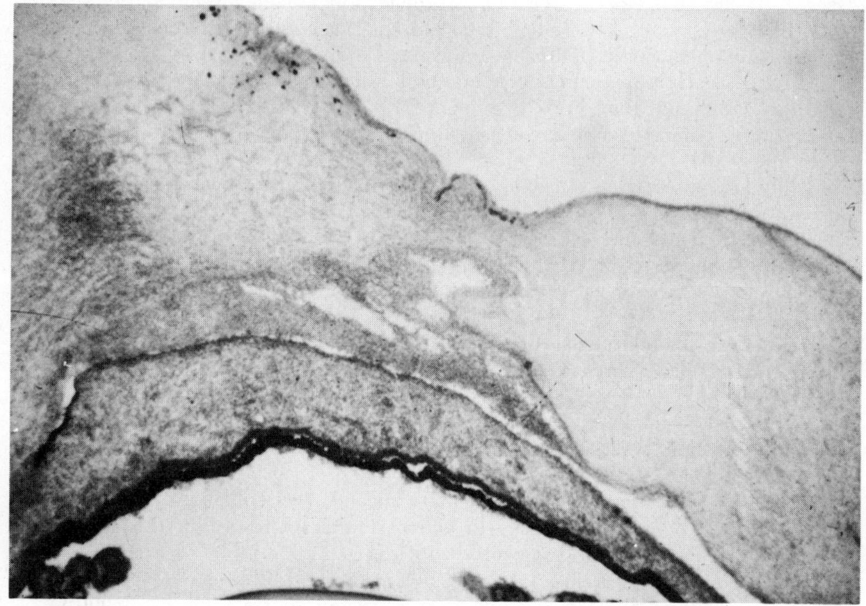

Fig. 41. Keratomalacia. The cornea has perforated.

so. In many cases corneal xerosis is transient and without sequelae, according to Paton. However, affected corneas must be considered in danger both from the threat of keratomalacia and from the increased likelihood of secondary infection.

Keratomalacia (Fig. 41) is characterized by clouding of the cornea from a sudden collequative necrosis of the stroma with whitening, softening, and sloughing of the tissue. Within a few hours, liquefaction of the cornea and prolapse of uveal tissue, with extrusion of intraocular contents and endophthalmitis, can lead to irremedial blindness.

Histologically, xerosis is a keratinization of the corneal epithelium commonly associated with a marked increase in the number of xerosis bacteria (corynebacteria), which are normally found in the conjunctival sac. Bitot spots are composed of masses of these bacilli with keratinized epithelial debris.

When corneal xerosis is followed by keratomalacia, remedial vitamin A therapy, including 100,000 units of vitamin A, 3 times a day, accompanied by a balanced diet must be initiated as quickly as possible.

References

Adler, F. H. Physiology of the Eye. Clinical Application, 3rd. ed. Mosby, St. Louis, 1959.
Allen, L., Burian, H. M., and Braley, A. E. The anterior border ring of Schwalbe and the pectinate ligament. Arch. Ophthalmol., 53:799, 1955.
Anderson, J. R. Hydrophthalmia or Congenital Glaucoma: Its Causes, Treatment and Outlook. Cambridge Univ. Press, London, 1939.
Armaignac, M. Almost complete congenital opacities of both corneas in two children of the same family. Arch. Ophthalmol., 31:468, 1911.
Axenfeld, T. L'etiologie du trachome. Acta 12th International Concilium Ophthalmologicum. Gustav. Fisher, Jena, 1914.
Ballentyne, A. J., and Michaelson, I. C. Textbook of the Fundus of the Eye. Williams & Wilkins, Baltimore, 1963.
Béal, R. Sur une forme particulière de conjunctivite aigue avec follicles. Ann. Ocul. (Paris), 137:1, 1907.
Beeler, A. Der heterotypische Conus, insbesondere der Conus nach unten und die Augbuchtung des angrenzenden Augenhintergrundes. Graefe Arch. Ophthalmol., 122:342, 1929.
Berens, C. The Eye and its Diseases. Saunders, Philadelphia, 1949, pp. 435–436.
Berliner, M. L. Lipid keratitis of Hurler's syndrome (gargoylism or dysostosis multiplex). Arch. Ophthalmol., 22:97,1939.
Bettman, J. W., and Cleasby, G. W. Congenital glaucoma. Pediatrics, 65:420, 1963.
Bickel, H. Cystine storage disease with aminoaciduria and dwarfism (Lignac-Fanconi disease). Acta Paediatr. 42, (Suppl. 90):9, 1952.
Smallwood, W. C., Smellie, J. M., and Hickmans, E. M. Clinical description, factual analysis, prognosis, and treatment of Lignac-Fanconi disease. Acta Paediatr. (Suppl. 90):27–28, 1952.
and Smellie, J. M. Cystine storage disease with aminoacidura. Lancet, 262:1093, 1952.
Bitot, P. Sur une lesion conjonctivale non encore decrit coincident avec l'hemerolopie. Gas. Hedb. Med. Chir., 10:284, 1863.
Block, B. Krankendemonstrationen aus der Dermatologischen. Klin. Zur., Schweiz Med. Wochen., 7:404, 1926.
Blum, J. D. Relations between heredito-familial degenerations and the congenital opacities of the cornea. A clinical and genaelogical study. Ophthalmologica, 109:123, 1945.
Boruchoff, A. S., and Dohlman, C. H. The Riley-Day Syndrome. Am. J. Ophthalmol., 63:523, 1967.
Brady, R. P., et al. Enzymatic defect in Fabry's disease, ceramide trihexosidase deficiency. New Eng. J. Med., 276:1163, 1967.
Braley, A. E., and Alexander, R. C. Superficial punctate keratitis. The isolation of the virus. Trans. Am. Ophthalmol. Soc., 49:283, 1951.
Brante, G. Gargoylism; a mucopolysaccharidosis. Scand. J. Clin. Lab. Invest., 4:43, 1952.
Braun-Vallon, S., et Bessman, N. La dysautonomie familiale a propos de 3 observations. Ann. Ocul. (Paris), 193:561, 1960.
Chandler, D. A., and Grant, W. M. Lectures on Glaucoma. Macmillan, Toronto, 1965.
Cogan, D. G. Syndrome of nonsyphilitic interstitial keratitis and vestibuloauditory symptoms. Arch. Ophthalmol., 33:144, 1945.
Ocular correlates of inborn metabolic defects. Can. Med. Assoc. J., 95:1055, 1966.
and Kuwabara, T. Ocular pathology of cystinosis. Arch. Ophthalmol., 63:51, 1960.
and Kuwabara, T. Ocular pathology of the 13–15 trisomy syndrome. Arch. Ophthalmol., 72:246, 1964.
Contino, F. Familial congenital opacities of the cornea. Ann. Ottal. Clin. Ocul, 69:438, 1941.

Costenbader, F. D., and Kwitko, M. L., Congenital glaucoma. Clin. Proc. Child. Hosp. (Wash.), 17:100, 1961.

and Kwitko, M. L. Congenital glaucoma, an analysis of seventy-seven consecutive eyes. J. Pediatr. Ophthalmol., 4:9, 1967.

Cullen, J. F., and Butler, H. G. Mongolism and keratoconus. Br. J. Ophthalmol., 47:321, 1963.

Dancis, J., and Smith, A. A. Familial dysautonomia. New Eng. J. Med., 274:207, 1966.

Dodge, P., cited by Smith, A. A., and Dancis, J. Physiologic studies in familial dysautonomia. J. Pediatr., 63:839, 1963.

Dohlman, C. H. Corneal edema and vascularization. In J. H. King and J. W. McTigue (Eds.), The Cornea. World Congress, Butterworth, Washington, D. C., 1965, pp. 80–95.

Duke-Elder, W. S. Textbook of Ophthalmology, Vol. II. Mosby, St. Louis, 1944, pp. 1822–1831.

System of Ophthalmology, Vol. III, Pt., 2. Congenital Deformities. Kimpton, London, 1964, pp. 509, 529, 539, and 883.

System of Ophthalmology, Vol. VII. Foundations of Ophthalmology. Kingston, London, 1962, p. 174.

System of Ophthalmology, Vol. X. Diseases of the Retina. Kimpton, London, 1967, p. 459.

Dunnington, J. H. Congenital alacrima in familial autonomic dysfunction. Arch. Ophthalmol., 52:925, 1954; and Trans. Am. Ophthalmol., Soc., 52:23, 1955.

Dunphy, E. B. Ocular conditions associated with idiopathic hyperlipemia. Trans. Am. Ophthalmol., Soc., 47:197, 1949.

Dupuy, F. I., et Madrigal, R. G. Hipertiroidismo en un mongol. Arch. Hosp. Univ., 9:389, 1957.

Eissler, R., and Longenecker, L. P., The common eye findings in mongolism. Am. J. Ophthalmol., 54:398, 1962.

El-Arabi, M. Coincidence of heredo-familial corneal dystrophy and primary pigmentary degenerations of the retina. Bull. Ophthalmol., Soc. Egypt, 46 (Pt. 1):223, 1953.

Falls, H. F. A gene producing various defects of the anterior segment of the eye. Arch. J. Ophthalmol., 32:41, 1949.

Ocular manifestations of the chronic renal tubular insufficiency syndrome. Arch. Ophthalmol., 62:188, 1959.

and Beall, J. G. Ocular varicella. Arch. Ophthalmol., 34:411, 1945.

Feigin, R. D., and Caplan, D. B. Corneal opacities in infancy and childhood. J. Pediatr., 69:383, 1966.

Fisher, F. P., and Ancona, S. Familial congenital opacities of the cornea. Acta Ophthalmol. (Kbh.), 14:406, 1936.

Forgacs, J., and Franceschetti, A. Histologic aspects of corneal changes; due to hereditary, metabolic and cutaneous affections. Am. J. Ophthalmol., 47:191, 1959.

Forsius, H. Arcus senilis corneae. Acta Ophthalmol. (Suppl.) (Kbh.), 42:1, 1954.

Franceschetti, A. Kurzes Handbuch der Ophthalmologie. Springer, Berlin, 1930, p. 712.

and Babel, J. A study of the anatomical classification of familial degenerations of the cornea. Ophthalmologica, 109:169, 1949.

Klein, B., Forni, D., and Babel, J. Clinical and social aspects of heredity in ophthalmology. Acta 16th Conc. Ophthalmol. Britannia, 1950, p. 157.

Francois, J., et Rabaey, M. Examen histochimique de la dystrophie cornéenne et étude de l'hérédite dans un cas de gargoylisme (Maladie de Hurler). Ann. Ocul. (Paris), 185:784, 1952.

Gardner, L. I., and Bergstrom, W. H. In W. E. Nelson, (Ed.), Textbook of Pediatrics, 8th ed. Saunders, Philadelphia, 1964, p. 1346.

Gellis, S. S. In W. E. Nelson, (Ed.), Textbook of Pediatrics, 6th ed. Saunders, Philadelphia, 1950, p. 1038.

Ginsberg, J., and Perrin, E. V. D. Ocular manifestations of 13–15 trisomy. Arch. Ophthalmol., 74:487, 1965.
Ginsberg, S. P. Familial Dysautonomia. The Riley-Day Syndrome. Clin. Pediat., 5:308, 1966.
Goldberg, M. F., and Duke, J. R. Ocular histopathology in Hunter's syndrome, systemic mucopolysaccharidosis Type II. Arch. Ophthalmol., 77:503, 1967.
Maumenee, A. E., and McKusick, V. A. Corneal dystrophies associated with abnormalities of mucopolysaccharide metabolism. Arch. Ophthalmol., 77:503, 1967.
Maumenee, A. E., and McKusick, V. A. Corneal dystrophies associated with abnormalities of mucopolysaccharide metabolism. Arch. Ophthalmol., 74:516, 1965.
Payne, J. W., and Brunt, P. W. Ophthalmologic studies of familial dysautonomia, the Riley-Day syndrome. Arch. Ophthalmol., 80:732, 1968.
Gorlin, R. J., and Pindborg, J. J. Syndrome of the Head and Neck. McGraw-Hill, New York, 1961.
Grayson, M. Edematous dystrophy of the cornea. Eye, Ear, Nose, Throat Mon., 47:441, 1968.
Gross, E. G. Beitrag zur Pathologischen Anatomie des Hydrophthalmus. Arch. Augenheilkd., 48:340, 1903.
Halberstaedter, L., and von Prowazek, S. Zur Aetiologie des Trachoms Berl. Klin. Wschr., 46:1110, 1909.
Hogan, M. J., and Bietti, G. Hereditary deep dystrophy of the cornea (polymorphous). Am. J. Ophthalmol., 68:777, 1969.
and Cordes, F. C. Lipochondrodystrophy (dysostosis multiplex; Hurler's Disease). Pathologic changes in the cornea in three cases. Arch. Ophthalmol.,
Howard, R. O Familial dysautonomia. Am. J. Ophthalmol., 64:392, 1967.
Hurler, G. Ueber einen Typ multipler Abartungen Vorwiegend am Skelettsystema. Z. Kinderh., 24:220, 1919.
Hutchinson, J. H., and Hamilton, W. Familial dysautonomia in two siblings. Lancet, 1:1216, 1962.
Jay, B., Blach, R. K., and Wells, R. S. Ocular manifestations of ichthyosis. Br. J. Ophthalmol., 52:217, 1968.
Jensen, V. J. Dermochondral corneal dystrophy. Acta Ophthalmol., (Kbh.), 36:71, 1958.
Jones, S. T., and Zimmerman, L. E. Macular dystrophy of the cornea. Am. J. Ophthalmol., 47:1, 1959.
and Zimmerman, L. E. Histopathologic differentiation of granular and lattice dystrophies of cornea. Am. J. Ophthalmol., 51:394, 1961.
Kaufmann, M. I. H. Herpes zoster ophthalmicus in a child. Unpublished data.
Keitch, C. G. Riley-Day syndrome, Br. J. Ophthalmol., 49:667, 1965.
Kenyon, K. R., and Artine, B. The pathogenesis of congenital hereditary endothelial dystrophy of the cornea. Am. J. Ophthalmol., 72:787, 1971.
Kielar, R. A., Cunningham, G. C., and Gerson, K. L. Occurrence of herpes zoster ophthalmicus in a child with absent immunoglobin A and deficiency of delayed hypersensitivity. Am. J. Ophthalmol., 72:555, 1971.
Komoto, J. Congenital hereditary opacities of the cornea. Klin. Monatsbl. Augenheilkd., 472:445, 1909.
Kressler, R. J., and Aegerter, E. E. Hurler's Syndrome (gargoylism). A summary of the literature and a report of a case with autopsy findings. J. Pediatr., 12:579, 1938.
Kroop, I. G. The production of tears in familial dysautonomia. Preliminary report. J. Pediatr., 48:328, 1956.
Kwedar, E. W. Hereditary nonprogressive deep corneal dystrophy. Arch. Ophthalmol., 65:127, 1961.
Kwitko, M. L. Congenital glaucoma, a clinical study. Can. J. Ophthalmol., 2:91, 1967.
Anterior segment anomalies, a clinical pathological report of conditions simulating congenital glaucoma. Can. J. Ophthalmol., 3:116, 1968.

Glaucoma in infants and children. Mod. Med. Can., 23:1, 1968; and Mod. Med. Aust., 12:3, 1969.
Wener, J., Simon, M. A., and Pintar, K. The inhibition of iris lipidosis in rabbits with oral magnesium. Can. J. Ophthalmol., 1:240, 1966.
Labirgall, G. S. Eye in hepatolenticular degeneration. Am. J. Ophthalmol., 55:1260, 1963.
Lamy, M., Aussannaire, M., Nezelof, C., Frezal, J., Jammet, M. L., Rey, J., and Labrune, B. Icthyosiform erythroderma of the newborn. Arch. Fr. Pediatr., 19:867, 1962.
Royer, P., and Nezelof, C. Presence of cellular inclusions in subjects with gargoylism. Presse Med., 67:1058, 1959.
Leith, A. B. Episceral venous pressure in tonography. Br. J. Ophthalmol., 47:271, 1963.
Lever, W. F. Histopathology of the Skin, 2nd ed. Lippincott, Philadelphia, 1961, pp. 326–336.
Liebman, S. D. Ocular manifestations of Riley-Day syndrome. Arch. Ophthalmol., 56:719, 1956.
Riley-Day syndrome (familial dysautonomia). Arch. Ophthalmol., 58:188, 1957.
Lieder, M. Practical Pediatric Dermatology, 2nd ed. Mosby, St. Louis, Chap. 12, 1961.
Manschot, W. A. Ocular anomalies in osteogenesis imperfecta. Ophthalmologica, 149:241, 1965.
Maumenee, A. E. Congenital hereditary corneal dystrophy. Am. J. Ophthalmol., 50:1114, 1960.
McGee, H. B., and Falls, H. F. Hereditary polymorphous deep degeneration of the cornea. Arch. Ophthalmol., 50:462, 1953.
McKusick, V. A. Heritable disorders of connective tissue. VII. The Hurler syndrome. J. Chron. Dis., 3:360, 1956.
Heritable Disorders of Connective Tissue, 2nd ed. Mosby, St. Louis, 1960.
McLaren, D. S. Malnutrition and the Eye. Academic Press, New York, London, 1963.
Meyer, K., et. al., P. Excretion of sulfated mucopolysaccharides in gargoylism. Proc. Soc. Exp. Biol. Med., 97:275, 1958.
Miller, et. al., A chromosomal anomaly with multiple ocular defects. Am. J. Ophthalmol., 55:901, 1963.
Morquio, L. Sur une forme de dystrophie osseuse familiale. Arch. Med. Enf., 32:129, 1929.
Nakanishi, I., and Brown, S. I. The histopathology and ultrastructure of congenital central corneal opacity (Peter's anomaly). Arch. Ophthalmol., 72:801, 1971.
Nelson, W. E. Textbook of Pediatrics, 6th ed. Saunders, Philadelphia, 1950, p. 231.
Textbook of Pediatrics, 8th ed. Saunders, Philadelphia, 1964.
Newell, F. W., and Koistinen, A. Lipochondrodystrophy (gargoylism). Pathologic findings in five eyes of three patients. Arch. Ophthalmol., 53:45, 1955.
Nizetic, B., et Sakic, D. Degeneration nodulaire de la cornée (Groenouw) liée a la couleur de l'iris (pedigree d'une famille). Acta Genet., 7, No. 2:274, 1957.
Norton, E. W. D., and Cogan, D. G. Syndrome of nonsyphilitic interstitial keratitis and vestibuloauditory symptoms. Arch. Ophthalmol., 61:695, 1959.
Oberman, W. J., et. al., Electrophoretic analysis of serum proteins in infants and children. I. Normal values from birth to adolescence. New Eng. J. Med., 255:742, 1957.
Oliner, L., et. al., Non-syphilitic interstitial keratitis and bilateral deafness (Cogan's syndrome) associated with essential polyangiitis (periarteritis nodosa). Review of syndrome with consideration of possible pathological mechanisms. New Eng. J. Med., 248:1001, 1953.
Paton, D. Keratomalacia, a review of its relationship to xerophthalmia and its response to treatment. Eye, Ear, Nose, Throat Mon., 46:186, 1967.
Peters, A. Ueber angeborene Defektibildung der Descemetschen Membran. Klin. Monatsbl. Augenheilkd., 44:27, 1906.

Ueber angeborene Staphylome. Cbl. Prak. Augenheilkd., 36:330, 1912.

Zur Frage der angelbornen Staphylome. Klin. Monatsbl. Augenheilkd., 76:803, 1926.

Pickard, R. Varicella of the cornea. Br. J. Ophthalmol., 20:15, 1936.

Pilger, I. S. Familial dysautonomia. Report of a case with stimulation of tear production by prostigmine. Am. J. Ophthalmol., 43:285, 1957.

Prangen, A. de H. The myopia problem. Arch. Ophthalmol., 22:1083, 1939.

Reese, A. B., and Ellsworth, R. M. The anterior chamber cleavage syndrome. Arch. Ophthalmol., 75:307, 1966.

Riley, C. M. Familial dysautonomia. Adv. Pediatr., 9:157, 1957.

Rochat, G. F. Die Corneauveranderungen bei der Dysostosis Multiplex. Ophthalmologica, 103:353, 1942.

Roger, F. C., et. al., Nutritional lesions of the external eye and their relationship to plasma levels of Vitamin A and the light thresholds. Acta Ophthalmol. (Kbh.), 42:1, 1964.

Rohner, M. A statistical study of the frequency of myopia. Schweiz Med. Wschr., 62:706, 1932.

Rosen, E. Interstitial keratitis and vestibuloauditory symptoms following vaccination. Arch. Ophthalmol., 41:24, 1949.

Rotth, A. Die Bedeutung der Verrucu des Lidrandes in der Aetiologie gewisser Bindehaut und Hornhautentzundungen. Klin. Monatsbl. Augenheilkd., 91:196, 1933.

Salleras, A. Bullous keratopathy. J. H. King and J. W. McTigue (Eds.), The Cornea. World Congress, Butterworth, Washington, D.C., 1965, pp. 292–299.

Scheie, H. G., Hambrick, G. W., Jr., and Barness, L. A. A newly recognized forme fruste of Hurler's disease (gargoylism). Am. J. Ophthalmol., 53:753, 1962.

Schub, M. Corneal opacities in Down's syndrome with thyrotoxicosis. Arch. Ophthalmol., 80:618, 1968.

Shinebourne, E., Sneddon, J. M., and Turner, P. Evidence for autonomic denervation in familial dysautonomia: the Riley-Day syndrome. Br. Med. J., 4:91, 1967.

Smith, A. A., Dancis, J., and Breinin, B. Ocular responses to autonomic drugs in familial dysautonomia. Invest. Ophthalmol., 4:358, 1965.

Farbman, A., and Dancis, H. Absence of taste-bud papillae in familial dysautonomia. Science, 147:1040, 1965.

Smith, J. L. Testing for congenital syphilis in interstitial keratitis. Am. J. Ophthalmol., 72:816, 1971.

Smith, R. S., Maddox, S. F., and Collins, B. E. Congenital alacrima. Arch. Ophthalmol., 79:45, 1968.

Snyder, W. B. Hereditary epithelial corneal dystrophy. Am. J. Ophthalmol., 55:56, 1963.

Sorsby, A. Systemic Ophthalmology, 2nd ed. Mosby, St. Louis, 1958, pp. 187–190 and 569–570.

Sourasky, A. Race, sex, and environment in the development of myopia (preliminary communication). Br. J. Ophthalmol., 12:197, 1928.

Spaeth, G. L., and Frost, P. Fabry's disease. Arch. Ophthalmol., 74:760, 1965.

Spencer, W. H., et. al., Late degenerative changes in the cornea following breaks in Descemet's membrane. Trans. Am. Acad. Ophthalmol. Otolaryngol., 70:973, 1966.

Stephenson, W. V. Anterior megalophthalmos and arachnodactyly. Am. J. Ophthalmol. 28:315, 1945.

Sulzberger, M. B. Uber ein bisher nicht beschriebene Congenitale Pigmentanomalie (Incontinentia pigmenti). Arch. Dermatol. Syph. (Berl.), 154:19, 1928.

Thomas, C. L. Cornea and sclera. Arch. Ophthalmol., 65:243, 1961.

Thygeson, P. Viral infection of the eye and adnexa. Trans. Am. Acad. Ophthalmol. Otolaryngol., 62:411, 1958.
Tost, M. Beitrag zur Dysplasia oculo-auriculo vertebralis. Klin. Monatsbl. Augenheilkd., 154:183, 1969.
Trevor-Roper, P. D. Diseases of the Cornea, Vol. II, No. 3. Int. Ophthalmol. Clin., Little, Brown, Boston, 1962, pp. 591–611.
Tucker, D. P. Blue sclerotic syndrome simulating buphthalmos. Am. J. Ophthalmol., 47:345, 1939.
Turpin, R., Tisserand, M., and Serane, J. Hereditary and congenital corneal opacities devised on three generations and involving two monozygotic twins. Arch. Ophthalmol., 3:109, 1939.
Vail, D. Megalophthalmus sine glaucoma. Arch. Ophthalmol. 6:39, 1931.
Von Noorden, G. K., Zellweger, H., and Ponseti, I. V. Ocular findings in Morquio-Ullrich's disease. Arch. Ophthalmol., 64:585, 1960.
Vossius, A. Beitrag zur Lehre von den angeborenen Conis. Klin. Monatsbl. Augenheilkd., 23:137, 1885.
Waardenburg, P. J. Genetics and Ophthalmology. Thomas, Springfield, Ill., 1963.
Wagner, F. Histologischer Befund der Hornhaut bei Dysostosis multiplex (Pfaundler-Hurler). Ber. Dtsch Ophthalmol. Ges., 55:371, 1949.
Wexler, D. Ocular histology in Hurler's disease (gargoylism). Arch. Ophthalmol., 46:14, 1951.
White, J. J. Corneal dystrophies. J. Mississippi Med. Assoc., 1:433, 1960.
Wirshing, L., Jr. Eye symptoms in acrodermatitis enteropathica. Acta Ophthalmol., (Kbd.), 40:567, 1962.
Wollensak, J. Charakteristische Augenbefunde beim Syndroma Block-Sulzberger (Incontinentia pigmenti). Klin. Monatsbl. Augenheilkd., 134:692, 1959.
Wong, V. G., Leitman, P. S., and Seegmiller, J. E. Alterations of pigment epithelium in cystinosis. Arch. Ophthalmol., 77:361, 1967.
Wright, J. C., and Meyer, G. E. A review of the Schirmer test for tear production. Arch. Ophthalmol., 67:564, 1962.
Yanoff, M., Frayer, W. C., and Scheie, H. G. Ocular findings in a patient with 13–15 trisomy. Arch. Ophthalmol., 70:372, 1963.
Zeeman, W. P. C. Gargoylismus. Acta Ophthalmol. (Kbh.), 20:40, 1942.
Zellweger, H., Giaccai, L., and Firzili, S. Gargoylism and Morquio's disease. Am. J. Dis. Child., 84:421, 1952.
Ponseti, I. V., et. al., Morquio-Ullrich disease. J. Pediatr., 59:549, 1961.
Zweifach, P. H. Incontinentia pigmenti, its association with retinal dysplasia. Am. J. Ophthalmol., 62:716, 1966.

11

Secondary Glaucoma in Infancy and Childhood

Secondary glaucoma in young children represents a distinct ophthalmologic entity which differs from buphthalmia in origin but may present with similar signs and symptoms.

A wide variety of conditions influence aqueous humor circulation in the child and give rise to an elevated intraocular pressure. In this chapter the pathogenesis of these conditions will be discussed.

INFLAMMATION

Inflammatory agents may damage the outflow apparatus of the eye and result in increased intraocular pressure.

Chemical

Caustic chemicals may scar the conjunctiva, sclerosing the filtration canals including the aqueous veins. Fig. 1 (See colorplate, frontis.) illustrates a tear gas burn of the eye involving the limbal area and adjacent structures. After the acute inflammation subsided, a dense sclerosis was present and an intraocular pressure of 60 mm Hg was recorded. Intensive glaucoma therapy was required. Other chemicals such as ammonia and french polish may produce an iritis and cyclitis and secondary glaucoma.

Infection

SYPHILIS. The *Treponema Pallidum* organism can be found in high concentrations in the clear cornea and otherwise histologically normal uvea of

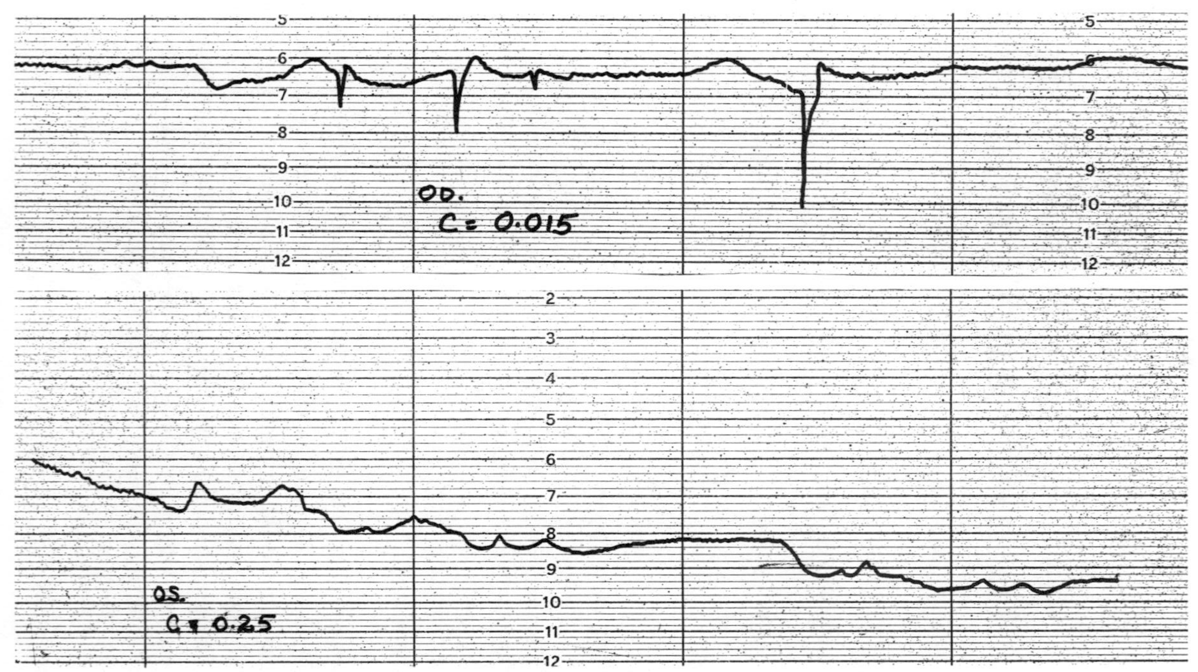

FIG. 1.B. Tear gas burn of eye. Tonography tracings. (Courtesy of R. Cordero Morino.)

the luetic fetus and newborn child. Present evidence would indicate that the spirochete may be found in the anterior chamber of syphilitic patients who have apparently undergone successful treatment. The most characteristic ocular disease associated with congenital syphilis is interstitial keratitis, which may be complicated by iritis and iridocyclitis. Secondary glaucoma may thus arise, causing an enlargement of the globe. An ectasia of the cornea results when the raised intraocular pressure is applied to an already diseased and weakened corneal stroma.

TUBERCULOSIS. Immunity is low or absent in the child but after infection, tissue hypersensitivity develops rapidly. Secondary glaucoma results when the tuberculous infection involves the anterior segment of the eye either by interference with the circulation of aqueous humor between the posterior and anterior chambers by inflammatory synechiae or by blockage of the iridocorneal angle with inflammatory debris.

OTHER BACTERIA. Various other bacterial agents may cause iritis and uveitis either by direct invasion or by an indirect immunologic response. These bacterial conditions include meningitis, typhoid fever, sarcoidosis, brucellosis, influenza, scrub typhus (tsutsugamushi disease), typhus fever, and scarlet fever.

SINUS DISEASE. A secondary ocular inflammatory response resulting in uveitis and secondary glaucoma may be associated with nonspecific sinus disease. Treatment of the sinus condition may alleviate the eye condition.

PROTOZOAL INFECTIONS. Toxoplasmosis (*Toxoplasma gondii*) is a common cause of uveitis and secondary glaucoma. Relapsing fever (*Spirochaeta recurrentis Obermeier*) and Weil's disease (*Spirochaetosis icterohaemorrhagica*) may also cause uveitis.

METAZOAN INFECTIONS. Onchocerciasis (*Onchocera volvulus* or *Onchocerca caecutiens*) may affect the anterior segment of the eye. A hypopion composed of dead microfilariae and chronic inflammatory cells causes a mechanical and inflammatory obstruction of the filtration angle, giving rise to secondary glaucoma.

PARASITIC CYSTS OF THE EYE. Hydatid disease of the eye (*T. echinococcus*) is associated with the formation of a thick-walled cyst beneath the retina, which may show great enlargement. The result is often a painful absolute glaucoma.

Rubella and Other Viral Diseases

After infection results in maternal rubella, the virus disseminates throughout the fetus, affecting developing tissues at a critical period in gestation. The formation of anterior chamber angle may be altered, leading to glaucoma (although cataracts are the most frequent abnormality found). The ocular pathology associated with maternal rubella infection has already been discussed (Chap. 1).

A wide variety of other viruses may cause iritis and uveitis; these include smallpox, herpes zoster, herpes simplex, mumps, and infectious mononucleosis. Peripheral anterior synechiae and posterior synechiae may be formed by the inflammatory reaction. Secondary glaucoma will follow if a significant portion of the filtration angle is involved. Yellow fever, another viral infection, results in extreme hemolysis. Hemorrhages may appear in the anterior chamber and the vitreous. The normal aqueous humor circulation is thus affected.

Nonspecific Inflammatory Diseases

Still's disease may be associated with uveitis and secondary glaucoma. Heterochromic iridocyclitis is another form of secondary glaucoma seen in young patients.

TRAUMA

Trauma to the eye may result in a variety of clinical manifestations, depending on the type of injury sustained and the structures involved.

Nonpenetrating Wounds

Nonpenetrating blunt injuries in young children are frequently followed by complications that lead to glaucoma. Trauma affecting the iris may cause injury and rupture of the sphincter muscle and iris root. This may result in mydriasis (Fig. 2, see colorplate, frontis), atrophy of iris stroma, and hemorrhage into the anterior chamber with glaucoma. Trauma affecting the ciliary body may produce a tear which begins at the anterior margin of the ciliary body and extends backward toward the major arterial circle, severing some of its branches. This type of injury often produces severe recurrent anterior chamber hemorrhage. Alper has described the gonioscopic appearance of this injury and noted the excessively deep recess of this portion of the filtration angle.

The histologic appearance has been described by d'Ombrain and by Wolfe and Zimmerman. Healing of the ciliary body tear (Fig. 3) results in

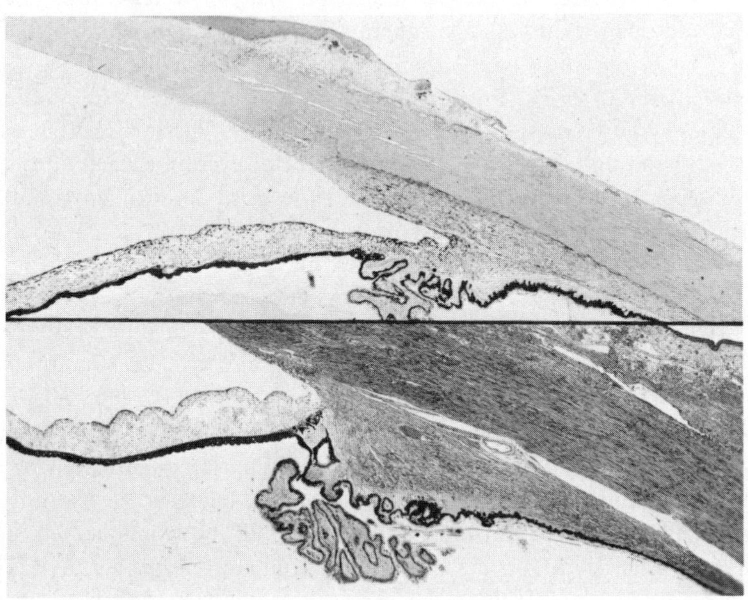

FIG. 3. Composite photograph illustrates postcontusion angle deformity (A. F. I. P. Neg. 61457, X 18.) compared with the normal angle (A. F. I. P. Neg. 814227, X 18.) (From Hogan and Zimmerman. **Ophthalmic Pathology**, 2nd ed., 1961. Courtesy of W. B. Saunders Company and the Registry of Ophthalmic Pathology of the Armed Forces Institute of Pathology.)

permanent damage to the aqueous outflow passages. If a large area is involved, glaucoma results. However, the onset is usually at a much later date, perhaps when the child has reached adulthood. Fig. 4 (See colorplate frontis.) illustrates the angle of a young child who sustained such an injury. Five years later a coefficient of outflow of 0.12 was recorded in the injured eye. The coefficient of outflow in the normal eye was 0.35.

Every case of uniocular glaucoma must be carefully examined with the gonioscope and slitlamp to determine any evidence of trauma to the iris and filtration angle. Iris atrophy and a deep recess in one portion of the iridocorneal angle are significant pieces of evidence of an earlier nonperforating ocular injury.

The scleral spur may also be torn by the blunt injury to the globe. The anterior ciliary vessels may be ruptured so that a hyphema is frequently seen in these cases.

Hemorrhages into the anterior chamber vary in quantity, clotting tendency, and recurrence. Small hemorrhages generally remain suspended in aqueous and diffuse through the aqueous outflow channels. Some of the red blood cells break down and degenerate. Large hemorrhages (Fig. 5, see colorplate, frontis) may fill the entire anterior chamber. Circulation in these cases is poor and clotting commonly occurs. The hemorrhage which results with the initial injury generally clears. However, in a small number of cases a secondary hemorrhage occurs on the third to fifth day, and this condition may be particularly resistant to treatment.

Persistent or recurrent hemorrhages may result in the formation of inflammatory membranes and adhesions between the iris, cornea, and lens—often involving the filtration angle. Secondary glaucoma occurs when the flow of aqueous is blocked. The injury may also affect the endothelium of the cornea so that hemoglobin passes into the corneal stroma, causing the so-called *blood staining* of the cornea.

The intraocular pressure must be determined frequently during this phase of the injury. A rise in pressure signals a blockage to the outflow channels. In this event intravenous urea should be administered intravenously in a dosage of 1 g/Kg body weight (run at 60 drops per minute), as advised by Kwitko and Costenbader. Acetazolamide (Diamox) should not be used as it decreases aqueous humor formation, which would reduce the normal aqueous flow required to irrigate the anterior chamber. Intravenous urea may be administered as many as three times as long as the nonprotein nitrogen level is normal.

If the intraocular pressure remains high, surgical intervention is indicated (Chap. 13).

Contusion of the globe may also dislocate the lens. When there is incomplete rupture of the zonular fibers, subluxation may result, but the lens, even though freely movable, remains in the hyaloid fossa. When the zonules are completely ruptured, dislocation may take place into the anterior chamber. The pupil and filtration angle are thus blocked, producing glaucoma (Fig. 6).

Penetrating Wounds

Following a penetrating injury to the eye, organization of the blood and fibrous tissue may occur with the formation of peripheral anterior synechiae. If the angle and pupillary region are involved, secondary glaucoma will follow (Fig. 7). When there is faulty wound healing, the surface epithelium may proliferate through the tract and into the eye, to line the filtration angle (epithelial downgrowth). Eventually glaucoma is produced.

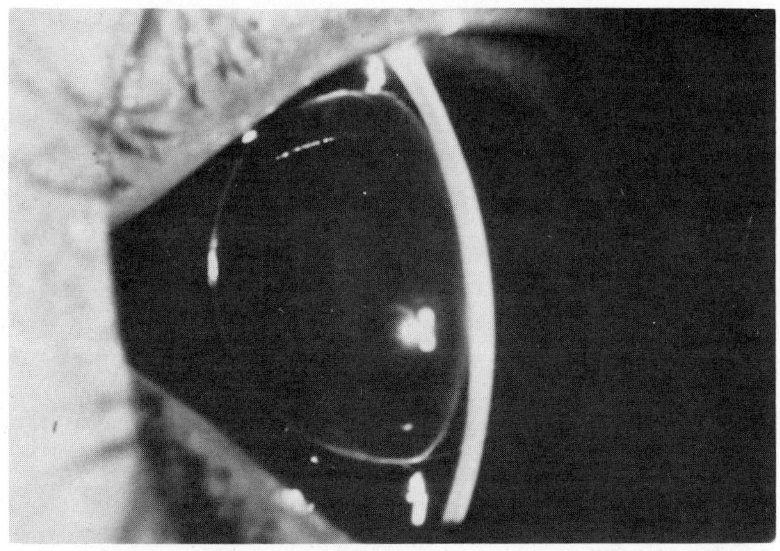

FIG. 6. Dislocation of lens into anterior chamber. (Courtesy of J. Barraquer.)

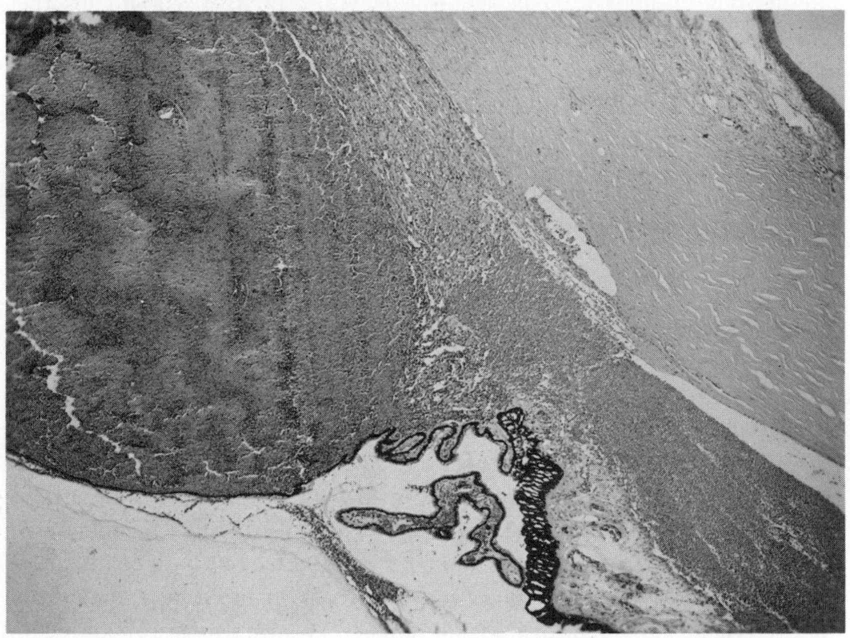

FIG. 7. Penetrating wound with hemorrhage into anterior chamber and ciliary body (A. F. I. P. Neg. 941796. (Courtesy of the Registry of Ophthalmic Pathology of the Armed Forces Institute of Pathology.) X 56.

Phacoanaphylactic Endophthalmitis

The term was introduced by Verhoeff and Lemoyne and Straub. This condition follows a perforating injury to the lens and usually affects only the injured eye. The inflammation may develop insidiously or acutely; the condition presents the usual appearance of uveitis with a hazy cornea, conjunctival congestion, white keratitic precipitates, and intense cellular exudation into the anterior chamber. Microscopically an intense infiltration of polymorphonuclear leukocytes is present. A zone of large mononuclear cells, epithelioid cells, and giant cells surrounds the area where the lens capsule is ruptured. The adjacent iris and ciliary body are intensely inflamed and infiltrated with lymphocytes and plasma cells. The iris is firmly bound to the lens by an inflammatory membrane.

Foreign Bodies

Lead and zinc are poorly tolerated in the eye. Copper may be oxidized and absorbed, leading to chalcosis. Iron may also be oxidized and absorbed after which it is distributed throughout the eye in an ionized form which is histochemically identical to hemosiderin. It combines with the proteins within the cells of the affected tissue to form insoluble salts, thus interfering with the metabolic activity of the cells. Signs of siderosis appear about one year following the injury. The iris epithelium, dilator muscle, ciliary epithelium, corneoscleral trabeculum, and uveal stroma may be involved. Glaucoma is a frequent complication.

Sympathetic Ophthalmia

Sympathetic ophthalmia may follow ocular injury with prolapse of iris or ciliary body tissue. The clinical picture is that of a typical granulomatous endopthalmitis which develops after an incubation period of two weeks or more. On microscopic examination a diffuse massive lymphocytic infiltration of uveal tissue is seen. Areas of epithelioid cells with occasional giant cells are superimposed on the lymphocytic infiltrate (Fig. 8). The inflammation, limited by Bruch's membrane, does not affect the choriocapilaris and the overlying pigment epithelium and retina. A massive exudate of epithelioid cells and lymphocytes with scattered cells and cell fragments from the

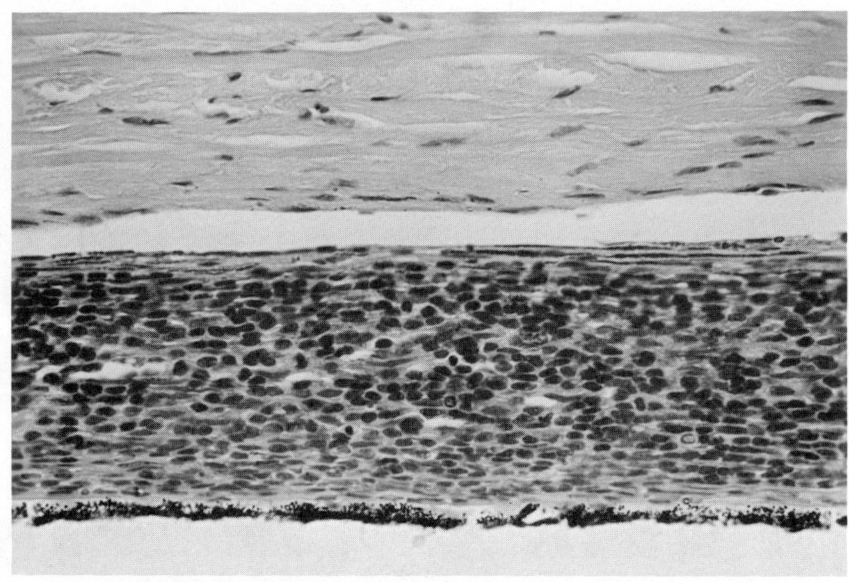

FIG. 8. Sympathetic ophthalmia (A. F. I. P. Neg. 940292. X 420.) (Courtesy of the Registry of Ophthalmic Pathology of the Armed Forces Institute of Pathology.)

pigment epithelium usually forms on the surface of the ciliary processes and in the space between the iris and the lens.

CAROTID-CAVERNOUS SINUS FISTULA

Spontaneous carotid-cavernous sinus fistula may occur from the rupture of a small aneurysm of the carotid artery. However, in general this condition follows an injury to the head and results from a tear of the carotid artery wall as it traverses the cavernous sinus. In this way arterial blood passes into the cavernous sinus and its tributaries. Engorgement and pulsation of orbital and retinal vessels results, leading to ocular throbbing. This is later followed by dilatation of conjunctival vessels (Fig. 9) and chemosis of the fornices. A hematoma is often present in the sinus. At an early stage the typical fundus picture is that of venous engorgement and pulsation. This is followed by arterial and venous thrombosis in long-standing cases. Proptosis is usually marked and may be bilateral because the two

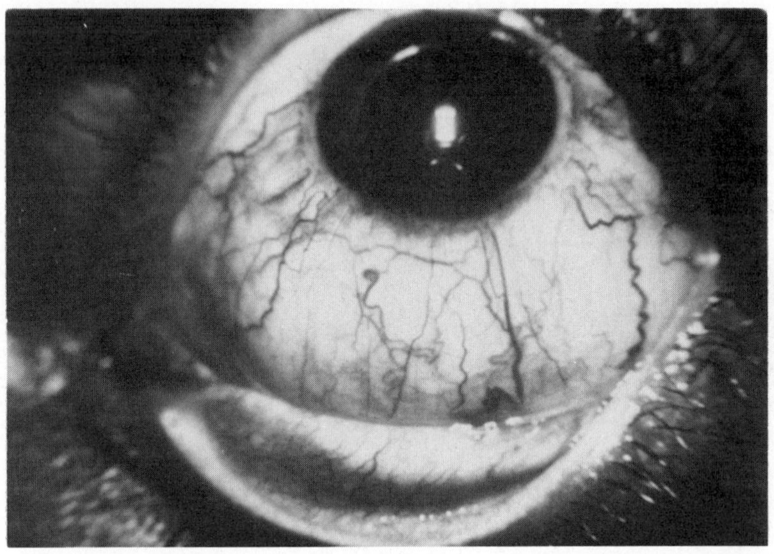

FIG. 9. Engorged conjunctival vessels following carotid-cavernous sinus fistula formation.

cavernous sinuses communicate with one another. The first and second divisions of the fifth nerve are often involved, resulting in ophthalmoplegia, pain, and hypalgesia. A systolic bruit, loudest over the affected eye and orbit, is usually present. The bruit may be diminished by compression of the appropriate internal carotid artery in the neck.

CONGENITAL TUMORS

An intraocular tumor may cause a rise in intraocular pressure by several means, namely: (1) hemorrhage resulting from the rupture of blood vessels supplying the neoplasm may block the trabecular spaces; (2) the tumor may become enlarged to the extent of causing an anterior displacement of the lens-iris diaphragm, and angle closure glaucoma; (3) tumor cells may invade the iris and filtration angle and cause an obstruction to aqueous outflow.

Retinoblastoma

Retinoblastoma is a congenital, inheritable malignant tumor that occurs almost exclusively in children. It arises from the nuclear layers of the retina and develops characteristically from multiple foci in one or both eyes. Although congenital, it is usually not recognized at birth (Fig. 10, see colorplate, frontis). The incidence of retinoblastoma is reported between one case in every 34,000 births and one in 23,000; one-third of all cases are bilateral. The tumor is composed of highly undifferentiated anaplastic cells which are uniformly small, round, or polygonal with a scanty and poor-staining cytoplasm. The cells' relatively large nuclei, rich in chromatin, stain deeply with hematoxylin and sometimes appear to be entirely free of cytoplasm or at the most to possess a tail-like process on each side, which makes the cell appear like an embryonic retinal cell. The characteristic histologic feature is the Flexner-Wintersteiner rosette formation. In true rosettes the columnar cells are arranged in a ring about a central circular lumen which is bordered by a fine limiting membrane. Sometimes protoplasmic processes from the individual cell bordering the lumen project into it, suggesting rudimentary rods and cones. Another feature is the pseudorosette. This effect may be seen as a perivascular growth of tumor cells surrounding a small blood vessel. A small group of tumor cells may degenerate, leaving a clear space that contains cellular debris surrounded by a ring of viable cells which will also give the pseudorosette appearance. Calcium deposition is another feature of this tumor that may be identified on radiologic examination. Metastases occur within the eye across the fluid-containing cavities. Debris containing tumor cells results from these metastases or from independent retinoblastic foci. This material is carried toward the filtration angle. Obstruction to the outflow apparatus may thus occur, giving rise to a secondary glaucoma (Fig. 11). Howard and Ellsworth reported a series of 235 patients with retinoblastoma. They noted the following presenting signs in order of frequency.

	No.	% of Total
White pupillary reflex	142	61.0
Strabismus	53	22.0
Decreased vision	11	5.0
Routine ocular examination (with known sibling)	6	2.0
Routine ocular examination (with no family history)	5	2.0
Orbital inflammation and proptosis	5	2.0
Red, painful eye (secondary glaucoma)	4	2.0
Unilateral dilated pupil	2	1.0
Spontaneous hyphema	1	0.5
Heterochromia iridis	1	0.5
Not recorded	5	2.0
Total	235	100.0

Secondary glaucoma was the seventh most common sign and comprised 2 percent of the total in this series.

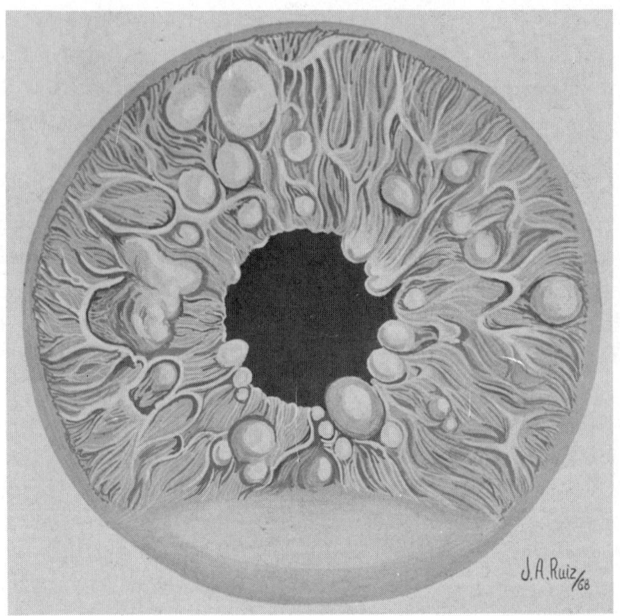

FIG. 11. Retinoblastoma. Metastases have spread to iris. Sterile hypopion is present, causing obstruction to flow of aqueous.

When the eye is obviously blinded by the tumor, an enucleation must be performed. However, small tumors are known to respond to radiation and chemotherapy. Photocoagulation has also been used as well as cryotherapy.

Neuroblastoma

This tumor (also known as sympathicoblastoma or Hutchinson's adrenal tumor), one of the most common malignancies of childhood, usually originates in the suprarenal medulla but may also develop in any part of the sympathetic nervous system including that portion within the orbit. Skeletal metastasis occurs in 74 percent of cases, particularly to the cranium. When the orbital bones are affected, the orbit becomes involved, producing exophthalmos (Fig. 12, see colorplate frontis). On histologic examination the cells are small, round, and undifferentiated, and are set in a fibrous framework. Necrotic areas may be present; fibrils are another feature.

Diktyoma

This tumor, first described in 1892, is observed most often at birth or becomes evident in early childhood when the parents note the peculiar pupillary reflex. The lesion is thought to be a choristoma. Diktyomas infilrate the zone around the lens and may spread forward into the angle and onto the cornea. If the tumor remains in the posterior cavity it may push the iris forward and obstruct the angle. All of these manifestations cause glaucoma. Histologically the tumors feature poorly differentiated neural tissue resembling embryonic retina. The masses also contain columnar epithelial cells arranged in sheets, tubes, or solid masses. Some areas resembling retinoblastoma may be seen. Ependyma-like spaces, cerebral tissue, and cartilage may be present. Frequent mitoses are noted in the marginal zone of the globe.

Leiomyoma

These tumors, which originate in the dilator and sphincter muscles of the iris, are true leiomyomas, indistinguishable histologically from smooth muscle tumors elsewhere in the body.

RETROLENTAL FIBROPLASIA (RETINOPATHY OF PREMATURITY)

In 1942 Terry described a fibrous tissue mass behind the lens in premature infants that was almost always bilateral, and coined the term retrolental fibroplasia. The disease is presently referred to as retinopathy of prematurity (Fig. 13, see colorplate, frontis.)

Eight-thousand children in the United States and six-hundred in Great Britain—that is, 30 percent of infants developing the disorder—were blinded before it was discovered that an exposure to oxygen administered in concentrations in excess of that in air for prolonged periods of time in premature infants was the sole and sufficient causative agent. There has been no documented instances of the condition occurring in infants with a gestational age of over 36 weeks. At a symposium on retrolental fibroplasia (RLF) held during the 1954 meeting of the American Academy of Ophthalmology and Otolaryngology, participants recommended (1) that routine administration of supplemental oxygen to premature babies be discontinued; (2) that it be given only if infants are cyanotic or show signs of respiratory distress; (3) that oxygen therapy be discontinued as soon as the respiratory distress is relieved. It was generally agreed that oxygen concentrations should not exceed 40 percent.

As the use of oxygen was drastically curtailed in nurseries throughout the world following this report, the incidence of retrolental fibroplasia dropped sharply, although some cases were still seen. In recent years a significant increase in the incidence of RLF has been noted. Kalina reported a series of 1,405 premature infants admitted to a special premature center. At admission 279 of them weighed 1,300 g or less. Of these 279 infants, 43 were given ophthalmic examination and six were found to have RLF with severe visual impairment; four with RLF weighed less than 1,000 g; only one of 911 survivors weighing more than 1,300 g had RLF.

Retrolental fibroplasia results from hyperoxia which causes an obliteration of the developing blood vessels of the immature retina owing to an excessively high ambient oxygen concentration. With adequate cardiovascular-respiratory function, dangerously high oxygen tensions may be achieved in the ocular circulation when a susceptible infant breathes oxygen-enriched air. Even concentrations below 40 percent are dangerous to some infants. On the other hand, in the presence of the respiratory insufficiency that occurs in the respiratory distress syndrome, 40 percent oxygen in the inspired air may be inadequate to achieve even a normal oxygen tension in the circulation. It is possible for such an infant to die of hypoxemia while breathing an oxygen mixture approaching 80 or 90 percent or even higher. There is no evidence that (in the absence of an elevated arterial blood oxygen tension) RLF can be caused by the direct diffusion of oxygen through the external surface of the eyes when they are exposed to high environmental oxygen concentrations.

In the disorder's earliest phase the sole manifestation is spasm and attenuation of the entire retinal vasculature. This is followed by tortuosity and dilatation of the vessels together with retinal hemorrhage and edema. Later there is a profuse growth of new vessels and fibrous proliferation which leads to the development of a retrolental membrane. Twenty-five percent progress to the cicatricial phase, usually in the third to fifth month.

Stages in RLF Development

STAGE I. The earliest sign is a transient threadlike attenuation of retinal blood vessels; later dilatation and tortuosity of the vessels occur. Hemorrhages may or may not be present. Early neovascularization, especially in the extreme periphery of the fundus, may be present. Often the histologic picture at this early stage of dilated retinal blood vessels (associated with an exudative detachment of the retina) resembles that of Coats' disease.

STAGE II. Neovascularization and some peripheral retinal clouding are seen in addition to changes already noted in Stage I. Hemorrhages are usually present. Vitreous clouding may or may not be present. Spontaneous regression may still occur at this stage.

STAGE III. In addition to the above changes, retinal detachment at the periphery of the fundus is seen. Spontaneous regression is unlikely at this stage.

STAGE IV. A circumferential retinal detachment is seen with elevation over a large area. Some retina remains in position.

STAGE V. Complete retinal detachment. The clinical picture at this stage is not unlike that of retinal dysplasia but the history will assist in distinguishing one disease from the other.

Grades of RLF in the Cicatricial Phase

GRADE I. A small mass of opaque tissue in the periphery of the fundus may be seen without visible retinal detachment. The fundus may have a pale appearance and the blood vessels may be attentuated.

GRADE II. A larger mass of opaque tissue in the periphery of the fundus is seen with some localized retinal detachment. The disc is distorted by traction toward the side of the tissue. These patients may still have useful vision.

GRADE III. A larger mass of opaque tissue is seen in the periphery which resembles a congenital retinal fold. Traction upon the retina produces a sharply demarcated elevated retinal septum which arches forward into the vitreous body, stretching from the disc to the extreme periphery of the fundus. Visual acuity in these patients varies from 20/50 to 5/200.

GRADE IV. Fibrovascular tissue originating near the temporal periphery of the retina extends toward the retrolental region. Dentate processes extend from the ciliary body to the retrolental tissue. The pupillary area is thus partially covered. Traction upon the retina temporally leaves an atrophic peripapillary conus nasally.

GRADE V. Retrolental tissue covers the entire pupillary area. No fundus reflex is present. In this advanced stage there is atrophy of the globe and orbit structures, posterior synechiae, and a shallow anterior chamber. The eyes usually remain small, lying deep-set in the orbits.

Complications

There are a number of other complications seen in these children. Some develop strabismic amblyopia; in others the amblyopia develops because of anisometropia, as the fundus pathology and degree of myopia are often asymmetrical. The combination of retinal edema and contraction of the retrolental fibrous connective tissue puts the ciliary processes on the stretch and forces the lens–iris diaphragm forward. The result is a shallow anterior chamber that may go on to angle closure, so that the most frequent complication is secondary glaucoma which is said to develop in 30 percent of severe cases. Cataracts develop only rarely.

Monitoring Arterial Tension P_{O_2}

Arterial blood gas measurements are helpful in determining the inspired oxygen concentration that will produce blood oxygen tensions high enough to support life but low enough to avoid the danger of RLF.

Arterial P_{O_2} measurement is a useful technique for monitoring oxygen therapy. The arterial blood may be sampled in the premature infant via the umbilical artery (by indwelling catheter), temporal artery (by percutaneous puncture), and radial artery (by percutaneous puncture). Arterialized capillary blood is not satisfactory for the determination of hyperoxic risks.

The technique of umbilical artery catheterization is performed as follows, under sterile precautions. A No. 5 French umbilical artery catheter (similar to a premature infant feeding tube but with an end hole and no side hole) is introduced through one of the umbilical arteries until its tip lies in the descending aorta. The path taken by the catheter can be demonstrated by anteroposterior and lateral radiographs. The distance of insertion can be estimated from the external dimensions of the baby. It is desirable to place the catheter tip well into the abdominal aorta. The catheter is taped to the abdominal skin and the cut end of the umbilical cord is covered with a sterile dressing. Arterial blood is sampled through a three-way stopcock attached to the end of the catheter. Between sampling periods, the catheter may be used for intravascular infusion of fluids, or it may be cross-clamped after it is filled with a measured volume of a solution of saline and heparin. Constant nursing observation is indicated so that any circulatory disturbance in the lower extremities, bleeding, or clotting of blood in the catheter can be detected. The catheter is left in place only as long as needed for monitoring oxygen therapy. Normal newborn babies breathing room air (20.94 percent oxygen) achieve an arterial P_{O_2} of 60 to 80 mm Hg on the average. Values higher than 110 mm Hg represent arterial hyperoxia. The magnitude of retinal risk has not been determined in the human premature infant for degree or duration of arterial hyperoxia. However, at the present time, studies would indicate the desirability of adjusting ambient oxygen concentration at frequent intervals (e.g., q 2 to 6 hrs) to maintain arterial P_{O_2} between 50 and 110 mm Hg.

Monitoring Ambient Oxygen

When determinations of oxygen tension are not available, the physician must be guided by the presence of generalized cyanosis, or cyanosis of the lips or the ears. It must be recognized that (1) such cyanosis may be relieved by a degree of oxygenation which is still not sufficient to achieve an arterial oxygen tension within the normal reported range and (2) cyanosis may be caused by hypothermia or peripheral vasoconstriction in the absence of hypoxemia. Thus, clinical judgment, meticulous care in recording oxygen levels, and a frequent review of current information must be exercised in order to determine the optimal percentage of oxygen enrichment.

Respiratory distress syndrome (RDS) is observed in roughly 10 percent of neonates born before 37 weeks of gestation. There is evidence which suggests that deaths associated with this disorder increased during the decade (1955 to 1965) of rigid oxygen restriction in nurseries for premature infants, and there is also evidence which suggests that the frequency of neurologic disorders—e.g., cerebral palsy—rose as the incidence of retrolental fibroplasia fell.

It is therefore recommended that oxygen therapy for newborn infants be guided by the following principles.

1. An infant who is not apneic and who has generalized or localized cyanosis (i.e., of the lips and ears), should be given sufficient oxygen to relieve this cyanosis. The inspired oxygen concentration should be 10 percent higher than that required to relieve the cyanosis (e.g., if cyanosis is overcome at 45 percent, the concentration should be increased to 55 percent). Such oxygen therapy should be authorized by a physician but may be instituted by an experienced nurse while the physician is being called.

2. The relief of cyanosis may require inspired oxygen concentrations

up to 40 percent, and rarely up to 60, 80, or even 100 percent before the arterial oxygen tension rises to an adequate level. Thus oxygen-limiting devices are inappropriate for infants requiring higher oxygen concentrations. Moreover, the performance of many of the devices in current use is erratic, especially in the absence of an active maintenance program for nursery equipment. Even a reliable limitation to 30 to 40 percent may result in hyperoxic retinal damage in susceptible infants. There is thus no substitute for frequent use of the oxygen analyzer, and no reliance should be placed on flow rates or limiting devices. If it becomes necessary to employ additional sources or devices to achieve very high oxygen concentrations, the additional oxygen must be passed either through the incubator heating and humidifying system or though an external heating-nebulizing system.

3. Oxygen administration should be curtailed as soon as improvement in the infant's condition permits. To avoid the deleterious effects created by a new episode of oxygen insufficiency in the bloodstream, the inspired oxygen concentration should not be reduced by decrements of greater than 10 percent each at intervals of 15 to 30 min, and even then only to the extent that such reduction does not precipitate clinical impairment (e.g., cyanosis, lethargy, grunting, decreased body temperature).

4. In small infants, periodic breathing is normal and needs no corrective management. However, apneic episodes should be corrected to avoid any duration beyond 20 sec, regardless of whether cyanosis occurs. Termination of an apneic episode may be accomplished with an auditory or tactile stimulus, or may require a few puffs of ventilation by face mask. A breathing bag which reinflates itself with air from within the incubator is recommended. The use of added oxygen as a substitute for close observation and ventilatory assistance when indicated may result unnecessarily in any of the deleterious effects ascribed to hyperoxia. Oxygen administration is not recommended as a means of preventing apneic spells. Thus the oxygen concentration that is considered adequate for an infant while he is breathing should not be increased simply to avoid the cyanosis which may result from a neglected apneic episode.

5. There are no clinical signs for detecting hyperoxia; and the signs of hypoxia as distinct from the safe range of oxygenation are generally unreliable. Therefore, an infant who is a candidate for prolonged (e.g., several days) oxygen therapy should be considered for transfer to a center in which arterial blood gas measurements are available.

6. An oxygen analyzer should be used to document the percentage of inspired oxygen required to meet the infant's needs, and thus to guide the oxygen flow adjustments. Frequency of oxygen analyses should be determined by the rate of change in the infant's condition, and by the amount of

random fluctuation of oxygen concentrations inherent in any particular incubator and oxygen system. In many instances, such analyses may be repeated at 2-hr intervals; however, the intervals may need to be shorter, especially in the early phase of management.

7. The oxygen analyzer should be checked at least once daily, to ensure that the reading is within 2 percent of true concentration when tested against both room air and 100 percent oxygen. When tested against 100 percent oxygen, the sample should be drawn from a 20-ml syringe barrel into which the oxygen is flowing at a rate of 1 liter per minute, rather than directly from an oxygen supply line. By testing in this way, falsely low readings from air leaks into the sampling system can be differentiated from calibration errors. In the case of an analyzer on which there are knob and/or screwdriver adjustments required by the variable output of the battery that powers the meter circuit, such testing should be carried out at least once at the start of each 8-hr shift, and even oftener to the point of recalibration with each analysis, until experience shows that once per shift is adequate.

8. Ophthalmoscopic examination of infants under 2,000 g birth weight who have received oxygen therapy should be performed through dilated pupils. The first examination should be carried out as soon as is practical, and certainly before discharge from hospital. In addition there should be another examination when the infant is three months of age. The child should be followed carefully over the first two years of life. Once RLF has become established, discontinuation of oxygen treatment does not guarantee an arrest of the condition.

JUVENILE XANTHOGRANULOMA (NEVOXANTHOENDOTHELIOMA)

Helwig and Hackney introduced the term juvenile xanthogranuloma in 1954. Hassenpflug considered the lesion to be a form of histiocytoma; however, the etiology remains unclear. There appears to be no sex differentiation. The typical skin lesion is a small nodule, slightly elevated, at first pinkish and eventually becoming yellow. It may be single or multiple, appearing at or shortly after birth. The disease is thought to be non-neoplastic and often subsides spontaneously over a period of years, leaving an umbilicated scar that usually disappears completely. The lesions are most commonly found on the scalp and head but sometimes they appear on the trunk and extremities. Similar nodules may be seen involving the conjunctiva, orbit, iris, and ciliary body. The iris lesion may appear as a diffuse

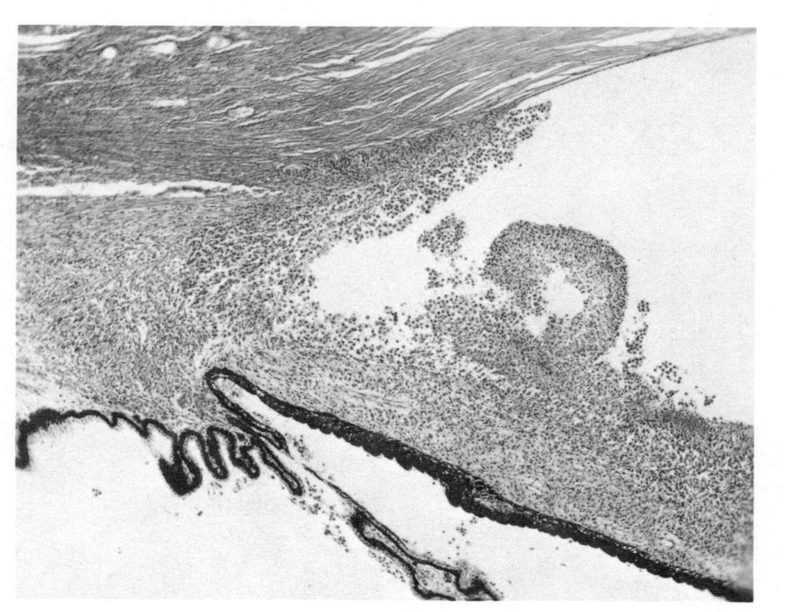

FIG. 14. Juvenile xanthogranuloma. (A. F. I. P. Neg. 916391.) (From Hogan and Zimmerman. **Ophthalmic Pathology**, 2nd ed., 1962. Courtesy of W. B. Saunders Company and the Registry of Ophthalmic Pathology of the Armed Forces Institute of Pathology.)

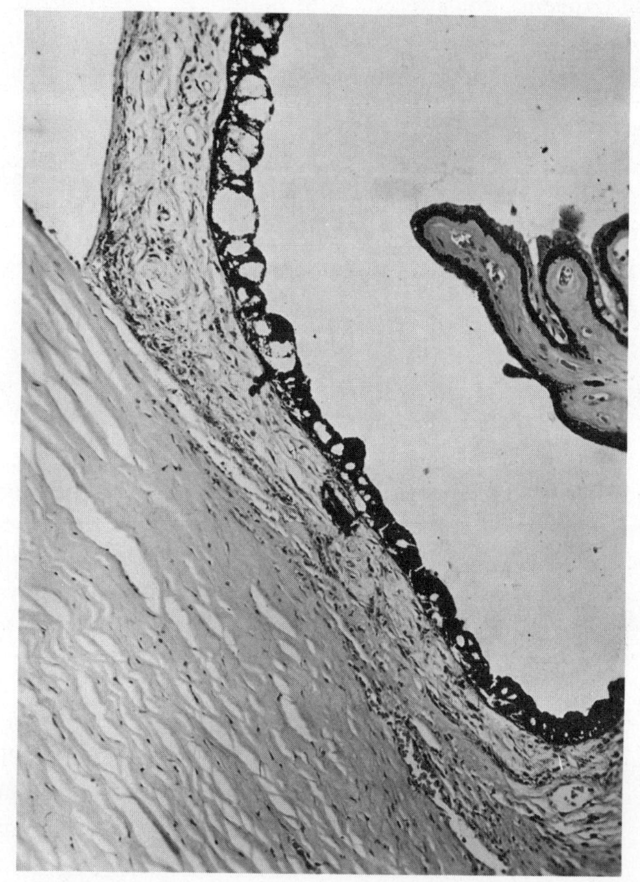

FIG. 15. Filtration angle in young diabetic. Note broad peripheral anterior synechiae blocking filtration angle. X 175.

yellow thickening and nodulation causing a heterochromia or the lesion may be entirely localized. Associated cutaneous nodules may or may not be present. The microscopic appearance of the iris is that of a diffuse or focally thickened infiltrate of large pale-staining mononuclear cells, multinucleated Touton giant cells, and eosinophils with associated large thick-walled capillaries. The ocular manifestation seen most often is a spontaneous unilateral hyphema which results with rupture of the capillaries. Blood and mononuclear cells block the filtration angle, causing glaucoma (Fig. 14). Peripheral anterior synechiae may form when the cells and blood become organized; this causes a permanent impairment of aqueous outflow.

The treatment of choice for this condition would appear to be radiotherapy when the lesion is diffuse and excision is not possible. The single dose should not exceed 200 r in order to avoid damage to the lens, with a total dose not to exceed 500 r. Topical and systemic steroids may preceed irradiation.

METABOLIC DISORDERS

Diabetes mellitus causes a form of iritis which features a marked perilimbal flush, an albuminous exudate in the anterior chamber, and numerous blood vessels on the iris surface (particularly around the pupil), with both anterior and posterior synechiae formation. Rubeosis iridis diabetica is seen especially in youngsters with severe diabetes who also suffer from systemic vascular disease, diabetic nephrosis, and hypertension. The small thin-walled blood vessels on the iris surface may rupture, causing a hyphema. Vitreous hemorrhage and retinitis proliferans are often present and the final result may be an uncontrolled glaucoma (Fig. 15). Other causes of spontaneous hyphema include: retinoblastoma, RLF, PHPV, iritis, unsuspected trauma, blood dyscrasias and juvenile xanthogranuloma.

DIETETIC DISORDERS

EPIDEMIC DROPSY. The alkaloid sanguinarine, a constituent of argemone oil, is a vasotoxic substance which produces a marked vasodilation with profuse transudation of fluid throughout the body—including the eye. This poison is ingested in contaminated mustard oil which is used for cooking in the Eastern Continents. The contaminant is argemone oil, which enters the cooking oil as argemone mexicana, a wild plant that grows among grain. The glaucomatous condition is slow in developing, with cupping of the disc and associated field loss occurring late in the disease. Often halos are the only symptom.

LENS-INDUCED GLAUCOMA

Those manifestations associated with trauma have already been discussed. Several generalized conditions such as Marfan's syndrome, sulfite oxidase deficiency, homocystinuria, Weill-Marchesani's syndrome, and Ehlers-Danlos syndrome feature a dislocated lens as part of the disease. Spherophakia and anterior lenticonus (Fig. 16) may also be associated with glaucoma.

Table 1 outlines a classification of lens-induced or phacogenic glaucoma. (Chap. 9).

TABLE 1

CLASSIFICATION OF LENS-INDUCED OR PHACOGENIC GLAUCOMA

PHACOS (the lens itself)

(1) Phacolytic glaucoma (glaucoma due to lens cortex): This condition is characterized by liquefaction of lens cortex in a hypermature lens, open iridocorneal angle, presence of large histiocytes containing engulfed liquefied lens material which obstructs the trabecular apparatus.

(2) Glaucoma capsulare (glaucoma due to pathology in lens capsule): pseudoexfoliation of the lens capsule occurs with obstruction of the intertrabecular spaces by desquamated particulate matter (hyaline flakes).

(3) Phaco-anaphylactic endophthalmitis (glaucoma due to secondary granulomatous inflammatory products from involved lens substance): anterior and/or posterior synechiae are present, with obstruction of the chamber angle by an inflammatory exudate.

PHACOMORPHIC GLAUCOMA (glaucoma associated with shape of lens)

(1) Intumescent cataract (senile or traumatic cataract): swelling of the lens may displace the iris forward and close the filtration angle or may interrupt aqueous circulation by blockage of the pupillary aperture (pupillary block).

(2) Microphakia (spherophakia): a small lens may obstruct the pupillary aperture (pupillary block).

(3) Anterior lenticonus: anterior aspect of the lens is congenitally misshapen and may "plug" the pupillary aperture (pupillary block).

PHACOTOPIC GLAUCOMA (glaucoma associated with location of lens)

For example, ectopia lentis.

*From Kwitko, M. L. Can. Med. Assoc. J., 89:569, 1963.

NORRIE'S DISEASE

This special form of congenital bilateral pseudotumor was first described by Norrie in 1927. The typical case is of X-chromosome recessive

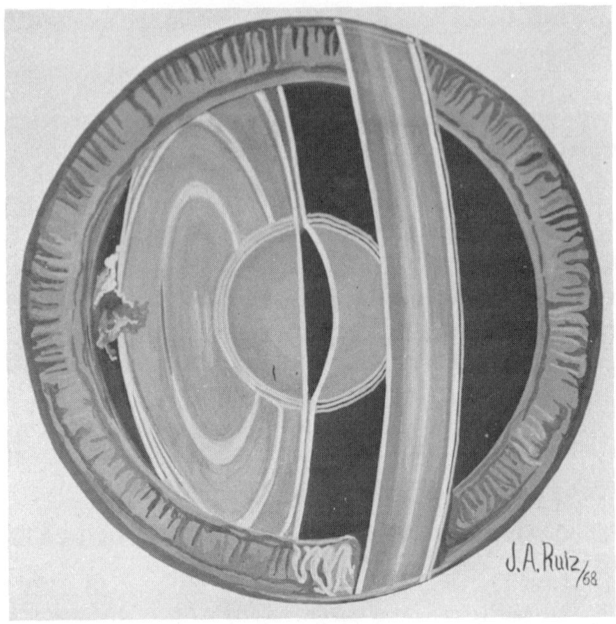

FIG. 16. Anterior lenticonus (composite slitlamp drawing).

inheritance. The histologic features include detachment of the retina with hypoplasia of the inner retinal layers, extensive synechiae, uveal ectropion, hyperplasia of the ciliary and retinal pigment epithelium, and ossification of the choroid. A retrolental mass is present, consisting of connective tissue, old hemorrhage, and persistent hyperplastic primary vitreous. Figs. 17A and B illustrate a case of bilateral blindness.

SPONTANEOUS RUPTURE OF THE EYEBALL

Goldzieher reported a massive intraocular hemorrhage in a nine-year-old girl, with elevation of the intraocular pressure leading to rupture of the globe. Pietruschka and Schill maintain that such ruptures occur because of previous degenerative inflammatory changes in the corneoscleral coat.

ADMINISTRATION OF STEROIDS

Steroid-induced glaucoma may be seen in infants and children. The disorder gives a clinical picture not unlike that of congenital glaucoma.

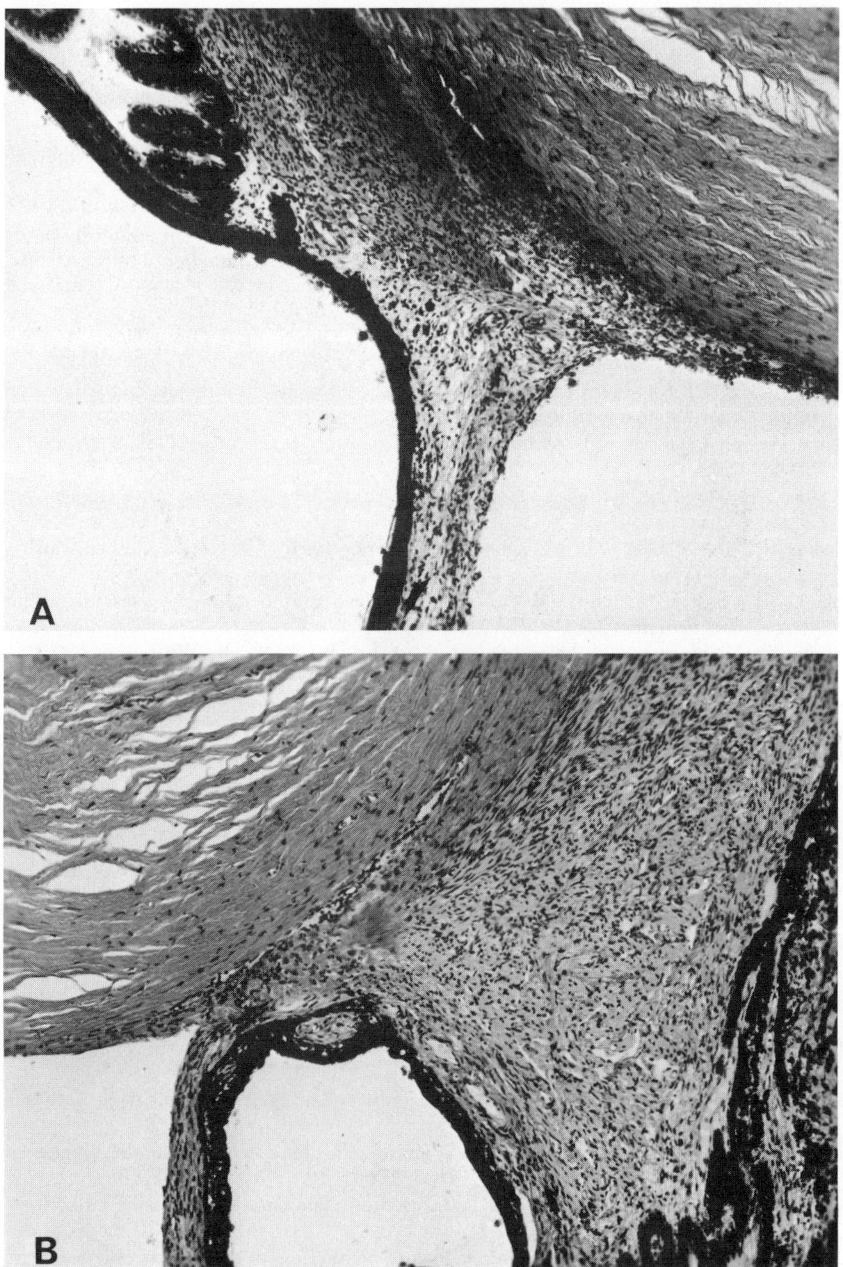

FIG. 17 A. and B. Case of bilateral blindness. Note anterior displacement of iris and insertion of longitudinal muscle fibers of ciliary body into trabeculum, anterior to scleral spur. (Courtesy of D. A. Rosen.) X 175.

Diagnosis is made when a history of topically administered cortisone is elicted. The condition usually subsides when the medication is discontinued.

References

Alfano, J. E. Steroid induced glaucoma simulating congenital glaucoma. Am. J. Ophthalmol., 61:922, 1966.

Alper, M. C. Contusion angle deformity and glaucoma. Arch. Ophthalmol., 69:455, 1963.

Anderson, S. R., and Warburg, M. Norrie's disease: congenital bilateral pseudotumor of the retina with recessive X-chromosome inheritance, Arch. Ophthalmol., 66:614, 1961.

Ashton, N., Ward, B., and Sperpell, G. Role of oxygen in the genesis of retrolental fibroplasia: a preliminary report. Br. J. Ophthalmol., 37:513, 1953.

Larval granulomatosis of the retina due to Toxocara. Br. J. Ophthalmol., 44:129, 1960.

Axenfeld, T. Über mildere und gutartige Metast. Aderhautentzündung. Ber. 25, Versl. Ophth. Ges. Heidelberg, 1896, p. 282.

Badal, A. and Lagrarge, F. Carcinome primitif des procès et du corps ciliare. Arch. Opht., 12:143, 1892.

Badtke, G. Die Missbildungen des Menschl. Auges. Der Augenarzt, IV. G. Thieme, Leipzig, 1961.

Becker, B., and Shaffer, R. N. Diagnosis and Therapy of the Glaucomas, 2nd ed. Mosby, St. Louis, 1965, p. 239.

Blank, H., Eglick, P. G., and Beerman, H. Nevo-xanthoendothelioma with ocular involvement. Pediatrics, 4:349, 1949.

Blodi, F. C. Systemic Ophthalmology, 2nd ed. Ed. by A. Sorsby. Butterworth & Co., London, 1958, p. 16.

Boniuk, M., and Zimmerman, L. E. Ocular pathology in the rubella syndrome. Arch. Ophthalmol., 77:455, 1967.

Brockhurst, R. J., Schepens, C. L., and Okamura, I. D. Uveitis: II. Peripheral uveitis: clinical description, complications and differential diagnosis. Am. J. Ophthalmol., 49:1257, 1960.

Schepens, C. L., and Okamura, I.D. Uveitis: III. Peripheral uveitis: pathogenesis, etiology and treatment. Am. J. Ophthalmol., 51:19, 1961.

Burian, H. M., and Allen, L. Histologic study of the chamber angle of patients with Marfan's syndrome. Arch. Ophthalmol., 65:323, 1961.

Byron, H. M. Ocular trauma, importance, prevention, therapy: Eye Ear Nose Throat Monthly, 42:48, 1963.

Campbell, K. Intensive oxygen therapy as a possible cause of retrolental fibroplasia: a clinical approach. Med. J. Aust., 2:48, 1951.

Coats, G. Forms of retinal disease with massive exudation. Roy. Lond. Ophthalmol., Hosp. Rep., 17:440, 1907-1908.

Uber Retinitis Exsudativa (retinitis haemorrhagiea externa). Graefs Arch. Ophthalmol., 81:275, 1912.

Cole, J. G., and Byron, H. M. Evaluation of 100 eyes with traumatic hyphema: intravenous urea. Arch. Ophthalmol., 71:35, 1964.

Costenbader, F. D., and Kwitko, M. L. Congenital glaucoma. Clin. Proc. Child. Hosp. (Wash.), 17:100, 1961.

and Kwitko, M. L. Congenital glaucoma: an analysis of seventy-seven consecutive eyes. J. Ped. Ophthalmol., 4:9, 1967.

Crosse, V. M., and Evans, P. J. Prevention of retrolental fibroplasia. Arch. Ophthalmol., 48:83, 1952.

d'Ombrain, A. Traumatic or "concussion" chronic glaucoma. Br. J. Ophthalmol., 33:495, 1949.
Duke-Elder, W. S. System of Ophthalmology, Vol. III, Pt. 2: Congenital Deformities. Henry Kimpton, London, 1964, p. 553.
System of Ophthalmology, Vol. IX: Diseases of the Uveal Tract. Henry Kimptom, London, 1966, pp. 656-661.
Dunn, P. M. Localization of the umbilical catheter by postmortem measurement. Arch. Dis. Child., 41:69, 1966.
Editorial. Oxygen therapy in the pre-term infant. Can. Med. Assoc. J., 99:564, 1968.
Falls, H. F., and Neil, J. V. Genetics of retinoblastoma, Arch. Ophthalmol., 46:367, 1961.
Friedenwald, J. C., Owens, W. C., and Owens, E. U. Retrolental fibroplasia in premature infants: III. The pathology of the disease. Trans. Am. Ophthalmol., Soc., 49:207, 1951.
Galin, M. A., Kwitko, M. L., Dodick, J. M., and Gitter, K. A.: Analysis of ocular pulse. Can. J. Ophthalmol., 4:37, 1969.
Ginsberg, S. Erkrankungen der Uvea. Hdnb. d. spez. pathol. Anat. u. Histol. IX/1. J. Springer, Berlin. 1928, p. 398.
Goldzieher, W. Zbl. prakt. Augenhk. 1904, Bd. 28, S. 257. Cited by Pietruschka, G., and Schill, H. Uber die spontane Bulbusruptur. Klin. Monatsbl. Augenheilk., 145:161, 1964.
Gyllensten, L. J., and Hellstrom, B. E. Retrolental fibroplasia, animal experiments: the effect of intermittingly administered oxygen on the postnatal development of the eyes of full term mice: a preliminary report. Acta. Paediat. (Uppsala), 41:577, 1952.
Hanssen, R. Drei Fälle von "Pseudotumor" des Auges, mit beiträgen Seltener befunde myopischer Veränderungen und zur frage der Retinitis Exsudativa Coats. Klin. Monatsblt. Augenheilk., 55:703, 1920.
Hassenpflug, I. Naevoxanthoendotheliom oder jugendlichen histiozystom. Dermat. Wochensch., 136:1345, 1957.
Helwig, E. B., and Hackney, V. C. Juvenile xanthogranuloma (Nevoxanthoendothelioma). Am. J. Pathol., 30:625, 1954.
Hogan, M. J., and Zimmerman, L. E. Ophthalmic Pathology. Saunders, Philadelphia, 1962, p. 438 and p. 449.
Howard, G. M., and Ellsworth, R. M. Differential diagnosis of retinoblastoma. A statistical survey of 500 children: I Relative frequency of the lesions which simulate retinoblastoma. Am. J. Ophthalmol., 60:611, 1965; II. Factors relating to the diagnosis of retinoblastoma. Am. J. Ophthalmol., 60:618, 1965.
Igersheimer, J. Systemic Ophthalmology, 2nd ed. by A. Sorsby. Butterworth, London, 1958, p. 19.
Ingalls, T. H., Tedeschi, C. G., and Helpern, M. M. Congenital malformations of the eye induced in mice by maternal anoxia: with particular reference to the problem of retrolental fibroplasia in man. Am. J. Ophthalmol., 35:311, 1952.
Syphilis und Auge. Handbuch der Hautund Geschlechtskrankheiten, Vol. XIII, ed. 2. Ed. by J. Jadassohn. Springer, Berlin, 1928.
Irvine, W. C., and Irvine, A. R., Jr. Nematode endophthalmitis. Toxocara canis. Report of one case. Am. J. Ophthalmol., 47:185, 1959.
Jolly, J. Glaucoma secundarium. Dia Med., 22:18, 1950.
Joyce, A., and Scott, R. K. Treatment of intraocular tumors with radon. 17th Intern. Cong. Ophthal. Acta., 1:453, 1954.
Kalina, R. E. Ophthalmic examination of children of low birth weight. Am. J. Ophthalmol., 67:134, 1969.
King, M. J. Retrolental fibroplasia: a clinical study of 238 cases. Arch Ophthalmol., 43:694, 1950.
Kinsey, V. E. Retrolental fibroplasia: a cooperative study of retrolental fibroplasia and

the use of oxygen. Arch. Ophthalmol., 56:481, 1956.
et al. Oxygen therapy and retrolental fibroplasia. Sight-Saving Rev., 38:131, 1968.
Kupfer, C. Retinoblastoma treated with intravenous nitrogen mustard. Am. J. Ophthalmol., 36:1721, 1953.
Kwitko, M. L. Genetic aspects of the anterior chamber cleavage syndrome. Exerpta Medica, No. 154. Amsterdam. Exerpta Medica Foundation, 1967, p. 80.
Anterior segment anomalies: a clinical pathologic report of conditions simulating congenital glaucoma. Can. J. Ophthalmol., 3:120, 1968.
Congenital anterior segment anomalies. Am. J. Ophthalmol., 64:477, 1967.
Congenital glaucoma: a clinical study. Can. J. Ophthalmol., 2:91, 1967.
Glaucoma due to hypermature cataract. Can. Med. Assoc. J., 89:569, 1963.
and Costenbader, F. D. Glaucoma due to secondary hyphema: a report of two cases treated with intravenous urea. Am. J. Ophthalmol., 53:590, 1962.
and Costendbader, F. D. Urea therapy in glaucoma due to secondary hyphema. Can. Med. Assoc., J., 86:447, 1962.
Laster, L. Sulfite oxidase deficiency. Am. Soc. for Clin. Invest. Meeting, Atlantic City, 1967.
Leber, T. Die Krankheiten der Netzhaut. Hdb. d. ges. Augenheilkd. Vol. XII, Part 2, Wilh. Engelmann, Leipzig, 1916, p. 105.
Levy, W. J., Neuroblastoma. Br. J. Ophthalmol., 41:48, 1957.
Locke, J. C. The prevention of retrolental fibroplasia. Postgrad. Med., 19:417, 1956.
Lubart, J. Sinusitis and nonspecific endogenous ocular inflammation. Arch. Otolaryngol., 67:334, 1958.
Maumenee, A. E., and Longfellow, D. W. Treatment of intraocular nevoxantho-endothelioma (juvenile xanthogranuloma). Am. J. Ophthalmol., 49:1, 1960.
Meyer-Schwickerath, G., and Helferich, E. Zur Therapie des Retinoblastomas. Klin. Monatsbl. Augenheilkd., 132:806, 1958.
Norrie, G. Causes of blindness in children: twenty-five years experience of Danish Institutes for the blind. Acta. Ophthal. (Kbh.), 5:357, 1927.
Nogle blindhedsaarsager: en oversigt. Hospitalstidende, 76:147, 1933.
Noyes, H. D. Glioma and pseudo-glioma. Trans. Am. Ophthalmol., Soc., 23:483, 1887.
Orzalesi, M. M., Mendicini, M., Bucci, G., Scalamandre, A., and Savignoni, P. G., Arterial oxygen studies in premature newborns with and without mild respiratory disorders. Arch. Dis. Child., 42:174, 1967.
Owens, W. C., Friedenwald, J. S., Silverman, W. A., Kinsey, V. E., Hemphill, F. M., Patz, A., Blodi, F. C., and Reese, A. B. Symposium: retrolental fibroplasia (retinopathy of prematurity) Trans. Am. Acad. Ophthalmol. Otolaryngol., 59:7, 1955.
and Owens, E. U. Retrolental fibroplasia in premature infants. Am. J. Ophthalmol., 32:1, 1949; Trans. Am. Acad. Ophthalmol. Otolaryngol., 53:18, 1948-49.
Patz, A., Hoech, L. E., and de la Cruz, E. Studies on the effect of high oxygen administration in retrolental fibroplasia: I. nursery observations. Am. J. Ophthalmol., 35:1248, 1952.
Eastham A., Higginbotham, D. H., and Kleh, T. Oxygen studies in retrolental fibroplasia: II. production of the microscopic changes of retrolental fibroplasia in experimental aminals. Am. J. Ophthalmol., 36:1511, 1953.
Phillips, R., Neuroblastoma. Ann. Roy. Coll. Surg. England, 12:29, 1953.
Rados, A. Uber Veranderungen im fruhstadium d. Retin. Exsudativa. Graefs. Arch. Ophthal., 105:973, 1920.
Reese, A. B. Heredity and retinoblastoma. Arch. Ophthal., 42:119, 1949.
Persistence and hyperplasia of primary vitreous: retrolental fibroplasia, two entities. Arch. Ophthal., 41:527, 1949.
Tumors of the Eye, 2nd ed. Harper & Row, New York, 1963.

Blodi, F. C., and Locke, J. C. The pathology of early retrolental fibroplasia: with an analysis of the histologic findings in the eyes of newborn and stillborn infants. Am. J. Ophthalmol., 35:1407, 1952.

and Blodi, F. C. Retrolental fibroplasia. Acta XVI Conc. Ophthal. (Britannia), 1950, p. 445.

Retrolental fibroplasia. Am. J. Ophthalmol., 34:1, 1951.

King, M. J., and Owens, W. C. A classification of retrolental fibroplasia. Am. J. Ophthalmol., 36:1333, 1953.

and Stepanik, J. Cicatricial stage of retrolental fibroplasia. Am. J. Ophthalmol., 38:308, 1954.

Problems encountered in an eye clinic for children. Am. J. Ophthalmol., 43:24, 1957. Hyman, G. A., Merriman, G. R., Jr., and Forrest, A. W. The treatment of retinoblastoma by radiation and triethylene melamine. Am. J. Ophthalmol., 43:865, 1957.

Ridley, H. Ocular onchocerciasis including an investigation in the Gold Coast. Br. J. Ophthalmol., Suppl. 10, 1945.

Systemic Ophthalmology, 2nd ed. by A. Sorsby. Butterworth, London, 1958, p. 258.

Rodger, F. C. Acute onochocerciasis and its treatment. Br. J. Ophthalmol., 41:544, 1957.

Scheie, H. G. Infantile and juvenile glaucoma. Trans. Am. Acad. Ophthalmol., Otolaryngol., 67:458, 1963.

Ocular changes associated with scrub typhus. Arch. Ophthalmol., 40:245, 1948.

Sichel, J. Uber das Encephaloid und Pseudonencephaloid der Netzhaut. Gax. Med., 29:30, 1857.

Sivasubramaniam, P. Systemic Ophthalmology, 2nd ed. Ed. by A. Sorsby. Butterworth, London, 1958, p. 261.

Smith, J. L., and Israel, C. W. Spirochetes in the aqueous humor in seronegative ocular syphilis, persistence after penicillin therapy. Arch. Ophthalmol., 77:474, 1967.

Sorsby, A. Systemic Ophthalmology, 2nd ed. Butterworth, London, 1958, p. 83.

Stallard, H. B. Glioma retinae treated by radon seeds. Br. Med. J., 2:962, 1936.

Stallard, H. B. Retinoblastoma treated by radio-active applications. Concil. Ophthal. (Belgian) Acta., 2:1360, 1958.

Straub, M. Inflammation of the eye caused by lenticular material dissolved in eye lymph. de Bussy, Amsterdam, 1919. Cited in Woods, A. C. Adventure in ophthamology. Am. J. Ophthalmol., 48:463, 1959.

Szewcyzyk, T. S. Retrolental fibroplasia: etiology and prophylaxis, a preliminary report. Am. J. Ophthalmol., 34:1649, 1951.

Terry, T. L. Extreme prematurity and fibroplastic overgrowth of persistent vascular sheath behind each crystalline lens: I. preliminary report. Am. J. Ophthalmol., 25:203, 1942.

Treacher Collins, E. Curators report on cases of pseudoglioma. Roy. Lond. Ophthal. Hosp. Rep., 13:361, 1892.

Tucker, D. P. Blue sclerotic syndrome simulating buphthalmos. Am. J. Ophthalmol., 47:345, 1959.

Verhoeff, F. H., and Lemoine, A. N. Endophthalmitis phacoanaphylactica. Trans. Intern. Cong. Ophthal., 1:234, 1922.

Vrabec, F. and Vrabec, J. K patogenezi obrazu ablatio falciformis retinae. Cas. Lek. C. 97/II; 1572, 1958.

Leukoconia-pseudoglioma. Eye Ear Nose Throat Monthly, 48:78, 1969.

Wachtel, J. G. The ocular pathology of Marfan's syndrome. Arch. Ophthalmol., 76:512, 1966.

Warburg, M. Norrie's disease (Atrofia bulborum hereditaria): a report of 11 cases of

hereditary bilateral pseudotumor of the retina complicated by deafness and mental deficiency. Acta. Ophthal. (Kbh), 41:134, 1963.
Welch, R. B., Maumenee, A. E., and Wahlen, H. E. Peripheral posterior segment inflammation; vitreous opacities and edema of the posterior pole. Pars planitis. Arch. Ophthalmol., 64:540, 1960.
Weller, C. V. the inheritance of retinoblastoma and its relationships to practical eugenics. Cancer Res., 1:517, 1941.
Wilder, H. C. Nematode endophthalmitis. Trans. Am. Acad. Ophthalmol. Otolaryngol., 55:99, 1950.
Toxoplasma chorioretinitis in adults. Arch. Ophthal., 48:127, 1952.
Williams, I. G. Radiation therapy in the treatment of retinoblastoma. Am. J. Roentgenol., 77:786, 1957.
Wilmer, H. A., and Scrammon, R. E. Growth of the components of the human eyeball. Arch. Ophthalmol., 43:599, 1950.
Wolfe, S. M., and Zimmerman, L. E. Chronic secondary glaucoma associated with retrodisplacement of iris root and deepending of the anterior chamber angle secondary to contusion. Am. J. Ophthalmol., 54:547, 1962.

12

Treatment of Congenital Glaucoma

> Whenever I approach a child,
> His presence inspires two feelings in me:
> Affection for the way he is now,
> And respect for what he may one day become.
> Louis Pasteur

It is generally acknowledged that surgery is the treatment of choice in infantile glaucoma. It is also accepted that angle surgery produces the highest incidence of intraocular pressure normalization, although procedures designed to bypass Schlemm's canal are known to be successful. There is no evidence in the literature of a favorable outcome without surgery, although some eyes present evidence of a spontaneous cure.

Nettleship, in 1888, stated that good results followed iridectomy in five patients seen at a very early stage. In 1905, Sattler reported the condition cured by iridectomy in two patients while in 1908, Germann reported a similar cure in two of 4 patients in a single family. Priestly Smith's report was discouraging. In 1914, Calhoun reported that results in patients with early involvement were gratifying and that the trephine operation was superior to iridectomy or to the Lagrange sclerectomy with iridectomy. Werner, in 1929, also expressed the opinion that a fistulizing operation was superior to iridectomy. In the 1931 Courtney and Hill report of 2 patients, one had an iridectomy performed 12 months previously and the other had a Lagrange sclerectomy with iridectomy. The glaucoma appeared to be under control but there was no improvement of vision or visual fields. Stokes's procedure of choice, when the patient was seen during the congestive stage, was a puncture of the anterior chamber followed in a few days by an iris inclusion operation. Sclerocorneal trepanation was preferred in those cases in which the eye was free from congestive signs.

Attempts to obtain fistulization in congenital glaucoma by means of a sclerectomy may therefore be traced back to the anterior and internal, single or multiple, sclerotomy as practiced by de Wecker and others. This technique consisted in puncturing the anterior chamber behind the limbus, crossing it, and counterpuncturing the other side through or under the conjunctiva. The openings were made of different sizes. These operations were largely ineffective and not without hazard.

De Vincentiis, in 1892, in his original operation of incision of the iridocorneal angle, did not counterperforate the sclera. His objective was a pure debridement of the angle. De Wecker combined with the de Vincentiis method a counterpuncture or sclerotomy, in the hope of adding the benefits of external fistulization to those of internal debridement. This combined method was called "internal sclerotomy." Rochon-Duvigneaud also used a restricted scleral puncture, calling the operation "reduced sclerotomy."

During the early years (1936–38), while performing the operation without a contact lens, Barkan added a limited counterpuncture of the sclera into the subconjunctiva in over 20 eyes, in the belief that external fistulization might improve the success rate of the operation. However, in none of these cases did permanent fistulization occur. In all cases normalization of pressure seemed to parallel the stripping of the angle. The punctures added additional hazards, which often led to adhesions of the iris to the corneo scleral wall, and were therefore abandoned.

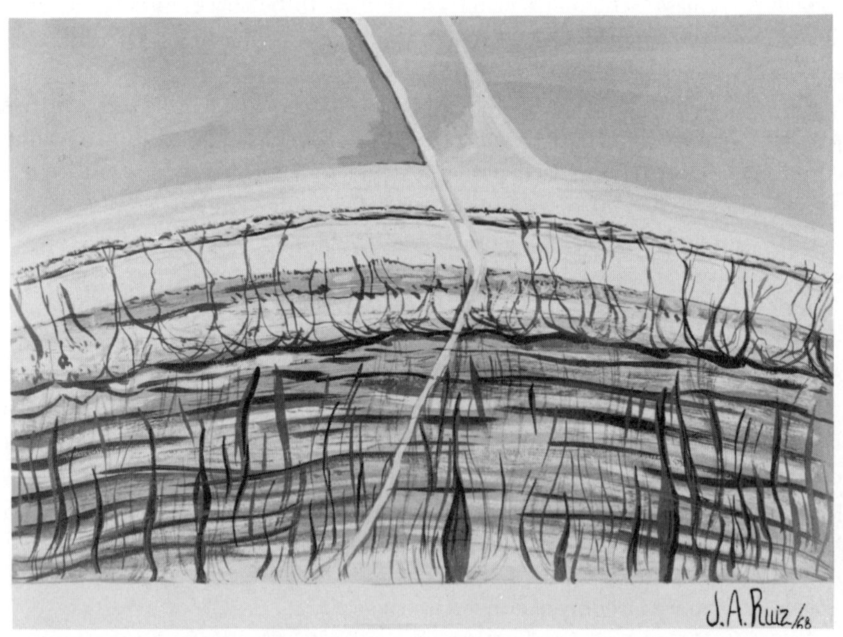

FIG. 1. Open angle glaucoma, filtration angle in the adult.

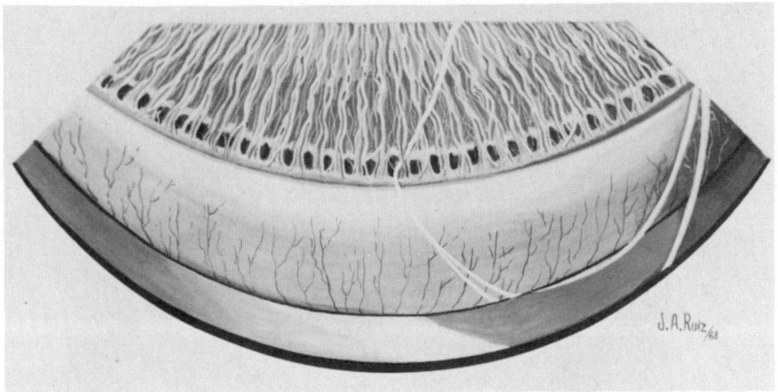

FIG. 2. Congenital glaucoma, filtration angle.

Interest in fistulization by means of internal, limited, or reduced sclerotomy has in recent times been revived by Scheie, who described the "goniopuncture" technique.

Results from iridencleisis, trephining, cyclodialysis, cyclodiathermy, and other operative procedures known to be effective in forms of glaucoma occurring in adults (Fig. 1), are often mutilating in the infantile type of the disease (Fig. 2). They not only fail to control pressure but are often associated with cataract formation, vitreous loss, hammock pupil, intraocular hemorrhage, subluxation of the lens, staphyloma (Fig. 3 A and B), permanent corneal opacity, atrophy of the globe, and on occasion, sympathetic ophthalmia. However, reports have appeared describing a success rate of up to 50 percent, including cases where the goniotomy failed.

Cyclodiathermy was popular in Europe for all stages of congenital glaucoma as a primary operation. However, this operation is not immune from the hazard of serious complications, e.g., detachment of the retina, atrophy of the globe, and sympathetic ophthalmia.

MEDICAL MANAGEMENT

Miotics such as pilocarpine, carcholin, eserine, prostigmine, and diisopropyl fluorophosphate have been used in the treatment of congenital glaucoma. Carbonic anhydrase inhibitors, e.g., acetazolamide, are well tolerated and cause significant lowering of intraocular pressure. Initially, some eyes are normalized, but none can be maintained or safely controlled.

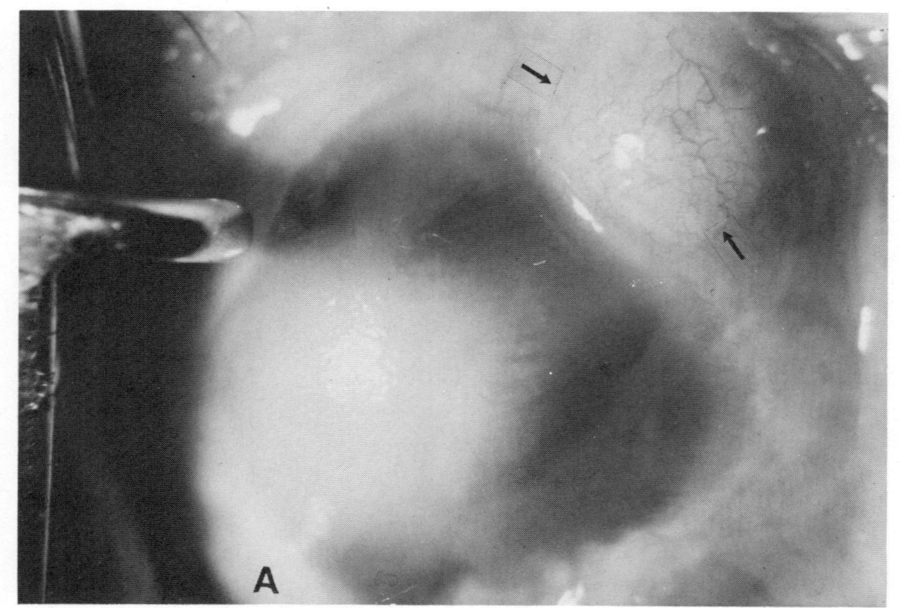

FIG. 3.A. Scleral staphyloma (arrows) following an iridenceisis operation in congenital glaucoma. The opaque cornea prevented visualization of the filtration angle.

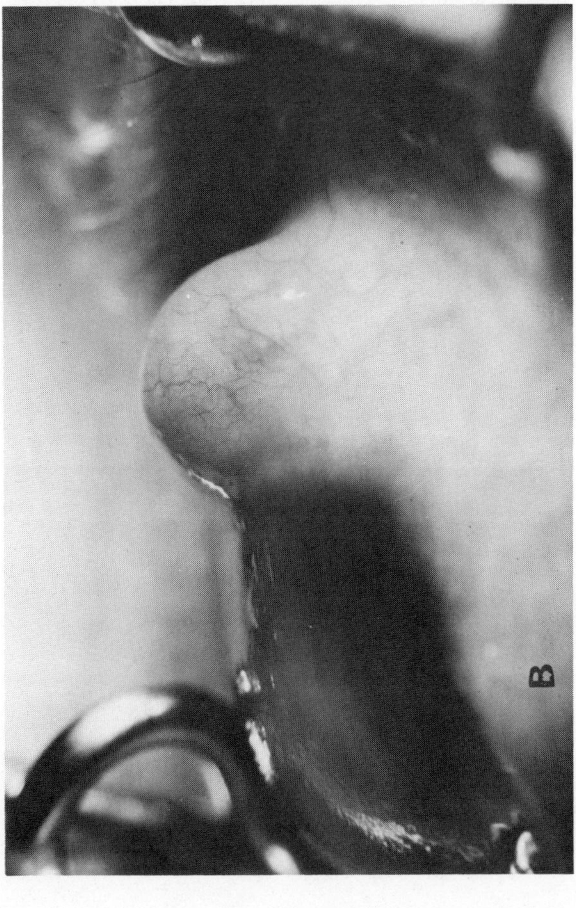

FIG. 3.B. Scleral staphyloma, profile view.

Medical therapy is useful primarily to reduce the tension, clear the cornea, and facilitate the surgery. When the tension persists after surgery, miotics are certainly indicated between operations. It must be emphasized that miotics are dangerous when they lead to the postponement of surgery. Another intriguing possiblity is that by controlling the tension by inhibiting the formation of aqueous with acetazolamide, further maturation of the eye will allow the so-called immature angle to proceed to its normal state. However, there is no clinical evidence to support this hypothesis. It must be noted that delay in treatment leads to ocular enlargement and decreases the probability of success.

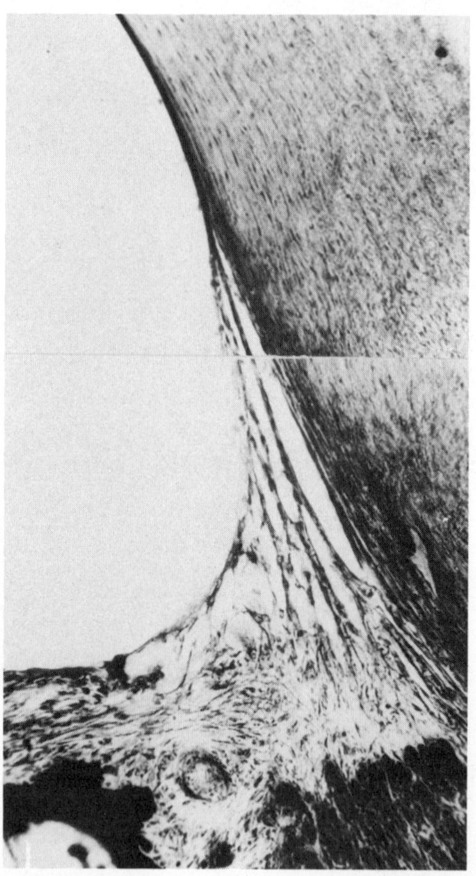

FIG. 4. Congenital glaucoma, filtration angle showing evidence of an impermeable membrane. (Courtesy of J. G. F. Worst.) X 200.

SURGICAL MANAGEMENT

One of the major advances in ocular surgery has been the development of goniotomy as the treatment for infantile glaucoma. It has proved to be the best procedure for this condition, with relatively little risk and generally gratifying results. The fact that the procedure may be repeated as often as 4 times is another important feature. Success seems to result from opening a route for aqueous flow into Schlemm's canal, by means of a partial or complete form of trabeculotomy. It is not presently known whether success is due to incising an impermeable membrane (Fig. 4), lowering the point of iris insertion on the trabecular meshwork, or interrupting an abnormal pull of the ciliary muscle on the trabecular fibers. A successful goniotomy increases the facility of aqueous outflow and normalizes the intraocular pressure. Goniopuncture, whereby an opening is made into the subconjunctival space independently or at the time goniotomy is performed, has been advanced by some surgeons.

External filtering operations should be reserved for those cases where the goniotomy operation has proven unsuccessful. New direct approaches to the trabeculum and Schlemm's canal offer another avenue of treatment. The surgical approaches for congenital glaucoma are summarized in Table 1.

TABLE 1

SURGERY FOR CONGENITAL GLAUCOMA

Trabecular Surgery

I. Trabeculotomy: the slitting open of the trabecular meshwork obstruction
   a. Internal transverse trabeculotomy (de Vincentiis, Barkan)
   b. Internal direct trabeculotomy, goniotripsy (Urrets-Zavalia, Kwitko and Galin)
   c. Trabeculotomy ab externo (Smith, Allen and Burian, Harms and Dannheim)
II. Trabeculectomy (Cairns, Dellaporta): the removal of a section of the trabeculum and the overlying Schlemm's canal

Nontrabeculum By-pass Surgery

I. Iridectomy with scleral cautery (Scheie)
II. Trephine

Combined Trabeculum and By-pass Surgery

I. Goniopuncture (Scheie)

PREOPERATIVE MEASURES

A thorough pediatric examination is performed as described in Chapter 7. In the case of infants, the usual diet is maintained up to 6 hrs preoperatively; sugar solution is forced up to 4 hrs preoperatively to avoid dehydration with the associated hyperpyrexia. Since it is important that the surgery will not be delayed, every effort must be made to prevent the infant from catching cold. On the day of surgery, pilocarpine 2 percent is instilled in the eye to be operated, 3 times at 10 min intervals, and chloromycetin drops 0.5 percent 6 times at 10 min intervals in the 2-hrperiod prior to the scheduled time of surgery.

ANESTHESIA

The onset of congestive symptoms which call attention to the condition is often rapid and may even be sudden. Barkan reported cases where cloudiness of the cornea was discovered by the mother when the infant was taken up in the morning (the eyes had been clear the previous night). In one instance the cloudiness was discovered when the infant was taken up from its afternoon nap. The lacrimation and photophobia may cause the child to

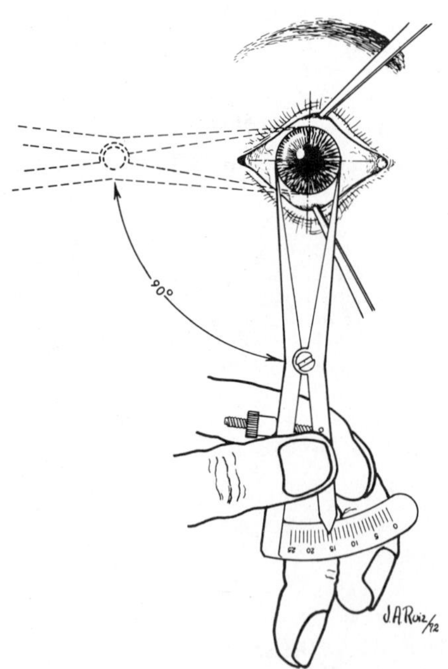

FIG. 5. Measurement of the corneal diameter. (Modified from Boyd. **Highlights Ophthalmol.** 8:4, 1966.)

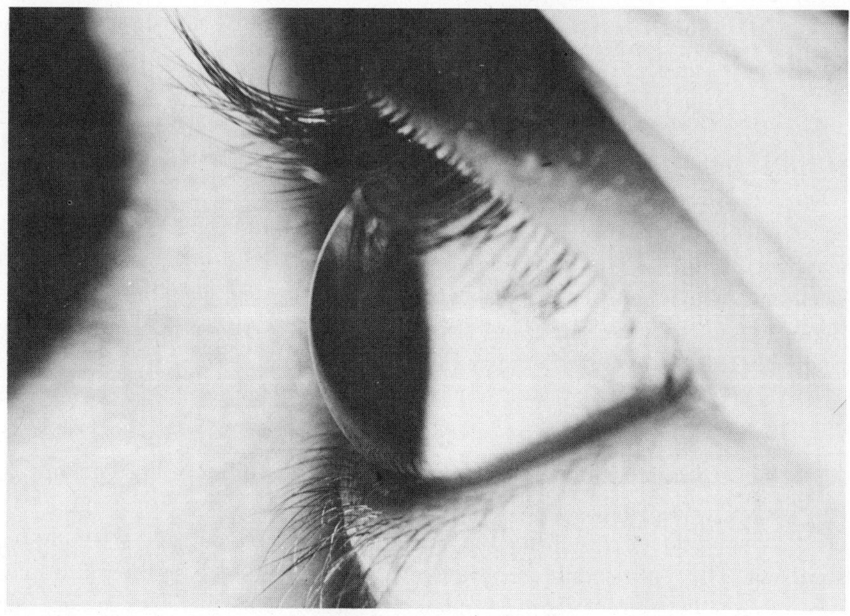

FIG. 6. Megalocornea. The enlarged cornea may be confused with the enlarged cornea of congenital glaucoma.

bury his face in the pillow. Upon entering a brightly illuminated room the head is often bowed with the eyes forcefully closed.

In view of the delicacy of the operation as applied to these children, who may be only a few days or weeks old, anesthesia is an important factor. Often the examination may not otherwise be performed.

No attempt should be made to give general anesthesia in one's office. This would subject the patient to unnecessary risks and could result in false readings. It is advisable to have the same anesthetist take part in each case in order to add to his experience. While the patient is being prepared, the lids must be kept closed with moist pledgets but without pressure, since the cornea in congenital glaucoma is extremely susceptible to exposure and pressure. For the same reason, the heat generated by the operating lamps should be avoided, by turning them aside after they are turned on and focusing them only when required. Anesthesia must be sufficiently deep at the moment of operation so there will be no movement of the patient. Topical anesthetic drops should be used in addition to the general anesthesia. Postoperative agitation is not harmful, since there is only a small, obliquely placed corneal puncture wound which does not permit egress of the ocular contents. The experienced anesthetist becomes aware of these facts.

Before the patient is draped a number of critical measurements are taken.

Corneal Measurements

The corneal diameter is measured horizontally with a millimeter caliper. When the horizontal endpoints are obscure, a vertical measurement should be included (Fig. 5). Measurements with reasonable accuracy to 0.25mm may be obtained. It is important to recall physiologic and familial corneal variations when considering a diagnosis of congenital glaucoma (Fig. 6). However, in infants with large eyes it is better to suspect congenital glaucoma than to overlook the possibility.

Tonometry

One of the most important confirmatory tests for infantile glaucoma is an elevated intraocular pressure, but one must be aware of the sources of error. These factors are outlined in Chapter 7. The tonometer base should be sterilized. The child should be at the level of deep surgical anesthesia so that the extraocular muscles are completely relaxed, and the eyes are in the primary position and not deviated upward or inward. Endotracheal intubation is the preferred method.

Differences in corneal diameter, in the range between 10 and 12 mm, do not appear to influence the intraocular tension. In eyes with corneal diameters of 13 mm and over, one gains the impression that the tonometric measurement is relatively too low. It seems likely that the readings in distended eyes are influenced by (1) a relative flattening of the central area of the cornea; (2) increased indentability of the thinned cornea; (3) decreased scleral rigidity; and (4) the fact that the amount of fluid displaced by the plunger has less effect on tonometer readings as the total volume of the eyeball increases. The low reading may indeed be a true one due to (1) increased outflow, caused by stretching of the region of the filtration angle; and (2) reduced functional integrity of the ciliary body.

Whereas a moderate elevation of the intraocular pressure may be well tolerated by an undistended eye for a considerable length of time, it is injurious to the more markedly distended buphthalmic eye (Fig. 7). In the absence of classical findings of infantile glaucoma, one should hesitate to operate on the basis of a single recording of elevated intraocular pressure. On the other hand, the finding of a normal pressure in an eye suspected of having infantile glaucoma should not lead to a false sense of security and exclusion of the diagnosis (Fig. 8). Whenever doubt exists repeated readings

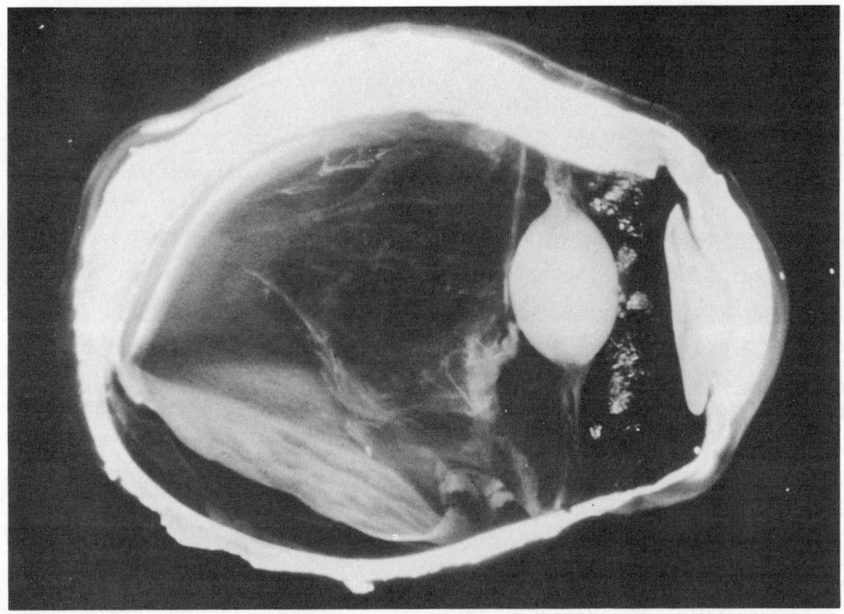

FIG. 7. Buphthalmic eye showing considerable distension.

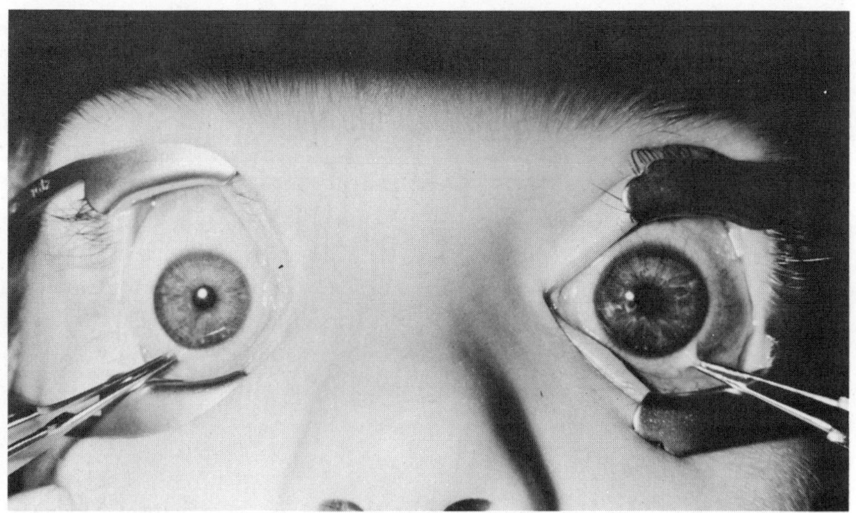

FIG. 8. Enlarged eye which showed a normal intraocular pressure on the first examination. A later examination confirmed the diagnosis of congenital glaucoma with an elevated tension.

should be taken. The price of a missed or delayed diagnosis is deterioration of the eyeball and loss of vision.

Slit Lamp Examination

The state of clarity of the cornea will determine the operative procedure, the anterior chamber examination will reveal the extent and location of iris and filtration angle vessels to be avoided, and the chamber depth will determine the manner of approaching the angle. The state and position of the lens must be determined to reveal lens opacities and ectopia lentis.

Ruptures or tears of Descemet's membrane, which are prominently referred to in the literature describing the pathological anatomy of hydrophthalmos, may not be present. It appears that these tears do not occur in infantile glaucoma before marked distention and degenerative changes have taken place. According to Barkan, rupture of Descemet's membrane plays no role in diagnosis at the time when diagnosis is of therapeutic importance.

Spencer et al. studied a group of congenital glaucoma cases which displayed early enlargement of the cornea with edema, and ruptures of Descemet's membrane. In each case the intraocular pressure remained at normal levels following surgery, with no further enlargement of the eye. The corneas cleared with the exception of areas of fine linear opacifications along the course of the breaks in Descemet's membrane. After an interval ranging from 12 to 31 years all of these patients developed corneal edema followed by bullous keratopathy of varying severity, despite the maintenance of a normal intraocular pressure. The end result was not affected by the type of glaucoma surgery (goniotomy, iridencleisis, trephine). Edema first developed adjacent to the sites of the breaks in Descemet's membrane and tended to spread peripherally as a diffuse haze. The edema fluctuated but slowly progressed to involve most of the cornea, leading to severe bullous keratopathy. This was not true in every patient, e.g., cases of bilateral Descemet's membrane ruptures were described where the condition advanced in one eye and remained stationary in the other.

Fundus Examination

When corneal irregularities obscure the fundus, it is helpful to view it through the goniolens. The optic nerve should be drawn and the relative size of the optic cup recorded. Glaucomatous cupping is not an uncommon occurrence as an early sign of congenital glaucoma.

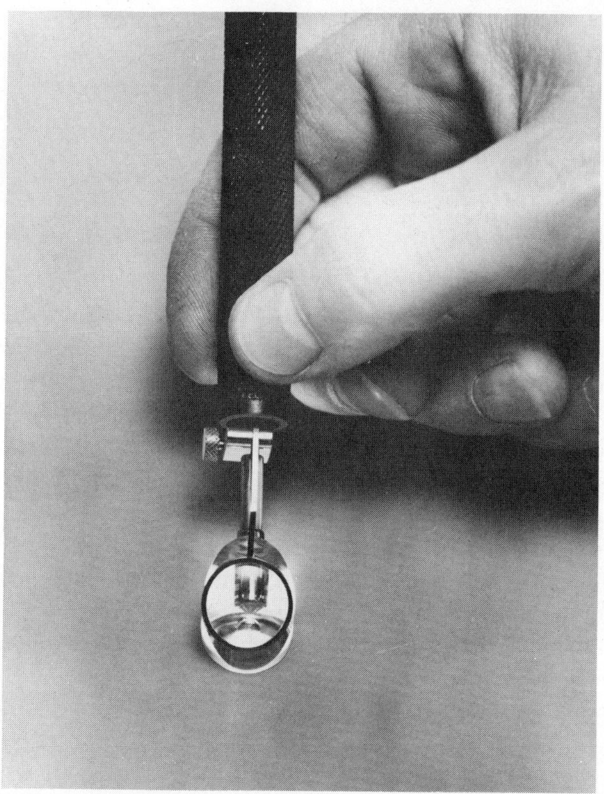

FIG. 9. Worst gonioscopy lens fitted with a fiber optic illumination system. The auxilliary lens is used to increase magnification.

Gonioscopic Findings

Gonioscopy is performed through the smooth-domed Koeppe lens of appropriate size or the infant diagnostic lens. The lens may be fitted with a fiber optic illumination system (Fig. 9). Using the binocular microscope, an estimation of the chamber angle width is made and the field of operation reconnoitered. The best site for the goniotomy is thus chosen, free from large vessels and peripheral anterior synechiae left from previous operations. Compression of the jugular venous drainage system may help with orientation within the angle, demonstrating a blood-filled Schlemm's canal as a circumferential red line deep to the surface of the trabeculum. This feature may be observed because of the marked translucency of the infant angle wall, and proves that Schlemm's canal is present in most early cases. The blood-filled canal may be hidden in those cases where the iris inserts close to the line of Schwalbe. In eyes with a corneal diameter greater than 14 mm, jugular compression does not produce the same effect because Schlemm's canal has become altered.

The Fellow Eye

Even though the appearance and ocular tension in the fellow eye are normal, careful observation should be maintained at regular intervals until adult life. Development of glaucoma in the fellow eye has been observed years after the first eye was affected.

Upon completion of the examination, a decision as to the type of treatment is made. Sometimes the decision can only be made at this time. Since the systemic effects of anesthesia make reliance upon the numerical values of tonometry or tonography uncertain, this decision is based upon the entire clinical picture, including symptomotology and physical findings. If there is any doubt as to the condition or indicated treatment, continued observation should be substituted for active therapy.

When the diagnosis is certain one should proceed with surgery. The position of the patient, operator, assistant, anesthetist, instrument table, and microscope are now arranged accordingly.

POSITION OF THE PATIENT

The infant's head is placed on a "donut," or another suitable headrest, for stability. The surgeon must place the operating table at a level giving him greatest comfort. The surgery will probably be performed in the standing position, even though the surgeon is normally seated for most other intraocular procedures. For goniotomy without use of a contact lens, the patient's eye should be lower than the normal position so that the operator may look more vertically downward.

PREPARATION AND DRAPING OF THE PATIENT

Lashes may be clipped with Steven's scissors covered with ointment, and wiped off with a cotton tip applicator after each clip. The ocular region is prepped in a manner usually used in the ophthalmic operating theater with the eyelids closed. After the patient is draped, a plastic eye sheet, which has a gummed surface allowing it to adhere to the skin, should be applied to the periocular region of the eye to be operated. A regular cloth eye drape taped to the skin with surgical masking tape serves equally as well. This draping has the advantage of being immobile during the critical operative movements.

MAGNIFICATION

The spherical surface of the Barkan type surgical goniolens (Fig. 10) tends to gather light and distribute it evenly over the chamber angle. The spherical goniotomy lens is therefore the surgical contact lens of choice to be used without an operating microscope. However, an operating loupe is still essential. The direct type goniotomy lens (Worst type), which has no intrinsic magnification of its own, requires the use of an operating microscope (Fig. 11 A and B.)

The microscope should have incorporated in it both very low magnification, for performing the preliminary surgical maneuvers, e.g., perforating the cornea with the goniotomy knife, and high magnification for

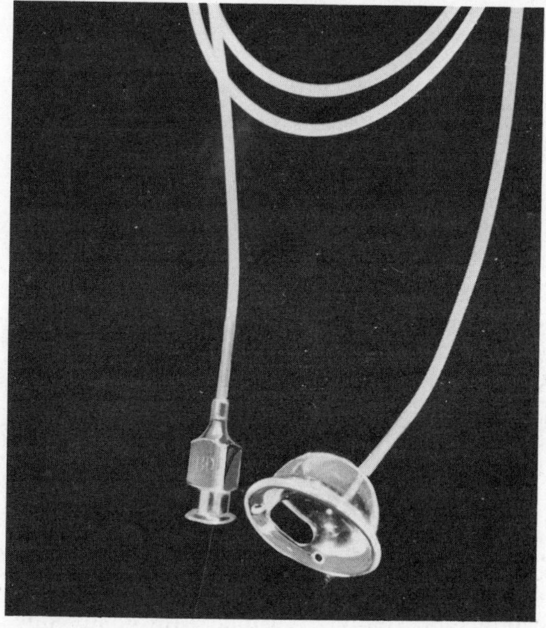

FIG. 10. The Medical Workshop spherical type goniotomy lens. This lens has a spherical surface, giving a gonioscopic image of the chamber angle with X 2 magnification. The lens is used with the binocular loupe. Special features include a scleral rim with 4 perforations, a lateral window, and a cannula.

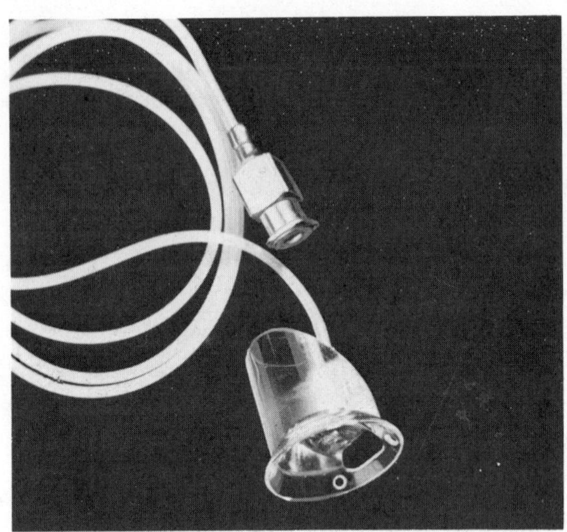

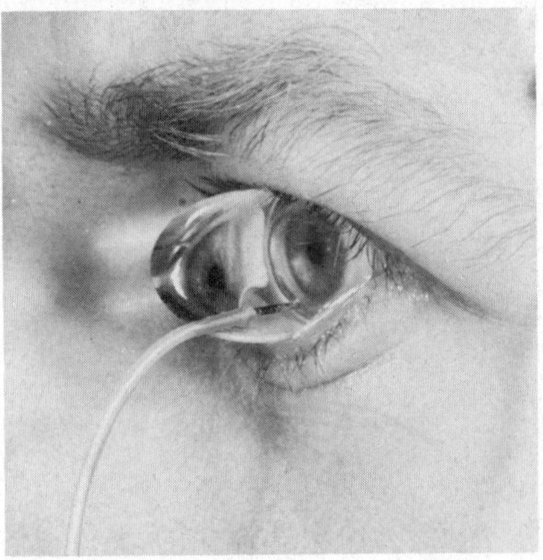

FIG. 11. **A.** The Medical Workshop (Worst) prismatic goniotomy lens. This lens has an oblique flat surface, through which nearly 180° of chamber angle is visible. The image is not enlarged so that an operating microscope must be used. **B.** The lens in position.

making the actual goniotomy incision. The Zeiss operating microscope, with zoom lens which tilts so that the filtration angle comes into focus, offers this variety of magnification options. Postoperative gonioscopy must also be performed with adequate magnification after the corneal epithelium has healed in and the cornea has cleared.

ILLUMINATION

The illumination of the chamber angle during goniotomy is the most essential single item. Using the Barkan lens, the room is placed in semidarkness. According to Barkan, proper illumination is obtained by placing the focused light close to the head of the operator.

As one often must visualize the chamber angle through a hazy cornea, the best illumination is provided by a strongly focused light, directed at nearly a right angle to the operator's line of vision immediately into the chamber angle, since the diffuse reflection from the hazy corneal surface deteriorates the degree of clarity of the chamber angle. Strongly focused, very oblique incidence of the light also produces a partial retroillumination, which brings out angle structures in "dark background" relief. As more of the cornea is available for observation, chances are better for more of the angle to be observed. This same type of perpendicular lighting with a strongly focused light may be used both with the Barkan-type spherical lens and the prismatic lens.

Since reflexes produced by any diagnostic contact lens originate to a large extent from its external surfaces, the light source should be inside the lens in order to eliminate these reflexes and provide the best illumination. This may be accomplished using a fiber optic system as designed by Worst and Cardona. In the Worst goniotomy lens (Fig. 12 A and B) the fiber beam is inserted in a cylindrical hole within the lens. A clear image without reflection is thus produced, with a superbly lighted chamber angle. The internally lighted contact lens is powered by a fiber optic source (Fig. 13). The field of operation is illuminated by the lighting system of the operating microscope. It is often helpful to close the overhead lights of the operating room.

EPITHELIAL EDEMA

The corneal epithelium must always be removed in chamber angle operations, even when corneal clarity seems sufficient for surgery. This is a preventative measure since epithelial edema has a tendency to increase rapidly, clouding over during some phase of the operation, and removal at that time is impossible.

The epithelium may be taken off by scraping with a round-bellied No. 15 Bard Parker blade (Fig. 14). However, several drops of 70 percent

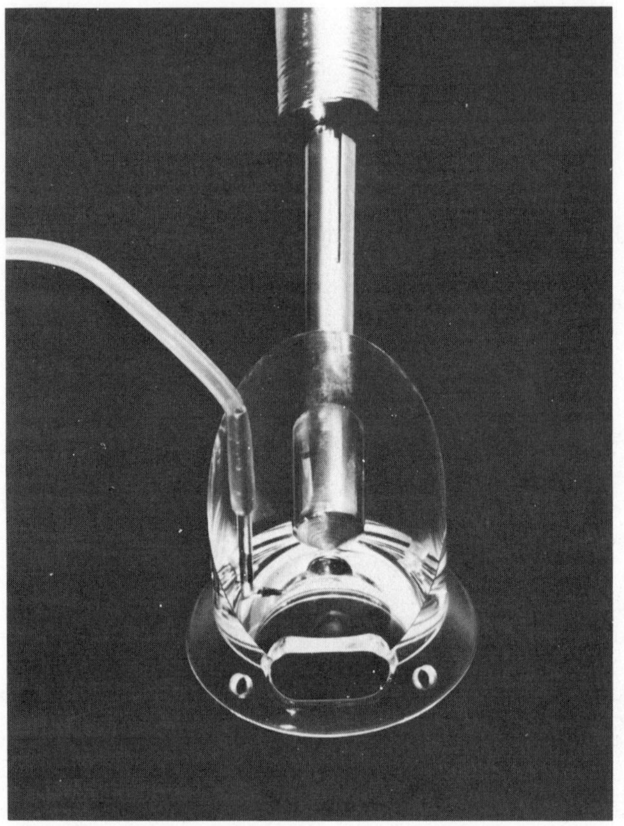

FIG. 12.A. The Medical Workshop (Worst) prismatic goniotomy lens with fiber optic illumination system.

alcohol, absorbed in a surgical microsponge, provides a more rapid and effective method. The epithelium is chemically coagulated and may be removed by simply wiping it off. Regeneration is not negatively influenced. Care should be taken, however, to leave an intact ring of peripheral epithelium (Fig. 15).

THE GONIOTOMY PROCEDURE

The goniotomy operation is one in which attention to detail is essential, and in which consistent success has come only after much practice.

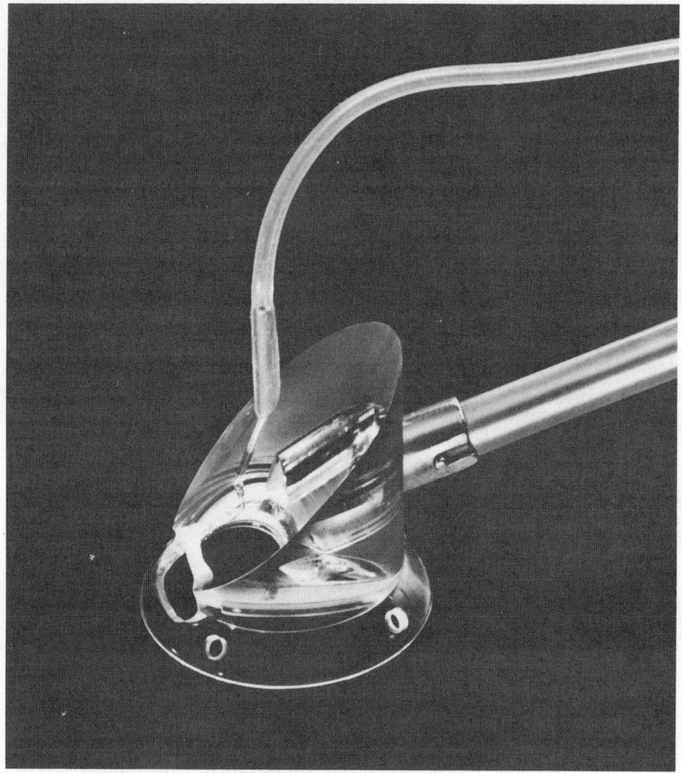

FIG. 12.B. Self illuminated prismatic goniotomy lens, side view.

Therefore, the best results are most likely to occur in the hands of those who make a special study of this disease and the surgical options available.

Choice of Cases for Goniotomy

Experience has shown that cases of congenital glaucoma fall into two groups: those in which the chances of success with goniotomy are high, and those in which failure is a frequent occurrence. The unsuccessful group includes neonatal cases (newborn glaucoma), those in which there are associated congenital abnormalities, and those eyes that have become grossly altered before treatment is begun. In the neonatal group, it appears wise to postpone the operation to at least 2 to 4 weeks of age, at which time the operation is easier to perform. The anterior chamber deepens, and the cornea may show some spontaneous independent clearing which may be aided with miotics and acetazolamide (Diamox).

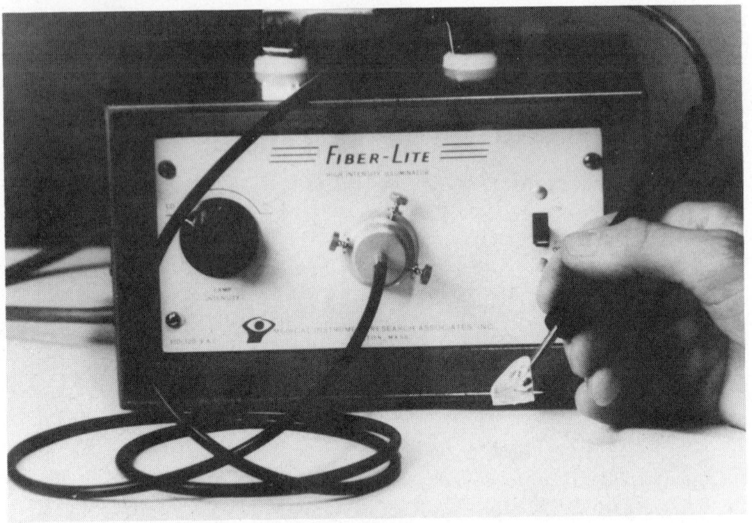

FIG. 13. Fiber optic illumination source.

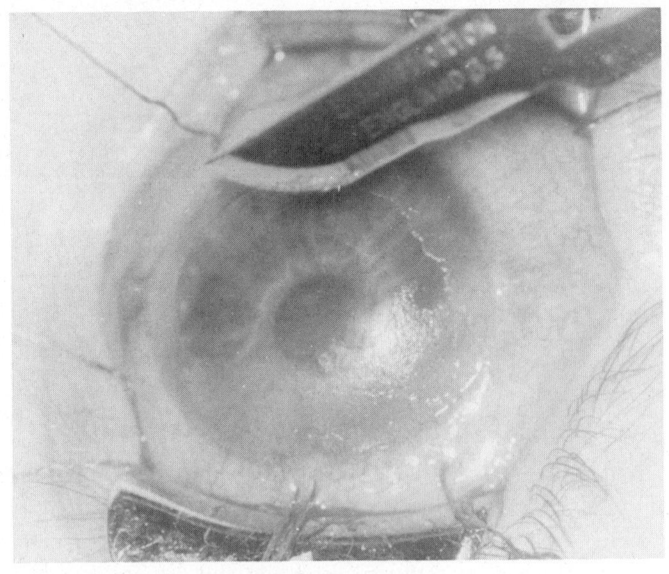

FIG. 14. Removal of the corneal epithelium with a Bard Parker No. 15 blade.

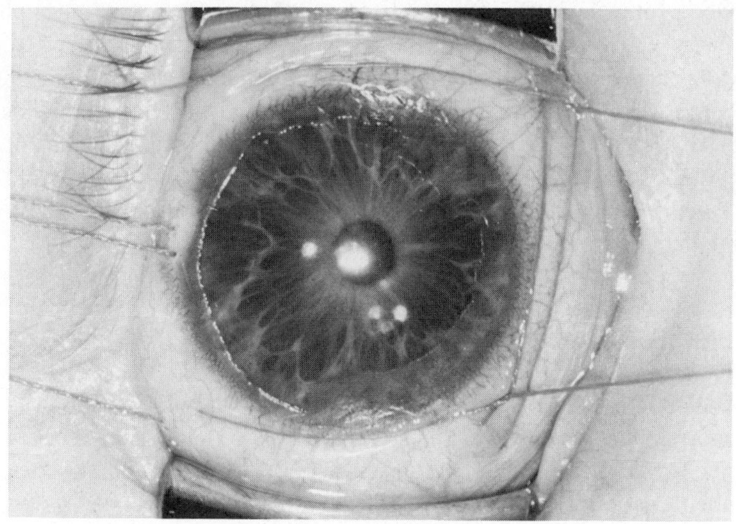

FIG. 15. Coagulation of the corneal epithelium with 70 percent alcohol, leaving the periphery intact.

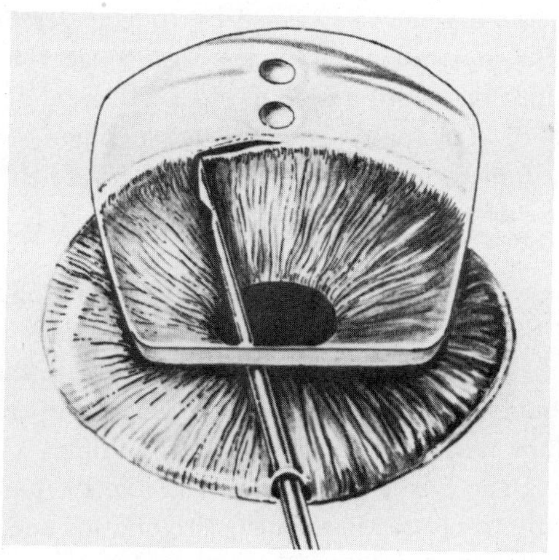

FIG. 16. The Barkan lens illustrating the two dimples on the surface.

Goniotomy is contraindicated in the late distended stage of buphthalmus because, by this time, Schlemm's canal has become obliterated. The operation may indeed be hazardous because of the presence of large dilated vessels. As with all perforating operations on the advanced buphthalmic eye, sudden loss of intraocular fluid may result in retinal detachment and dislocation of the lens.

To the successful group belong those cases where the disease has become manifest after the age of 3 months.

Instruments

GONIOTOMY LENSES. The perfect lens acts as if the cornea has been automatically removed. The spherical type of gonioscopy contact lens has the advantage of inherent magnification and can be used on the recumbent patient, but has the disadvantage of not being corrected for optical errors. At higher magnifications obtained with the operating microscope, a loss of resolving power occurs. For this reason contact lenses that have no inherent magnification are probably better for high power observation. The increase in magnification is provided by the microscope itself.

Poor angle visibility may be caused by folding Descemet's membrane. The pressure of the contact lens on the eye with congenital glaucoma, which has a relatively thin cornea but a well developed Descemet's membrane, may produce a series of transverse highly refractile ridges, which reduce the resolving power of the gonioscopic system. All hand-held gonioscopy and goniotomy lenses suffer from this defect. Lenses separated from the cornea by a fluid layer exert less pressure on the cornea.

Barkan Lens. The original Barkan lens has two dimples (Fig. 16) and is supported by the fingers (Fig. 17) or forceps. This lens (Fig. 18) has a disadvantage in that it is not easy to hold in place with the tip of the index finger. If an air bubble leaks under the lens during the operation, surgery has to be abandoned, or carried on under adverse conditions.

Lister Lens. The Lister lens is shown in Fig. 19 A and B. The original two dimples on the top of the Barkan lens are omitted and the lens has been piped with a small silver cannula (also employed in the Worst lens) which is connected via a fine polyvinyl chloride (PVC) tube to a syringe containing saline. During the operation the lens is held by the projecting end of the cannula, and the saline meniscus between lens and cornea is maintained from the reservoir in the syringe. The problem of having air bubbles appear under the lens is therefore largely overcome.

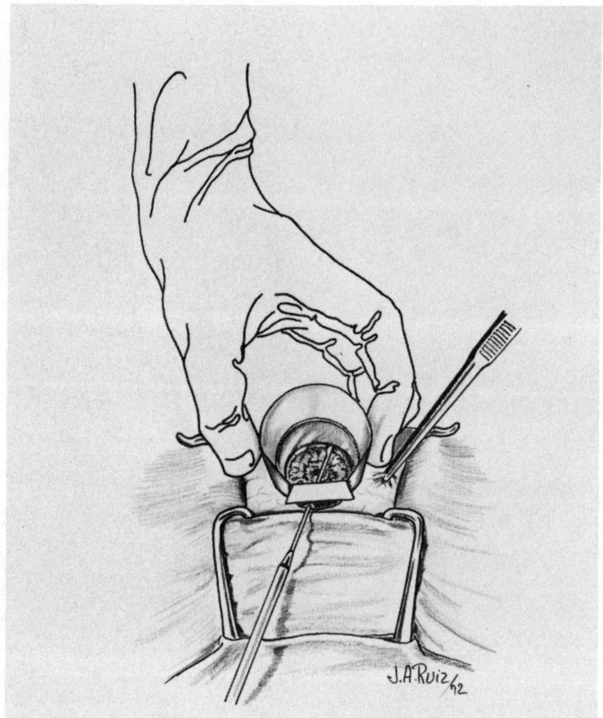

FIG. 17. The Barkan lens hand held.

FIG. 18. The Barkan lens side view.

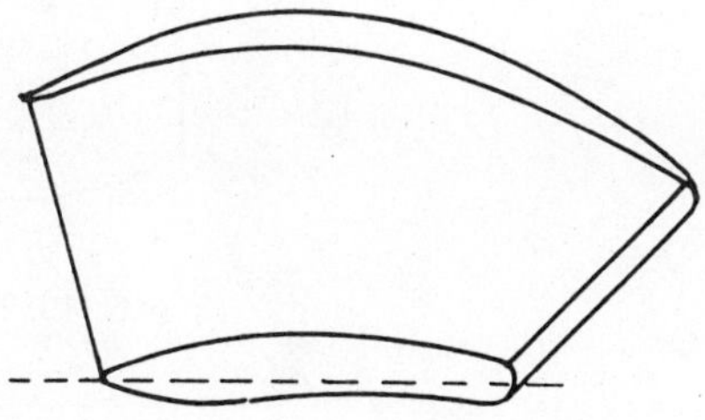

Worst Lens. SPHERICAL GONIOTOMY LENS. Features include a scleral rim and cannula (Fig. 20 A and B). This lens provides an enlargement of X 2, allowing the operation to be performed with only a binocular loupe for magnification.

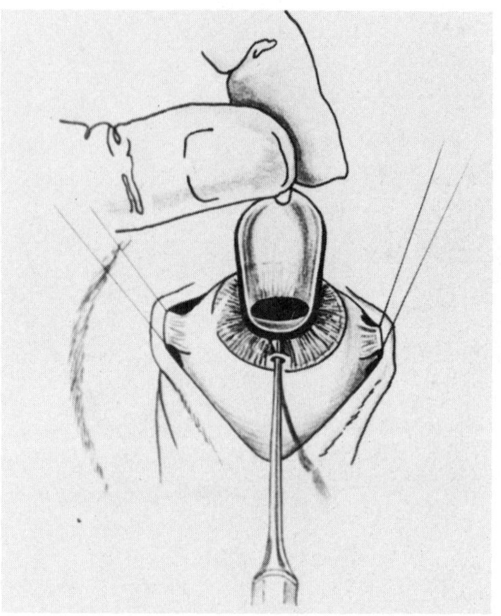

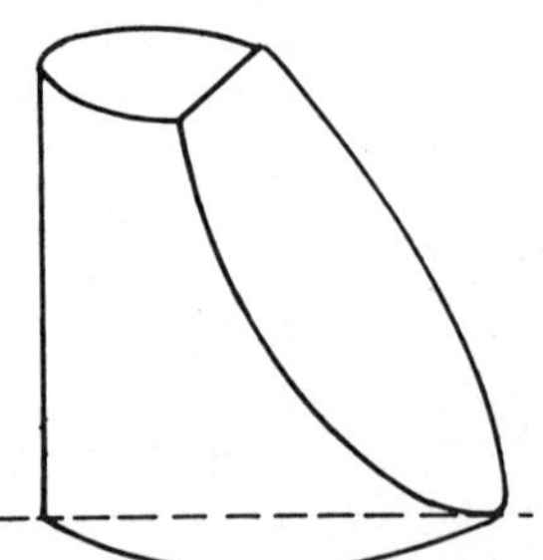

FIG. 19. The Lister lens.

PRISMATIC GONIOTOMY LENS. This lens, with scleral rim and cannula is shown being used in Fig. 21. The image formed by this lens is not magnified. A binocular operating microscope is therefore required. These goniotomy lenses are made in two sizes: regular, for children older than 3 months of age, and small, for children under 3 months of age. It is the width of the

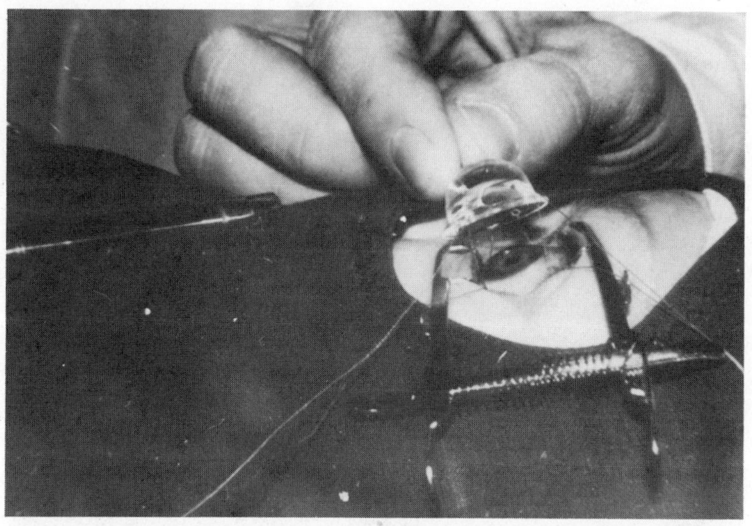

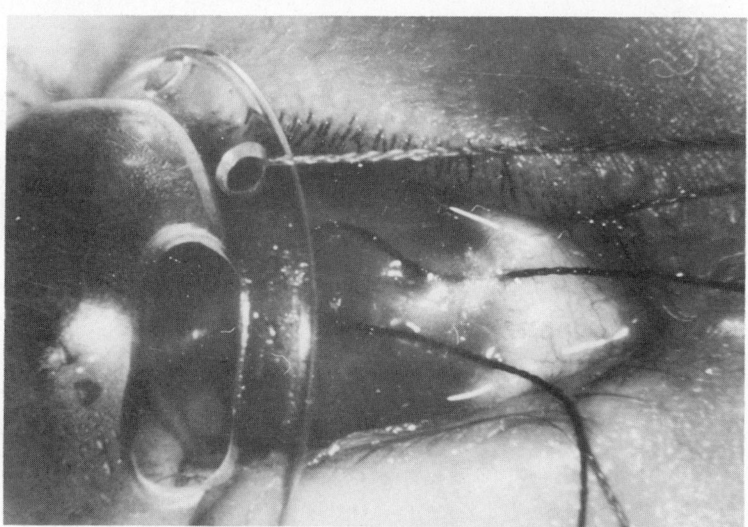

FIG. 20. The spherical lens modified for attachment to the globe.

palpebral aperture, not the size of the eye, which determines the choice of the size of the lens. The regular size lens should be used whenever possible. The special features of the lens include (1) a scleral rim with 4 holes in it, through which 4 episcleral sutures are passed and tied to give fixation (Fig.

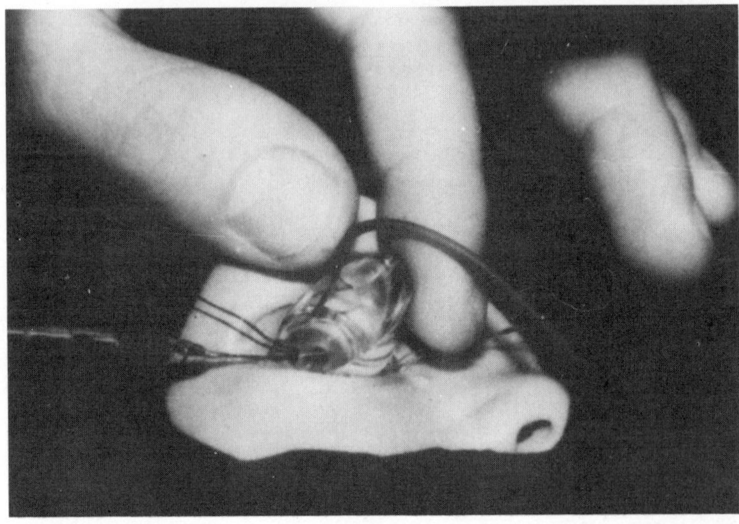

FIG. 21. The prismatic goniotomy (Worst) lens attached to the globe during a goniotomy procedure.

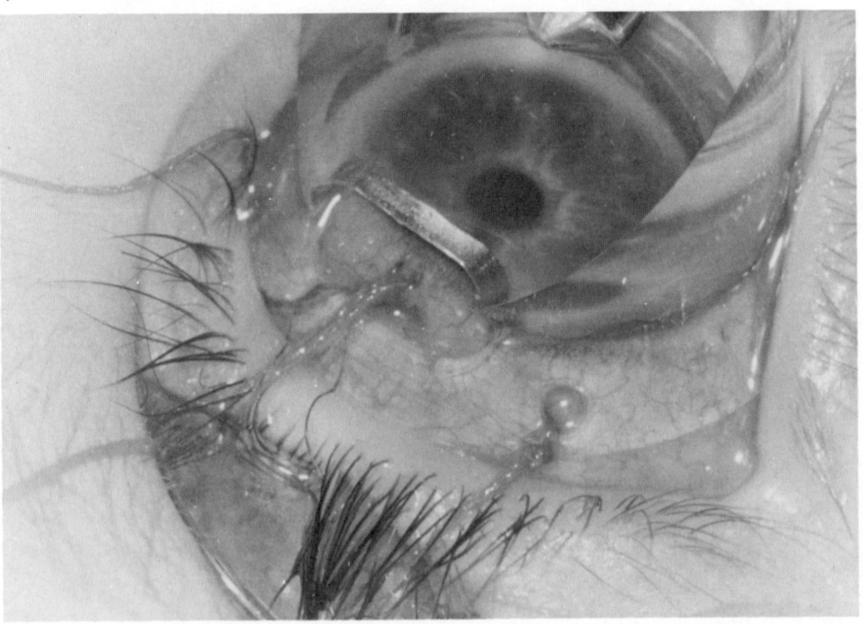

FIG. 22. The prismatic goniotomy (Worst) lens showing the perforated scleral rim through which sutures are passed, fixing the lens to the eye.

22); (2) a vertical cannula which is attached to a 5 or 10 cc syringe by means of a polyvinyl chloride (PVC) tubing (Fig. 23A). The space between the lens and the cornea is filled with saline at the beginning of the operation and if necessary during the most critical phases of the operation (Fig. 23B). This fluid cushion prevents the lens from exerting pressure on the cornea. Folds in Descemet's membrane induced in this way are largely eliminated: (3) a lateral hole which permits introduction of the goniotomy knife (Fig. 23B); (4) A flat anterior surface at right angles to the line of observation of the chamber angle. This provides nearly a 180° view of the angle in its normal anatomical relationship without mirror inversion. The flat anterior surface guarantees that no optical errors are present because of spherical aberration. If care is taken to keep the anterior surface perpendicular to the line of observation, prismatic errors may also be excluded and (5) The contact lens allows for its own illumination by means of a fiber optic system (Fig. 12 A and B).

Swan-Jacob Lens. Swan has designed a gonioprism which is used with the magnification of a microscope. The microscope is least awkward to use when it is placed directly over the eye, so that it needs to be focused only up and down. Therefore, the Swan gonioprism is shaped with a curved front surface angled to minimize distortion, so that the surgeon may stand at the head of the table and see a large area of the angle even without magnification. The operation can therefore be performed with the patient's head in the conventional operating position. The lens is small enough that a speculum may be used and canthotomy, as recommended by Barkan, is unnecessary. The fluid space has been eliminated so that the lens may be placed on the cornea with only a drop of solution lubricating the corneal surface. This may be a disadvantage, since the direct contact of the lens on the cornea may cause folding of Descemet's membrane in the thin cornea of congenital glaucoma, decreasing visibility.

The gonioprism has a handle which allows the lens to be manipulated by the operator without having his fingers in the surgical field (Fig. 24). The lens can also be placed on the cornea after the knife has entered the globe and has been passed across the chamber angle. This is simpler than to have the surgeon pass the knife across the pupillary area with the lens in place, except, perhaps, with the Worst lens which is attached to the globe itself. According to Swan, goniotomies have been performed on the temporal and vertical areas as well as the nasal side, since the lens makes the entire circumference of the chamber angle accessible.

GONIOSCOPIC FLUIDS. *Saline.* Saline is readily available in the operating room and can be used with the Lister and Worst canulated lenses.

Methyl Cellulose. Haag-Streit gonioscopic fluid (methocel) is thick,

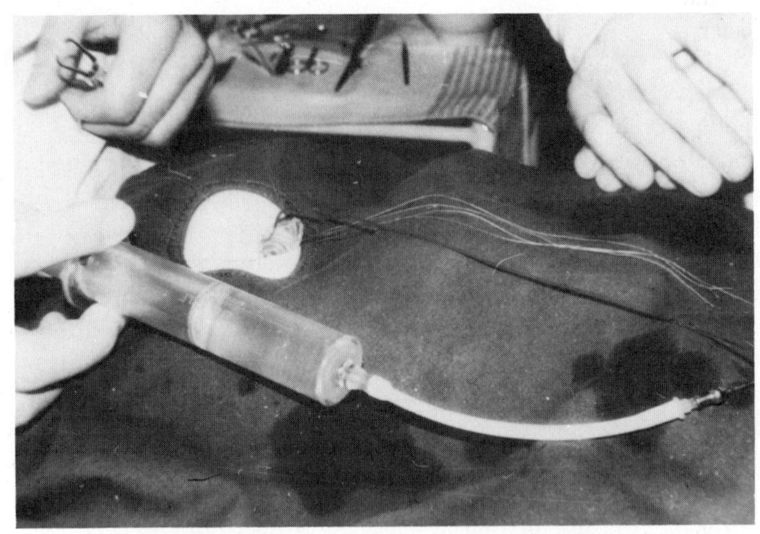

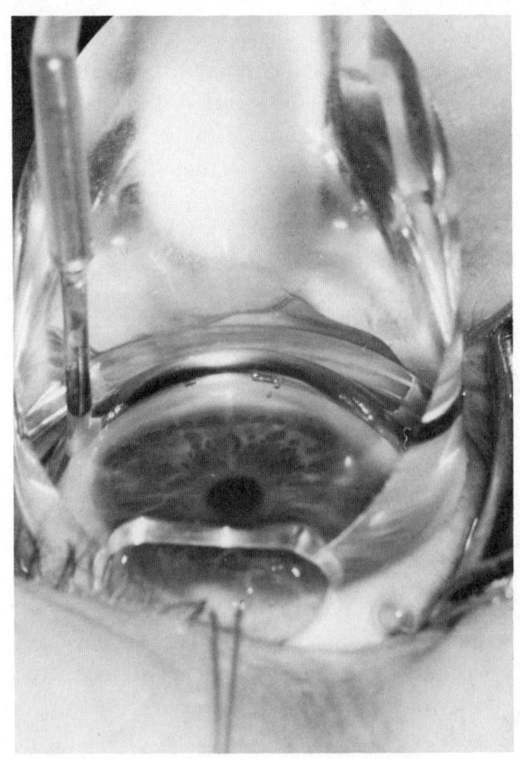

FIG. 23. The prismatic goniotomy lens.

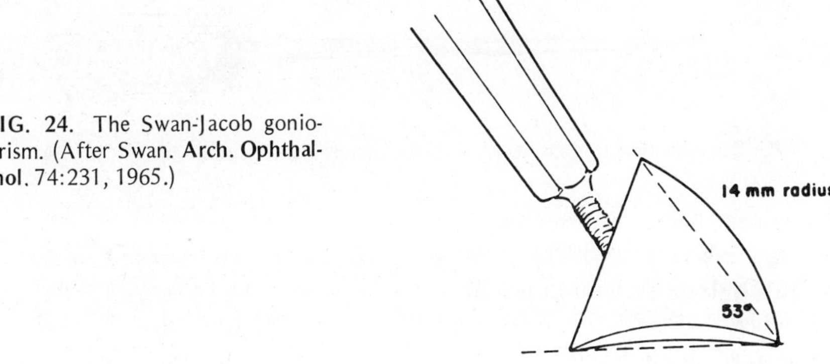

FIG. 24. The Swan-Jacob gonioprism. (After Swan. **Arch. Ophthalmol.** 74:231, 1965.)

viscid yet extremely clear, and gives excellent suction between lens and eyeball. The frequent appearance of air bubbles at crucial times in the operation, when less viscid fluids are used, is thus avoided. Care must be taken to clear away all excess fluid so that none will be carried into the anterior chamber with the goniotomy knife.

GONIOTOMY KNIVES. The selection of a knife for goniotomy is important because of the preciseness of the operation, which must be performed with minimal trauma and without loss of the anterior chamber.

The relationship between the blade and the taper of the shaft must be such as to allow easy passage of the knife across the anterior chamber, but must provide adequate plugging of the entry wound to prevent loss of aqueous before the goniotomy has been completed. The blade tip must be handled with great care and tested on a drum before each procedure, insuring the integrity of the point and sharpness of the blade.

Barkan Knife. The Barkan knife has a relatively wide blade and a

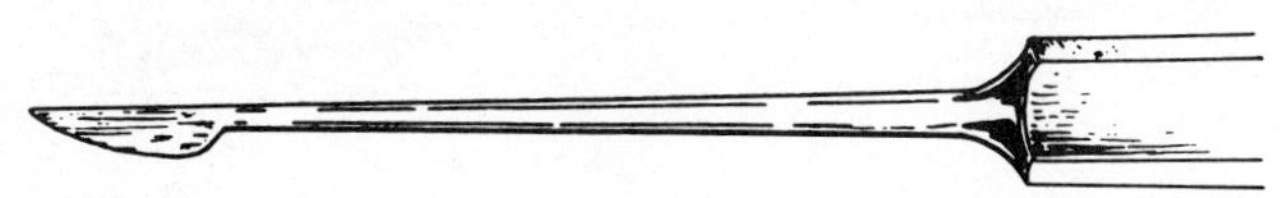

FIG. 25. The Barkan knife. (After Swan. **Arch. Ophthalmol.** 74:231, 1965.)

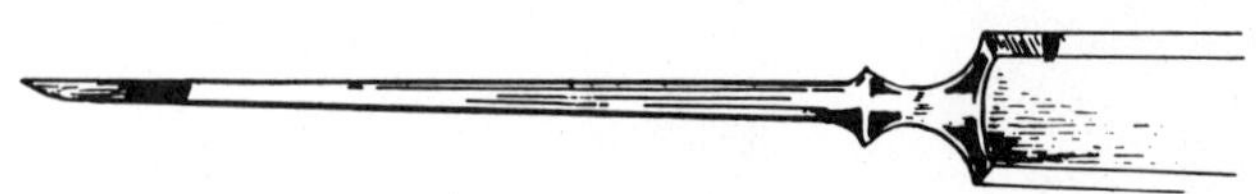

FIG. 26. The discission knife. (After Swan. **Arch. Ophthalmol.** 74:231, 1965.)

prominent heel, which makes a large hole on penetration and is apt to catch on the iris (Fig. 25). The shaft is slightly conical and tapered to fill the relatively large puncture opening as the knife is advanced across the anterior chamber. This makes it increasingly difficult to slide the shaft through the cornea when approaching the chamber angle. A dimple may form at this critical moment, sucking air under the contact lens. For reaching more lateral regions of the chamber angle the knife must be slightly retracted, thus giving the aqueous a chance to escape along the now less well-closed puncture. Aqueous may also be lost as the knife is withdrawn.

Discission Knife. The small, delicate knife which was designed for the discission operation (Fig. 26) eliminates most of the disadvantages of the Barkan knife. The blade is smaller than the shaft, so that the aqueous does not escape when the knife is being manipulated in the anterior chamber or even when the blade is withdrawn. This knife has a relatively short shaft, so that in large eyes it may be difficult to reach completely across the anterior chamber. The knife also has the disadvantage that it cuts in only one direction and, therefore, must be turned over if the surgeon desires to cut in the opposite direction.

Swan Knife. Because of the difficulties described for the Barkan and discission knives, Swan designed a knife with a spade-shaped blade (Fig. 27) which permits cutting in both directions without having to be rotated. The shaft is narrower than the other blades so that only a small puncture wound is made at the point of entry into the globe, and this is blocked by the shaft.

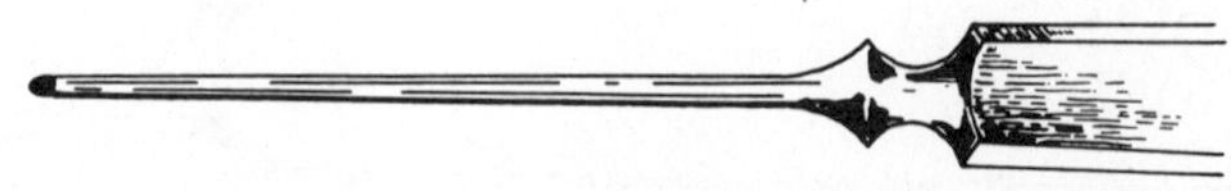

FIG. 27. The Swan knife. (After Swan. **Arch. Ophthalmol.** 74:231, 1965.)

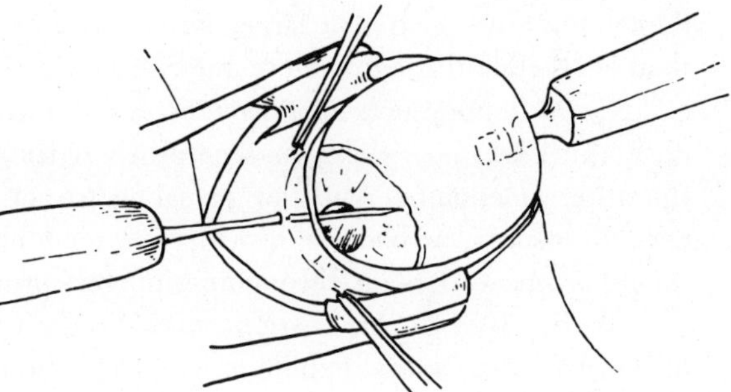

FIG. 28. The Swan-Jacob gonioprism and Swan knife. Puncture is made under a conjunctival flap. (After Swan. **Arch Ophthalmol.** 74:231, 1965.)

Although the knife is usually introduced through clear peripheral cornea, Swan prefers to slant the blade through the limbus under a conjunctival flap, as shown in Fig. 28. Any leak of aqueous around the shaft of the knife is promptly blocked by the conjunctiva reducing the risk of a shallow chamber, or, at worst, resulting in a temporary filtration similar to that sought by goniopuncture. Another important advantage of making a

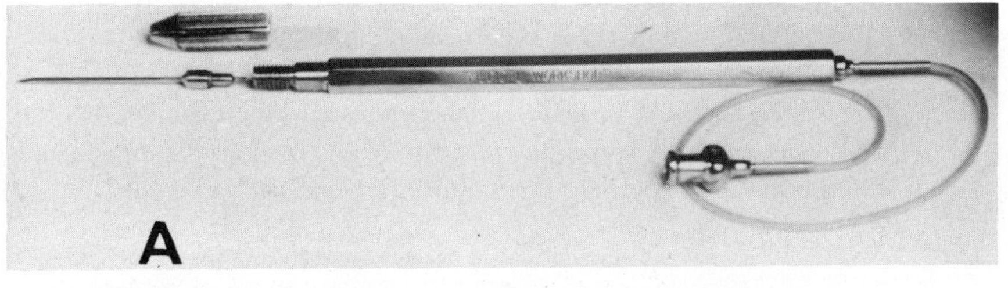

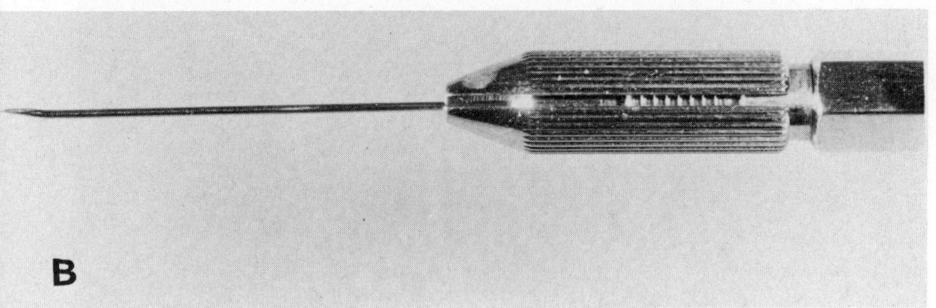

FIG. 29. The Worst hydrostatic goniotomy needle.

limbal puncture is that a larger circumference of the angle can be reached than is possible through a more anterior point of entry.

Corneal punctures made under conjunctiva are often difficult to find once the knife is withdrawn. Therefore, if the surgeon would prefer to fill the anterior chamber with air or saline to act as a tamponade because of excess bleeding, or because of a shallow chamber, it may not be as easy as if the puncture were made through peripheral cornea.

Worst Hydrostatic Goniotomy Needle. The goniotomy needle is inserted in the hollow handle (Fig. 29A). The needle is passed through the slit in the knurled nut and the nut is screwed on the handle (Fig. 29B). The tip of the needle has a sharpened bevel. A cannula is attached to the end of the handle, which in turn is connected via a polyvinyl chloride (PVC) tubing to a saline-filled 5 cc syringe or an intravenous infusion bottle. Care must be taken to wash out all air bubbles from the system before introducing the needle into the eye. The bottle is hung at least 100 cm above the eye, thus creating hydrostatic pressure which maintains the depth of the anterior chamber. Adjustments in pressure are made, after observing the position of the lens-iris diaphragm, by raising or lowering the bottle after the needle has been introduced into the anterior chamber. Although a slightly deepened chamber is preferable because it places angle structures on the stretch, too much deepening causes an increase in corneal edema.

The simpler preferred method is to attach the cannula to a 5 cc syringe filled with saline. Pressure is maintained in the anterior chamber by the assistant, who can carefully watch the position of the iris-lens diaphragm and deepen the chamber by injecting some saline when necessary (Fig. 30).

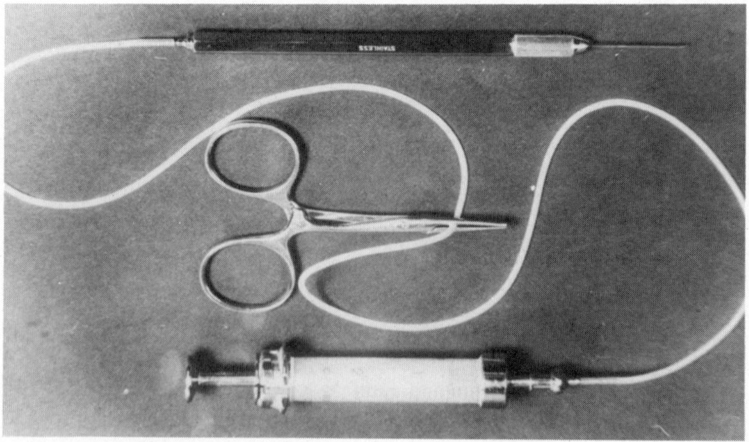

FIG. 30. The Worst hydrostatic goniotomy needle attached to syringe via a polyvinyl chloride (PVC) tubing.

OTHER INSTRUMENTS. The other instruments required include a small speculum; two pairs of curved, self-locking fixation forceps; 2 cc, 5 cc, and 10 cc Luer lock syringes, and an iris spatula to provide pressure over the entry wound during the injection of air or saline. When performing the delicate maneuvers of the goniotomy operation dependable fixation of the head is of great importance: an adequate headrest should be employed. Worst has designed an air cannula with a safety stop that limits the entry of the sharp point into the anterior chamber. This can be used to inject air as well as saline into the anterior chamber following goniotomy, although a blunt narrow gauge needle serves equally as well. A blunt punctum dilator may be used when the iris is caught in the corneal puncture although injection of air or fluid usually accomplishes this task.

Preparation of Instruments

The goniotomy lens should be soaked in a sterilizing solution (Zephiran, or an equivalent solution). Plastic lenses cannot withstand boiling or autoclaving. The other instruments should be sterilized by the same method used for other eye instruments.

SPONTANEOUS GONIOTOMY

With careful gonioscopy, it can often be shown that many apparently normal second eyes in unilateral congenital glaucoma show some signs of the disease. A spontaneous goniotomy may have saved these eyes from the fate of buphthalmia. Other cases show definite signs of congenital glaucoma, e.g., corneal distension, either with or without rupture of Descemet's membrane but with normal tension. In some cases the rupture in Descemet's membrane may be found to extend into the chamber angle, possibly causing a disruption in the angle which allows filtration to take place.

PRACTICE GONIOTOMY

Goniotomy requires a certain expertise in manual skills which differ in several respects from the normal surgical routine. It is therefore desirable for the beginner to practice this type of microsurgical intervention before actually performing the operation. This practice goniotomy may be done with any of the lenses and knives already described in order that the surgeon determines, as with other surgical procedures, which instruments best suit his own talents. Both the cat eye and pig eye are suitable. The use of the cat eye

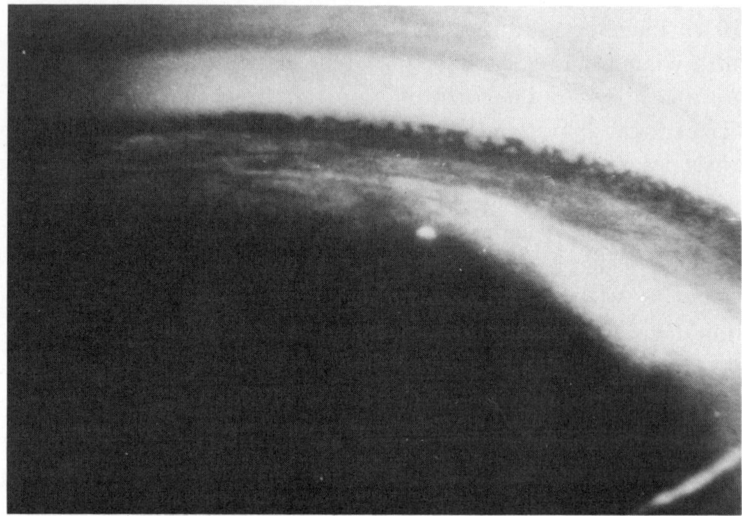

FIG. 31. Pig's eye, chamber angle.

requires the sacrifice of laboratory animals. The pig eye serves equally well, is more easily obtainable from any abbatoir, and bears many apparent physical similarities to those encountered in the chamber angle of congenital glaucoma. The chamber angle of a pig's eye is shown in Fig. 31 with its typical pectinate ligament. The goniotomy knife is introduced into the anterior chamber and the pectinate ligaments are severed from their attachment (Fig. 32 A and B), resulting in a downward movement of the iris root not unlike that seen after stripping of the chamber angle in congenital glaucoma.

AIR GONIOTOMY

It has been demonstrated by animal experimentation that a distinct view of the anterior chamber angle can be obtained if air is substituted for the aqueous humor. Experimentally, a fine, sharp, no. 27 gauge hypodermic needle, mounted on a tuberculin syringe, is inserted into the anterior chamber of a rabbit eye through an oblique puncture at the limbus. The experiment has also been performed in the dog. The needle is directed to a point slightly peripheral to the margin of the pupil, so that the lens is protected. The aqueous is withdrawn, collapsing the chamber. The syringe is removed from the needle and replaced with a second, empty one, with the plunger drawn back halfway. Two cc of air are injected, filling the anterior chamber and pushing the iris-lens diaphragm from the collapsed position to one slightly back than normal. The angle of the anterior chamber becomes visible, and with a binocular loupe details are readily identifiable by direct observation without the aid of a gonioscopy lens.

It was proposed that goniotomy could be carried out under these conditions, since the absence of a contact lens would greatly simplify the procedure. It would also be possible to perform a goniotomy in cases of glaucoma with a shallow anterior chamber, as well as in those with a wide angle. However, visualization is often disturbed by reflections from the anterior and posterior corneal surfaces, and the appearance of folds in Descemet's membrane produced by the fixation forceps when the intraocular pressure is lowered. Moreover, the size of the image is smaller than when seen through the system of cornea and aqueous or cornea and saline solution. The magnifying power with these fluids, for oblique observation, is approximately X1.15. When combined with the power of a contact lens, the total magnification when seen through the lens, cornea, and fluid system amounts to about X1.73, depending on the type of lens, whereas there is no magnification when seen through air.

DEEPENING AND MAINTENANCE OF THE ANTERIOR CHAMBER

Preliminary deepening of the chamber is rarely indicated because of the increased depth normally found in congenital glaucoma. However, in cases where the chamber is shallow and the angle unusually narrow, as in very young infants, or when cloudiness of the cornea reduces visibility for surgery, preliminary deepening of the chamber is helpful. This maneuver minimizes the hazard of picking up the root of the iris with the tip of the knife, and permits a more accurate anteroposterior placement of the incision. Even in the ideal case, much of the difficulty in the goniotomy and goniopuncture operation is a result of the loss of the anterior chamber depth at a critical moment, and consequent disappearance of the angle landmarks leading to failure or only partial success of the intended surgery. Deepening of the chamber is indicated postoperatively to act as a tamponade where there is excessive bleeding, and also to prevent contact with the formation of adhesions between the iris and the raw surfaces of the angle wall incision.

Continuous control of the anterior chamber depth can be attained by use of the following method described by Wong and Collier.

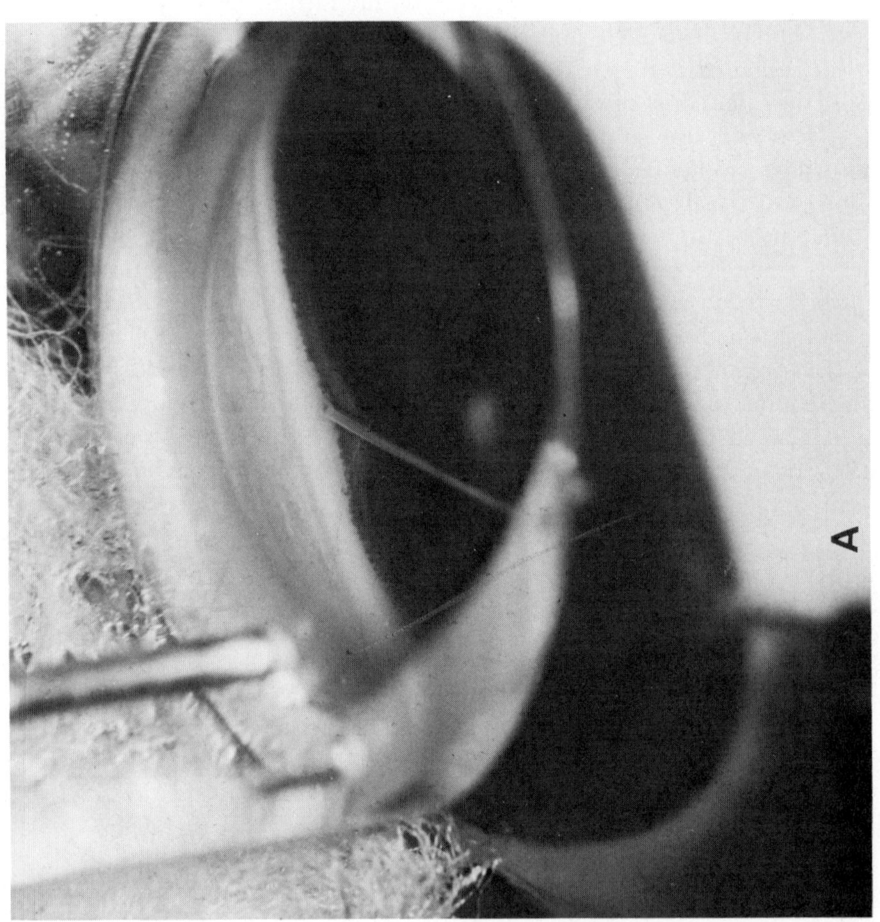

FIG. 32.A. Pig's eye, practice goniotomy.

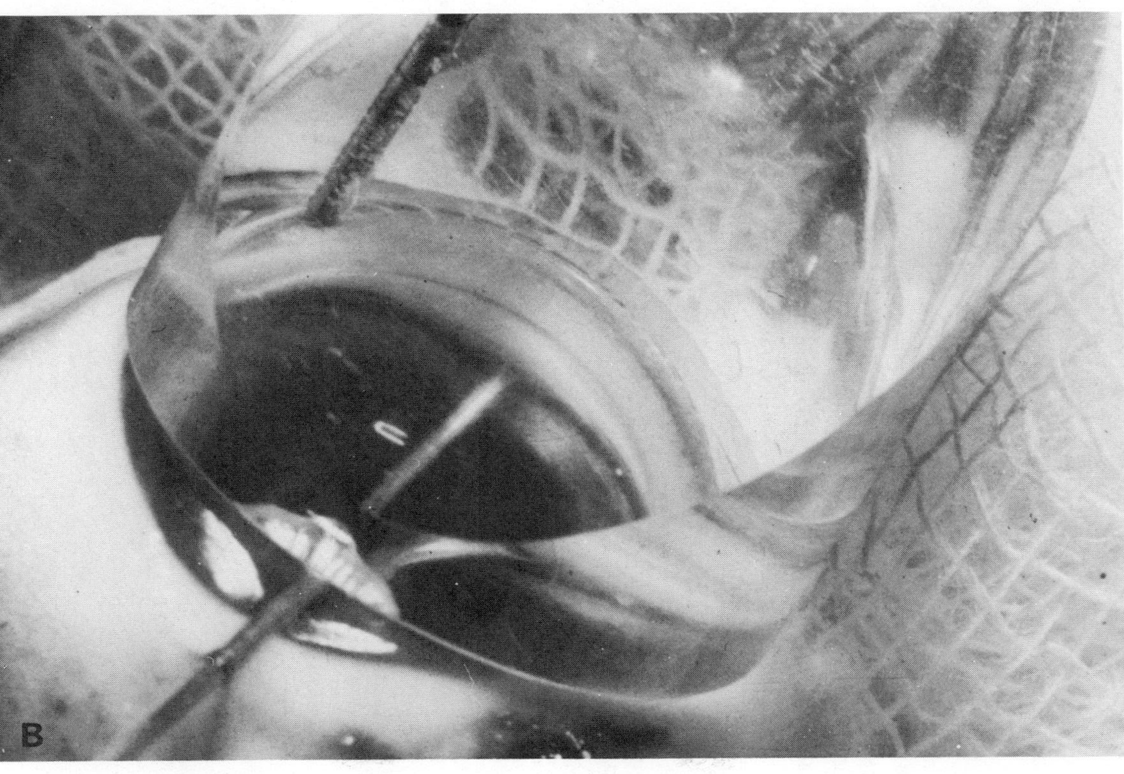

FIG. 32.B. Pig's eye, pectinate ligaments being cut with goniotomy knife. (Courtesy of J. G. F. Worst.)

Technique

A 27-gauge, 0.5-in long hypodermic needle attached to a 10 cc saline-filled syringe is inserted into one end of a No. 20 polyethylene tube (approximately 12 in in length). A second 27-gauge needle is broken from its attachment to the hub, and the blunt end inserted into the opposite end of the PE tube (sterilized by immersion in 70 percent ethyl alcohol for 24 hrs). The tubing is then irrigated with gentle pressure on the syringe plunger to eliminate air and to insure against leakage within the system. At the time of operation, the eye is fixed with forceps at the opposite limbus. Using a discission knife, previously dipped in fluorescein, a tangential incision is made into the anterior chamber, one mm axial to the corneoscleral border and parallel to the surface of the iris, at 6:30 in the right eye and 5:30 in the left eye (Fig. 33). The wound canal should be at least 3 mm long, and the tip of the knife should barely perforate Descemet's membrane as observed through a X 5 magnifying binocular loupe. It may be necessary to tip the knife backward slightly in order to perforate this membrane. The needle tip from the end of the polyethylene tubing is then inserted into the anterior chamber through the wound canal (Fig. 34). The tubing should be fixed either with a towel clip, or by placing it under the lid speculum. Control of the anterior chamber depth can now be maintained by the assistant during the surgical procedure, with slight positive or negative pressure on the

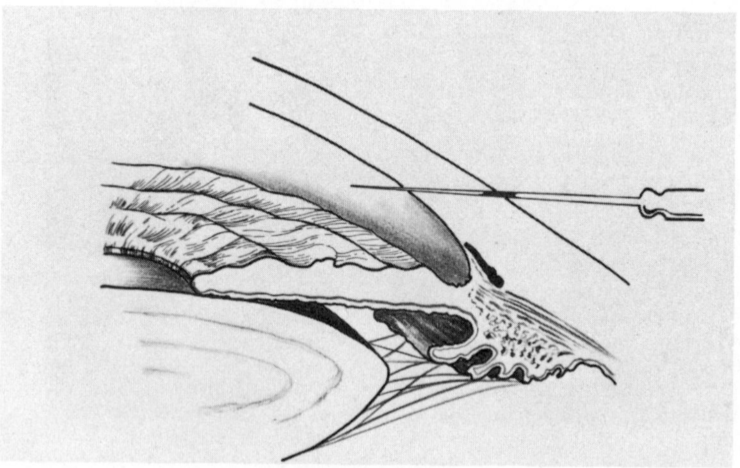

FIG. 33. Maintaining and deepening of the anterior chamber, limbal puncture. (After Wong and Collier. **Arch. Ophthalmol.** 77:384, 1967.)

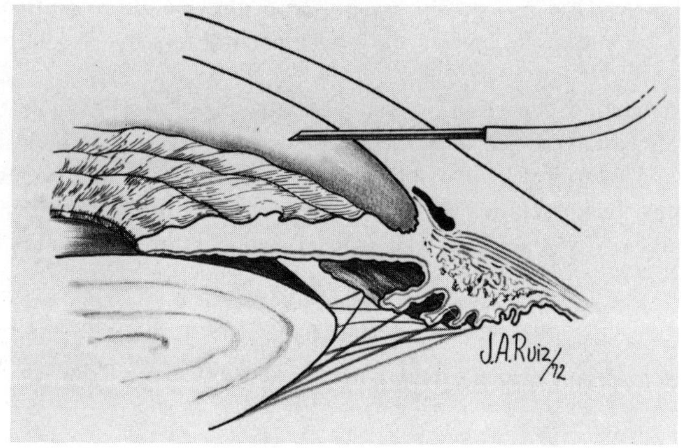

FIG. 34. Maintaining and deepening of the anterior chamber. Introduction of the 27-gauge needle attached to the polyethylene tubing. (After Wong and Collier. **Arch. Ophthalmol.** 77:384, 1967.)

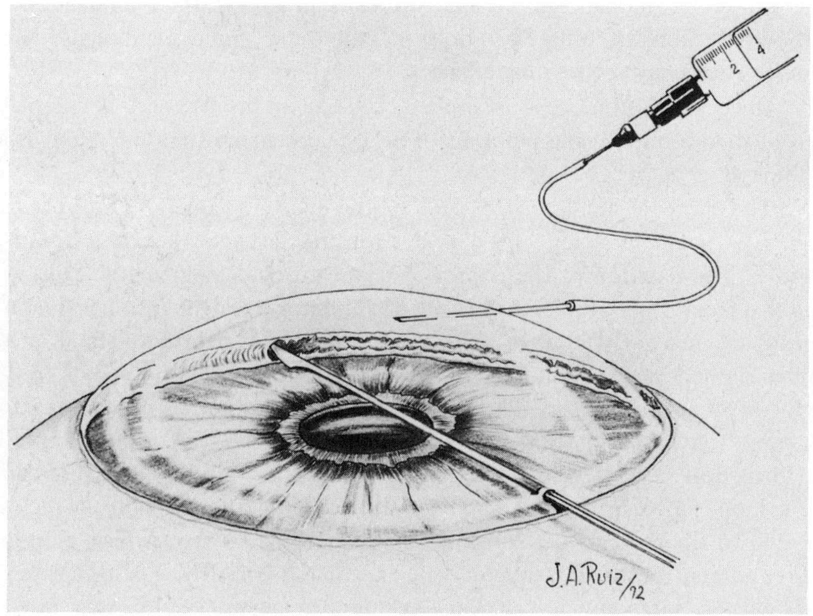

FIG. 35. Maintaining and deepening of the anterior chamber during a goniotomy procedure. (After Wong and Collier. **Arch. Ophthalmol.** 77:384, 1967.)

syringe plunger (Fig. 35). At the conclusion of the operation, gentle pressure is applied on the syringe while the surgeon withdraws the needle from the eye.

Deepening of the anterior chamber introduces another delicate technical detail which, if not adequately performed, may result in leakage of aqueous and postponement of the operation. However, if the surgeon feels that he must have facilities available to deepen the anterior chamber at will, the cannulated Worst knife, as well as the above method, satisfies these needs adequately.

GONIOTOMY TECHNIQUES

The Barkan Technique

Goniotomy Using the Contact Lens

Most of the techniques described by Bietti, Swan, Lister, Shaffer, Kwitko, and others are simply adaptations of the original Barkan technique. His description of the operation is still valid today, although some modifications have proven beneficial.

Once the contact lens is applied, time is of the essence. A complete check, therefore, is made beforehand in order to assure that everything is in readiness.

The surgeon stands on the side of the eye to be operated on; for the right eye between 9 and 11 o'clock; for the left eye, between 3 and 4 o'clock. The position of the *fixator* assistant (at 3 o'clock for the right eye and 9 o'clock for the left) and of the *illuminator* assistant (at the surgeon's right) are checked. Either or both may require a platform to stand on to obtain a good view of the field of operation. The scrub nurse stands to the right of the *illuminator.* The instruments are tested (e.g., syringes for patency) and placed where they are easily reached. A canthotomy is performed, if necessary, with straight scissors. The contact lens is dried and placed on gauze in a small bowl on the small instrument table, which is located to the right of the surgeon. The goniotomy knives are placed on the table, points toward the surgeon. The anesthetist is on the side opposite to that of the surgeon, i.e., at 5 o'clock for the right eye, in order not to interfere with the *fixator* assistant standing at 3 o'clock. The positions are changed appropriately for the left eye. The speculum is now inserted. The corneal epithelium is removed as described, and the cornea moistened with physiological saline solution applied by means of a glass rod or irrigator. The eye is fixated 2 to 3 mm posterior to the corneoscleral border, at 12 and 6 o'clock, by means of two self-locking forceps. Care must be taken not to touch the locks, to prevent them from springing open during the operation.

When operating on the right eye, the *fixator's* right hand holds the forceps at 12 o'clock, the left at 6. The left hand must be in such a position that it does not obstruct the view of the *illuminator* as he moves counterclockwise. When operating on the left eye, the right hand is at 6 o'clock and the left at 12. Regardless of the side under operation, the *fixator,* unless tall, should stand on a platform in order to assure comfortable visibility of the eye throughout the procedure, and to prevent the tendency (arising from poor visibility) to retract or dimple the eye with the forceps.

If a speculum is not used, the forceps are better applied to the insertions of the superior and inferior recti; or they may be applied to other meridia and the eye rotated, according to the area of the filtration angle chosen for surgery. An alternate method is to use superior and inferior rectus bridle sutures (Fig. 36).

The surgeon grasps the eye in the horizontal meridian at the nasal limbus with a fixation forceps. A preliminary oblique knife-needle puncture may be made in the upper temporal quadrant to permit restoration of the anterior chamber following surgery. At this moment the surgeon may choose to perform a horizontal temporal puncture to provide a track for the

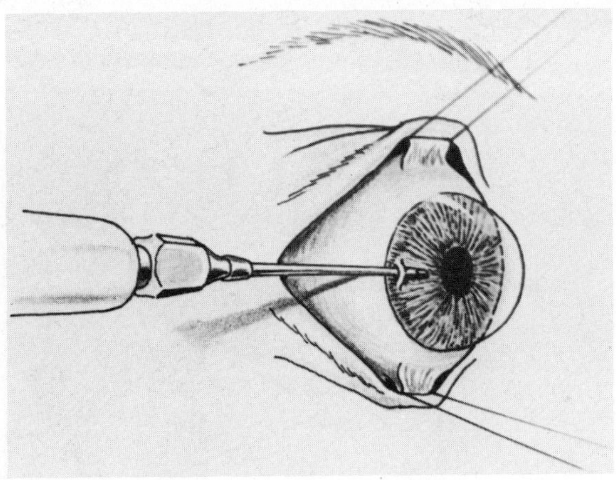

FIG. 36. Creation of a tract for the goniotomy knife.

goniotomy knife (Fig. 36), although a sharp knife should make this maneuver unnecessary. The head and eye are rotated away from the surgeon, who applies the contact lens by injecting either methyl cellulose or physiological saline solution between it and the cornea. The Swan-Jacob lens may be applied after the knife has entered the anterior chamber. The lens is manipulated and the height of the table and lights are adjusted until the optimum view of the operative field is obtained. The operator may apply the end of a cotton swab, previously dipped in an antibiotic solution, to the intended site of puncture. The surgeon supports the lens with the index finger of his left hand (Fig. 37). The two indentations on top of the lens cause friction, helping to prevent the finger from slipping, or they may be used with a forceps for fixation (Fig. 38). The *fixator* rotates the eye slightly to expose the temporal limbus where the puncture is to be made. The goniotomy knife is then passed to the operator, by the instrument nurse. She retracts the instrument table and the *illuminator* assumes his position on a platform immediately to the operator's right, sufficiently removed from him to provide room to sway counterclockwise. The *illuminator* must stand with feet well apart, to be able to sway in unison with the counterclockwise movement of the surgeon without having to take a step. He maintains the lamp in contact with the temple of the surgeon, at the same time looking down the line of the lamp to have the same view of the angle and blade of the knife as the surgeon.

The eye is punctured obliquely, either at the limbus or under

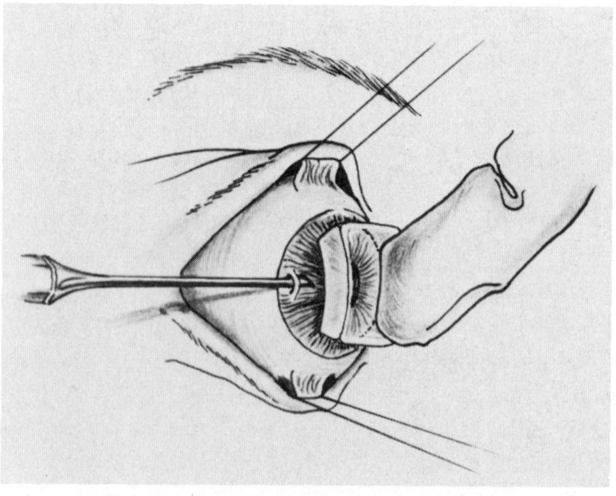

FIG. 37. Barkan lens held by index finger.

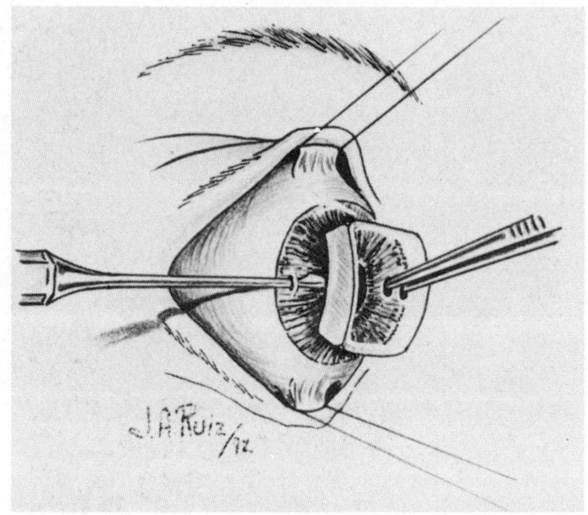

FIG. 38. Barkan lens fixated with forceps.

conjunctiva opposite the region to be operated. At the moment of puncture, extra pressure on the contact lens is exerted by the operator's index finger in the direction of the optic axis, to prevent ingress of air under the lens. For the same reason the lens must not be tilted and dimpling of the sclera with the fixator's forceps must be avoided.

The operator slides the knife with the blade flat across the pupil and parallel to the iris plane to the opposite side.

Placement of Incision

Since extensive stripping is associated with a greater hazard of hemorrhage, it is well to consider allocating the area of the first incision in such a way that another untouched area of the angle can be stripped on a second occasion. For this purpose, it is advisable to start with the eye rotated 2 hrs in a counterclockwise direction. Rotation is necessary because the excursion in the right eye is limited by the brow, and in the left by the cheek bone. The right eye is rotated so as to bring the area between 3 and 6 o'clock of the nasal angle within operative reach. If a later examination shows that this procedure was not sufficient to normalize the pressure, stripping of a neighboring area of the angle (from 3 to 12) may be undertaken. In the latter case, the right eye is rotated 2 hrs in a clockwise direction to make the area accessible. It is possible, therefore, by means of two goniotomies, to strip the angle up to one-half of its circumference.

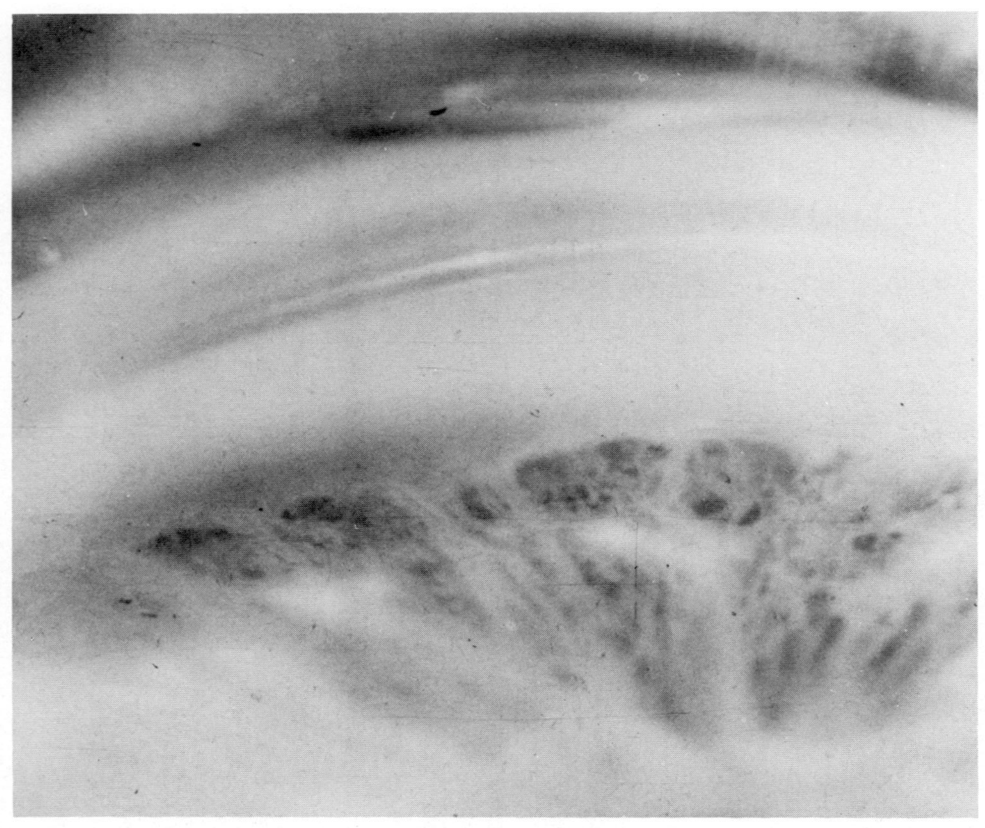

FIG. 39. Filtration angle in congenital glaucoma illustrating the semiopaque band of tissue just posterior to Schwalbe's line. (Courtesy of J. G. F. Worst.)

If the incision is superior to the trabeculum the operation will be nonfunctional. If the incision is placed inferior to the trabeculum, only pectinate fibers and iris root are affected, causing a peripheral iridotomy which can be the source of considerable hemorrhage and goniosynechiae as the blood organizes.

In infants only a few days old where there has been no distention, the corneal diameter may be no more than 10 mm and the anterior chamber relatively shallow. The small size of the anterior segment makes goniotomy technically difficult, so that a preliminary deepening of the anterior chamber, as already described, facilitates the operation.

Since most infants have blue eyes with a transparent iris stroma, the scalloped, serrated edge of the pigment segment of the epithelial layer at the iris root is a prominent feature on gonioscopy and makes an excellent landmark by which to judge placement of the point of the blade, i.e., in the anterior aspect of the middle third of the trabeculum, the semiopaque band of tissue just posterior to the line of Schwalbe (shown in Fig. 39). The iris structure moves posteriorly, and a membranous interface seems to cleave.

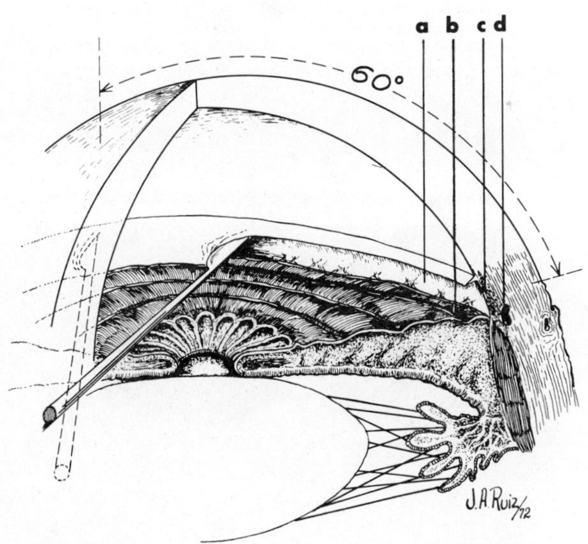

FIG. 40. Goniotomy. Incision placed at the anterior aspect of the middle third of the trabeculum. (A) Filtration angle; (B) iris; (C) trabeculum; (D) Schlemm's canal. (Modified from Boyd. **Highlights Ophthalmol.** 7:5, 1966.)

The iris root is seen to retract behind the blade, leaving a white wake (Fig. 40). Great care must be exercised to avoid blood vessels at the iris root which are usually clearly visible. During the stripping, some resistance is felt in the form of a slight grating sensation which gives the operator a feeling of guidance and deliberate movement; the fixator must recognize the need to exert slight resistance.

The blade is moved counterclockwise, dividing the tissue in this plane as long as adequate visibility permits. The point is then disengaged, the blade rotated and brought back to the starting point, and swept in the opposite direction. One-quarter to one-third of the circumference of the angle is treated in this way at one sitting, unless an unusual number of vessels present a risk of excessive hemorrhage. The treated arc should then be shorter. It has been confirmed in some cases, as shown by postoperative gonioscopy, to strip the angle over almost one-half its circumference at one operation. However, it is better to repeat the operation than to tempt a major hemorrhage by too extensive a stripping.

It seems remarkable that exposure of a relatively small area of trabeculum, provided that this area is normally permeable and has not

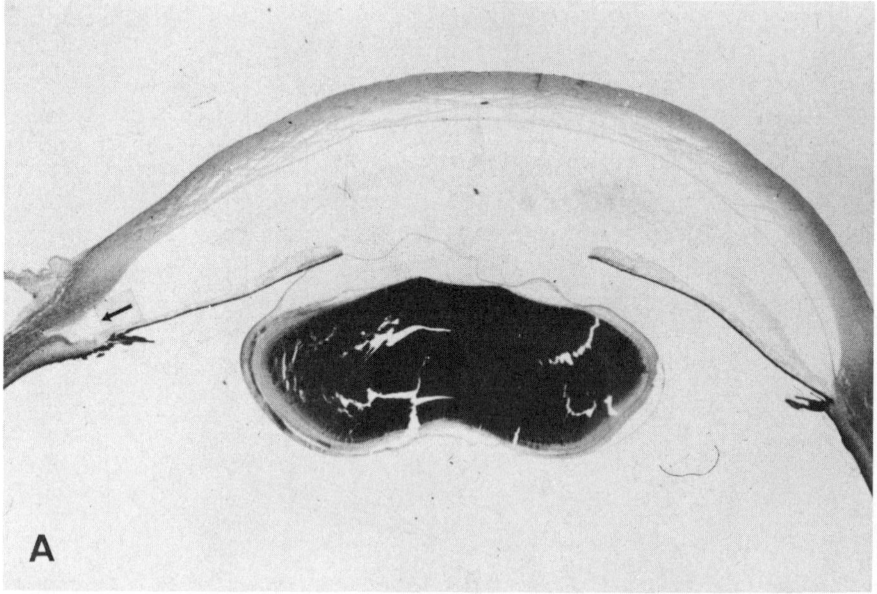

FIG. 41.A. Congenital glaucoma. The one side has been successfully operated (arrow). (Courtesy of F. D. Costenbader.) X75.

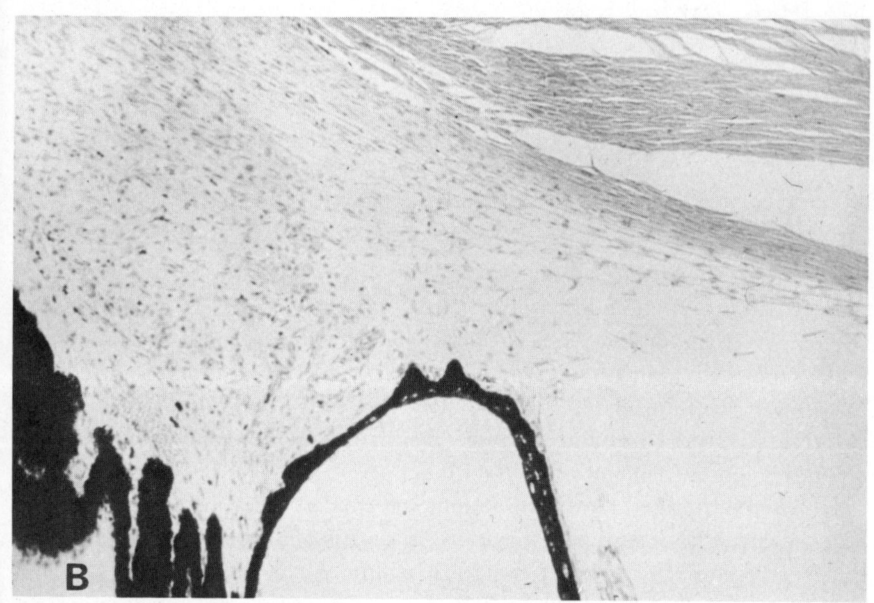

FIG. 41.B. Congenital glaucoma. The unoperated angle. (Courtesy of F. D. Costenbader.) X300.

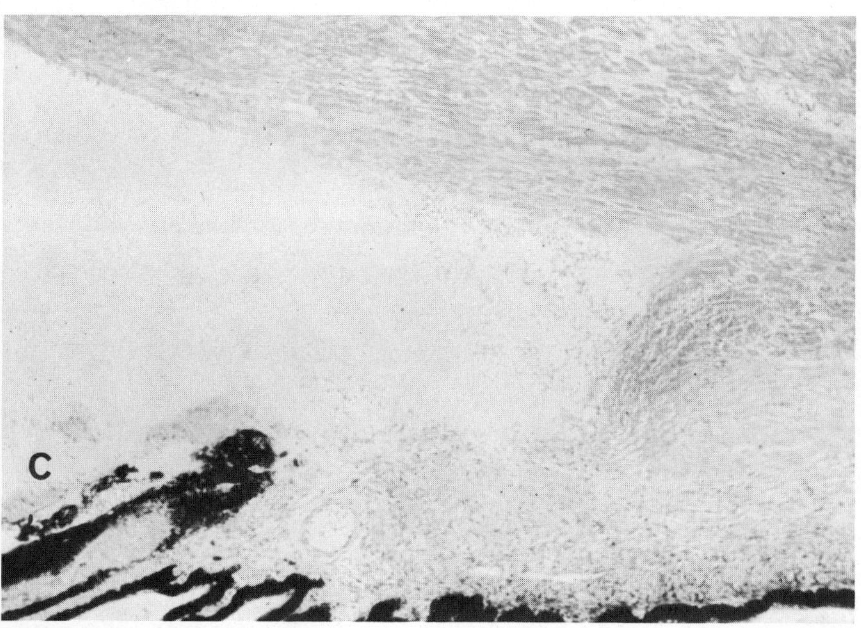

FIG. 41.C. Congenital glaucoma. The operated angle. (Courtesy of F. D. Costenbader.) X 300.

become scarred as the result of surgical trauma or the condition itself, is sufficient to normalize tension. The explanation may be that the trabeculo-Schlemm's canal mechanism has a much greater potential capacity for outflow than is necessary for normal physiologic demands. It may also be that access to aqueous flow is given to adjoining areas beyond the ends of the incision.

Fig. 41 illustrates a case of congenital glaucoma where the angle was incised, normalizing the intraocular pressure.

If the stripping has been properly placed, some blood of venous color quite commonly, but not invariably, begins to ooze from several points along the line of stripping, a few seconds after removal of the knife. When a small arteriole is severed bleeding is more extensive, and may follow immediately upon the commencement of the incision.

When stripping has been completed the contact lens and fixation forceps are withdrawn and the knife is gently removed. Care is taken to avoid enlarging the corneal puncture wound by exerting slight pressure against the back of the blade during its removal with an iris spatula. Often some aqueous humour escapes from the entry wound. Should the pupil remain eccentric after removal of the knife, the cornea is tapped near the puncture site with a spatula, or the tip of a blunt punctum dilator is inserted to remove the iris adhesion. It is essential to reform the anterior chamber with saline, acetylcholine solution (Miochol), or air (Fig. 42) to maintain the

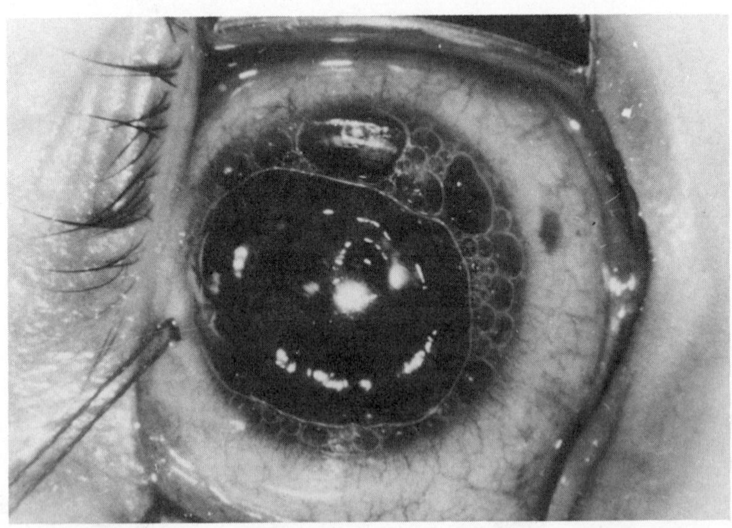

FIG. 42. Postoperative goniotomy with air in anterior chamber.

patency of the goniotomy cleft and to prevent, as far as possible, the formation of peripheral anterior synechiae. Acetylcholine (Miochol) is probably the most effective agent since it also constricts the pupil, thus withdrawing iris tissue from both incision and puncture sites. This maneuver is carried out by means of a 2 cc syringe and narrow-gauge blunt cannula inserted through the puncture site. Light pressure should be maintained with the iris spatula over the entry wound for about 10 sec after withdrawal of the cannula, to seal the wound and prevent escape of the solution. Sometimes the cannula cannot be inserted through the entry wound; then the small oblique peripheral corneal puncture made earlier in the procedure can be used. If this was not done, the puncture may not be made easily at this time because of the softness of the eyeball.

Removal of blood from the anterior chamber is usually unnecessary, since bleeding often stops in several minutes. The blood itself acts as a tamponade. Blood that may fill over one-half or more of the chamber at the end of the procedure is usually absorbed within 24 to 48 hrs. Secondary bleeding rarely occurs.

The speculum is removed; the canthotomy need not be closed with sutures (and still heals adequately). Pilocarpine 1 percent eye drops and chloramphenicol drops are instilled into the conjunctival sac. Binocular pads are applied, the pad over the operated eye being covered with a rigid shield. The child is placed in bed on the operated side, so that the blood present may settle on the opposite side of the anterior chamber. Arm cuffs may be applied if deemed necessary. In older children, restraints are usually not required.

Elixir phenobarbitol may be indicated to sedate the child. After 24 hrs the patches are removed and the eye examined. The hyphema has usually cleared. Chloramphenicol ointment is applied to the operated eye with an eye pad and shield. The dressings are removed after 48 hrs.

Goniotomy without Contact Lens

Barkan and Scheie have outlined the following procedure for use when *goniotomy using the contact lens* is not feasible. It must be emphasized that operating under the contact lens is desirable whenever possible, and that a description of the "blind goniotomy" is included only for the sake of completeness. It has been described by experienced goniotomists who themselves have emphasized the need for diligent practice before attempting this procedure.

The preparatory measures already outlined for goniotomy using the contact lens are carried out. The height of the eye should be such that the operator looks vertically down upon it. Illumination is provided by a high intensity lamp, placed in a position so that the light falls as nearly vertically from above as possible. The *illuminator* stands opposite the surgeon, at 4 o'clock for the right eye, and 8 o'clock for the left eye. The bulbus is fixated with two forceps held by the assistant, in the same manner as for the operation with the contact lens. The forceps should be held vertical to the sclera and must include episcleral tissue, to permit the *fixator* to offer resistance or counterpressure during stripping. Additional fixation at the contralateral limbus by the operator, with a forceps held in his left hand, is helpful. If the assistant is not sufficiently experienced with this operation, it is best for the surgeon to divide the functions of fixation with him. In this case the surgeon fixates with the locking forceps in his left hand at 12 o'clock on the right eye and at 6 o'clock on the left, while the assistant fixates with his left hand at 6 o'clock on the right eye and at 12 o'clock on the left. The head is rotated toward the surgeon and the eye slightly abducted to bring the nasal limbus into a frontal plane with the surgeon's line of sight. In the case of a greatly enlarged eye this lateral movement may be limited because the temporal limbus disappears behind the lateral canthus as the result of even slight abduction.

The puncture in the cornea is made as already described, either just within the temporal limbus or just beyond the limbus under conjunctiva in the horizontal meridian, making certain that it is oblique (valvelike) to encourage retention and reformation of the anterior chamber. The blade of the knife is carried across the anterior chamber, avoiding the pupil in transit. The tip disappears behind the limbus on the opposite side in a plane just anterior to that of the iris. According to Scheie, a correct position of the knife in the angle is insured if the knife is carried across the anterior chamber in such a way that the tip is directed at the junction of clear cornea and sclera, "as if making a counterpuncture for a cataract section that would be too deep."

When seen through the cornea, the knife appears about 0.5 mm further anterior (shallower) than it is in actuality. This appearance must not influence the surgeon to guide his knife deeper in the anterior chamber, as a posterior position of the blade is the greatest hazard of the operation. It is better to err on the conservative side by maintaining a more anterior plane at the risk of not stripping the angle. The operation can always be repeated. As the blade engages the angle and starts its excursion in a counterclockwise direction slight resistance is felt, associated with a grating feeling as the knife is guided somewhat by the inner scleral sulcus. The absence of this feeling is an indication that the blade is placed too far posteriorly. In the right eye, the knife is inserted in the 9 o'clock meridian and the sweeping incision started in the angle at the 5 o'clock position. It is extended upward as nearly as possible to the 1 o'clock meridian. Rotation of the knife clockwise, after sweeping in one direction is completed, around its own axis helps to prevent it from being guided or from slipping into a more posterior position. The knife is then withdrawn over the iris, keeping the blade away from the pupillary space. The remainder of the procedure is completed in a fashion already described for *goniotomy with the contact lens.*

Air Block

If the miotic pupil is completely covered by air some degree of air seclusion may be observed, producing a transitory bombé of the iris while the child is still on the operating table. The seclusion can be relieved by removing some air, or aqueous will eventually enter the anterior chamber and the bombé relieved by shifting the air bubble from the pupil, by means of external pressure exerted on the cornea with the tip of a glass rod.

If air again gets behind the miotic pupil a pupil block results and the air must be removed. Manipulation with the glass rod is often effective in causing the air to come forward, even through a small pupil. If not, the pupil must be dilated with strong mydriatics, e.g., 10 percent neosynephrine and cyclogel (R) used in combination. Because of this complication, the author no longer uses air following anterior segment surgery for infantile glaucoma. Instead acetylcholine solution (Miochol), which is highly effective in constricting the pupil, drawing the iris away from the puncture and incision sites and deepening the anterior chamber, is used.

The Worst Technique

The Worst technique, consisting of a special lens, knife, and surgical procedure, has been designed to allow high magnification of the angle during surgery (Fig. 43A), and to avoid some of the pitfalls inherent in the other techniques.

The lens is attached to the sclera by means of sutures. In this way the lens forms a support for the eye, preventing deformation and providing the surgeon with a hold on the eye so that he can steady it and move it into the desired postions. The cannula attachment allows the surgeon to inject fluid under the lens, thus providing a perfect optical continuity between the lens cornea, anterior chamber, and filtration angle (Fig. 43B), particularly during

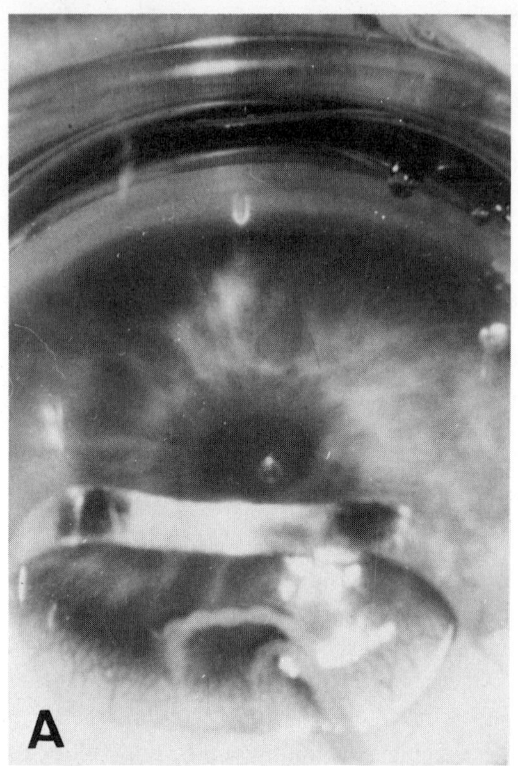

FIG. 43.A. The Worst lens, during a goniotomy operation. The U-suture is present in the lens opening.

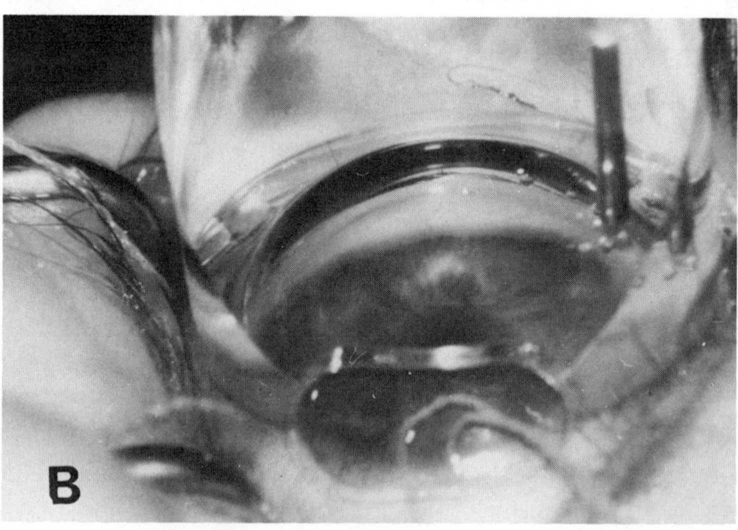

FIG. 43.B. The Worst lens. Fluid may be injected between the lens and cornea through the cannula.

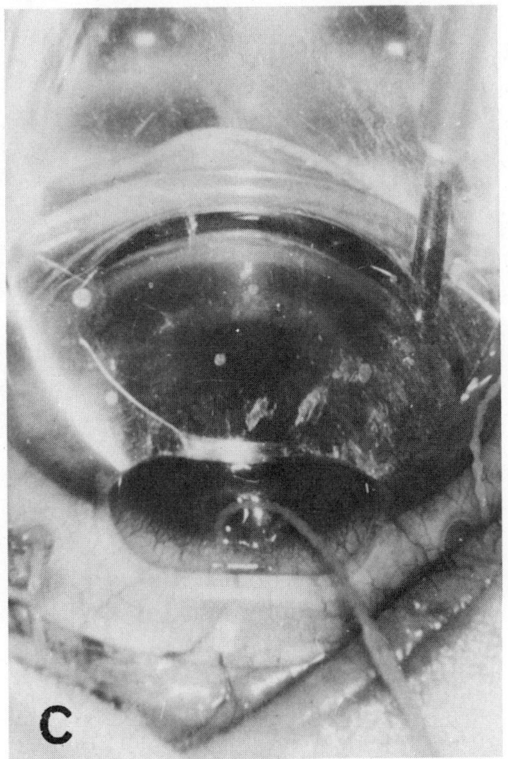

FIG. 43.C. The Worst lens in position.

the most critical phases of the operation (Fig. 43C). This method is the preferred choice of the author.

The lens with its scleral rim is brought under the eyelids. Sometimes a spatula must be used to ease the eyelids progressively over the rim. The holes in the scleral rim are marked on the sclera by pressing the tip of a punctum dilator through them. Their distance to the limbus varies from one eye to the other. The first goniotomy should be planned for the nasal side, so that the lateral opening in the lens through which the goniotomy needle is introduced (Fig. 43B) should be on the temporal side. For this position the 4 holes in the scleral rim are located in the 4 intermuscular oblique quadrants.

These positions may be adapted to the chamber angle area to be incised. For less accessible locations such as the temporal region, the eye would be rotated laterally and the goniotomy knife introduced over the bridge of the nose. Once the sclera is marked, the lens is removed and a

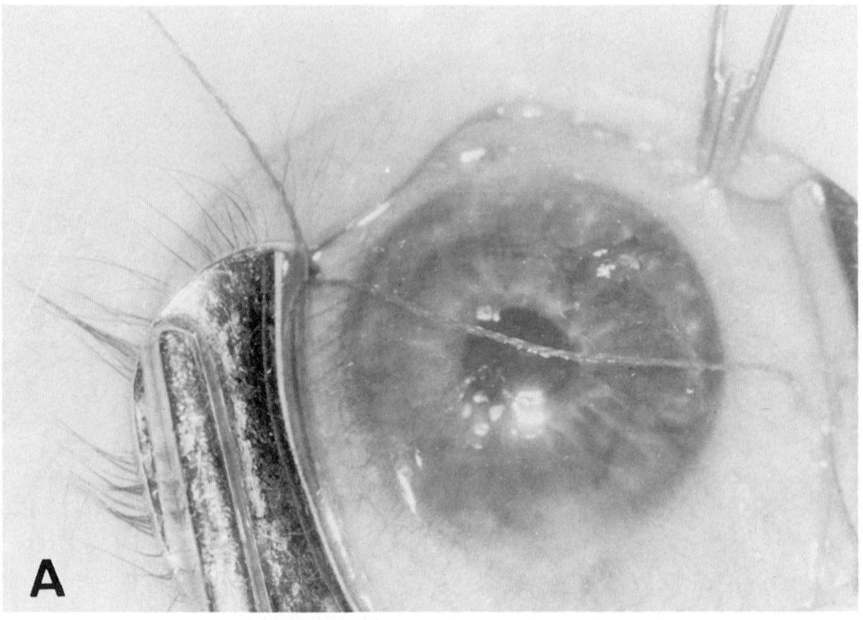

FIG. 44.A. Sutures of 4-0 black silk are inserted into conjunctiva-episcleral tissue.

speculum inserted. Sutures of 4-0 silk are inserted through the conjunctiva and the episclera at the 4 marked places (Fig. 44A and B). Where the sutures cross (Fig. 45) they are cut (Fig. 46), giving 4 loops of sutures which will be used to attach the lens to the globe. The ends are not cut, so as to serve as traction sutures.

A U-suture of 4-0 silk is passed through the limbus at the site of the planned puncture site (Fig. 47). This suture is an essential element of this technique and must not be omitted. The suture must be inserted deeply, using a simple round-pointed needle. (Cutting needles should be avoided as the suture will cut out.) The puncture site should be framed in a small square as the two ends of the suture emerge above the conjunctival limbus (Fig. 48). Since the tip of the Worst goniotomy knife cuts an opening with a slightly smaller diameter than the shaft of the needle, the introduction of the needle into the limbus requires some force; the suture acting as a bridle is a most effective aid to steady the cornea and act as counterpressure. The surgeon actually pulls the limbus onto the needle instead of pushing the needle into the anterior chamber. The U-suture will also serve to close the puncture site at the end of the operation, so that the 4 points where the suture emerges from the sclera must be close together. The corneal epithelium must be

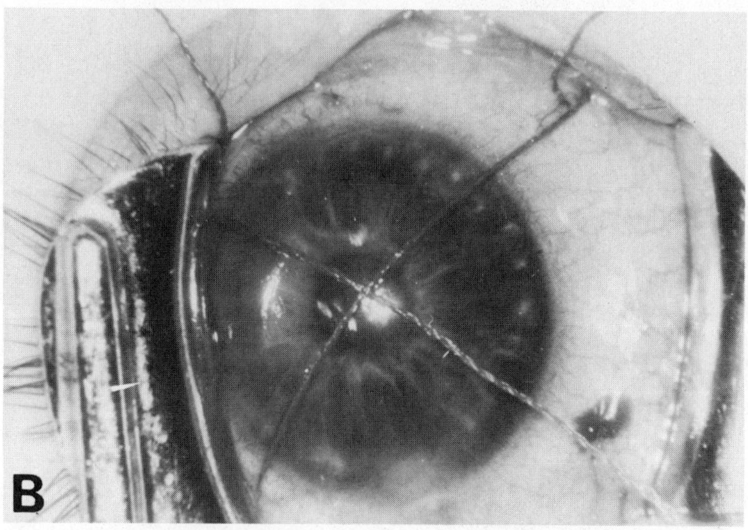

FIG. 44.B. Four 4-0 black silk sutures are inserted crossing at the pupil.

abraded. One end of each episcleral suture is drawn through the corresponding hole of the scleral rim of the lens. The corneal U-suture is passed through the lateral hole (Fig. 49). The speculum is removed and the lens is

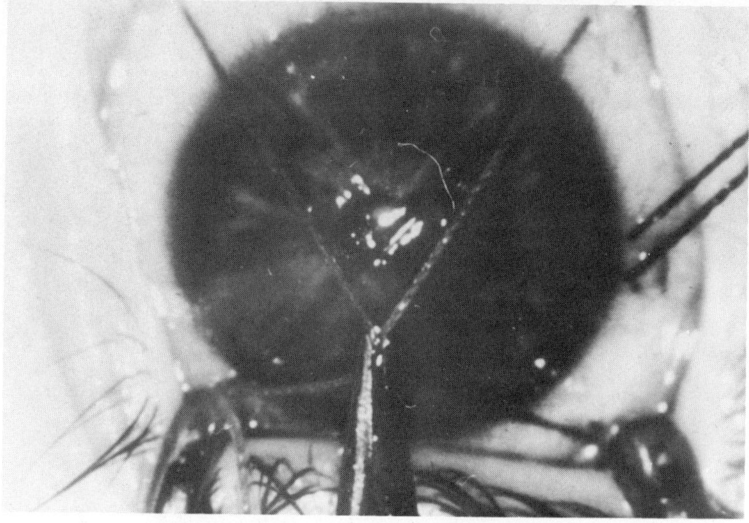

FIG. 45. The sutures are brought together.

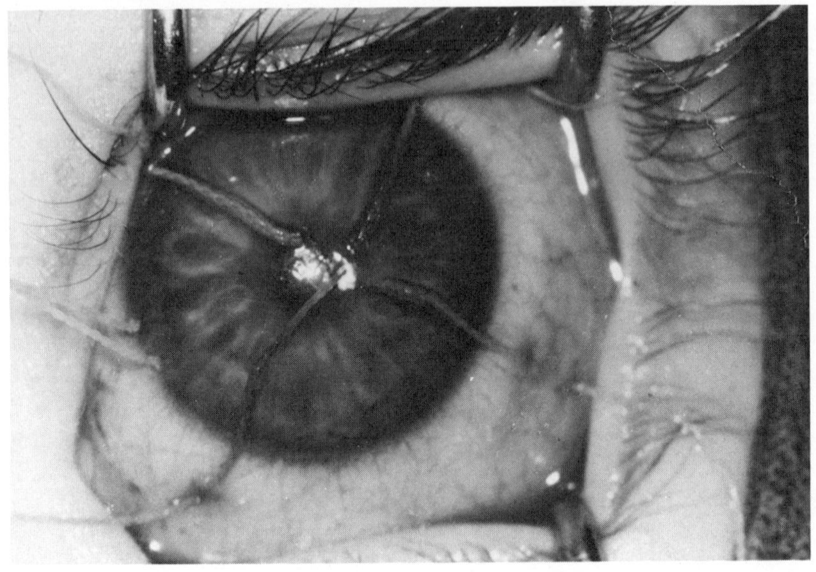

FIG. 46. The sutures are cut.

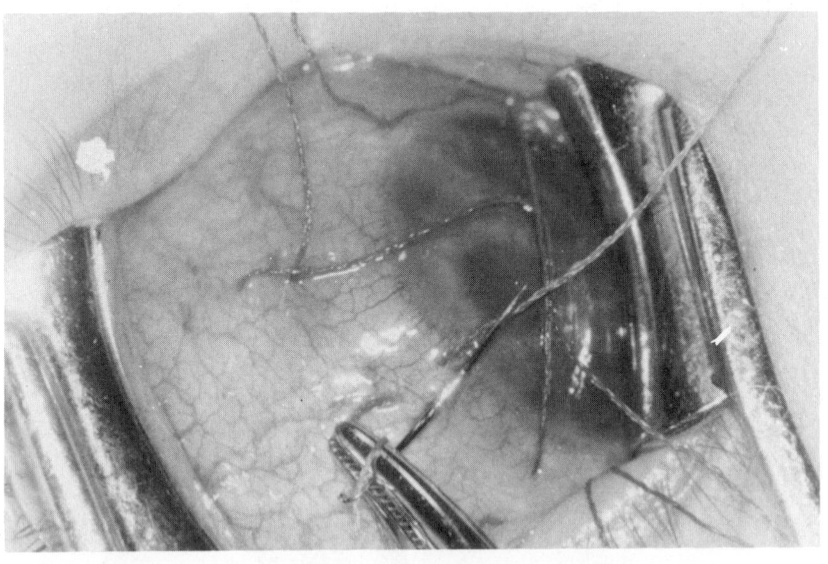

FIG. 47. The U-suture inserted at the puncture site.

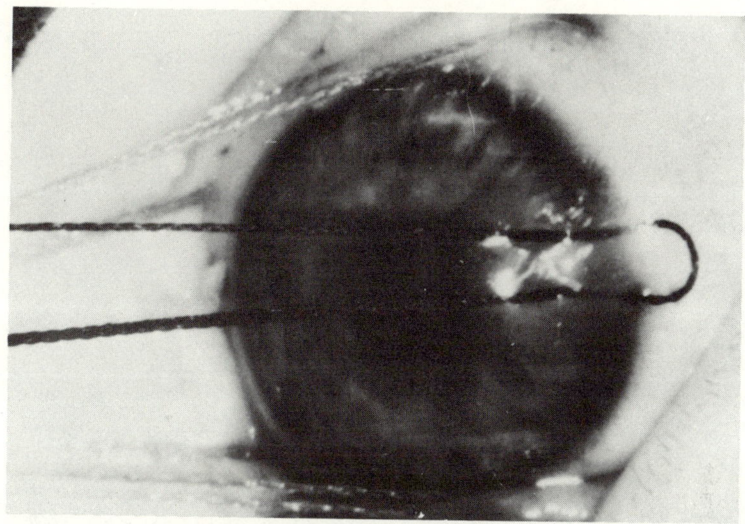

FIG. 48. The U-suture forming a small square through which the goniotomy knife will be introduced.

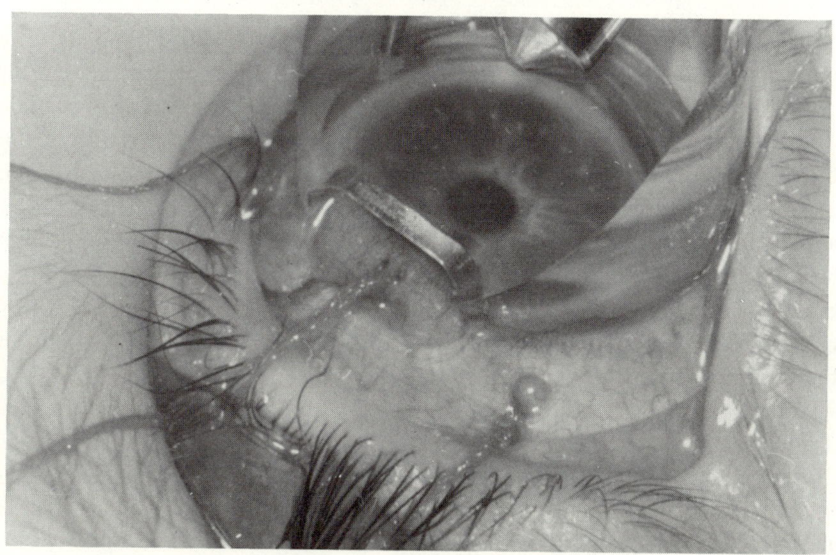

FIG. 49. The Medical Workshop Worst prismatic lens.

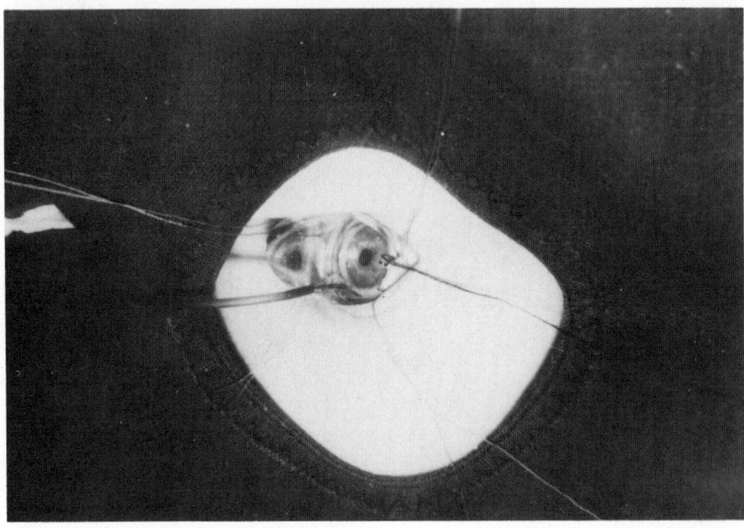

FIG. 50. The episcleral sutures of the Worst lens being used as traction sutures.

replaced on the eye. The sutures are knotted lightly and left uncut. The upper and the lower sutures are united in pairs. These will now serve as bridle sutures for the assistant, to steady and direct the eye (Fig. 50). The head of the patient, which is supported on a headrest, is rotated away from the surgeon. This brings the lateral hole in the lens to its highest position, and allows a larger working approach to the chamber angle. This position also facilitates the expulsion of stray air bubbles, which may enter under the lens during the manipulations. The assistant constantly watches for these bubbles and expels them via the cannula in the lens. The goniotomy needle is placed in the center of the 4 points of the U-suture. With a steady pull on the suture, the needle is pushed slowly into the anterior chamber (Fig. 51). When the tip of the knife has entered the anterior chamber, the anterior chamber is injected, via the 2 cc syringe, so as to bring the iris-lens diaphragm slightly below its normal level (Fig. 52). This artificial deepening of the anterior chamber is an effective way to protect the pupillary area. It also stretches the chamber angle structures which are thus more easily severed and, finally, it acts as an effective tampon against hemorrhage. It should be noted that too much deepening can cause corneal clouding which is reversible. As the chamber angle is approached, the U-suture pulls the cornea outward so that no dimple forms to suck air under the lens.

The goniotomy incision is started directly opposite the site of incision

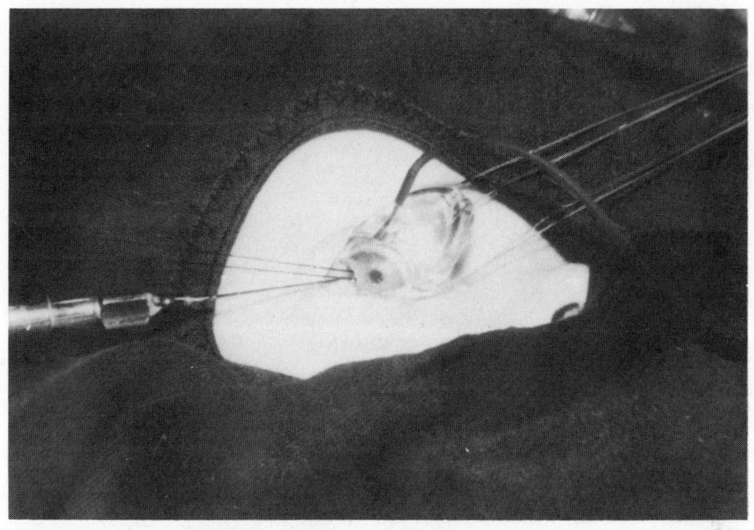

FIG. 51. Worst goniotomy knife puncturing cornea.

(Fig. 53). The incision should be made as in the description of the Barkan technique (Fig. 54A). The iris drops and a white scleral area comes into view.

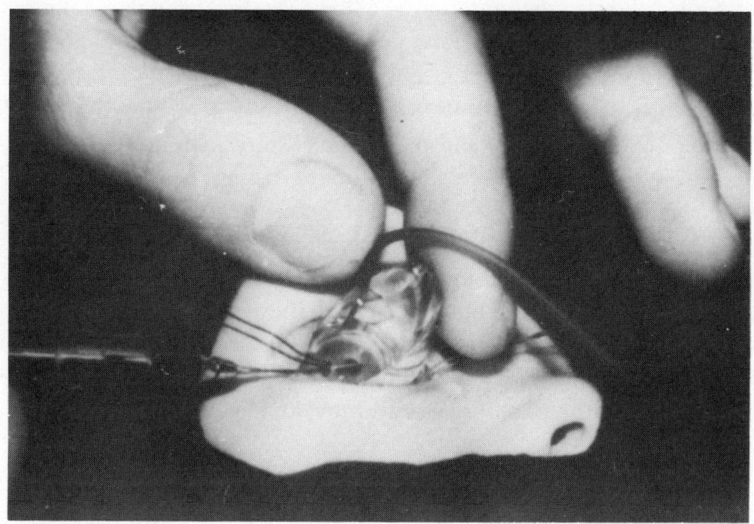

FIG. 52. Worst lens in position with goniotomy knife crossing anterior chamber.

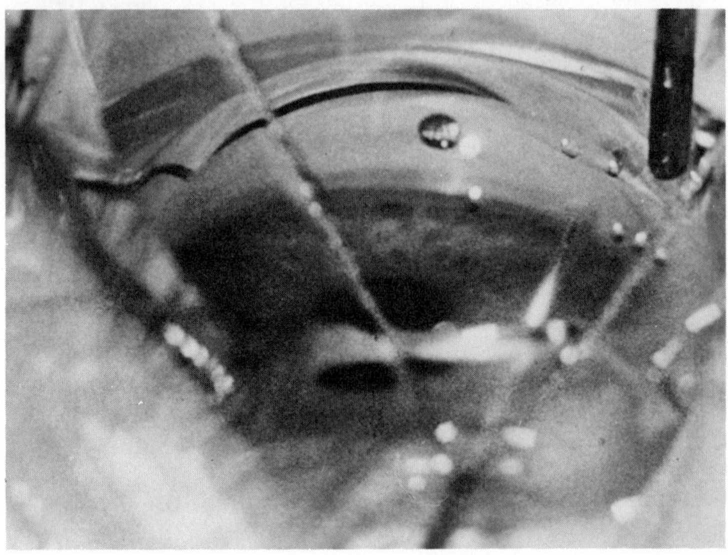

FIG. 53. The goniotomy incision.

When proceeding with this stripping action along the apparent Schwalbe's line, a typical white line may become visible (Barkan's white line) (Fig. 54B). A slight oozing of blood may occur, which can be arrested by increasing the amount of fluid in the anterior chamber via the cannulated knife and syringe, which raises the intraocular pressure.

The incision is first made in one direction. The needle is brought back to the original spot and a cut made in the opposite direction. At least one-quarter can be stripped, and possibly one-third with this technique. The needle is now withdrawn, preferably without crossing the pupillary area. The anterior chamber may be deepened just before removing the needle. The U-suture is tied once to prevent the escape of fluid. If the chamber is still shallow and blood is oozing, more saline or air may be injected through the puncture site (Fig. 55). The compression of the perforation by the U-suture is usually so effective that the suture may be removed after a few minutes. Sometimes the limbal area is so thin that a 10-0 or virgin silk suture is necessary to close the puncture site to prevent the escape of air or aqueous.

POSTOPERATIVE GONIOSCOPIC FINDINGS

Postoperative gonioscopy shows that as the result of goniotomy the iris root has drooped backward (Fig. 56 A and B). The operated portion of the angle appears cleared of obstructing tissue, and the true angle wall or trabeculum becomes exposed. If the incision is sufficiently superficial, a clean separation of the tissue from the underlying trabeculum results without damage to surrounding structures.

In many cases, the scleral spur can be identified in the stripped area. In several instances of successful normalization of tension, the blood-filled Schlemm's canal is plainly visible with its characteristic undulating outline adjacent and anterior to the spur, indicating that the trabeculo-Schlemm's canal mechanism is undisturbed. It is evident that injury to this mechanism must be avoided. This emphasizes the importance of stripping the tissue superficially by operating with a contact lens, i.e., under gonioscopic control.

Goniotomy, even when unsuccessful, does not damage the globe and other procedures can be subsequently applied without disadvantage.

GONIOPUNCTURE

The goniopuncture procedure was first described and popularized by Scheie. The operation was developed after he observed a fistula, through the corneoscleral wall, which had been caused while performing a goniotomy upon a 19-year-old girl with advanced glaucoma. Noting that the tension had been controlled as a result of aqueous flow through the fistula, an operation was developed to create a similar opening by a puncture from within the anterior chamber.

The initial and later reports have indicated that the operation is of no value in the patient over age 30, because the fistula fails to remain patent. However, the operation has proved to be useful for the management of both infantile and juvenile glaucoma in individuals up to that age.

The operation possesses the virtues of its simplicity, its relative safety, and the fact that the eye is relatively unmutilated. The operation can be repeated as many as 2 or 3 times. If failure results from this many punctures, more conventional procedures can be attempted, since goniopuncture does not interfere with the outcome of filtering or other operations.

Technique

The operation is performed under general anesthesia (Fig. 57). A speculum is inserted. An oblique puncture may be made at the upper temporal margin of the cornea for injecting air or fluid into the anterior chamber (Fig. 57A and B) at the end of the operation, bearing in mind that the thinned limbal area, in buphthalmia, may not retain the injected

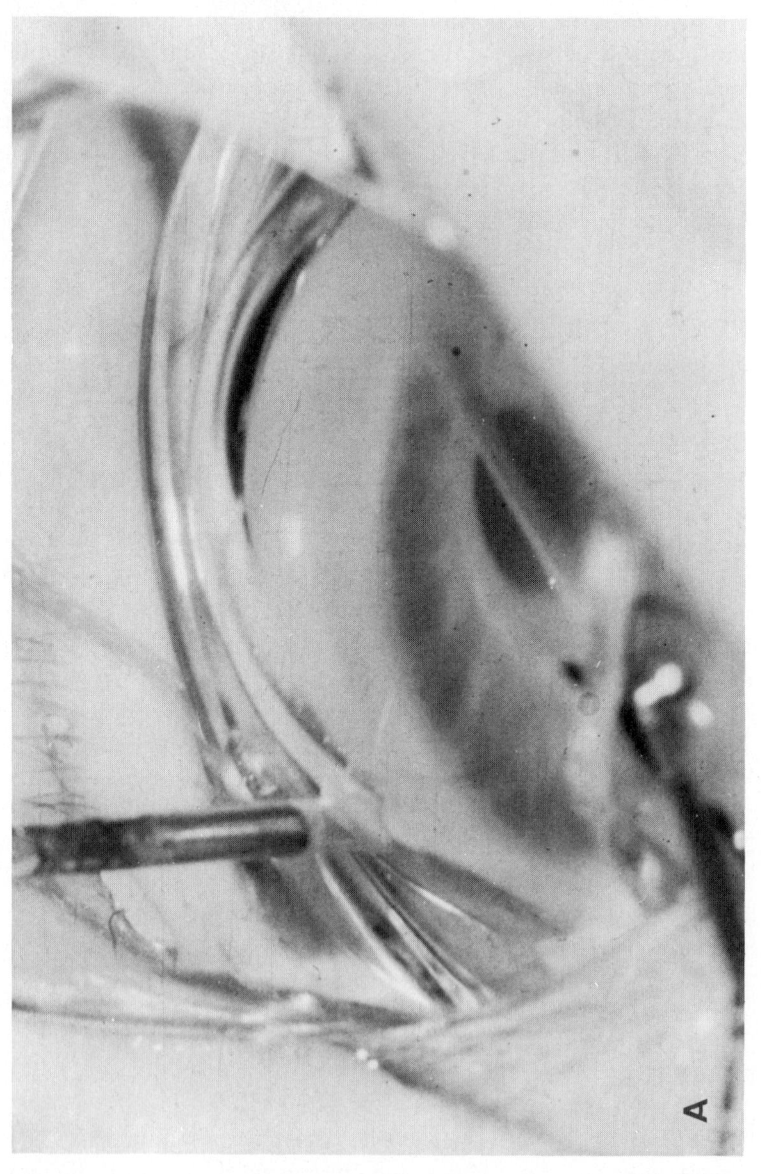

FIG. 54.A. The goniotomy incision.

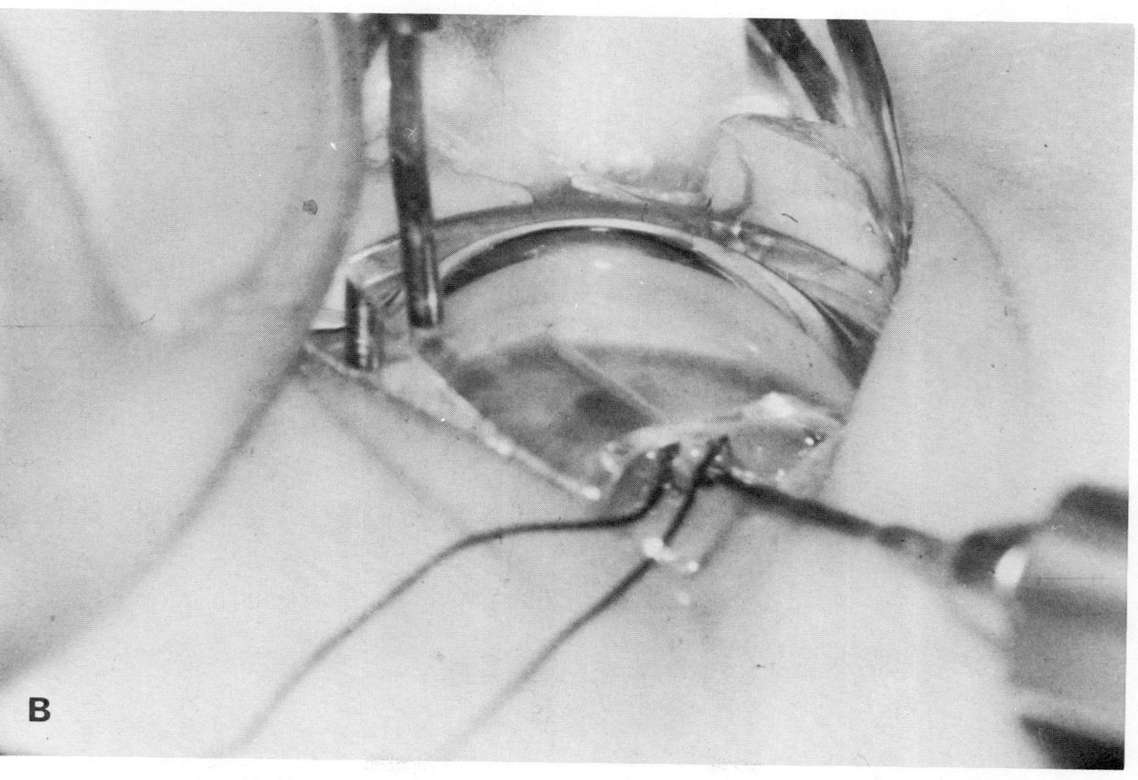

FIG. 54.B. The goniotomy incision showing Barkan's white line. (Courtesy of J. G. F. Worst.)

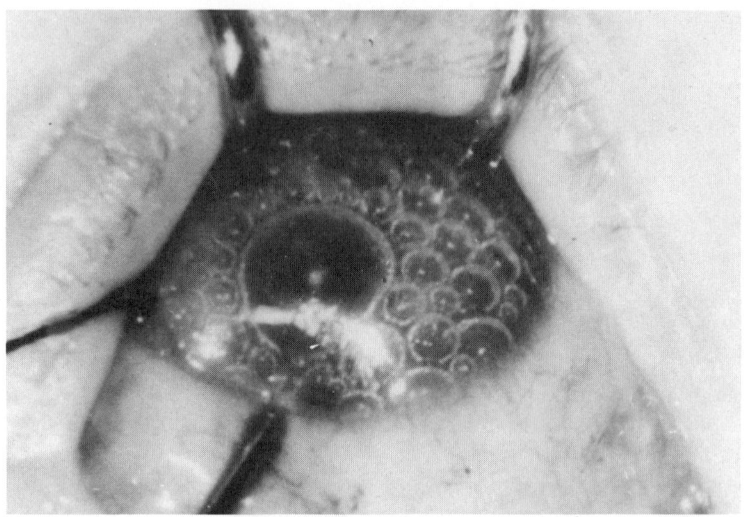

FIG. 55. Injection of air following goniotomy procedure.

substances. The conjunctiva overlying the area where the puncture is to be made is ballooned outward away from the globe by the subconjunctival injection of saline solution (Fig. 57C). This helps to prevent perforation of the conjunctiva by the knife.

An inferior goniopuncture is preferred in order to keep the upper portion of the globe unscarred for subsequent possible filtering operations. Nothing is lost by attempting this safe procedure as an initial operation, according to Scheie.

A goniopuncture or goniotomy knife is introduced through clear cornea, 1 to 1.5 mm within the limbus at approximately 9:30 o'clock in the right eye, or at 2:30 o'clock in the left eye, and directed nasally toward the 6 o'clock meridian. The blade is introduced flat on a plane parallel with the iris, and the tip is carried across the chamber until it reaches the trabecular region of the opposite angle slightly behind Schwalbe's line in the anterior trabeculum. It is then thrust forward through the corneoscleral wall into the subconjunctival space, until the blade of the knife is visible beneath the previously ballooned conjunctiva (Fig. 5D). The blade is then pulled back into the anterior chamber and withdrawn from the eye. The fistula produced permits escape of aqueous. A small opening in the corneoscleral wall is desirable in glaucomatous infant eyes because of the thinness of the wall. Furthermore, to insure a small puncture opening, the knife should not be rotated in the subconjunctival space, as shown in Fig. 57E, **except** in older patients to permit a rapid reformation of the anterior chamber. Temptation to enlarge the opening (Fig. 58A and B) as the knife traverses the corneoscleral wall must be resisted. A larger opening leads to incarceration of the iris, with plugging of the fistula. Occasionally, bleeding occurs at the time of the puncture but, as in goniotomy, it usually causes no difficulty. Air or saline may be injected through the preformed temporal tract in juvenile glaucoma if bleeding is excessive, although Scheie advises that in infants (infantile and newborn glaucoma), especially, no attempt be made to re-form the anterior chamber, because the air or saline flows into the subconjunctival space and builds up external pressure on the eye, delaying re-formation of the anterior chamber. Chloramphenicol drops are applied and pilocarpine 1 percent instilled to retract the iris away from the site of the puncture. Both eyes are covered for 24 hrs.

Complications are unusual. The anterior chamber usually re-forms promptly. Scheie reports that one eye was lost from a massive intraocular hemorrhage on the third postoperative day, which he attributed to a rupture of a choroidal vessel. The patient suffered severe pain with immediate loss of light perception.

COMBINED GONIOTOMY-GONIOPUNCTURE PROCEDURE

Detailed description of this technique is unnecessary. The operation is accomplished simply by performing a goniopuncture upon completion of the sweeping incision of a goniotomy maneuver (Fig. 59). The operation can be simply performed, and is accompanied by no more complications than with either operation alone. The combined procedure is undertaken to obtain the benefits of each type of operation. This seems logical because goniotomy theoretically exerts its effect through debridement of the angle, allowing access of aqueous to the canal of Schlemm, while according to Scheie goniopuncture exerts its effect by creating a fistula.

POSTOPERATIVE MANAGEMENT

The anterior chamber has usually re-formed the morning after surgery, and no further dressings are needed following goniotomy and/or goniopuncture operations. Local steroid drops combined with an antibiotic are instilled 4 times daily for a few days, to help prevent infection and to allay

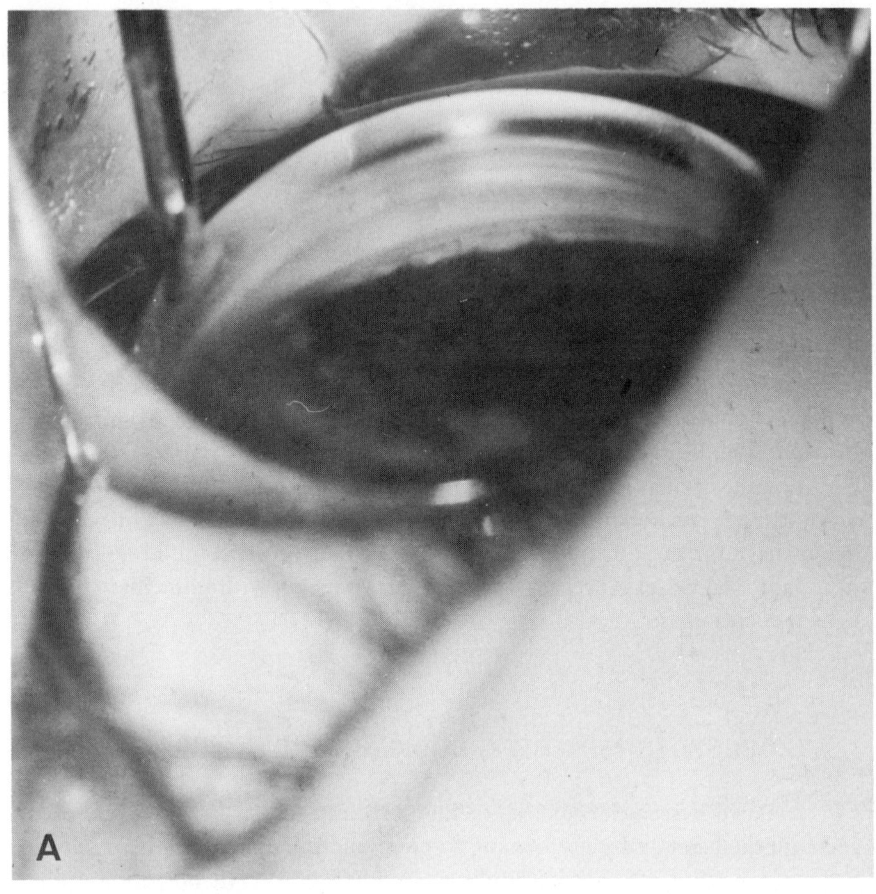

FIG. 56.A. Postoperative goniotomy site, the trabeculum is exposed.

postoperative reaction. Atropine is used only if the eye shows marked reaction but this is rarely indicated because it permits the iris root to relax toward the angle wall and could help promote peripheral anterior synechiae formation. The two most worrisome postoperative complications are hyphema and infection. Although some hemorrhage into the anterior chamber is the rule at the time of surgery, recurrent hyphema is rare. The patient is usually discharged from the hospital on the fifth postoperative day.

During the immediate postoperative period when surgery is successful there is usually a rapid subsidence of symptoms including loss of photophobia, decreased tearing, as well as a return of the normal corneal

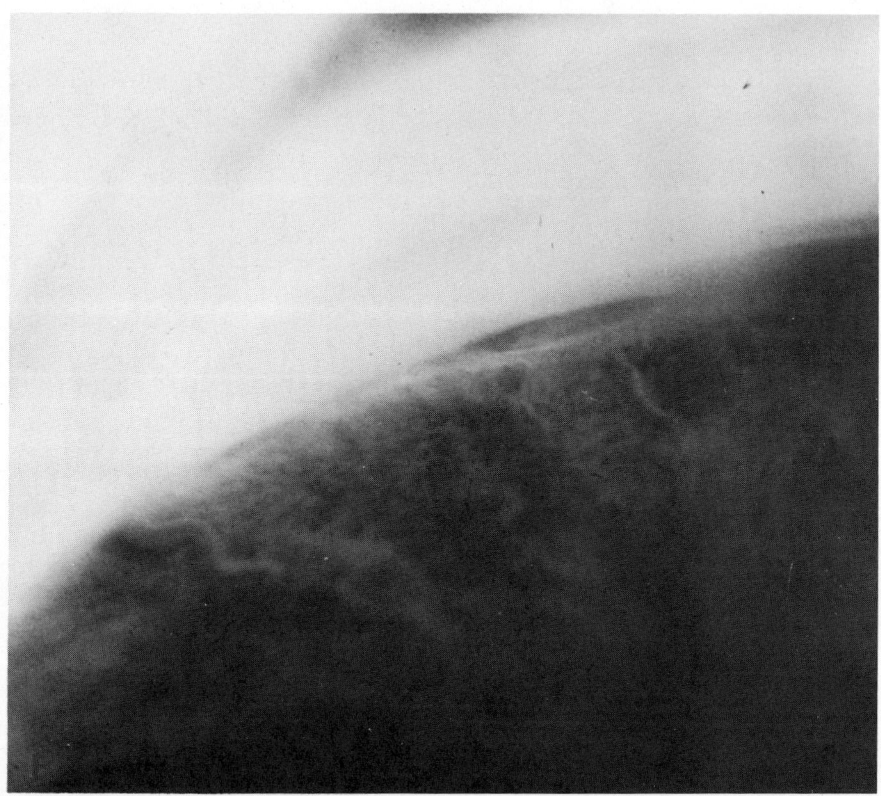

FIG. 56.B. Postoperative goniotomy site.

luster, except that tears in Descemet's membrane, previously unnoticed in the generalized corneal edema, now become obvious. It may take 3 to 4 weeks for all the symptoms to subside. With the pressure normalized, further treatment is unnecessary. If the presenting symptoms persist, the anti-glaucomatous medication should be reinstituted and the case reassessed. The eye must be carefully observed for bacterial inflammation.

Approximately 6 weeks following surgery the patient is reexamined under general anesthesia, to observe the operative site, measure the intraocular pressure, observe evidence of further corneal enlargement, and look for regression of disc cupping. If a progression of signs has occurred and symptoms persist, another goniotomy, with or without goniopuncture, should be repeated in another sector at this time.

When normalization of intraocular pressure is obtained, the child is

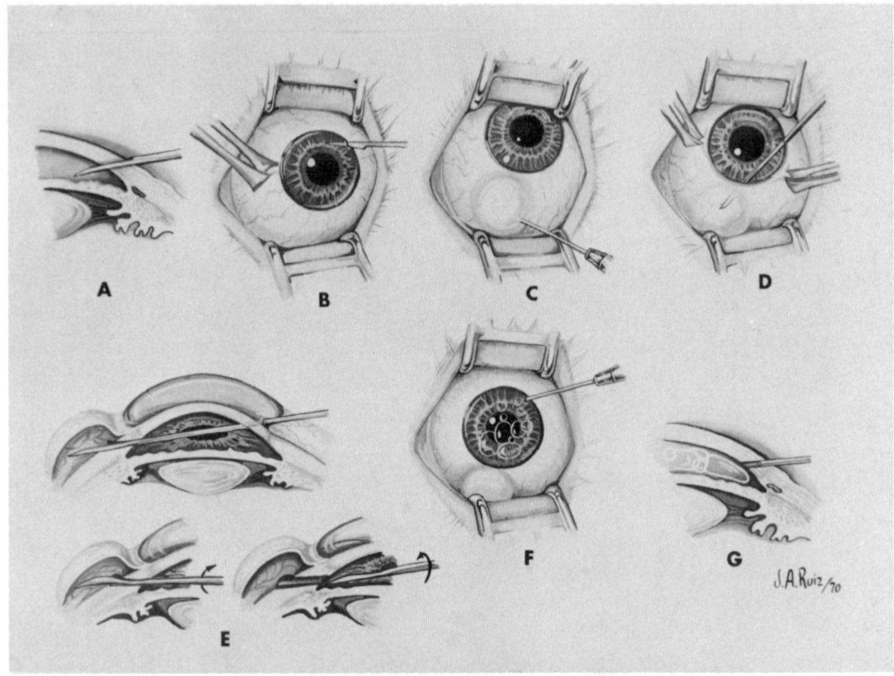

FIG. 57. Goniopuncture operation of Scheie. (A and B) Temporal perforation for injection of air or saline; (C) subconjunctival injection of saline over goniopuncture site; (D) the thrust of the goniotomy knife visible under the conjunctiva; (E) twisting of goniotomy knife performed only in older patients; (F and G) injection of air through temporal perforation with blunt needle. (From Scheie. **Trans. Am. Acad. Ophthalmol. Otolaryngol.** 67:458. 1963.)

reexamined in 8 weeks, and if still normalized, 12 weeks later. It does not appear that intervals longer than 4 months should be utilized, for recurrence of the glaucoma may occur rapidly and with fewer than the original symptoms. For those cases which do not respond to an initial stripping of the chamber angle, filtering procedures or the microsurgical techniques should not be performed until a full 360° goniotomy has been attempted. For though one part of the angle may be so underdeveloped as to be without a Schlemm's canal, other areas of the angle may have attained sufficient maturity to start functioning after a goniotomy.

There is indeed a remarkable asymmetry in the degree of retardation of various parts of the chamber angle in congenital glaucoma. After a goniotomy several weeks may elapse before the tension is normalized, while in others it may take a shorter period or no time at all. The pressure can be

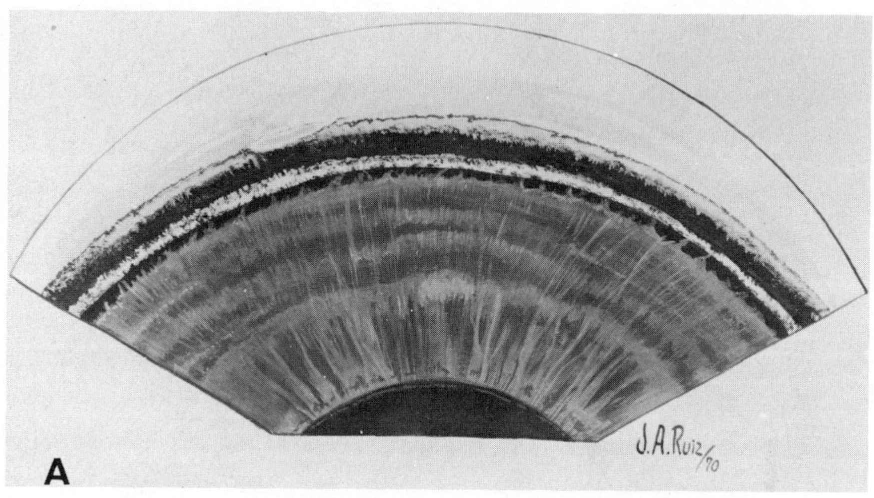

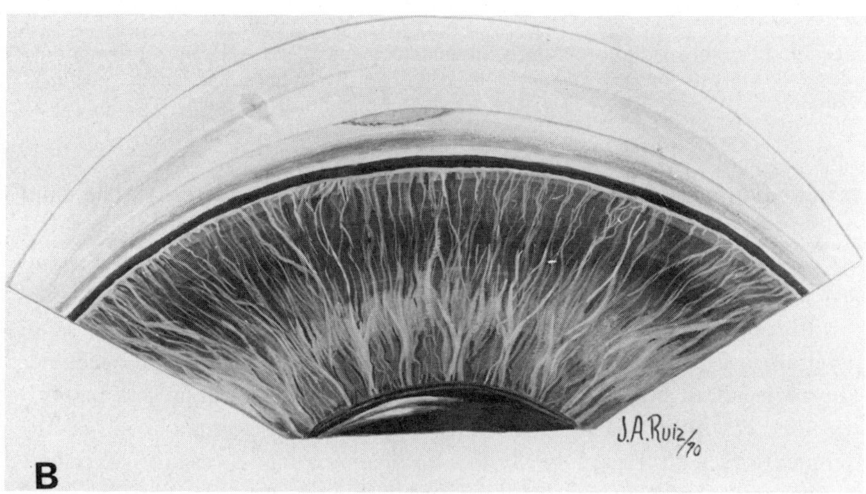

FIG. 58. Goniopuncture sites. (After Scheie. **Arch. Ophthalmol.** 65:38, 1961.)

elevated simply on the basis of ocular irritation and probably by increased protein in the aqueous, according to Scheie.

When the patient reaches a cooperative age (usually about 4 years),

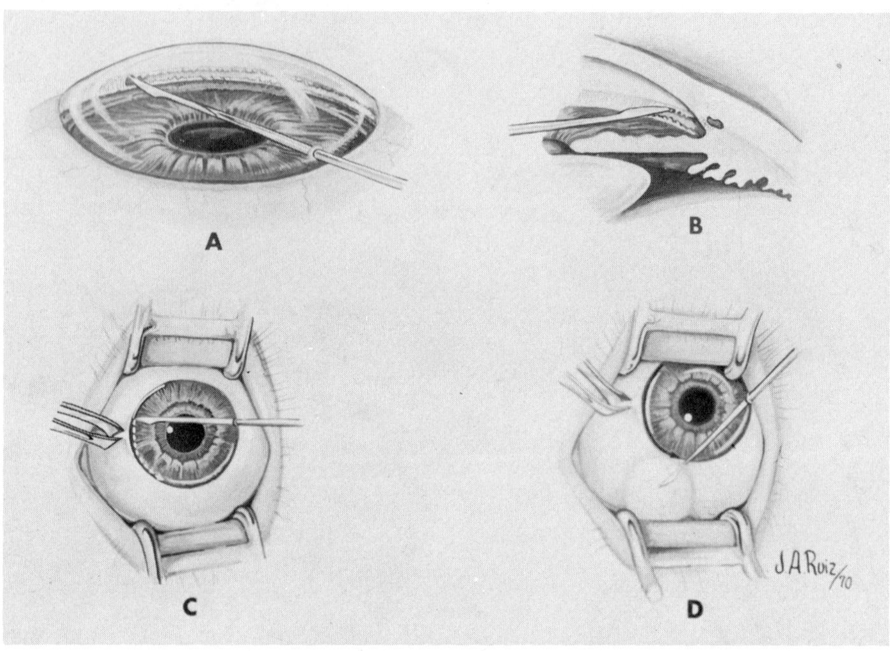

FIG. 59. Combined goniotomy and goniopuncture operation. (A, B, and C) Goniotomy sweep; (D) thrust forward of blade in region of Schwalbe's line under ballooned conjunctiva. (After Scheie. **Trans. Am. Acad. Ophthalmol. Otolaryngol.** 67:458, 1963.)

examination can be performed in the office quite satisfactorily. The child should be followed periodically for the rest of his life. There is evidence that occasional patients who have been well controlled for many years develop increased tension in later life.

Repeated general anesthesia after one year of age presents formidable psychological problems. To allay fear, the child should be heavily sedated. The advice of an anesthetist experienced with such cases will be very helpful. If not carefully managed, severe psychological trauma can result. Cooperation with regard to follow-up examination is usually excellent because of the great concern of the parents.

DIRECT GONIOTOMY (GONIOTRIPSY)

The classical goniotomy is curative with good visualization through a clear cornea in from 70 to 80 percent of cases, when a formed and potentially functional anterior drainage system is present. Otherwise a much

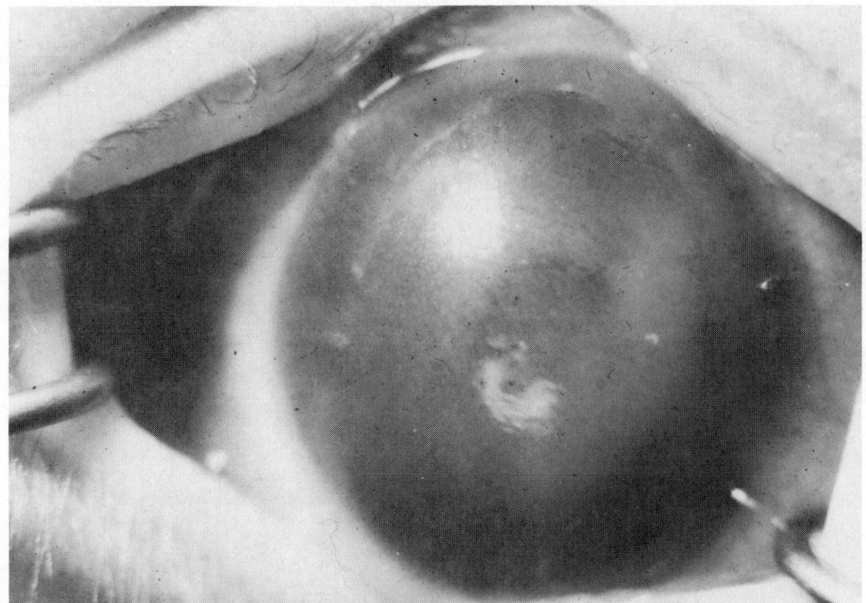

FIG. 60. Opaque cornea of congenital glaucoma. The pupil may be distinguished.

more complex problem exists. In 1960, Urrets-Zavalia described the goniotripsy operation. Studies by Kwitko and Galin have shown this operation to be a worthwhile procedure in congenital glaucoma cases where visualization of the filtration angle is not possible because of an opaque cornea (Fig. 60).

Technique

Cases are selected where the opaque cornea precludes visualization of the angle, either after dehydration of the cornea or removal of the epithelium. There are some cases where anterior segment structures cannot be distinguished at all (Fig. 61). The procedure is carried out under general anesthesia.

A suspensory ring may be sutured to the sclera (Fig. 62), but this is not essential in all cases. A limbal incision is made temporally, approximately 5 mm in length (Fig. 63A), in an absolutely perpendicular manner. This is often difficult with an edematous soft cornea. The ends of the incision are extended at a right angle, using a fine sharp scissor (Fig. 63B), to reach the filtration angle. A flap of cornea is thus elevated, which affords a direct view

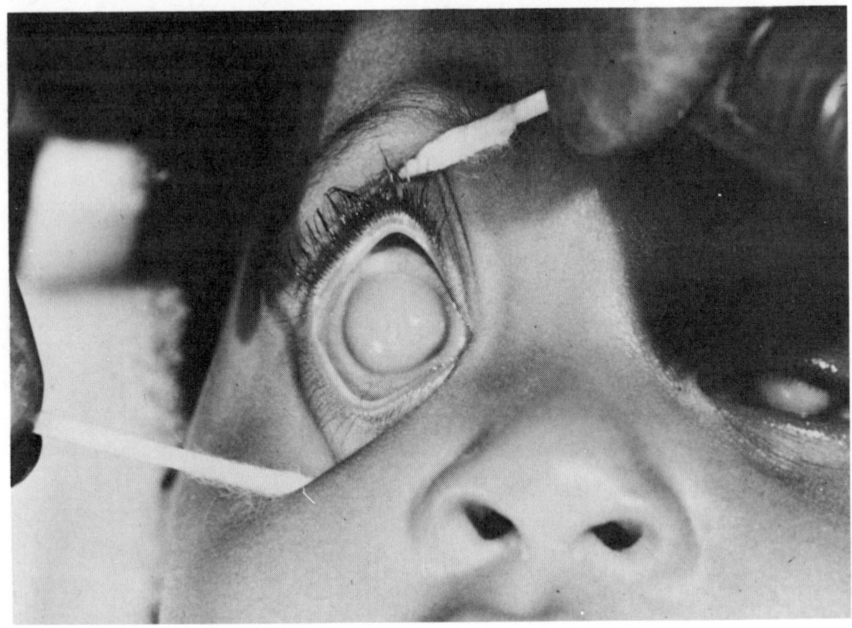

FIG. 61. Opaque cornea of congenital glaucoma. No anterior segment structures may be distingushed. (Courtesy of M. A. Galin.)

of the angle when reflected posteriorly. A small iridectomy or iridotomy is performed deep to the corneal flap, since the iris frequently prolapses at this point in the operation. The iris diaphragm now falls back. A suture is placed in the margin of the corneal flap which encompasses two-thirds of the thickness of the cornea. (Fig. 63C). This allows for a complete evaluation of the angle by elevating the corneal flap.

At this point, under direct microscopic visualization, a goniotomy is carried out using the standard goniotomy knife. With a direct view of the angle, one can truly incise just the superficial tissue in the anterior part of the middle third of the trabecular area (Fig. 63D-F). After the angle is incised the iris is seen to fall backward (Fig. 63G).

The filtration angle in the recesses of the incision may also be incised by lifting the peripheral ends of the incision and extending the goniotomy blade into the angle (Fig. 63E), giving a 60° goniotomy. The edges of the corneal incision are closed with multiple 10-0-sutures, since the peripheral cornea in these children is thin and aqueous leakage is a problem. A conjunctival flap may be pulled over the wound. Air or saline is injected to reconstitute the anterior chamber (Fig. 63H).

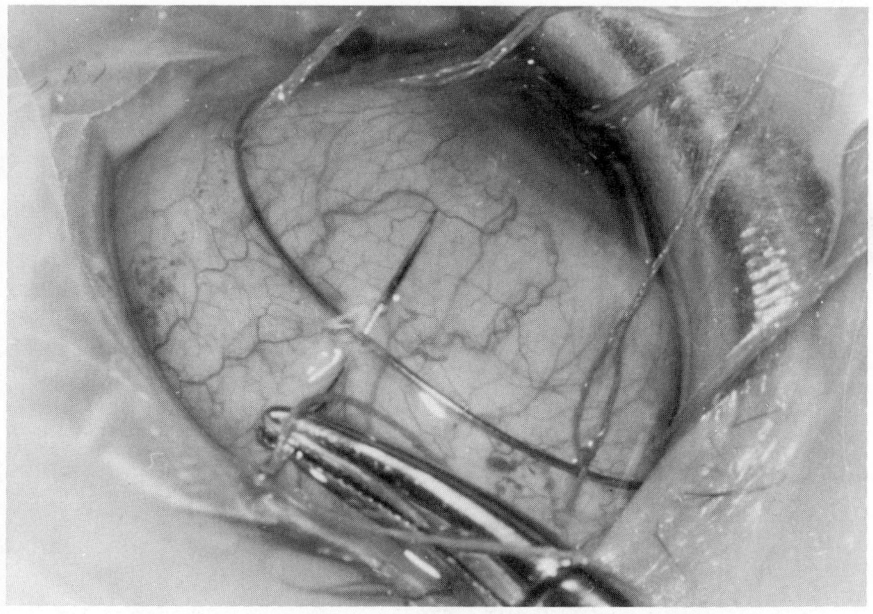

FIG. 62. Goniotripsy operation; suturing of suspensory ring.

In the series of Kwitko and Galin, 7 out of 12 children with opaque corneas responded to this treatment. Two of the failures were reoperated, but despite perfect visualization and placement of the goniotomy incision the cases were still unsuccessfully controlled, suggesting an abnormality beyond the trabeculum.

Postoperatively the wound heals leaving a wide scar (Fig. 64) which varies in extent (Fig. 65A and B). Later the corneal scar fades and often the iridectomy is the only visible evidence of surgery (Fig. 66).

TREPHINE

Recent work by Sugar with the limboscleral trephination operation has shown the value of this approach in some cases of congenital glaucoma.

The limboscleral trephination is essentially a return to the original type of so-called scleral trephination used by Fergus and Elliot, independently, in 1909. The complications of this operation include (1) lens trauma at the time of surgery; (2) production of a thin bleb and relatively high incidence of bleb rupture and late infection: (3) an excessively large limboscleral

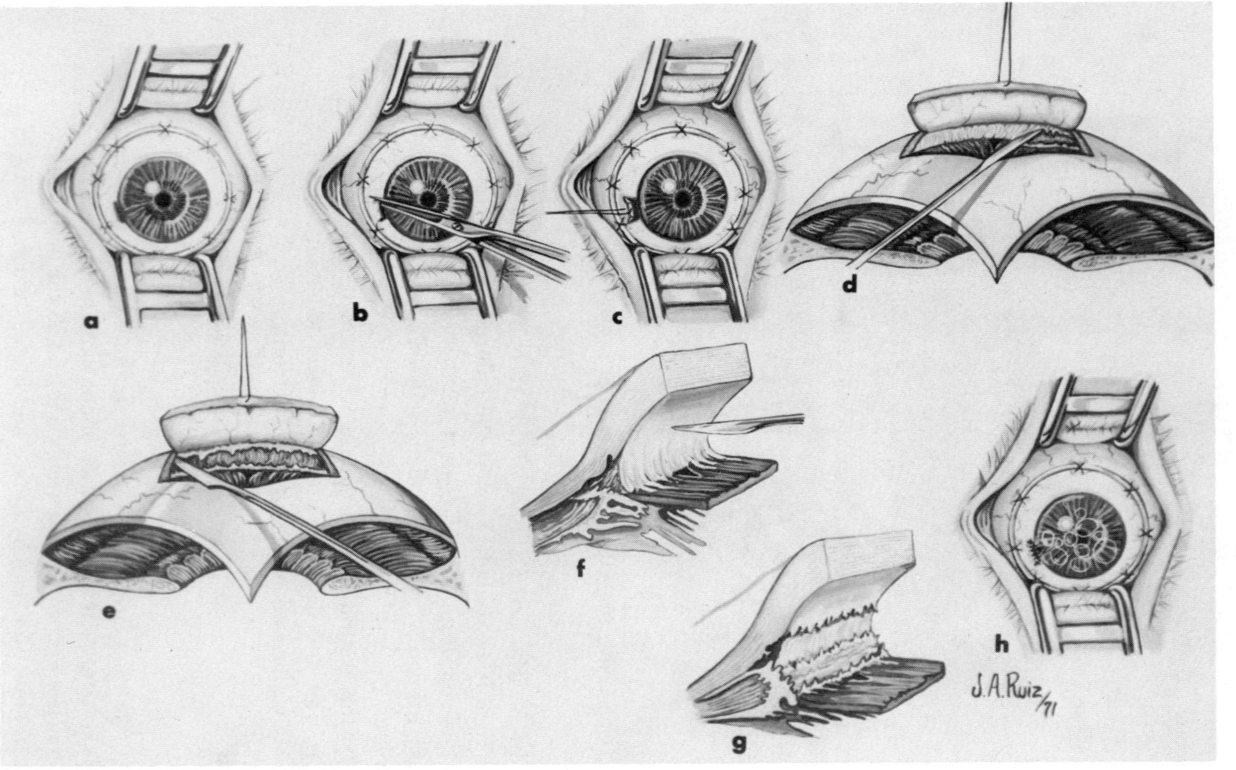

FIG. 63. The direct goniotomy-goniotripsy operation. (A) the limbal incision; (B) the extremities of the incision are extended at right angles into the filtration angle; (C) a 10-0 or virgin silk suture encompassing two-thirds of the width of the cornea is inserted; (D) (E) and (F) the flap is elevated and angle incised using the microscope; (G) the iris diaphragm falls back; (H) the wound is closed with multiple sutures, and air or saline is injected to reconstitute the anterior chamber.

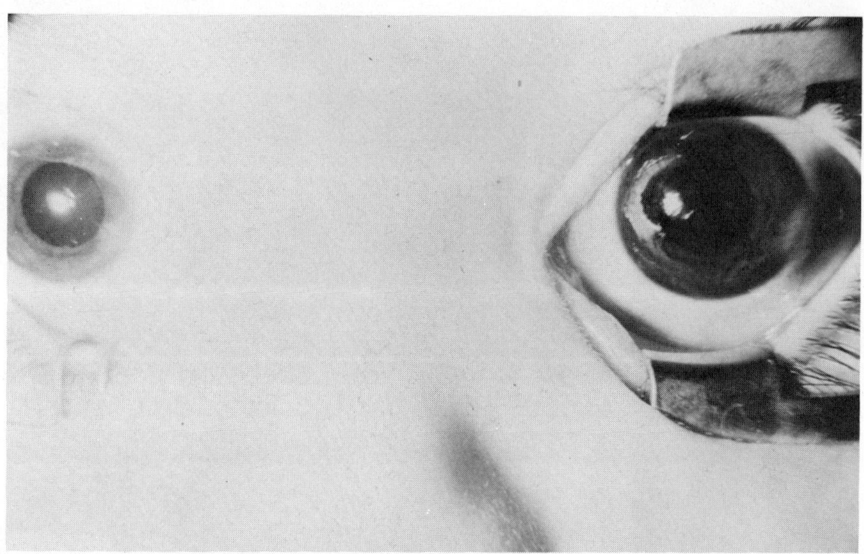

FIG. 64. Direct goniotomy-goniotripsy operation, 3 months postoperative appearance.

opening, and (4) a leaking conjunctival flap. Sugar introduced several modifications to correct these problems.

Technique

The procedure is carried out under general anesthesia (Fig. 67). The conjunctiva above the cornea is ballooned out with 1/2 cc of anesthestic solution. This will determine the site of least scarring.

A narrow knife needle blade, its tip dipped in fluorescein solution, is introduced obliquely at the limbus of the lower temporal quadrant of the cornea into the anterior chamber, to act as a tract for future anterior chamber injections.

A conjunctival incision about 12 to 16 mm long is made, concentric with the limbus beginning just above the level of the superior rectus insertion (Fig. 67A). An incision of the same dimensions is made separately in Tenon's capsule in order to bare the sclera, anterior to the superior rectus insertion. The flap is turned back over the cornea and the sclera is bared to the limbus. Blunt-tipped scissors may be used to free the deeper layers of Tenon's capsule. The toe of a Desmarres knife (Fig. 67B) or the belly of a #15

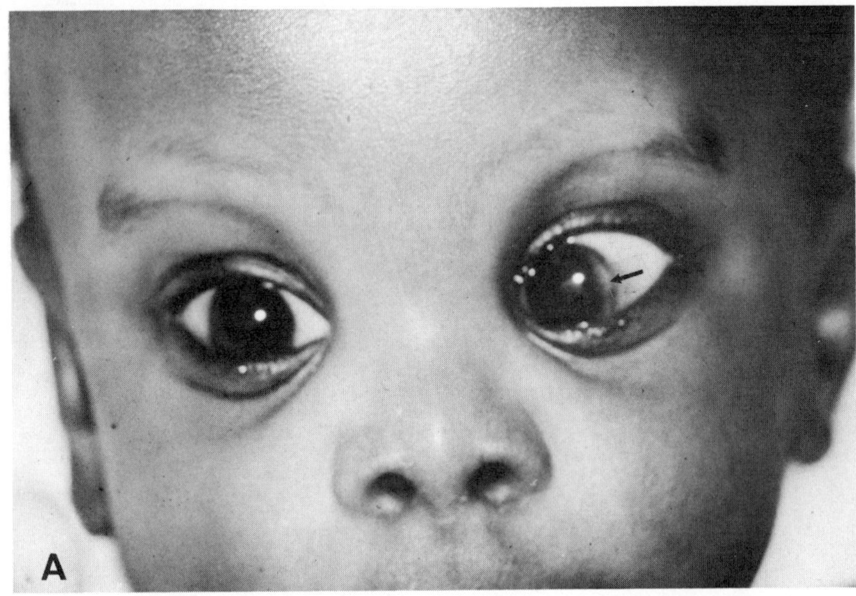

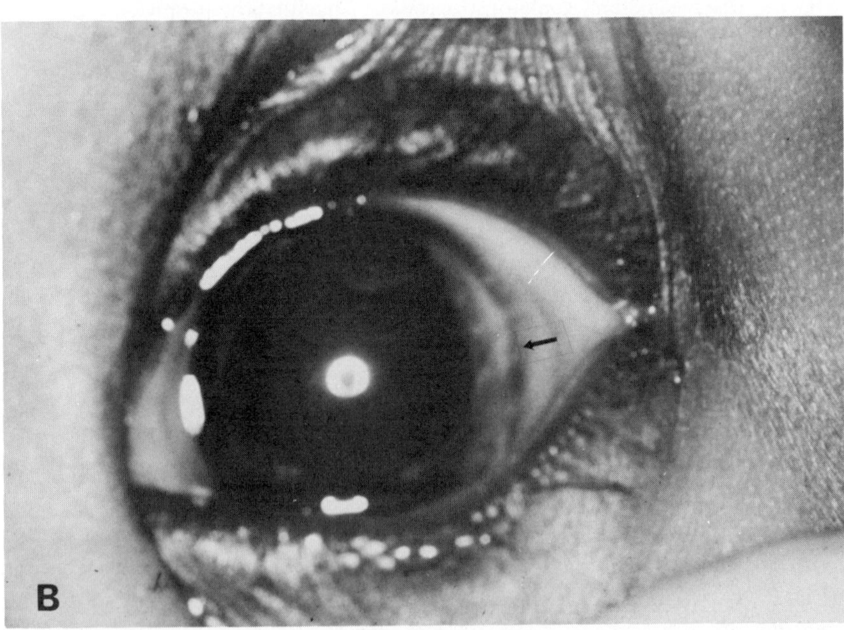

FIG. 65. Direct goniotomy-goniotripsy operation (arrow). (Courtesy of M. A. Galin.)

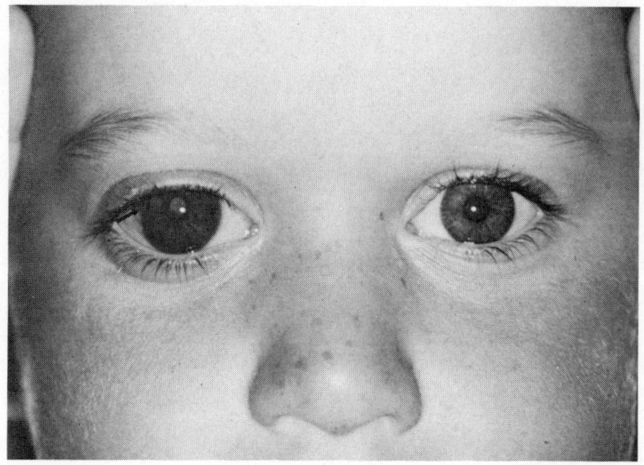

FIG. 66. Direct goniotomy-goniotripsy operation. Iridectomy (arrow) is visible in right eye.

Bard-Parker scalpel blade is used to scrape the sclera and limbus area to within a half mm of the corneolimbal junction, for a distance of about 3 to 4 mm, leaving the area of fusion of Tenon's capsule with the conjunctiva intact. Tenon's capsule tissue is often very thick in children, and a layer of the innermost Tenon's condensation is excised with blunt scissors in the area which is to become the bleb. The trephine (1.5 or 2.0 mm) is applied with its anterior margin about a third or half mm behind the corneolimbal junction (Fig. 67C). A turn of the trephine is made so as to mark its position and the trephine is then removed. The conjunctival flap is then replaced to ascertain the correctness of the trephine location. The flap is reflected back again and the trephine reapplied at the corrected position. The trephine is tilted slightly forward so that the limboscleral disc will be hinged on its scleral side (Fig. 67D). The moment the trephine cuts through into the anterior chamber there is a sudden upward jerk of the upper pupil border, producing a pear-shaped pupil. When the trephination is made slowly and the trephine groove observed frequently a slow leak is produced, and this prevents spontaneous iris prolapse. On the other hand care must also be taken, with a newly sharpened trephine, to observe the depth of the trephine's cut so as not to go through the sclera too rapidly. Bleeding is controlled with superficial applications of the cautery. After the trephine is removed, the unhinged portion of button of sclera is usually pushed upward by the prolapsed iris. A

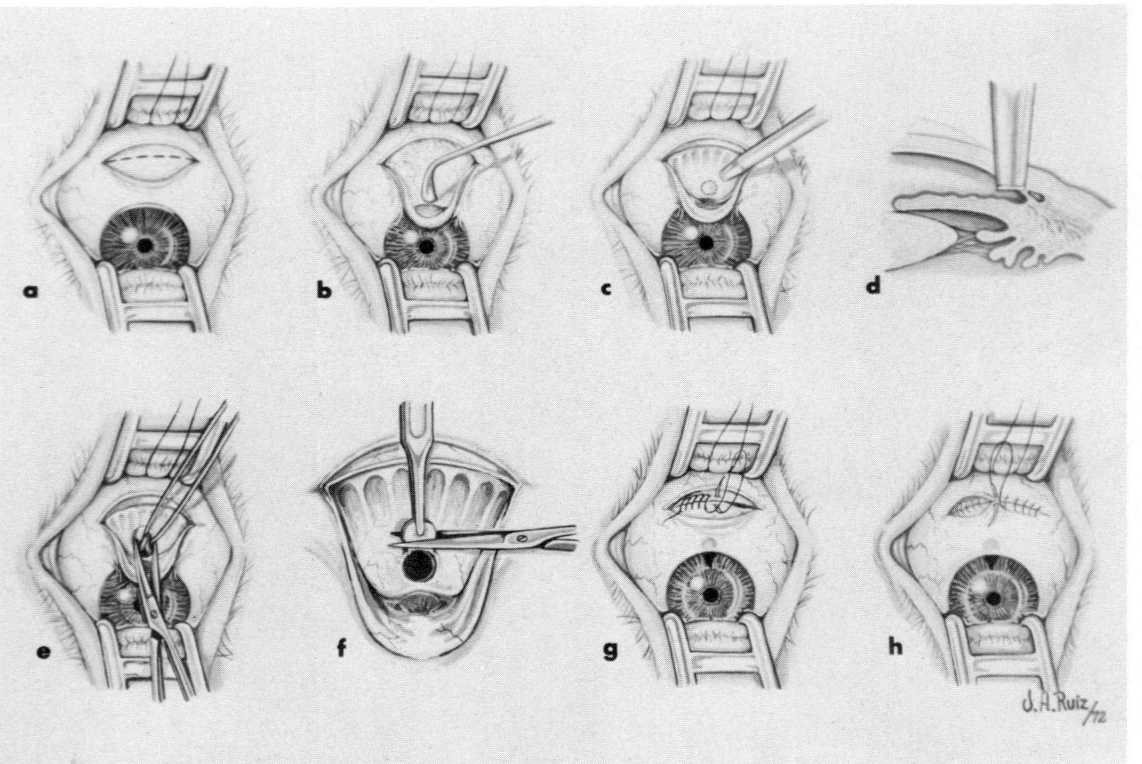

FIG. 67. The limboscleral trephanation operation. (A) Conjunctival incision; (B) the limbal area is cleared; (C) the trephine groove is made; (D) perforation takes place; (E) iridectomy; (F) a portion of the plug is excised; (G) Tenon's capsule is sutured; (H) the conjunctiva is sutured.

peripheral iridectomy is done (Fig. 67E), at this point if it can be performed with technical ease. If the 1.5 mm trephine was used, the entire button is removed. With a 2-mm trephine, the button is cut transversely in half, removing only the anterior, unhinged portion (Fig. 67F).

The size of the opening may be limited by cutting across the button at any desired level, leaving the hinged fraction in place. It may be more convenient at this stage to grasp the prolapsed iris and perform the iridectomy. It is important that the round shape of the pupil be restored. This is done by gently lifting the anterior lip of the fistula to release the iris, and by using a steady stream of saline solution on the sclerectomy site, or by massaging the cornea with a cyclodialysis spatula, if necessary. The conjunctival flap is replaced, and a running 6-0 catgut suture is used to close Tenon's capsule (Fig. 67G). It may be locked at regular intervals during the suturing and should catch the episclera at one place to prevent prolapse of the conjuctiva. Interrupted virgin or 10-0 silk is used to unite the conjunctival edges (Fig. 67H). It is not necessary to remove these sutures postoperatively. The blunt-end #30 needle is introduced through the previously placed, fluorescein-stained puncture tract in the lower temporal quadrant of the cornea, to fill the anterior chamber with saline. If the limboscleral fistula is patent, the bleb balloons out indicating that the flap is adequately sutured. Atropine and chloramphenicol ointments are instilled and only the one eye is patched. Atropine is used for about 10 days postoperatively. Local steroids are begun on the third day and continued for one to two weeks together with antibiotic drops.

Results

Sugar reported a 7-year follow-up of 25 patients under 20 years of age (Table 2). Of the 25 limboscleral trephinations 12 were done for primary congenital glaucoma, and 13 were done for cases with associated abnormalities. The success rate was 58 percent in the primary group and 61 percent in the second group.

Sixteen trephinations were done in patients between 20 and 35 years of age. This group included 7 cases with pigmentary glaucoma. Seventy-seven percent of the operations done were successful, while the success rate in patients with pigmentary glaucoma was 43 percent.

Postoperative complications in 156 limboscleral trephinations are summarized in Table 3, and include delay in reformation of the anterior chamber and the occurrence of postoperative hyphema. Hypotony with visual decrease occurs temporarily in the early postoperative period. Failure

TABLE 2

25 LIMBOSCLERAL TREPHINATIONS ON YOUNG PATIENTS UP TO AGE 20*

		No.	Percent Success
Primary glaucoma		12	58
Infantile	1		
Childhood and adolescent	11 (5 failed)		
Secondary glaucoma		13	61
Axenfeld syndrome	3 (2 failed)		
Rieger's syndrome	2		
Sturge-Weber syndrome	3		
Postcataract (aphakic)	1 (failed)		
Aniridia (2 with dislocation of lens)	3 (2 failed)		
Posttraumatic hyphema	1		

*After H. S. Sugar, Eye, Ear, Nose, Throat Mon., 47:165, 1968.

of bleb formation occurs in the immediate postoperative period in young patients, while in the 30 to 35 age group, it was often delayed for months or, sometimes, years. Other complications include cataract formation, hyphema, postoperative uveitis, and ciliary process incarceration into the fistula. Leakage of the conjunctival wound leads to collapse and delayed formation of the anterior chamber.

TABLE 3

POSTOPERATIVE COMPLICATIONS IN 156 LIMBOSCLERAL TREPHINATIONS*

1 postoperative uveitis
1 incarceration of ciliary process
18 delayed reformation of anterior chamber
11—2 days
5—4 days
1—7 days
1—10 days
1 temporary hypotony
16 postoperative hyphema—none significant
2 cataracts (20-year-old patient)

*After H. S. Sugar, Eye, Ear, Nose, Throat Mon., 47:165, 1968.

IRIDECTOMY WITH SCLERAL CAUTERY

Iridectomy with scleral cautery was originally developed as a method of producing a fistula in the wall of the anterior chamber angle, by causing retraction of the lips of the scleral incision. Heat is applied to the line of the incision and once again after entering the anterior chamber, causing shrinkage of tissue with separation of wound edges and the formation of a permanent fistula through which aqueous could escape into the subconjunctival space. The technique for infantile and juvenile glaucoma differs somewhat from that used in the adult. The difficulties encountered, and the poor visual result anticipated, in operating upon eyes with advanced changes of infantile glaucoma, suggest that iridectomy with cautery should be used, whenever possible, earlier in the course of the disease. At present, if 2 or 3 goniotomy-goniopunctures have failed, Scheie employs iridectomy with cautery, at a time when useful vision can be salvaged. As Haas has pointed out, success from surgery in infantile glaucoma cannot be evaluated by measurements of visual acuity. Only whatever visual function remains at the time of operation can be salvaged.

Technique

Infantile Glaucoma

The operation is carried out under general anesthesia. A lid speculum is placed and a superior rectus suture is inserted (Fig. 68). The conjunctiva and Tenon's capsule are ballooned outward over one-third of the globe at the operative site, by the injection of 0.5cc of local anesthetic (Fig. 68A). This will determine the site of least scarring. The conjunctiva and Tenon's capsule are incised directly down to the sclera, about 7 mm from the limbus (Fig. 68B). The blade of a scissors is inserted between Tenon's capsule and the sclera and the incision is enlarged parallel to the limbus (Fig. 68C). Both Tenon's capsule and the conjunctiva are cut simultaneously. This thick flap, consisting of both layers, is then reflected forward to its true limbal insertion, exposing the limbus, using blunt dissection. The cornea is not split. Tenon's capsule is often very thick in children and a layer of the innermost Tenon's condensation may be excised using blunt scissors.

Because the volume of the anterior chamber is unusually large and the corneoscleral wall quite thin in congenital glaucoma, aqueous will flow profusely after the perforation is made, making cauterization extremely difficult, because of the cooling effect of the aqueous. Therefore, contrary to the adult procedure, cautery alone is applied with a sweeping motion along the sclera, parallel and adjacent to the junction of clear cornea and opaque limbus, or about 1 mm back of the limbus, much as a scalpel would be used in making a scratch incision for an iridectomy. With repeated sweeps

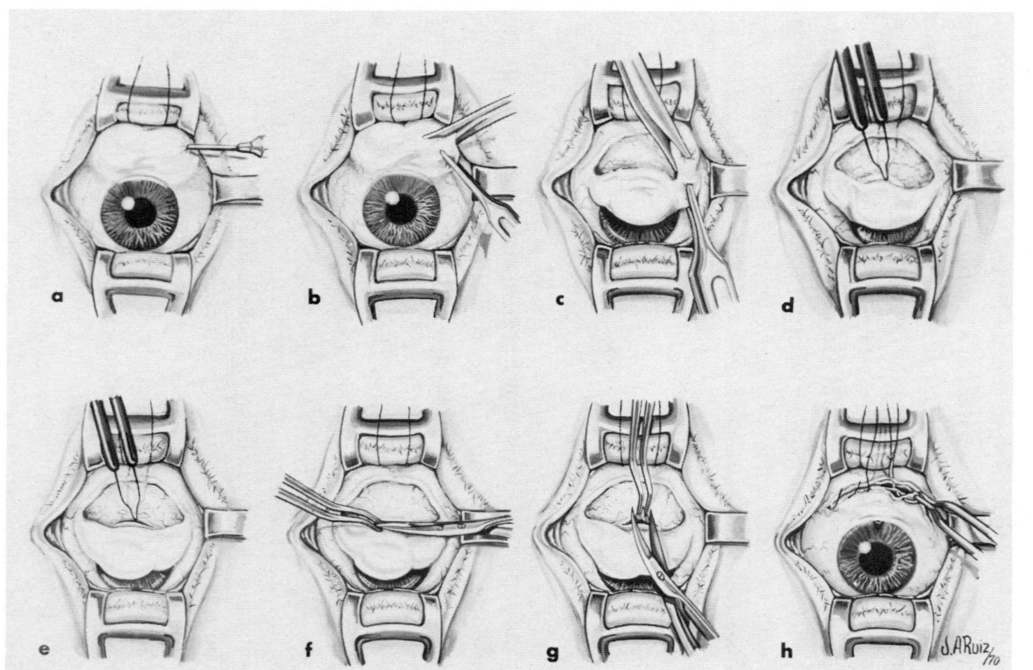

FIG. 68. Iridectomy and scleral cautery operation. (A) Ballooning of conjunctiva; (B) and (C) incising of conjunctiva; (D) scleral cautery; (E) perforation as indicated by gush of aqueous; (F) excision of anterior lip of fistula; (G) iridectomy; (H) wound closure.

of the cautery, over a line approximately 4 mm long, a gaping vertical groove one mm wide is deepened (Fig. 68D). A sudden gush of aqueous indicates perforation has taken place (Fig. 68E). This renders the cautery less effective; therefore, the field must be kept as dry as possible.

The posterior lip is usually cauterized more extensively than the anterior because it is more accessible, and because it reduces the hazard of perforating the conjunctiva. The opening is enlarged with the tip of a scalpel or blunt tonotomy scissors, over the length of the cauterized area.

A portion of the anterior lip may be excised (Fig. 68F), but again there is the hazard of conjunctival perforation. In most instances a peripheral iridectomy can be performed with ease, because as the wound gapes open from the cautery, the iris ordinarily prolapses. However, when this does not take place, it usually can be made to do so by gentle pressure on the posterior lip of the wound (Fig. 68G). Occasionally, especially in eyes with very wide angles, it may be necessary to enter the chamber with a forceps and withdraw the root of the iris.

Extreme care must be taken in performing the iridectomy because of the danger of vitreous loss. This occurs mainly because the anterior segment of the buphthalmic eye is enlarged with the lens occupying a disproportionately smaller volume. This allows the vitreous to fill a greater area in the anterior portion of the eye, whereas it would normally be displaced posteriorly by the lens mass. The zonule is greatly stretched and may present in the wound, resembling iris tissue and suggesting an inadequate iridectomy. All temptation to further manipulate the eye or to excise more iris tissue should be resisted. This is especially true in markedly enlarged eyeballs.

Following iridectomy the iris is reposited, usually with a saline stream from the irrigator. The conjunctival flap is closed with interrupted virgin or 10-0 silk sutures approximately both Tenon's capsule and the conjunctiva in separate layers (Fig. 68H). Atropine and an antibiotic ointment are instilled. Only the eye operated on is covered. Postoperative reaction is usually slight and atropine and local antibiotic-steroid drops are used for about 6 days. Massage is used as soon as the anterior chamber is formed.

Juvenile Glaucoma

Since the scleral wall is thicker in the older patient, the adult technique for iridectomy with scleral cautery may be used. If the eye is greatly distended it is better to use the technique already described for infantile glaucoma. A series of cautery applications is made along the site of the incision, adjacent to the junction of clear cornea and opaque limbus. A partially penetrating scratch incision, approximately 5 or 6 mm long and perpendicular to the surface of the globe, is then started through the cauterized area and another series of applications of the cautery is made along the lips of the incision. This process can be repeated once or twice as the incision is deepened. The anterior chamber is entered with a sweep of the scalpel that opens the length of the incision. It may be completed with blunt scissors. An iridectomy is then performed; no further cautery is needed. The application of the cautery as the incision is deepened avoids the necessity for using cautery after the eye is opened, when it is less effective because of the cooling effect of escaping aqueous. Excessive application of the cautery can result in a delayed reformation of the anterior chamber, or an excessive postoperative reaction. Only enough cautery should be used to separate the wound edges. The remainder of the procedure is carried out as described above. The filtering bleb tends to be thicker than when the operation is performed on the adult eye.

Results

Infantile Glaucoma

Scheie reported 57 eyes (40 patients) with infantile glaucoma which were operated on, using iridectomy with scleral cautery. All were reoperations, except two eyes of one patient with bilateral aniridia. The large majority of the eyes had been operated on at least twice, and some of the eyes had been subjected to 5 and 6 procedures, which ranged from simple goniopuncture or combined goniotomy-goniopuncture to various conventional filtering procedures and cyclodiathermy.

Associated anomalies treated included congenital aniridia, plexiform neurofibromatosis involving the eyelids and the temporal region, and Sturge-Weber's syndrome. The corneal diameters ranged from normal to as large as 17 mm. The ages ranged from 10 days to 14 years. The intraocular pressure was controlled in 31 eyes (54 percent).

The operation is considerably more hazardous than goniotomy or goniopuncture. The most serious and frequently encountered complication was vitreous loss, especially in eyes with a large corneal diameter. When vitreous loss did occur in Scheie's series, it was usually synonymous with loss of the eye, at least for visual purposes.

Juvenile Glaucoma

Scheie reported 15 eyes (12 patients) with juvenile glaucoma which were operated on using iridectomy with scleral cautery, with control of intraocular pressure in 13 eyes. All but 3 of these eyes had been operated on previously by goniopuncture or by conventional filtering procedures. It was used as a primary procedure in one eye of a patient who was 37 years of age. He had been aware of glaucoma for 15 years. The corneal diameter was 14 mm, yet no ruptures in Descemet's membrane were present. This was classified as juvenile glaucoma but, because of his age, iridectomy with cautery was employed. Associated abnormalities included essential iris atrophy, Sturge-Weber's syndrome, and aniridia. The age of the patients ranged from 5 to 37 years. Follow-up ranged from 6 months to 5 years. No serious complications were encountered in this group.

TRABECULOTOMY AB EXTERNO

In the trabeculotomy ab externo operation, a portion of the inner wall of Schlemm's canal and the corresponding trabecular meshwork are opened directly, interiorizing the aqueous veins to the anterior chamber.

In 1959, Dellaporta developed in eye bank eyes the trabeculodialysis procedure, in which he effected the complete detachment of a section of the trabecular meshwork from its bed by a special spatula. This causes a section of Schlemm's canal to become part of the anterior chamber. The method was not tried in glaucomatous eyes. In 1960, Smith and Burian described the trabeculotomy ab externo procedure, an operative technique designed to provide a direct avenue for aqueous humor to enter the canal of Schlemm by rupturing its inner wall and adjacent trabecular meshwork.

In 1962, Smith described the utilization of a nylon fiber threaded through Schlemm's canal and then pulled tight at each end to effect this disruption. At the same time, Allen and Burian devised a fine semicircular spatula to accomplish this aim. The principle of this technique has been variously modified, and culminated in the development of a successful microsurgical procedure by Harms and Dannheim, and Lynn.

Deviating from the principle of trabeculotomy, Cairns, in 1968, described a clinically successful trabeculectomy procedure by which he removed a 4-mm section of the corneoscleral trabeculum and overlying Schlemm's canal.

While goniotomy opens the trabecular meshwork at an unspecified level from the anterior chamber approach, trabeculotomy ab externo opens the anterior chamber from the side of Schlemm's canal. Performance of trabeculotomy is predicated upon the presumption that the case has an obstruction to outflow between the anterior chamber and Schlemm's canal. Aqueous is less viscous than blood, and there are no valves in the outflow system of the eye. If blood can flow retrograde through the episcleral and aqueous veins into the canal of Schlemm and aqueous enters the canal from the anterior chamber, aqueous should be able to leave the eye with minimal resistance, except when an obstruction is present. Proven reflux of blood into Schlemm's canal, therefore, strengthens the argument for trabeculotomy in a given case. Other features suggesting a blockage at the level of the inner wall of Schlemm's canal include the absence of pigment in the trabecular area, and the absence of aqueous flow through the trabecular meshwork when Schlemm's canal is opened at surgery. This is indeed the case in congenital glaucoma, since the canal can be made to fill with blood with moderate jugular compression, and is visible in front of the scleral spur in a high percentage of cases.

Instruments

The universal problem with the available methods for trabeculotomy is the lack of easy, accurate control of the instruments, both for localization and insertion into the canal of Schlemm above its course, and for horizontal lysis of the inner wall of Schlemm's canal and the trabecular meshwork.

Trabeculotome Probes

ALLEN-BURIAN TRABECULOTOME'. The blade of the Allen-Burian trabeculotome measures 0.5 by 0.2 mm at the tip and enlarges to 0.7 by 0.4 mm farther back along the blade. The instrument has a number of disadvantages. The operator's hand and the instrument may move between the microscope and the surgical field, or may enter the path of illumination so that the blade may stray out of the canal of Schlemm even if the instrument is started in the proper location.

Since the handle of the Allen-Burian trabeculotome, which should be kept parallel to the visual axis, cannot be totally visualized through the microscope, scrub and circulating nurses must be trusted to judge parallelism of the visual axis and trabeculotome handle, and direct the surgeon to tilt right, left, forward, and back.

LYNN-ALLEN TRABECULOTOME. The Lynn-Allen trabeculotome, shown in Fig. 69, uses the same blade specifications as the Allen-Burian trabeculotome. The instrument consists basically of a large complete ring, a smaller partial (incomplete) ring, and a blade (Fig. 69C). The smaller partial ring serves both as a support and a guard. One-eighth of this guard ring is absent, which permits the cornea over the blade tip to remain convex while the blade is rotated horizontally into the anterior chamber from Schlemm's

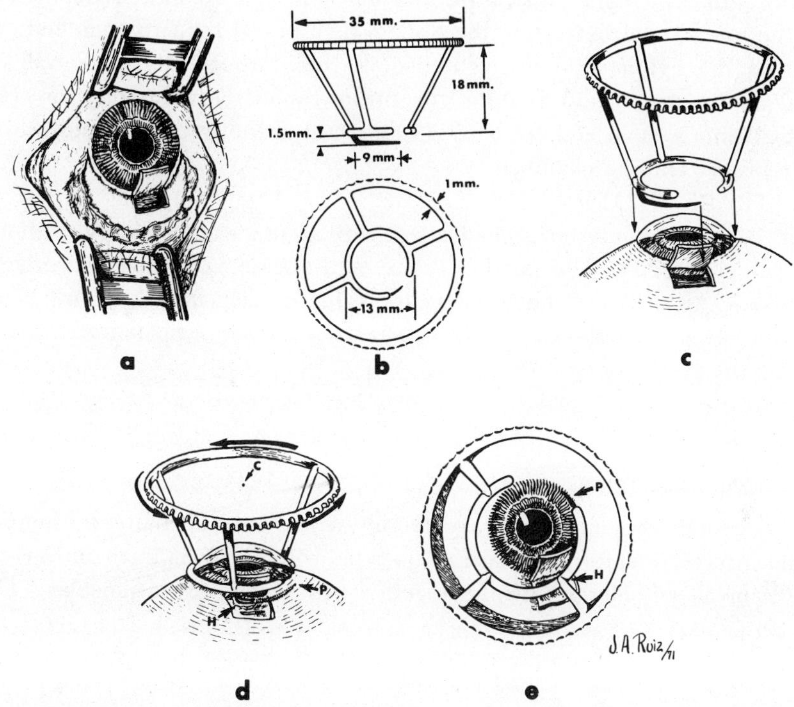

FIG. 69. The trabeculotome of Lynn-Allen. (A) The scleral flap; (B) trabeculotome; (C) positioning of the instrument; (D and E) inserting the blade into Schlemm's canal. (After Lynn and Berry. **Am. J. Ophthalmol.** 68:430, 1969.)

canal, as shown in Fig. 69D and E. The open segment of the ring also permits visualization of the blade tip. The 1.5-mm vertical separation between blade and guard provides sufficient space to allow horizontal entry into the anterior chamber, yet protects deeper structures. The upper larger knurled ring serves as a handle which is easy to grasp, no matter what limbal location is chosen for trabeculotomy, and does not obstruct either illumination or visualization with the microscope. The upper and lower rings are 18 mm apart so that fixation forceps or any other desired instruments may be inserted between the struts. The instrument may therefore be used in enophthalmic eyes. Right and left hand models are used for maximum trabecular cleavage through one scleral opening.

MONOFILAMENT NYLON SUTURE OF REDMOND SMITH. Redmond Smith effected a trabeculotomy by inserting a monofilament nylon suture into Schlemm's canal, threading it around a part of the circumference of the cornea and extracting the tip. He then pulled the two ends taut, so that as the nylon suture straightened, it tore through the inner wall of Schlemm's canal. Unfortunately, the suture cannot be accurately directed in Schlemm's canal and tends to ride forward in the trabecular meshwork, entering the anterior chamber.

TRABECULOTOME OF HARMS. The "warped hairpin" of Harms (Fig. 70) may be inserted and advanced with accuracy and delicacy, without impeding visibility. The parallel limbs of the Harms instrument are both curved so that as one limb enters the canal of Schlemm the other rides outside, over the limbus, acting as a guard against posterior penetration from within the canal.

Other Instruments

An operating microscope, preferably with zoom capability, is essential. Fine corneoscleral forceps (Castroviejo type) with 0.12-mm teeth and a razor blade breaker holder are helpful together with a standard intraocular set of instruments.

Localization and Identification of Schlemm's Canal

Strachan has measured the largest dimension of the canal of Schlemm in celloidin-mounted eyes and found it to be only 0.25 mm. Harms and Dannheim, and Smith, emphasize the difficulty of finding landmarks so that the canal of Schlemm can be properly identified and entered. The use of a radial incision at the limbus is associated with the hazard of perforating into the anterior chamber (Fig. 71E[A]). For this reason it is better to identify Schlemm's canal by probing in the bed of a scleral flap (Fig. 70A, B and C; Fig. 71E[B]). Since the cut edge of sclera offers impassable resistance to a blunt, flexible probe, Harm considers ease in passage good evidence that the probe lies in Schlemm's canal. However, any other opening, e.g., the supraciliary body space, which is located near the canal, may allow easy passage of a blunt probe and may thus be mistaken for the canal of Schlemm.

Lynn has devised a 3-0 nylon monofilament suture, with the end thermally blunted, to locate and probe the canal and the supraciliary body space. The diameter of a 3-0 monofilament nylon suture is 0.22 mm, while the nylon probe tip measures about 0.33 mm. The probes are made from 2- or 3-in lengths of 3-0 suture material and are reusable. While the tip is

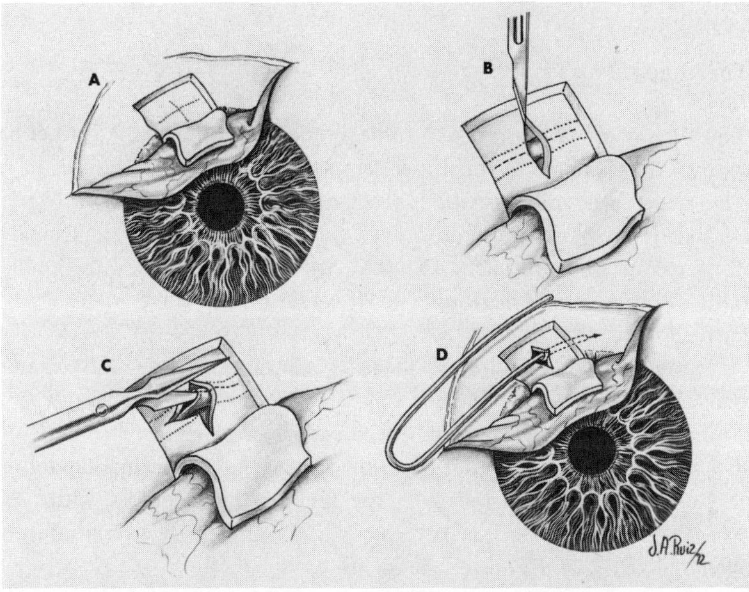

FIG. 70. The trabeculotome of Harms. (A) Localizing Schlemm's canal; (B and C) incision into the canal; (D) insertion of trabeculotome. (After Dannheim. **Trans. Am. Acad. Ophthalmol. Otolaryngol.** 76:375, 1972.)

observed under the microscope, each piece of suture is slowly moved to within one-quarter in of the red-hot tip of a disposable cautery. As soon as the suture end begins to melt, it must be withdrawn promptly. Singeing the suture tip in this way results in a small terminal knob, which helps prevent the probe from cutting through delicate tissues.

Choice of Procedure Site

Final preoperative evaluation helps in the selection of the site, for trabeculotomy may be accomplished with equal facility at any location around the limbus. The evaluation involves a knowledge of earlier surgery, gonioscopy, and slit lamp examination of the anterior chamber. Previous operative sites, especially the area within or adjacent to a sector iridectomy, should be avoided. If the patient has had no previous surgery, the upper quadrants are preferred, so that during the postoperative period the patient may sit and simultaneously allow residual blood to flow from the trabeculotomy site.

Technique

The operation is carried out under general anesthesia. A limbal-based conjunctival flap is made in the upper temporal quadrant.

The two rectus muscles which bracket the proposed trabeculotomy site are isolated in the peritomy region with muscle hooks, and a half-length of 4-0 silk is passed beneath each. The two sutures are anchored to the drapes for stable fixation and positioning of the eye during the remainder of the procedure.

A corneal-based scleral flap, measuring approximately 3 by 3 mm, is made at the corneoscleral border. The lamella consists of two-thirds to three-fourths of the thickness of the corneoscleral tissue. The bed of the scleral flap should resemble that of a scleral buckling for retinal detachment. As the flap dissection progresses to the limbus, the racemose white scleral fibers (with moderate vascularity) give way anteriorly to a circumferential, homogeneous, dark blue colored glassy zone.

The Lynn technique for localization of Schlemm's canal is carried out as follows. After the blue zone has been demonstrated across the anterior extent of the scleral bed, a 2.5 mm incision is made into the supraciliary body space parallel to the limbus in the middle of the scleral bed (Fig. 71C). A blunt nylon probe, held with tying forceps, is passed into the incision, then pushed anteriorly through the supraciliary body space (Fig. 71D). When modest resistance to the anterior passage of the probe is encountered, indicated by a springy movement of the nylon probe without the exertion of undue forward pressure by the tip of the probe, the end point is reached.

Care is taken to hold the nylon suture well back from the incision, so that lateral movement of the probe can be recognized. The resistance to forward passage is offered by the fragile attachment of the ciliary muscle to the scleral spur. Penetration of the muscle would allow the probe to enter the iris stroma, the anterior chamber, or the posterior chamber. If the scleral flap is not thick enough to allow visualization of the probe through its bed, the probe should be accurately grasped at a known exterior location. The probe is then withdrawn and replaced on top of the scleral bed. External landmarks indicate the extent of its forward progress. Three trials are made and the passage which meets resistance most posteriorly is used as a landmark for incision into Schlemm's canal.

Incision into Schlemm's Canal

A vertical incision is made about 0.33 mm anterior to the point where

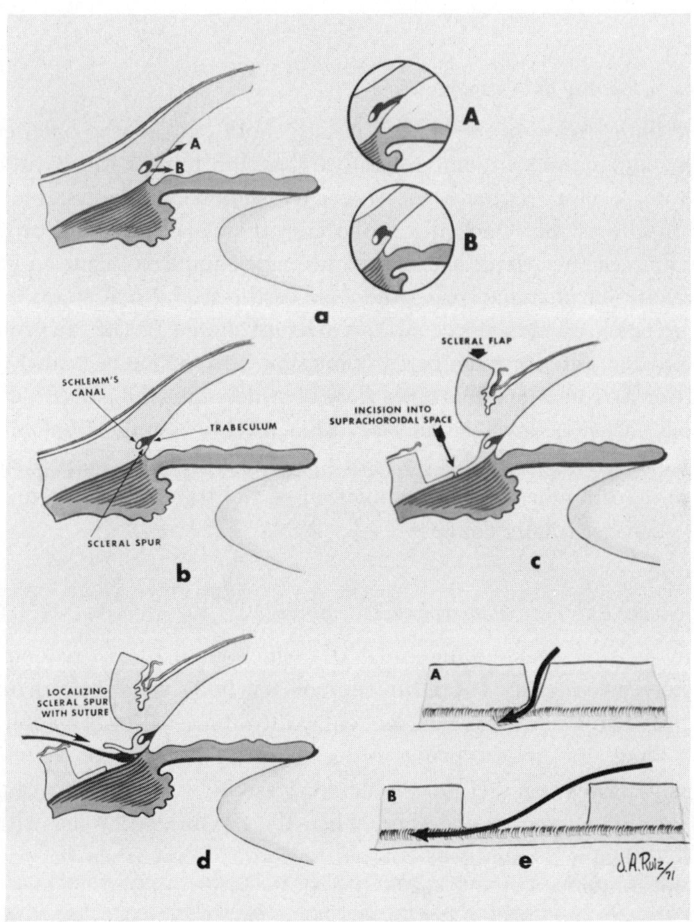

FIG. 71. Trabeculotomy ab externo (Lynn). A (A) Undesirable long posterior flap which tends to close if chamber becomes shallow or blood clot organizes in the chamber angle, (B) Preferred trabeculotomy. B, C and D, localizing Schlemm's canal with nylon probes. E (A), probe may be misdirected if inserted into Schlemm's canal via a vertical incision, (B), Probe will find its way with greater accuracy into Schlemm's canal if inserted from the bed of a scleral flap. (After Lynn and Berry. **Am. J. Ophthalmol.** 68:430, 1969.)

the probe resisted further forward passage. The incision enters the canal of Schlemm, a structure with finer texture than the nearby iris. The open canal of Schlemm varies in appearance, primarily because of differences in pigmentation. The canal is carefully opened from one side of the scleral bed to the other, avoiding perforation into the trabecular meshwork (Fig. 70C).

Proving Identity of Schlemm's Canal

The blunt nylon probe is inserted into both ends of the open canal of Schlemm, and passed circumferentially along the limbus for a distance of about 8 or 9 mm. Virtually no resistance should be encountered during passage of the probe. Once the probe is in the canal, it should be grasped well back from the scleral bed and an attempt should be made to rotate it into the anterior chamber, using the edge of the scleral bed as a fulcrum. If the probe lies in Schlemm's canal, this attempt should fail. If the probe does rotate into the anterior chamber, the incision into Schlemm's canal was too far anterior or too deep. The rapid flow of aqueous, as the anterior chamber is entered, usually serves as an early clue to this complication. Moderate aqueous leakage through the trabecular meshwork occurs fairly frequently and is no contraindication to completion of the trabeculotomy, unless the anterior chamber totally collapses.

Erroneous Entry Into Supraciliary Body Space

The incision seeking the canal of Schlemm, made as recommended above, may erroneously enter the supraciliary body space. Unfortunately, this complication simulates a correct entry into the canal of Schlemm in two regards. First, the nylon probe is easily inserted into the opening and effortlessly passed parallel to the limbus; secondly, the probe cannot be rotated into the anterior chamber. When the flexible probe lies within the canal of Schlemm it cannot be rotated posteriorly, but when the probe lies within the supraciliary body space, it may be easily rotated backward. This posterior rotation serves to differentiate between the two positions. Another early clue to this mislocation is the unexpected texture and color when comparing the bed of the original entry to the supraciliary body space with the presumed incision into Schlemm's canal.

As the surgeon gains clinical experience with the surgical anatomy of this area, he becomes increasingly aware of the different qualities of color and texture of the structures.

Positioning for Lysis of Trabecula

After the identity of Schlemm's canal has been proven, low power magnification is used to verify that the trabeculotome (in this case the Lynn-Allen) placed on the outside of the eye can be advanced into the canal, rotated into the anterior chamber, and withdrawn without interfering with illumination or visibility of the pertinent structures. Repositioning of the eye is frequently necessary at this stage. Once the eye is adequately positioned and a "golfer's practice swing" has been negotiated successfully, high power magnification is again advised, so that the tip of the trabeculotome blade may be accurately directed into Schlemm's canal.

Passage of the Trabeculotome into Canal

Traction at the edge of the scleral bed is obtained with medium-sized corneoscleral forceps, and the trabeculotome blade tip is started into the canal of Schlemm. The magnification is then reduced to the limit and the trabeculotome is passed gently and gradually around the chamber angle until it lies completely within Schlemm's canal, up to the heel of the trabeculotome blade (Fig. 69D and E). The rotation for insertion of the blade into the canal is around the center of the rings (Fig. 69C). If the nylon probe passed properly, the trabeculotome blade should not meet much resistance during entry of the canal. If definite resistance is met, a false passage should be suspected. Careful recheck of landmarks should confirm that the blade has actually started in Schlemm's canal, and the ring guard should be nearly centered over the cornea. If one side of the canal accepts the probe and the other does not, a constriction of Schlemm's canal may be suspected. In this case, an abbreviated trabeculotomy is performed on that side, opening the canal to whatever extent possible. A full trabeculotomy is performed in the other direction.

Lysis of Trabecula

After the blade is inserted into Schlemm's canal the rotation continues, but the axis of rotation is changed to the heel of the blade (Fig. 69E,point H). The blade point labelled "P" Fig. 69E is allowed to enter the anterior chamber for a distance of only 2 mm. If the blade has been inserted into the canal of Schlemm without difficulty and the attempted rotation into the anterior chamber meets definite resistance, the trabeculotome should not be forcefully rotated. The trabeculotome should be partially withdrawn along the canal, reversing the rotation of the instrument around the center point, "C," to retract the point a distance of about 1 mm. A second attempt should then be made to rotate the blade into the anterior chamber around the axis "H." This maneuver usually frees the tip from its presumed entrapment in a pocket of sclera and allows easy rotation into the anterior chamber. As the blade is withdrawn, the position of the tip is maintained 2 mm inside the limbus. When the tip lies opposite the edge of the scleral flap, it is then

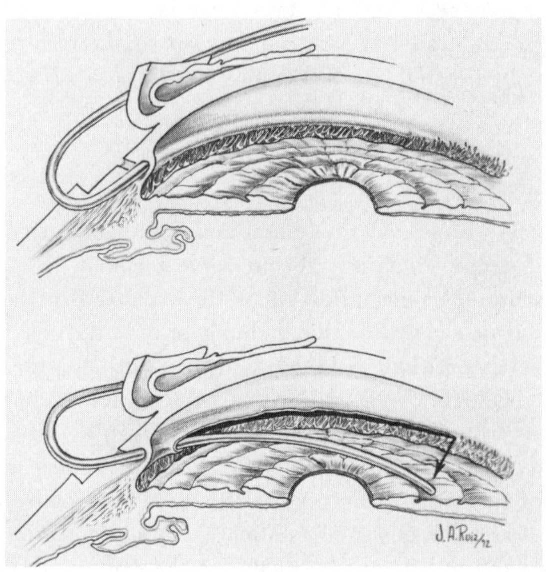

FIG. 72. Harms-Dannheim trabeculotomy ab externo. (After Dannheim. **Trans. Am. Acad. Ophthalmol. Otolaryngol.** 76:375, 1972.)

withdrawn directly. After lysis of the inner wall of Schlemm's canal and trabecular meshwork in one direction, the same procedure should be promptly performed in the opposite direction.

Harms uses a U-shaped warped hair pin probe which is introduced into the canal on one side (Fig. 72). The tip of the probe is rotated into the anterior chamber, rupturing the inner wall of Schlemm's canal and trabecular meshwork as described above. The meshwork in the bed of scleral access is spared to avoid emptying of the anterior chamber or prolapse of iris tissue.

The problems of passing the Harms probe along Schlemm's canal with accuracy is no less critical than with the Lynn-Allen trabeculotome. In Fig. 73 we see how the probe may pass superficial (Fig. 73A) or deep to, (Fig. 73C) as well as within, Schlemm's canal (Fig. 73B). These mislocations have all been observed histologically on autopsy eyes.

Hyphema During Surgery

Blood often enters the anterior chamber in variable amounts after the first unidirectional passage of the probe, and the amount usually increases

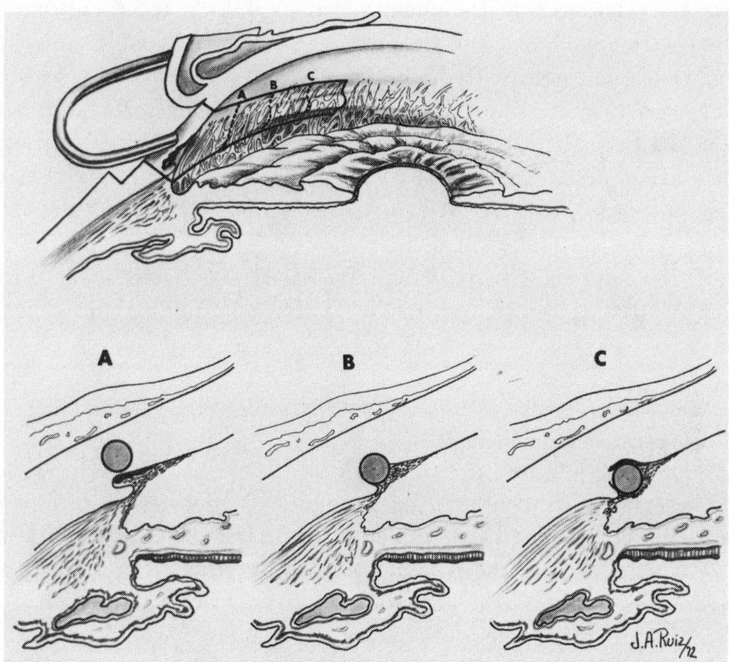

FIG. 73. Harms-Dannheim trabeculotomy ab externo. (A) The probe superficial to Schlemm's canal; (B) the probe within Schlemm's canal; (C) the probe in the trabeculum deep to the inner wall of Schlemm's canal. (After Spenser. **Trans. Am. Acad. Ophthalmol. Otolaryngol.** 76:389, 1972.)

considerably with the second passage. No attempt to irrigate the anterior chamber with saline is advisable because of the possibility of prolapsing the iris. The blood is usually resorbed during the first few days following surgery.

While blood in the anterior chamber may be used as a criteria for a successful trabeculotomy, the blood may actually become organized and cause the flap of trabecular tissue to seal down. The scleral flap is closed with 7 to 9 interrupted sutures of 8-0 white silk. By pressing on the globe, it can be shown that the fistula is watertight and aqueous will not leak from the wound. Usually the anterior chamber is not lost during the operation. If the eye is still soft and tends to fill with blood after the wound is closed, a knife-needle incision may be made at the limbus for the injection of saline into the anterior chamber, as a tamponade against further bleeding. The traction sutures are then removed and the limbal-based conjunctival flap is sutured using virgin or 10-0 silk.

In the Harms and Dannheim's series of 196 trabeculotomies, 28 attempts were abandoned and the surgeon changed to a more conventional form of glaucoma surgery. Redmond Smith found it necessary to change the type of operation in 13 of 39 cases because he penetrated the anterior chamber or had difficulty in localizing the canal. In Lynn's series, one patient's attempted trabeculotomy had to be converted to a conventional filtering procedure, because of the surgeon's inability to find the canal of Schlemm. Lynn has stated that since the relationship between the anterior limit of the supraciliary space and the canal was established, using his method of nylon probes, no further failures in finding the canal have occurred.

Postoperative Management

Pilocarpine 2 percent and an antibiotic corticosteroid ointment are instilled (the pilocarpine keeps the cleft in the trabecular meshwork open). The eye is patched, and the patient is sent to the recovery room with orders to position his eye, with the new trabeculotomy cleft high enough that the blood may settle into some other part of the chamber angle. Starting the day after surgery, 1 percent pilocarpine, 1 percent paredrine, and an antibiotic corticosteriod ointment are instilled 5 min apart, every 8 hrs.

Although microscopic hyphemata were commonly seen in the Lynn series and Strachan has noted reflux from the trabeculotomy site on slit lamp examination, gross secondary hyphemas are uncommon in the postoperative trabeculotomy patient.

Gonioscopy, in the follow-up period, revealed no visible cleft in 30 percent of Harms and Dannheim's successful cases. In Lynn's series, gonioscopy did not reveal clefts in certain cases whose intraocular pressure was far better controlled following surgery. One of Smith's pigmentary glaucoma patients also showed no clinical cleft on gonioscopy.

Trabeculotomy suffers from the disadvantage of being difficult to perform. Precise localization of the canal of Schlemm, followed by the passage of an instrument into its lumen, requires a degree of skill which is not easily attained. However, if it is accepted that the obstruction is in the trabeculum, it is the most rational of procedures.

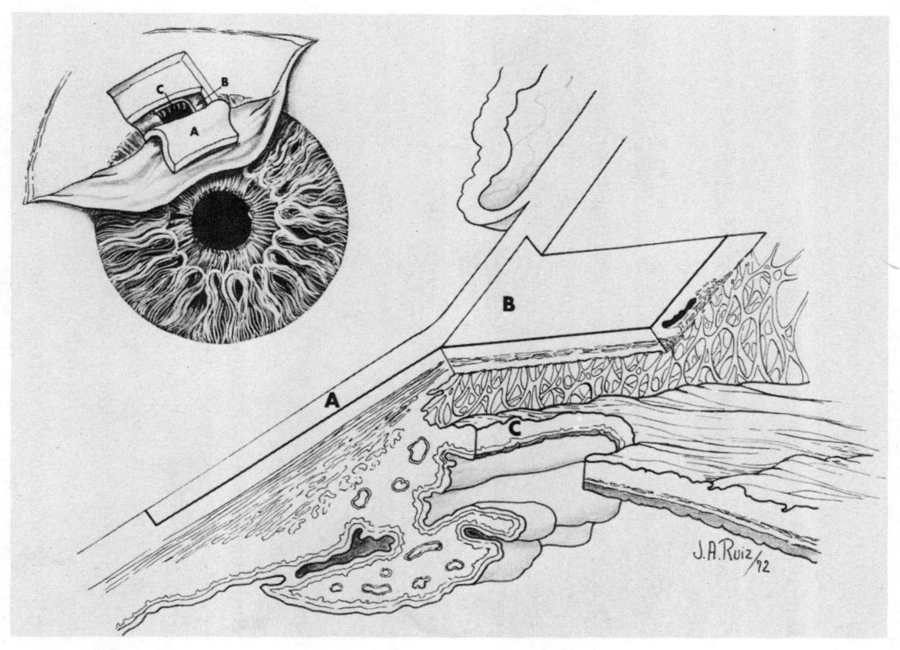

FIG. 74. Trabeculectomy. (A) Scleral flap; (B) excised segment of trabeculum, Schlemm's canal, deep cornea, and sclera; (C) iridectomy. (After Cairns. **Trans. Am. Acad. Ophthalmol. Otolaryngol.** 76:384, 1972.)

TRABECULECTOMY

The principle of the trabeculectomy procedure is to perform, underneath a sclerocorneal flap, a trephination of the surgical limbus which will effect the excision of a corresponding section of the corneoscleral trabeculum and the overlying Schlemm's canal. The position of the canal is inferred from its relationship to the trabeculum, which may be visualized during the procedure. The result of this operation is the establishment of two openings in Schlemm's canal, and thereby direct communication between its lumen and the anterior chamber.

Indications

A trabeculectomy is indicated for eyes in which the resistance to the aqueous outflow is assumed to lie in the trabecular meshwork. Prerequisites for technical success of the operation are an open angle, at least in the vicinity of the surgery; a patent Schlemm's canal; and patent outflow channels to the episcleral vessels. Types of glaucoma for which this operation is appropriate are primary glaucoma in phakic or aphakic eyes, congenital glaucoma, and glaucoma secondary to obstruction of the trabeculae by cellular debris.

Technique

The technique of trabeculectomy is shown in Fig. 74. The patient is placed under general anesthesia. The pupil is constricted and the eye rendered normotensive by the administration of acetazolamide, the dose determined by body weight (See Chap. 7). A superior rectus bridal suture is inserted. A paracentesis puncture is made at a site remote from the 12 o'clock position to facilitate re-formation of the chamber at the end (if this should prove to be necessary). A large, 8-mm, wide, limbal-based flap of Tenon's capsule and conjunctiva is reflected over the cornea. Excess subconjunctival tissue, commonly found in young children, should be excised to give a thinner flap. A half-thickness, limbal-based sclerocorneal lamellar flap, 5 by 5 mm, is raised. The anterior chamber is then entered along a line parallel to, and in front of, Schwalbe's line in the cornea. Peripheral iridectomy may be performed through this incision as a guard against iris prolapse. Parallel incisions are made backward from the extremities of this incision, and the deep flap thus created is turned back

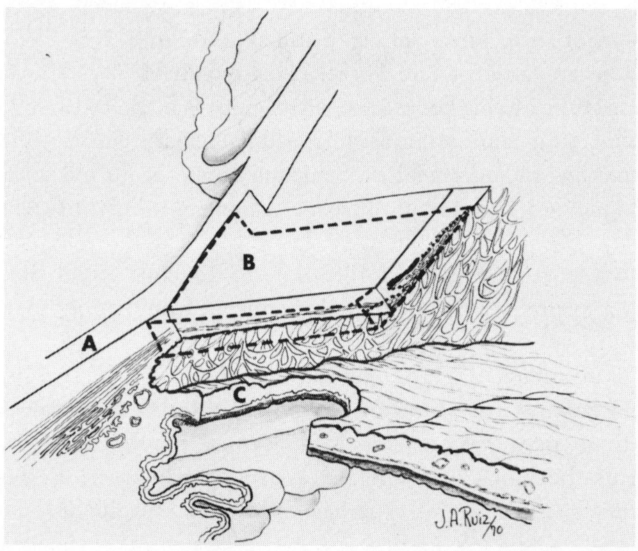

FIG. 75. Trabeculectomy. (A) Scleral flap, (B) dotted, excised segment including scleral spur, anterior longitudinal ciliary muscle, trabecular meshwork, Schlemm's canal, deep cornea, and sclera, (C) iridectomy. (After Spenser. **Trans. Am. Acad. Ophthalmol. Otolaryngol.** 76:389, 1972.)

toward the sclera until the trabecular band is seen on its upper surface. This flap, now containing trabeculum, Schlemm's canal, deep cornea and sclera, is cut off by scissor behind the trabecular band.

The defect may be fashioned with a sharp, 2-mm diameter, Elliot trephine involving two-thirds sclera and one-third cornea. In most instances, the trephine button is completely cut at the first attempt and is pushed outward slightly by the bulging uvea. It is grasped with fine forceps, but may not be removed until the delicate connections between the corneoscleral trabeculae and the uveal meshwork are either cut with fine, blunt-tipped scissors or stripped off with a spatula. Two open ends of the canal of Schlemm are now in direct communication with the anterior chamber, as are, presumably, the aqueous veins and collector channels in the area of the excision. Cautery is not used in this procedure, the vessels being left to bleed until spontaneous thrombosis occurs, aided by instillations of 1:1,000 adrenalin.

The outer scleral lamella is replaced and closed with 4 or more 8-0 white silk sutures. The chamber usually re-forms spontaneously by this time, but if it does not, it is reformed with saline through the previously placed paracentesis puncture. The conjunctival flap is replaced and sutured. Chloramphenicol eye ointment is instilled and only this eye patched. Atropine drops are used for 2 to 4 weeks postoperatively.

In a variation of this procedure, an attempt is made to excise a portion of the scleral spur and anterior longitudinal ciliary muscle, along with trabecular meshwork and canal of Schlemm (Fig. 75, dotted outline). The latter technique may possibly produce an opening, not only into the canal of Schlemm, but also into the potential space between the sclera and ciliary body, so that posterior internal filtration of aqueous could theoretically occur, as in a cyclodialysis. Whether this concept would apply to congenital glaucoma is not yet established.

The disadvantage of the operation is that despite the use of the operating microscope, the surgeon attempting a trabeculo-canalectomy for the first time may experience difficulty in precise localization and orientation of the block of tissue to be excised. However, as the surgeon gains experience errors of this type become less of a problem, according to Cairns.

A measure of controversy surrounds the exact manner in which the trabeculectomy functions. A successful operation may permit increased aqueous outflow via several pathways. The aqueous may gain direct access through the patent cut ends of Schlemm's canal (Fig. 76A), but histologic evidence at present casts doubt on this route. Aqueous may leave via the ostia of the intrascleral outflow channels, or may permeate the thinned outer scleral lamellae (Fig. 76B). It may filter externally along the course of the scleral scar (Fig. 76C), producing a bleb which may or may not be visible clinically. Finally, it is possible that aqueous filters internally via a surgically produced cleft between the sclera and the ciliary body (Fig. 76D).

It is generally felt that trabeculo-canalectomy appears, in most instances, to work by producing localized external filtration. In the patient in whom external filtration is not evident, yet intraocular pressure is effectively reduced, we need to determine whether pressure has been lowered by inadvertent cyclodialysis associated with an incision posterior to the scleral spur detaching the ciliary muscle, or whether it has been reduced by some other mechanism.

SINUSOTOMY

Krasnov's operation (Fig.77) consists of removing a narrow segment of sclera external to Schlemm's canal, based on the theory that

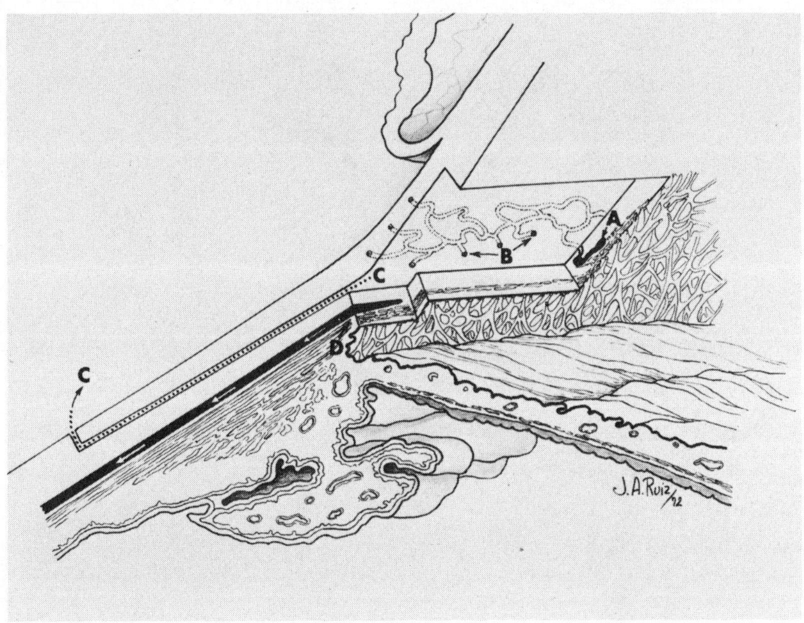

FIG. 76. Trabeculectomy. (A) Cut end of Schlemm's canal; (B) ostia of intrascleral outflow channels; (C) filtration taking place along the course of the scleral scar; (D) scleral-ciliary body cleft. (After Spenser. **Trans. Am. Acad. Ophthalmol. Otolaryngol.** 76:389, 1972.)

channels located in the excised tissue play a role in causing glaucoma. Although this concept does not apply directly to congenital glaucoma, certain observations are pertinent.

Experiments have been performed in which Schlemm's canal was exteriorized in enucleated human eyes over as much as half of the circumference. This increased the facility of outflow more than would be predicted from the internal trabeculotomy experiments. The increase in facility of outflow was roughly proportional to the circumferential extent of Schlemm's canal exteriorized. Making an opening of less than an hour of circumference from the canal to the outside, without damaging the inner wall, had such a slight effect that the rest of the circumference of the canal could not have drained through this opening.

Removing the scleral and outer wall of Schlemm's canal may be considered to remove the tissue against which the trabecular meshwork and inner wall of Schlemm's canal may be compressed, by the intraocular

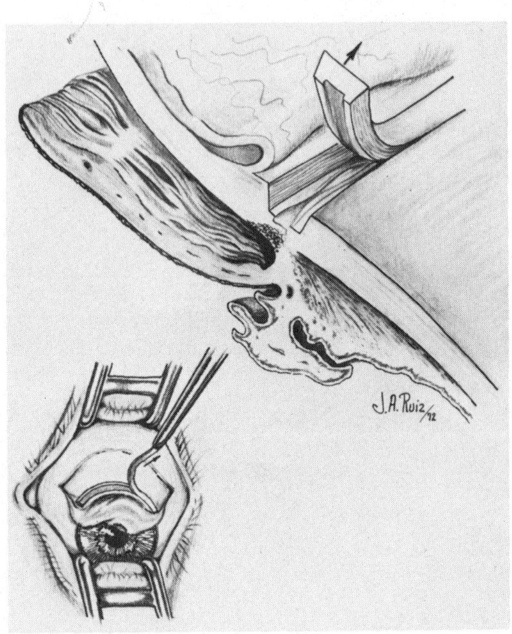

FIG. 77. Sinusotomy. (After Krasnov. **Trans. Am. Acad. Ophthalmol. Otolaryngol.** 76:368, 1972.)

pressure, thus giving rise to glaucoma. The raised pressure may also be relieved by removing blocked channels in the excised tissue, or by simple filtration.

FAILURE IN FISTULIZING SURGERY

Fistulizing procedures are notoriously poorly tolerated in the infant eye. For this reason meticulous care must be taken at each step of the operation.

On comparing the success rates in the primary glaucoma groups in the various age categories described, it becomes evident that success is directly proportional to increasing age. Most ophthalmologists feel this is associated with the fact that the Tenon's capsule is thicker in younger people and atrophies with increasing age. However, there may be other factors which account for the poor results in young people. These may be related, not only to the quantity of subconjunctival tissue, but to its vascularity and, perhaps, to chemical constituents about which we know very little.

Choice of Site

There is the greatest chance of success if the site is located where conjunctival scarring from the original operative procedure is minimal, and is located as close to the 12 o'clock position as possible. The site of least scarring is determined by ballooning out the subconjunctival tissue with a local anesthetic solution. The area which apparently has the least adherence to the limbosclera and sclera is the site of choice.

Preventing Closure from Adhesion of the Flap

Preparation of the Flap

The incision should be made 7 to 8 mm above the limbus after the conjunctiva has been ballooned out with a 0.5 cc injection of a local anesthetic (adrenalin added). The latter will aid in hemostatis. Healing of such an incision, with fibrosis and scar formation, will therefore occur a considerable distance from the filtering area. The incision is made to the sclera through both Tenon's capsule and the conjunctiva, which permits the reflection of these layers to the limbus, using only blunt dissection. During dissection, the flap and the surface of the sclera should be traumatized as little as possible. Scleral bleeding points should be controlled by mild cautery or by pressure upon the bleeding points with a microsponge applicator (which may be dipped in adrenalin); hemorrhage beneath the flap can lead to fibrosis. In addition, episcleral bleeding under the flap may leak into the anterior chamber, causing a severe hyphema which would accentuate the postoperative reaction. Cotton fibers or other foreign material deposited beneath the flap may also contribute to fibrosis.

There is usually an ample amount of subconjunctival tissue present in the infant eye which should be excised in the area of the fistula.

Closure of the Flap

The cut edges of both Tenon's capsule and the conjunctiva should be closed, using interrupted or continuous lock-type virgin or 10-silk sutures, by suturing them in separate layers or as a single layer. Otherwise the raw edge of Tenon's capsule would retract into the area of the fistula, causing an adherence. Catgut sutures should not be used because of the reaction they evoke compared to silk. Closure of the conjunctival incision should be as watertight as possible to retain and accumulate aqueous beneath the flap; thus avoiding the development of a firm contact between Tenon's capsule and the sclera.

Perforation of the Flap

Since it is necessary to excise the excess subconjunctival tissue adjacent to the fistula near the limbus, perforation may occur even when extreme care is exercised. Small holes often pass unnoticed and repair themselves spontaneously. If the hole is noticed at the time of surgery, regardless of its size, it should be repaired. The flap is everted and virgin or 10-0 silk sutures are used on the inner aspect, inserted through the edges of the hole to provide a watertight closure. The knot is tied on the deep side of the flap. Catgut sutures should be avoiced because of the reaction they evoke. Some surgeons prefer to move the fistula to another area, but this is probably unnecessary.

The filtering bleb may rupture spontaneously or as a result of trauma, months or years after a successful filtering operation. Symptoms may be mild if at all present. The patient should have both eyes patched and be given systemic and local antibiotics. Most of these ruptures seal spontaneously. If the anterior chamber does not reform in 2 or 3 days the hole should be covered by a flap of conjunctiva and Tenon's capsule. Failure of filtration may occur as a result of the rupture and its repair.

Postoperative Care

Postoperative reaction predisposes to fibrosis of the flap and should, therefore, be reduced as much as possible. Atropine and local steroids should be used routinely. If the eye becomes very irritable, systemic steroids can be added, as soon as possible, to obtain a white eye. When a postoperative infection is suspected, systemic local and subconjunctival antibiotics, in an adequate dosage, should be administered immediately.

Massage of the eye is very helpful in promoting filtration. It should be instituted as soon as the anterior chamber is formed and continued until an adequate bleb has developed. The patient is often too young to follow instructions, so that simple pressure to the eyeball through the upper eyelid is all that is possible. Light pressure is applied alternately with two fingers by the parent, while the eye is still very soft following surgery, but heavier pressure is used as the eye becomes more firm. Massage is used for 1 min, 3 times daily.

The anterior chamber may remain flat for a considerable period. Several causes are responsible including (1) hyposecretion of aqueous. This is seen most commonly in older persons and in cases of advanced glaucoma; there is no bleb present. (2) choroidal detachment. Posterior sclerotomy with drainage of subchoroidal fluid and air injection into the anterior chamber may be necessary; there is no bleb present. (3) maximum drainage through the fistula; a large bleb is present. Treatment is unnecessary as the fistula narrows down.

Management of Adhesion of Flap

Filtration may never occur or fail several months after an apparent successful operation because of the development of flap adhesions. The filtering area loses its edematous aspect in spite of massage. It becomes solid in appearance and frequently shows newly-formed blood vessels. Treatment includes (1) transfixation of the filtering area and elevation of the bleb with a knife-needle or Graefe knife; and (2) redissection of the flap, excision of excess subconjunctival tissue, and enlargment of the fistula.

Lack of aqueous humor formation and circulation into the bleb can result in the disappearance of a filtering cicatrix, so that acetazolamide (Diamox) and related drugs are contraindicated after filtering operations.

Preventing Closure from Operative Difficulties

The introduction of saline, at the end of the surgical procedure, through the previously placed corneal incision, serves to start the bleb area in its future function. This maneuver is often omitted.

Location of Scleral Incision

The fistula should be placed on the angle wall just behind the opaque limbus to enter the anterior chamber through the trabecular area posterior to Schwalbe's line. If care is not taken to dissect the flap of Tenon's capsule and conjunctiva to its true insertion into the limbus, the incision may be placed too far posteriorly. The flap may be firmly adherent to the sclera in the area 3 or 4 mm distal to the limbus, especially when there has been repeated surgery and cyclodiathermy. Such adhesions may simulate a true limbus and lead the surgeon to make the incision too far posteriorly, causing injury to the ciliary body. Vitreous may be lost when the iridectomy is performed. Filtration may fail because of incarceration of the ciliary body, ciliary processes, and even vitreous. The ciliary processes continue to secrete aqueous into the conjunctival flap and Tenon's capsule when they are incarcerated in the fistula, leading to the appearance of a filtering cicatrix in the face of an uncontrolled tension.

Great care must be taken to remove the entire thickness of a trephine button because the inner layers may peel off, remain in place, and plug the opening. When corneal splitting is too far forward into the cornea, the flap over the fistula is too rigid and tends to seal the opening. The incision for iridectomy and scleral cautery should be made perpendicular to the surface of the cornea. Postoperative gonioscopy is essential to determine the cause of failure and act as a guide to management.

Preventing Closure from Vitreous Loss

Vitreous loss, which can occur with any of the filtering procedures, renders the prognosis for filtration poor, especially in the buphthalmic eye, although occasionally, a filtering cicatrix may still develop. A hypotensive eye, a properly placed incision, and gentle technique are important preventive measures.

Preventing Closure by the Iris

An inadequate iridectomy may result in blockage of the fistula. This may result from a sudden escape of aqueous during massage, which can carry the iris into the scleral opening. If the iris has plugged the fistula, the flap should be reflected at once and the iridectomy enlarged. Unfortunately this cannot be done without hazard, since vitreous often lurks in the iridectomy site and may be lost with excessive manipulation.

Preventing Closure by the Lens

The equator of the lens may come forward, plugging the fistula. This is more apt to occur with ectopia lentis if the pressure was not lowered before surgery. This complication is often not recognized at the time of surgery. However, when the diagnosis is made injection of air into the anterior chamber may relieve the condition, but more often a lens extraction is necessary. Injury to the lens during glaucoma surgery leads to lens swelling and blockage of the fistula. If the capsular opening is large, lens material may escape into the anterior chamber and through the fistula. A very tiny nick in the lens capsule may lead to an inflammatory reaction which appears as a low grade iritis.

Reoperation after Failure of Filtration Operation

If the glaucoma remains uncontrolled, further surgery should be advised. The eye must have useful vision, however, because of the ever-present danger of sympathetic ophthalmia. When useful visual function is not present, no operation or reoperation, except enucleation, is justified, and often a retrobulbar injection of alcohol will serve as well.

If the first filtering operation (after several goniotomies) has been uncomplicated except for failure of filtration, another filtering procedure should be done, usually of another type. The peripheral iridectomy with scleral cautery causes little further injury to the eye and another such operation can be done elsewhere on the globe; nasally, temporally, or even over the inferior portion of the limbus. It can be performed to one side or another of a previously performed trephine or the surgeon may prefer to do a trabeculotomy ab externo or a trabeculectomy. Should these procedures all fail cyclodiathermy must be the next operation. It is rarely permanently effective but is relatively safe and can be repeated. Cryosurgery, as a treatment for congenital glaucoma, is not presently used.

SURGICAL RESULTS

There is a great difference in prognosis for those cases occurring during the first two months after birth and those occurring later, owing to a difference in the severity of the disease. The goniotomy operation rarely succeeds in eyes with a corneal diameter greater than 14 mm. In fact, goniotomy is not recommended in the late distended state of buphthalmus with corneal diameters greater than 15 mm.

Barkan's original reports are summarized in Tables 4 and 5. According to Haas, in 69 eyes in which the onset of glaucoma occurred before the third month after birth, the total cure was only effected in 55 percent. Cure required 149 goniotomies to normalize the tensions in the eyes of 38 patients. When onset occurred after the second month, 97 percent were normalized and the incidence of success per goniotomy had risen to 72 percent (Table 6). In another series Haas reported control of tension below 28, in 194 of 253 eyes (77 percent) (Table 7). Bietti stated that 82 percent of 321 eyes were normalized with a recurrence rate of 10 percent. Scheie summarized his results in infantile glaucoma and found that when performed

TABLE 4

GONIOTOMY IN CONGENITAL GLAUCOMA*

Number of infants and children	51
Eyes operated on by goniotomy	76
Successful (pressure normalized; vision maintained or restored)	66
Unsuccessful	10
Eyes on which goniotomy was not applicable	11

*After O. Barkan, Br. J. Ophthalmol., 32:701, 1948.

as a primary procedure, goniotomy successfully controlled the tension in infantile glaucoma in 62 percent of eyes and goniopuncture in 48 percent. However, when the two were combined into one procedure the results from a single operation improved to 76 percent, in a series of 153 eyes of which 117 were controlled.

To determine the relative value of goniotomy and goniopuncture in infantile glaucoma, a goniotomy was done on one eye and a goniopuncture on the other. The goniopuncture was done when any difference existed, on the eye with the higher tension and the larger corneal diameter. Goniotomy was done as a primary procedure on 21 eyes and successfully controlled the pressure on 13 eyes (62 percent). Goniopuncture was done as a primary procedure on 52 eyes with control of pressure resulting in 27 eyes (52 percent).

The results from goniopuncture in juvenile glaucoma showed that the tension was normalized in 19 of 35 eyes (57 percent), by one or more goniopunctures. The longest follow-up period was 11 years and the shortest, one year. The appearance of the eyes was impressive, since it was difficult to tell that they had been operated on. Hypotony did not occur. No late complications occurred.

TABLE 5

GONIOTOMY IN CONGENITAL GLAUCOMA*

Number of infants and children operated	121
Eyes operated on by goniotomy	196
Successful (pressure normalized; vision maintained or restored)	152
Unsuccessful	36
Results not yet certain (incomplete)	8
Recurrence	10

*After O. Barkan, Am. J. Ophthalmol., 36:1523, 1953.

TABLE 6

THE RESULTS UPON INTRAOCULAR PRESSURE OF THE GONIOTOMY OPERATION

	No. of eyes	No. normalized	% normalized	No. goniotomies to normalize	% success per goniotomy
From birth through 2 months	69	38	55	149	25
From 2 months through 4 months	38	36	97	50	72

From J. Haas, Invest. Ophthalmol. 7:140, 1968.

Shaffer reported 67 eyes of 44 patients. The results are summarized in Table 8.

Richardson et al. traced 54 operated-upon congenital glaucoma patients (88 eyes), whose ages ranged from 5 to 26 years. All of these patients had goniotomy as a primary procedure within 6 months of the onset of symptoms. Filtering surgery or cyclodiathermy was only used if 3 or 4 goniotomies were unsuccessful. All cases had normal intraocular pressures.

Tension control was obtained in a large majority of patients irrespective of the amount of surgery necessary. All those requiring only one goniotomy had satisfactory tension control; those requiring two or more goniotomies, but no diathermy or filtering procedure, maintained good intraocular pressure in 90 percent of eyes. Even those requiring filtering procedures, or cyclodiathermy in addition to goniotomies, had controlled tension in 82 percent.

Tonography analysis of 32 goniotomized eyes with tensions below 20

TABLE 7

NUMBER OF EYES IN WHICH TENSION WAS NORMALIZED BY ONE OR MULTIPLE GONIOTOMIES (253 CASES)*

Goniotomies Required	Eyes Normalized
1	114
2	52
3	10
4	10
5	8
Total	194 or 77 percent

*After J. Haas, Trans. Am. Acad. Ophthalmol. Otolaryngol., 59:333, 1955.

TABLE 8

PRESSURE CONTROL BY GONIOTOMY*

Sixty-seven eyes of 44 patients below the age of 12 months at the time of onset.

Bilateral cases		29	(73%)
Male patients		28	(71%)
Tension controlled by goniotomy 1 to 10 years		57	(85%)
Number of goniotomies per eye:	1 Goniotomy	44	(77%)
	2 Goniotomies	10	(18%)
	3 Goniotomies	3	(5%)
10 Failures:	1 eye tensions 21—24, 6 years, perfect disc.		
	1 eye tension 24, C 0.09, 2nd goniotomy, result unknown.		
	1 eye tension 15 after multiple operations.		
	7 eyes of 4 patients: No useful vision.		

*After R. N. Shaffer, Can. J. Ophthalmol., 2:243, 1967.

mm Hg showed a facility of outflow of 0.19 or above in 23 eyes (72 percent). The results are summarized in Table 9.

Costenbader and Kwitko made the following observations in their series of 77 eyes. In the group "birth to 5 days," 55 surgical procedures were carried out including 26 goniotomies, 7 goniotomies with goniopuncture, 12 cyclodialyses, 5 iridencleises, 2 Scheie procedures, 2 cyclodiathermies, and 1 trephine. The greatest number of operations performed on an individual patient was 9 procedures in one eye and 7 in the other eye. Another patient had 7 procedures in one eye and 6 in the opposite eye, while another infant had 4 procedures in each eye.

In the group "5 days to 6 months," 68 surgical procedures were carried out including 26 goniotomies, 27 goniotomies with goniopuncture, 6

TABLE 9

TONOGRAPHIC ANALYSIS OF PRESSURE CONTROL BY GONIOTOMY*

Thirty-two goniotomized eyes with tension of 20 mm Hg or below. Follow-up 1 to 25 years.

C of 0.19 or higher, 23 eyes (72%)	Tension: 7-20 (mean, 15 mm Hg) Facility of outflow: 0.19-0.37 (mean, 0.25) Po/C ratio: 30-84 (mean, 57)
C below 0.19, 9 eyes (28%)	Tension: 14-18 (mean, 16 mm Hg) Facility of outflow: 0.10-0.18 (mean, 0.14) Po/C ratio: 55-126 (mean, 93)

*Twenty-two eyes followed 1 to 10 years, augmented by 10 eyes from offices of O. Barkan and W. Ferguson, followed 10 to 25 years. Tonography by J. Hetherington and N. Ballin. After R. N. Shaffer, Can. J. Ophthalmol., 2:243, 1967.

iridencleises, 3 Scheie procedures, 2 goniopunctures, 2 trephines, 1 cyclodialysis, and 1 cyclodiathermy. Three patients had 4 procedures performed in one eye and 3 in the opposite eye.

In the group "6 to 36 months," 34 surgical procedures were performed including 14 goniotomies, and 16 goniotomies with goniopuncture. There were, in addition, 2 iridencleises, 1 cyclodialysis, and 1 Scheie procedure. One patient had 2 procedures in one eye and 5 in the other eye. Another patient had 3 operative procedures in each eye.

Recurrence of Increased Pressure.

Once successfully normalized for one year, the recurrence rate is between 10 and 20 percent. Recurrence of pressure is unlikely when (1) the tension is normalized without drops for 3 months after operation, (2) gonioscopy shows the angle cleanly stripped, and (3) the iris is recessed over one-quarter of the circumference.

In the case in which the exposed area is too small, it may be sufficient to normalize the pressure for a few weeks; but this often proves to be insufficient to satisfy later demands made upon the area for drainage. These cases may therefore be regarded as incompletes rather than recurrences. A correctly placed superficial goniotomy, performed on another sector, may be expected to normalize the pressure.

VISUAL RESULTS

Vision is an unacceptable guide for an evaluation of congenital glaucoma surgery, since the postoperative vision is a result of the lack of treatment as often as of the treatment. All available data, however, is in agreement that surgical success and functional success are far from synonymous in infantile glaucoma. A comparison of the visual results related to the amount of surgery necessary shows a striking picture, according to the study by Richardson et al. In those eyes requiring just one goniotomy, 51 percent (20 out of 39) had vision recorded as 20/50 or better, so that more than one goniotomy decreases the chance for a good visual result. Those requiring more than one goniotomy, but no other procedure, had 45 percent of cases with vision greater or equal to 20/50, while in those 17 eyes requiring filtering procedures or cyclodiathermy, only two were able to see better than 20/200.

Costenbader and Kwitko made the following observations in their series of 77 eyes. In their group "birth to 5 days," vision in terms of fixation was recorded in 4 patients out of 16 as central and maintained. In the group "5 days to 6 months," a visual acuity was obtained in 25 eyes out of 37. One eye had 20/50, one had 20/20, and 18 had central and maintained fixation. A vision 20/200 or less was recorded in 5 eyes. In the group "6 to 36 months," it was possible to obtain a visual acuity in only 13 eyes out of 20. Of these, one case had 20/50 vision, one had 20/30, 3 had 20/20, 4 had central and maintained fixation, and 4 had 20/200 or less.

Richardson et al. also observed that adequate tension and visual control are both directly related to the age of onset of symptoms. Those eyes with symptoms at birth had adequate tension control in 14 of 17 eyes, but the visual results in the same group showed only one of 17 eyes with 20/50 or better, and 12 of 17 with less than 20/200 vision.

As already mentioned, ocular conditions such as amblyopia, astigmatism, and anisometropia have an important negative effect on visual acuity as well as the elevated intraocular pressure. In the Richardson study there was a significantly high incidence of anisometropia (65 percent) and heterotropia (58 percent) within the group of patients with perfectly normal tension in both eyes. It would appear that in many surgically-controlled congenital glaucomas, anisometropia leads to amblyopia ex anopsia and a resultant heterotropia.

An interesting statistical relationship was noted between the visually poorer eye in bilateral cases and the involved eye in unilateral cases. In each of these groups vision of better than 20/50 was obtained only one-fourth of the time in contrast to the visually better eye in bilateral cases, where 20/50 was exceeded two-thirds of the time.

When the comparison of the visually poorer eye in bilateral (controlled tension) cases with the unilateral involved eye was pursued further, and only those eyes with less than 20/50 vision were considered, it was apparent that each of these groups demonstrated a similar and very high percentage of anisometropia (81 to 90 percent). Disc changes were present (40 percent) in each of these groups.

Filtering procedures or cyclodiathermy, after unsuccessful goniotomies, offer a suprisingly good chance for tension control, but an extremely poor chance for visual salvage.

Less than 50 percent of infantile glaucoma eyes with surgically normalized tension had good visual acuity (20/50 or better), yet fewer than half of the congenital glaucoma eyes with good tension control but poor vision had significant organic damage to the optic nerve head.

In the total series of 88 eyes, 97 percent had excellent pressure control, but less than 40 percent had visual acuity in the 20/20 to 20/50 range. Forty percent had vision below 20/200. In many eyes with very poor vision, excellent optic discs could be seen and fields of vision were full. An anisometropia of at least 2 diopters of sphere or 1.5 diopters of astigmatism was found in all the poor-visioned eyes, with an obvious strabismus noted in up to 60 percent of cases. Patching the better eye may convert some of these cases into alternating strabismus with equal vision, if the occlusion is instituted before the child is 5 years old.

Other cases suffer from poor visual acuity (see Chap. 8) owing to the presence of permanent corneal haze and scarring; opacification in the lens, secondary changes due to surgical trauma, metabolic alterations, or unknown causes; and late detachment of the retina following vitreous loss during surgery. In cases where stronger miotics have been employed, cyst formation at the pupillary border may occlude the pupillary space and obstruct vision. Alfano reported one case where the pupillary cysts were of sufficient size to occlude the pupillary opening. This occlusion was sufficient to produce amblyopia and subsequent exotopia. Following cessation of the miotic the cyst regressed, the vision returned to almost normal levels, and the exotropia disappeared.

As in adult open-angle glaucoma, optic nerve cupping, when present, does not correlate with and is not a legitimate index of damage to visual acuity but with peripheral field loss. It is well known that patients may have marked cupping but retain normal central visual acuity. Data on field loss cannot always be given, since visual fields are often impossible to obtain in young children.

In 1959, Scheie reported a series of patients whose pressure was normalized by surgery. Of 53 eyes operated 32 (60 percent) had vision of 20/50 or better. At that time he stated, "If the patient is operated on prior to corneal enlargement and marked ocular damage . . ." good vision could be expected. Visual acuity would be severely affected with the increasing corneal diameter because as the cornea stretches, the amount of corneal scarring increases. The correlation of visual acuity seems to be with corneal diameter rather than optic nerve cupping.

ANALYSIS OF UNSUCCESSFUL CASES

A review of the unsuccessful cases suggests that failure to normalize pressure is due either to congenital absence, or a marked insufficiency of Schlemm's canal, postoperative fibrosis, and scarring of the angle wall. The latter is often the result of cloudiness of the cornea, which makes it necessary to operate under adverse conditions.

In some eyes the incision is made too deeply, causing a split in the sclera. Incision or scraping of the angle wall should be avoided, since they cause fibrosis in the region of the trabeculum and Schlemm's canal, and result in adhesions of the iris to the wall. Postoperative fibrotic tissue covering a blood-filled Schlemm's canal, which can be seen in its characteristic positon, has been observed, and indicates that the lack of result is not due to the absence of Schlemm's canal. The tissues of the infant eye appear to be more prone to form adhesions than those of the adult, which may be a reason for the ineffectiveness of cyclodialysis in infants.

Although angle surgery is the operation of choice, the success rate decreases in the older child and adolescent. Filtration or the newer microsurgical techniques, i.e., trabeculotomy ab externo and trabeculectomy, then become increasingly necessary, but fortunately are better tolerated as the patient's age increases.

There is still that group of unfortunate cases that fail to respond to treatment carried out without technical difficulty, in experienced hands, under generally good conditions. The last word on the treatment of congenital glaucoma has not been written; there is still much to learn.

Some patients who, as children, had successful operations for monocular infantile glaucoma, develop open-angle glaucoma in the uninvolved eye 20 years later! It is therefore obvious that these patients' intraocular pressures require close supervision for the rest of their lives.

COMPLICATIONS

One hundred sixty-two surgical procedures were performed in the Kwitko and Costenbader series (Table 10). The most frequent complication of angle surgery is hyphema, which is usually innocuous. However, it may occasionally fill the entire chamber and cause blood staining earlier than in the usual case, owing to the preexisting corneal damage. It must be noted that these eyes are predisposed to anterior chamber hemorrhage, even from trivial injuries. Three of the cases in this series of 77 eyes developed hemorrhages that required intensive treatment. One patient suffered a total hyphema following the second goniotomy procedure. The anterior chamber was irrigated on two occasions after the intraocular pressure rose above 60 mm Hg. The cornea became blood-stained, vascularized, and later opacified. The pressure remained above 50 mm Hg and the eye was finally enucleated. A hyphema developed in another patient when the child fell out of bed following a goniotomy. The blood was evacuated surgically. The final result was 20/20 vision in the operated eye with an intraocular pressure of 18.5 mm Hg. Another patient developed a hyphema which could not be

TABLE 10

CONGENITAL GLAUCOMA COMPLICATIONS

162 Surgical Procedures.

Gross Hyphema	3 eyes
Endophthalmitis	1 eye
Dislocation of lens	1 eye

*After F. D. Costenbader and M. L. Kwitko. J. Pediatr. Ophthalmol., 2:9, 1967.

controlled. The final result was a soft phthisical eye with no light perception. In a total of 247 operations for infantile glaucoma, massive hyphema with bloodstaining of the cornea occurred in only three eyes in Scheie's series. This is significant in view of the frequency of recurrent hemorrhage following traumatic hyphema.

In one eye the lens dislocated spontaneously into the anterior chamber after a goniotomy. It is known that as the pressure remains elevated, limbal enlargement takes place, stretching the zonular ligaments. This results in iridodenesis and even subluxation of the lens. The surgical procedure in this eye probably precipitated the dislocation.

One patient developed an intraocular infection following surgery, which responded well to antibiotic therapy. The final result was a clear ocular media and good fixation with a normal intraocular pressure. The child was too young to obtain an accurate visual acuity.

The goniotomy performed without a contact lens is said to be simplified because the knife is guided by the scleral sulcus. However, if the knife does not cut at the proper depth or if an undiagnosed high insertion of the iris is present, tearing of the iris root, rupture of the major arterial circle, and cutting into the ciliary body occurs. If the knife enters the angle too high it cuts the cornea. The knife may cut deep and damage the corneoscleral system and Schlemm's canal. Other postgoniotomy findings noted in eyes operated without good visualization of the angle, reveals peripheral synechiae, iridotomies, corneal scarring, and even injury to the lens.

References

af Ursin, K. V. The fate of infantile and juvenile glaucoma patients. Acta. Ophthalmol., (Kbh.), 25:345, 1947.

Algan, B. Le Traitment du Glaucoma Infantile. Thomas, Nancy, France, 1951.

Le traitment du glaucoma infantile. Med. Diss. (Nancy), 1957.

Allen L. Model built under Grant B-1392 (C-3) from the National Institute of Neurological Diseases and Blindness and exhibited at the 65th Annual Meeting of the A. M. A., Miami Beach, Fla., June, 1960.

and Burian, H. M. Trabeculotomy ab externo. Am. J. Ophthalmol., 53:19, 1962.

Allen, T.D. The history and development of the iris inclusion operations. Am. J. Ophthalmol., 27:964, 1944.

and Ackerman, W. G. Hereditary glaucoma in a pedigree of three generations. Arch. Ophthalmol., 27:139, 1942.

Amoils, S.P., and Simmons, R.J. Goniotomy with intraocular illumination, Arch. Ophthalmol., 80:488, 1968.

Anderson, J.R. Hydrophthalmia or Congenital Glaucoma. Its Causes, Treatment and Cure. Cambridge Univ. Press, London, 1939.

Bailliart, P. Conduite a tenir dans un cas de glaucoma infantile. Bull Soc. Ophtalmol. Fr., 642:1949.

Ballantyne, A.J. Buphthalmos with facial naevus and associated conditions. Br. J. Ophthalmol., 24:65, 1940.

Barkan, O. A new operation for chronic glaucoma. Restoration of physiological function by opening Schlemm's canal under direct magnified vision. Am. J. Ophthalmol., 19:951, 1936.

Glaucoma. Classification causes and surgical control. Am. J. Ophthalmol., 21:10, 1938.

Technic of goniotomy. Arch. Ophthalmol., 19:217, 1938.

Operation for congenital glaucoma. Am. J. Ophthalmol., 25:552, 1942.

Goniotomy, preliminary deepening of the anterior chamber with air or saline solution. Am. J. Ophthalmol., 28:1133, 1945.

Goniotomy for congenital glaucoma; urgent need for early diagnosis and operation. J. A. M. A., 133:526, 1947.

Technic of goniotomy for congenital glaucoma. Trans. Am. Acad. Ophthalmol. Otolaryngol., 52:210, 1948.

Goniotomy for the relief of congenital glaucoma. Br. J. Ophthalmol., 32:701, 1948.

The technique of goniotomy for congenital glaucoma. Arch. Ophthalmol., 41:65, 1949.

Surgery of congenital glaucoma. Am. J. Ophthalmol., 36:1523, 1953.

Present status of goniotomy. Am. J. Ophthalmol., 36:445, 1953.

Symposium: Congenital glaucoma. Goniotomy. Trans. Am. Acad. Ophthalmol. Otolaryngol., 59:322, 1955.

Pathogenesis of congenital glaucoma. Gonioscopic and anatomic observation of the angle of the anterior chamber in the normal eye and in congenital glaucoma. Am. J. Ophthalmol., 40:1, 1955.

Cyclogoniotomy. Am. J. Ophthalmol., 42:63, 1956.

Becker, B., Podos, S. M., and Asseff, C. F. Microsurgery of the outflow channels, clinical research. Trans. Am. Acad. Ophthalmol. Otolaryngol., 76:405, 1972.

and Shaffer, R.N. Diagnosis and Therapy of the Glaucomas, 2nd ed. Mosby, St. Louis, 1965, pp. 218-240.

Benner, R. La ponction diathermique du corps ciliare, resultats abtenus avec operation antiglaucomateuse de Vogt. Ann. Ocul. (Paris), 180:89, 1947.

Bettmen, J. W., and Cleasby, G. W. Congenital glaucoma. Pediatrics, 32:420, 1963.

Bietti, A. Osservazioni oftalmometriche sopra occhi operati per glaucoma con speziale riguardo all'incisione dell'angolo iridio (de Vincentiis). Ann. Ottalmol., 25:319, 1896.

Bietti, G.B. Sui risultati di interventi goniolitici nell'idroftalmo. Saggi Microchirurg., 23:1, 1952.

Beitrage zur chirurgische Behandlung einiger Glaukom formen. Klin. Monatsbl. Augenheilkd., 139:737, 1961.

Contribution a la connaissance des resultats de la goniotomie dans le glaucome congenital. Ann. Ocul. (Paris), 199:481, 1966.
Blaickner, J. Uber Iridenkleisisoperationen. Z. Augenheilkd., 72.265, 1930.
Bocchi, A. L'incisione del tessuto dell'angolo irideo (de Vincentiis) nell'idrottalmo Ann. Ottalmol., 25:319, 1896.
Cairns, J. E. Trabeculectomy. Trans. Am. Acad. Ophthalmol. Otolaryngol., 76:384, 1972.
Calhoun, F. P. Hereditary glaucoma (simplex), Sect. Ophthalmol. A. M. A., 1914, pp. 101-121.
Callahan, A. A. A frequently overlooked cause of blindness in infants. Congenital glaucoma. Trans. Med. Assoc. Alabama, 19:13, 1949.
Surgery of the Eye. Thomas, Springfield, Ill., 1956.
Chandler, P. A. Treatment of glaucoma. Arch. Ophthalmol., 32:23, 1944.
Chavez, E., Galin, A. M., and Kwitko, M. L. Surgery of congenital glaucoma. 21st Consilium Ophthalmologicum, Mexico, 1970, Pt. 2, Exerpta Medica, Amsterdam, 1971, p. 1041.
Costenbader, F. D., and Kwitko, M. L. Congenital glaucoma. Clin. Proc. Child Hosp. (Wash.), 17:100, 1961.
and Kwitko, M. L. Congenital glaucoma, an analysis of seventy-seven consecutive eyes. J. Pediatr. Ophthalmol., 2:9, 1967.
Courtney, HR. H., and Hill, E. Hereditary juvenile glaucoma simplex. Trans. Sect. Ophthalmol. A.M.A., 1931, pp. 47-68.
Dalsgaard-Nielson, E. Buphthalmia, a survey of buphthalmic patients admitted to the eye clinic of Rigshopital in the period of 1910-1943. Acta Ophthalmol. (Kbh.), 23:49, 1945.
Dannheim, R. Trabeculotomy, Trans. Am. Acad. Ophthalmol. Otolaryngol., 76:375, 1972.
Dellaporta, A. Evaluation of anterior and posterior trabeculodialysis. Am. J. Ophthalmol., 48, No. 3, Pt. 2:294, 1959.
and Fahrenbruch, R. C. Trapano-trabeculectomy. Trans. Am. Acad. Ophthalmol. Otolaryngol., 75:283, 1971.
De Vincentiis, C. Incisione del L'angolo irideo Nel glaucoma. Ann. Ottalmol., 22:540, 1893.
Sulla considetta "sclertomie interne." Lav. Clin. Ocul. Napoli, 4:227, 1895.
de Wecker, L. La sclerotomie interne. Ann. Ocul. (Paris), 113:95, 1895.
Dieter, W. Zur Technique der Iridectomie (subconj. Messer-Iridektomie). Ber. Zusa Dtch Ophthalmol. Ges., 53:282, 1940.
Douglas, D. H. Results after goniotomy. Trans. Ophthalmol. Soc. U. K., 80:627, 1960.
Ellingsen, B. A., and Grant, W. M. Trabeculotomy and sinusotomy in enucleated human eyes. Invest. Ophthalmol., 11:21, 1972.
Eroshevsky, T. I. Surgery of congenital hydrophthalmos. 21st Concilium Ophthalmologicum, Mexico, 1970, Pt. 2. Exerpta Medica, Amsterdam, 1971, p. 1509.
Gallenga, R. Il trattamento operatiorio dell'irdoftalmo. Rasseng. Ital. Ottalmol., 15:161, 1946.
Germann, D. Fall von juvenilem Glaukom, Klin. Monatsbl. Augenheilkd., 46:95, 1908 cited by Courtney and Hill.
Goulding, H. B. Chronic glaucoma (buphthalmos) goniotomy. Trans. Ophthalmol. Soc. U. K., 65:412, 1945.
Grant, W. M. Microsurgery of the outflow channels, laboratory research. Trans. Am. Acad. Ophthalmol. Otolaryngol., 76:398, 1972.
Guinan, P. M. Peripheral iridectomy with scleral cautery. Scheie's operation for glaucoma. Trans. Ophthalmol. Soc. U. K., 81:713, 1961.
Haas, J. Symposium: Congenital glaucoma. End results of treatment. Trans. Am. Acad. Ophthalmol. Otolaryngol., 59:333, 1955.

Principles and problems of therapy in congenital glaucoma. Invest. Ophthalmol., 7:140, 1968.
Harms, H. Glaukom–Operationen am Schlemm'schen Kanal. Sitzungsber der 114. Versammlung des Vereins Rhein-Westf. Augenarzte, 1966.
and Dannheim, R. Trabeculotomy, results and problems. In Symposium: Microsurgery of the Eye. Buergenstock, Switzerland, June 13-15, 1968.
Heinz, K. Traumatische luxation einer Komplizierten Kataract in den Glasskorper mit wesentli cher Besserund des Sehvermogens ohne Reigerscheinungen Wiener Klin. Wochensch., 59:819, 1947.
Netzhautabhebung mach Anlegen einer Lindnerschen Bulbusfistel und iner Elliotschen Trepanation. Wiener Klin. Wochensch., 59:819, 1947.
Hertzberg, R. Goniotomy for congenital glaucoma. A review with report of 3 cases. Med. J. Aust., 2:357, 1951.
Hobbs, H. E. The trabecula in chronic simple glaucoma, with special reference to the gonioscopic appearance of blood in the canal of Schlemm. Br. J. Ophthalmol., 34:489, 1950.
Holst, J. C. The results of iridencleises subconjunctivalis cum iridotomia meridionali (Holth) in the period 1928-1939. Acta Ophthalmol. (Kbh.), 25-271, 1947.
Hoskins, H. D., and Shaffer, R. N. Evaluation technique for the congenital glaucomas. J. Pediatr. Ophthalmol., 8:81, 1971.
Hughes, W. L., and Cole, J. G. Technical uses of air in ophthalmology. Arch. Ophthalmol., 35:525, 1946.
Jaensch, P. A. Anatomische und Klinische untersuchungen zur Pathologie und Therapie des Hydrophthalmus Congenitus. Graefe's Arch. Ophthalmol., 118:21, 1927.
Jauernig, U. Primarer und secundarer Hydrophthalmus. Klin. Monatsbl. Augenheilkd., 99:542, 1937.
Johnson, G. J., Corey, P. W., and Morin, J. D. Tonography in infants and children. Can. J. Ophthalmol., 6:24, 1971.
Kalt, M. L'hydrophthalmie congenitale. Ann. ocul. (Paris), 170:97, 1933.
Kluyskens, J. Le glaucome congenital. Arch. Ophtalmol., 11:574, 1951.
Koster, W. Beitrag zur Kenntnis der Dauererfolge bei der Operativen Behandlung des Kalukoms. Arch. Ophthalmol., 64:400, 1906.
Krasnov, M. M. Microsurgery of glaucoma. Am. J. Ophthalmol., 67:857, 1969.
Externalization of Schlemm's canal (sinusotomy) in glaucoma. Br. J. Ophthalmol., 52:157, 1968.
Sinusotomy, foundations, results and prospects. Trans. Am. Acad. Ophthalmol. Otolaryngol., 76:368, 1972.
Kwitko, M. L. Congenital glaucoma, a clinical study. Can. J. Ophthalmol., 2:77, 1967.
and Galin, M. A. Direct goniotomy for congenital glaucoma. Exerpta Medica, in press.
Lagrange, P. Traitment du glaucome infantile. Bull. Soc. Opthalmol. Fr., 38:1, 1925.
Leydhecker, W. Operationsergebniss bei hydrophthalmus unter besorderer Berucksichtibung der Goniotomie. Klin. Monatsbl. Augenheilkd., 142:650, 1963.
Lister, A. Surgery of congenital glaucoma. Trans. Ophthalmol. Soc. Aust., 11:39, 1952.
Some aspects of congenital glaucoma. Trans. Ophthalmol. Soc. U. K., 79:136, 1959.
Technique of goniotomy. Br. J. Ophthalmol., 49:594, 1965.
Lohlein, W. Glakom als Erbleiden in Gutt's hb. d. Erkrankeiten, Vol. 5. Theime, Leipzig, 1939, p. 35.
Lynn, J. R. An improved trabeculotomy ab externo. Presented at Proctor Meeting, Glaucoma Problems in Research, San Francisco, Dec. 5, 1968.
and Berry, P. B. A new trabeculotomy. Am. J. Ophthalmol., 68:430, 1969.
Maggiore, L. Struttora, comportamento e significato del canale di Schlemm Nell'occhio

umano in condizione normali e pathologiche. Ann. Ottalmol. e Clin. Ocul., 40:317, 1917.
Magitot, A. Étude anatomique sur le glaucome infantile. Ann. Ocul. (Paris), 147:241, 1912.
Maumenee, A. E. Indications for surgery in the glaucoma; congenital, and infantile glaucoma. Highlights Ophthalmol., 8:2, 1966.
McArevey, J. B. Trabeculectomy as a method of operative procedure for the treatment of buphthalmos or infantile glaucoma. Trans. Ophthalmol. Soc. U. K., 65:406, 1945.
The treatment of congenital glaucoma. Br. J. Ophthalmol., 69:568, 1950.
McKinney, J. W. Goniotomy for glaucoma. Am. J. Ophthalmol., 30:1175, 1947.
Goniotomy for congenital glaucoma. A case report. Am. J. Ophthalmol., 33:132, 1950.
McLean, J. M. Personal communication.
Atlas of Glaucoma Surgery. Mosby, St. Louis, 1967.
Meyer, S. J. Symposium: congenital glaucoma. Review summary and conclusions. Trans. Am. Acad. Ophthalmol. Otolaryngol., 59:342, 1955.
Moore, M. C. A case of buphthalmos treated by goniotomy. Med. J. Aust., 1:800, 1951.
Nettleship, E. On the prognosis of chronic glaucoma. Glaucoma in early life. Roy. London Ophthalmol. Hosp. Rep., 12:220, 1888.
Paufique, L. Le glaucome congenitale, contexte clinique, et indications therapeutiques. Ann. Ocul. (Paris), 189:27, 1956.
Treatment du glaucome infantile, Bull. Soc. Ophtalmol. Fr., 39:1958.
et Etienne, R. Examen clinique d'un glaucoma infantile. Indications therapeutiques. Ann. Ocul. (Paris), 187:305, 1954.
Pesme, P. Necessité d'un traitement chirurigal présose dans le glaucome infantile. Bull. Soc. Ophtalmol. (Paris), 654, 1947.
Poulard, et Lavat La sclerecto-iridectomie dans le glaucome infantile. Ann. Ocul. (Paris), 496, 1925.
Preziosi, L. The electrocautery in the treatment of glaucoma. Br. J. Ophthalmol., 8:414, 1924.
Comments on a case of buphthalmos cured by the galvanocautery puncture (Preziosi's operation) with special reference to a modification in its technique. 17th In. Congs. Opthalmol., 1954.
Redslos, M. E. Le traitment de l'hydrophthalmie. Bull. Acad. Med., 130:650, 1946.
Remky, H. Atropin als druksenkendes Mittel bei Kindlichem Glaucom. Klin. Monatsbl. Augenheilkl., 115:539, 1949.
Renard, M. G. A propos du traitment du glaucome infantile. Bull. Soc. Ophtalmol. Fr., 656, 1949.
Richardson, K. T., Jr., Ferguson, W. J., Jr., and Shaffer, R. N. Long term functional results in infantile glaucoma. Trans. Amer. Acad. Ophthalmol. Otolaryngol., 71:833, 1967.
Robertson, E. N., Jr. Goniotomy in congenital glaucoma. J. Oklahoma Med. Assoc., 43:409, 1950.
Surgical treatment of congenital glaucoma. Arch. Ophthalmol., 47:611, 1952.
Therapy of congenital glaucoma. Arch. Ophthalmol., 54:55, 1955.
Rochon-Duvigneaud, X. Traitement du glaucome. Gaz. Hop., 72:746, 1895.
Roussel, F. Le traitement du glaucome infantile par l'enclavement du l'iris. Bull. Soc. Belge Ophtalmol., 88:317, 1948.
Royer, J. Les glaucomes congenitaux chez l'enfant. Conf. Lyon Ophtalmol., 71:1, 1958.
Sattler, R. Juvenile glaucome. Trans. Am. Ophthalmol. Soc., 10:519, 1905.
Scalinci, N. La incisione del tessuto dell'angolo irideo nell idrottalmo. Ann. Ottalmol., 29:324, 1900.

Scheie, H. G. Goniotomy in treatment of congenital glaucoma. Arch. Ophthalmol., 42:266, 1949; and Trans. Am. Ophthalmol. Soc., 47:115, 1949.

Goniopuncture. A new filtering operation for glaucoma, preliminary report, Arch. Ophthalmol., 44:761, 1950.

Symposium: Congenital glaucoma. Diagnosis, clinical course, and treatment other than goniotomy. Trans. Am. Acad. Ophthalmol. Otolaryngol., 59:309, 1955.

Surgery in congenital glaucoma. Am. J. Ophthalmol., 45:936, 1958.

Retraction of scleral wound edges, as a fistulizing procedure for glaucoma. Am. J Ophthalmol., 45:220, 1958.

The management of infantile glaucoma. Arch. Ophthalmol., 62:35, 1959.

Goniopuncture, an evaluation after eleven years. Arch. Ophthalmol., 65:38, 1961.

Filtering operations for glaucoma. A comparative study. Am. J. Ophthalmol., 53:571, 1962.

Results of peripheral iridectomy with scleral cautery in congenital and juvenile glaucoma. Trans. Am. Ophthalmol. Soc., 60:116, 1962; and Arch. Ophthalmol., 69:13, 1963.

Infantile and juvenile glaucoma. Trans. Am. Acad. Ophthalmol. Otolaryngol., 67:458, 1963.

Closed fistula and reoperations for glaucoma. Trans. 8th Congreso Panamericano de Oftalmologia, 1968, p. 137.

Seefelder, R. Klinische und anatomische untersuchungen zur Pathologie und Therapie des Hydrophthalmus congenitus. Graefe's Arch. Ophthalmol., 63:205, 1906.

Sgrosso, P. Contribuzione clinica alla cura del glaucoma merce l'incisione dell tessuto dell'angolo irideo. Lav. Clin. Ocul. Napoli, 4:236, 1894-1896.

Shaffer, R. N. Goniotomy in congenital glaucoma. Am. J. Ophthalmol., 47:90, 1959.

Genetics and the congenital glaucomas. Am. J. Ophthalmol., 60:981, 1965.

New concepts in infantile glaucoma. Can. J. Ophthalmol., 2:243, 1967.

Microsurgery of the outflow channels, conclusions. Trans. Am. Acad. Ophthalmol. Otolaryngol., 76:411, 1972.

Smith, P. On the pathology and treatment of glaucoma. Churchill, London J & A, 1891.

Smith, R. A new technique for opening the canal of Schlemm. Br. J. Ophthalmol., 44:370, 1960.

Nylon filament trabeculotomy in glaucoma. Trans. Ophthalmol. Soc. U. K., 82:439, 1962.

Soby Bey, M. and Gindi, W. A modified form of Lagrange's sclerectomy. Bull. Ophthalmol. Soc. Egypt, 36:129, 1943.

Spencer, W. H. Histological evaluation of microsurgical techniques. Trans. Am. Acad. Ophthalmol. Otolaryngol., 76:389, 1972.

Stallard, H. B. Eye Surgery. Williams & Wilkins, Baltimore, 1958.

Strachan, I. M. A method of trabeculotomy with some preliminary results. Br. J. Ophthalmol., 51:539, 1967.

Sugar, H. S. The Glaucomas. Hoeber, New York, 1957.

Further experience with limboscleral trephination. Highlights Ophthalmol., 8:19, 1966.

Further experience with limboscleral trephination. Eye, Ear, Nose, Throat Mon., 47:31, 1968.

Swan, K. C. Goniotomy, a modified lens and technique. Arch. Ophthalmol., 47:231, 1965.

Tartar, J. Erfahrungen mit der Iridenkleisis cum iridotomia lobulair nach Holth gegen das infantile und juvenile Glaucom. Graefe's Arch. Ophthalmol., 143:403, 1941.

Taylor, U. Sulla incisione del tessuto dell'angolo irideo. Ann. Ottalmol., 2:117, 1891-2.

Sull'incisione del tessuto dell'angolo irideo contribuzione alla cura del glaucom. Lav. Clin. Ocul. Napoli, 3:125, 1891.

Sull'incisione dell'angolo irideo. Lav. Clin. Ocul. Napoli, 4:197, 1894.

Teng, C. C., Katzin, H. M., and Chi, H. H. Primary degeneration in the vicinity of the chamber angle. Am. J. Ophthalmol., 43:193, 1957.

Thomas, C., Cordier, J., et Algan, B. La cyclodiathermie perforante de Vogt dans le traitement du glaucome infantile. Bull Soc. Ophtalmol. Fr., 661, 1949.

Thomas, M. C., et Beissel, M. Un cas d'ophtalmie sympathique apres cyclodiathermie perforante. Bull. Soc. Ophtalmol. (Paris), 605, 1947.

Torok, E. Iridectomy in glaucoma, a new technique. Arch. Ophthalmol., 52:574, 1923.

Troncoso, M. U. Surgical treatment of congenital glaucoma. Am. J. Ophthalmol., 35:463, 1952.

Tyner, G. S., and Swets, E. J. Report on 13 eyes treated by goniopuncture. Arch. Ophthalmol., 54:59, 1955.

Urrets-Zavalia, A. Goniotripsy. An operation for congenital glaucoma. Ophthalmologica, 140:14, 1960.

Valude et Duclos. Debridement d'l'angle irideen. Ann. Ocul. (Paris), 98:119, 1898.

Van der helm, F. G. M. Hydrophthalmia and its treatment. A general study based on 630 cases in the Netherlands. Bibl. Ophthalmol., 61:64, 1963.

Van Wesemael, M. Traitement chirurgical du glaucome infantile. Bull. Soc. Belge Ophtalmol, 83:53, 1946.

Vogt, A. La ponction diathermique du corps ciliare. Arch. Ophtalmol., 3:1071, 1940.

Walker, W. M., and Kanagasundaram, C. R. Surgery of the canal of Schlemm. Trans. Ophthalmol. Soc. U. K., 84:427, 1964.

Webster, D. H. Management of Infantile glaucoma. Am. J. Ophthalmol., 31:95, 1948.

Weekers, L. Resultat de l'enclavement de l'iris dans les diverses formes du glaucome. Bull. Soc. Ophtalmol. (Paris), 491, 1939.

et Fanchamps, J. Resultats tensionels elvignes obtenue par l'enclavement de l'iris dans les diverses formes du glaucome. Arch. Ophtalmol., 1:585, 1937.

et Weekers, R. Technique de al cyclodiathermie non perforante Ann. Ocul. (Paris), 180:76, 1947.

et Weekers, R. Les fondements physiopathologiques et la technique de l'iridencleisis. Ophthalmologica, 117:305, 1949.

Werner, S. Zur Kenntnis des erblichen juvenilen Glaukoms. Act Ophthalmol. (Kbh.), 7:162, 1929.

Wilson, W. A. Congenital glaucoma. Ann. West. Med. Surg., 5:221, 1951.

Wong, V. G., and Collier, R. H. Maintenance of the anterior chamber depth during anterior segment surgery. Arch. Ophthalmol., 77:384, 1967.

Worst, J., and Otter, K. Low vacuum diagnostic contact lenses. Am. J. Ophthalmol., 51:410, 1961.

Worst, J. G. F. Goniotomy, an improved method for chamber angle surgery in congenital glaucoma. Am. J. Ophthalmol., 57:185, 1964.

The cause and treatment of congenital glaucoma. Trans. Am. Acad. Ophthalmol. Otolaryngol., 68:766, 1964.

Congenital glaucoma, remarks on the aspect of chamber angle ontogenetic and pathogenetic background and mode of action of goniotomy. Invest. Ophthalmol., 7:127, 1968.

Zaky, M. Lagrange's sclerectomy. Bull. Ophthalmol. Soc. Egypt, 36:132, 1943.

Zentmayer, W. Hydrophthalmos with a histologic report of two cases, one of which presented a congenital coloboma. J. A. M. A., 61:1103, 1913.

13

Treatment of Other Types of Glaucoma Seen in Young Patients

The surgical treatment of congenital glaucoma and the various operative options available has been outlined in Chapter 12. Treatment for the other types of glaucoma seen in young patients may be far more complex, for it often involves both medical and surgical therapy and a decision must frequently be made as to when to discontinue one and begin to consider the other.

The aim of treatment in glaucoma is to preserve visual field and visual acuity. Loss of these senses is directly related to an elevated pressure owing to the damage it causes to vital ocular structures, primarily the cornea and the optic nerve.

The intraocular pressure depends on the balance between the rate of aqueous secretion at the ciliary body and the facility of aqueous outflow at the trabeculum. It has not yet been determined at exactly what pressure ocular damage takes place. All that can be said is that there appears to be a highly individualistic susceptibility. Some eyes are damaged with pressures of 20 to 24 mm. Hg while others remain free of impairment with pressures in the 30's. However, it can generally be stated that sustained elevated pressures will lead to damage to most eyes, young and old.

It is difficult to differentiate, from a therapeutic point of view, between adolescent glaucoma, presenile glaucoma, pigmentary glaucoma, and adult open-angle glaucoma, except that the latter occurs in an older age group. These may well be the same disease. Therefore, treatment of glaucoma in the young patient is patterned after open-angle glaucoma in the adult, using all the medical armamentarium available and resorting to surgery only when the disease process is continuing in spite of a rigorous medical regime.

Since the anatomy of the young eyeball differs significantly from the adult, the physical response to glaucoma is not the same (see Chaps. 4 and 6). Thus, medical management must be carefully supervised to prevent ocular impairment, and even more so after it has occurred. Once the optic nerve is damaged it is far more susceptible to further damage than the normal disc, so that the intraocular pressure must be maintained at an even lower level.

The reliability factor is also much more important in the young patient. Whether it is a lack of self-interest, laziness, or an absence of responsibility, the youngster with glaucoma is often less observant of his needs than the adult (who may have little else to do). Since glaucoma is associated with ocular damage by chronic erosion rather than a cataclysmic visual loss (except for angle closure which is rare in children), he may not realize the seriousness of missing his eye drops for one, two, ten days or longer, since visual loss is hard to appreciate on a day-to-day basis. This reason alone may result in earlier surgical intervention than in the adult.

MEDICAL MANAGEMENT

Miotic Therapy

Miotic drugs consist of eye drops which increase the facility of aqueous outflow in normal as well as glaucoma patients, by a mechanism which remains obscure and thus lowers the intraocular pressure. These solutions are intended solely for local corneal instillation and should never be used orally or by injection; such use is dangerous and may be fatal. There are two types.

Parasympathomimetic (Cholinergic) Drugs

These eye drops presumably act directly on the parasympathetic motor endplate in the iris, in the same manner as acetylcholine.

There are two kinds of parasympathomimetic eye drops.

PILOCARPINE HYDROCHLORIDE, OR PILOCARPINE NITRATE (0.5 to 6 percent water soluble solution). The drops are used every 4 to 8 hrs. The drug acts directly on parasympathetic end organs. Miosis begins in 10 to 15 min and lasts 4 to 8 hrs. The aqueous solutions are stable and easily penetrate the cornea. A 2 percent solution of pilocarpine alkaloid in castor oil is indicated for treatment throughout the night. Injection and follicular formation in the conjunctiva are possible with pilocarpine.

CARBACHOL (carbamoylcholine chloride; Carbacel; Carcholin; Carbamiotin) (0.75, 1.5, 3 percent aqueous solution). The drops are used every 4 to 8 hrs. Carbachol should be administered with caution if the epithelial barrier of the conjunctiva and cornea has been weakened or removed by topical anesthetics, tonometry, or trauma, or if the patient is subject to bronchial asthma. Undesirable side effects may be countered by atropine sulfate given parenterally in a dosage of 0.4 to 0.6 mg (1/150 to 1/100 g). The dosage may be repeated if necessary.

When indicated, pilocarpine is the treatment of choice with carbachol being used when resistance, intolerance, or sensitivities develop. Although somewhat stronger than pilocarpine, it does not penetrate the intact cornea as well. Gentle corneal massage through the lids enhances the absorption of carbachol.

Anticholinesterase Drugs

These eye drops reversibly or irreversibly inhibit the enzyme cholinesterase, which permits acetylcholine to accumulate at the parasympathetic nerve endings, augmenting parasympathetic nervous system activity. There are two types of solutions, short acting and long acting. The short-acting anticholinesterase drugs include:

PHYSOSTIGMINE (eserine salicylate) (0.25 to 1 percent aqueous solution, 0.5 percent oil solution, and 0.25 percent ointment). Eserine temporarily inactivates cholinesterase and produces miosis in about 30 min. The drops are used every 4 to 8 hrs and last from 12 to 36 hrs. The drug is sensitive to light and heat, resulting in discoloration of the solution. When this occurs the solution should be discarded. Conjunctival congestion and follicular hypertrophy, as well as iritis, may occur following the use of eserine. Eserine may produce twitching of the lid, by increasing the tonus of the skeletal muscle and hyperreactivity of the pupillary and accommodative reflexes with resultant temporary decrease in visual acuity.

PROSTIGMIN (neostigmine) (used as a bromide in 3 to 5 percent solution). The drops are administered every 4 to 8 hrs. It is more stable than eserine and causes less conjunctival irritation.

The long-acting anticholinesterase drugs include the following.

ECHOTHIOPHATE IODIDE (Phospholine iodide; 217 MI) (0.06, 0.125, 0.25 percent water soluble solutions). Phospholine iodide is more stable than Floropryl but must be refrigerated. The drops are used every 12 to 24 hrs. It induces miosis in about 30 min and lasts several days to weeks. Phospholine iodide is a potent and relatively irreversible inhibitor of cholinesterase.

DIISOPROPYLFLUOROPHOSPHATE (Floropryl; DFP) (0.01 to 0.1 percent solution in peanut oil; 0.025 percent ointment). The drops are used every 12 to 72 hrs, preferably before retiring. This drug is easily inactivated by hydrolysis to form hydrofluoric acid, so that tears and water must be avoided. The eye dropper must therefore be kept away from the eyelids and eyelashes, and the solution must not be diluted. Its main action is against the nonspecific or pseudocholinesterases; it is extremely potent.

DEMECARIUM BROMIDE (Humersol; Tosmilen; BC-48) (0.125 to 0.25 percent water soluble solution). The drug is long-acting and shows a marked specificity for acetylcholinesterase. It is stable and does not require refrigeration. The drops are used every 12 to 72 hrs.

In general, the long-acting anticholinesterase agents cause more side effects and are less well tolerated than the parasympathomimetic (cholinergic) drugs. Diisopropylfluorophosphate, which is marketed as an ointment and drops prepared in a peanut oil vehicle, may cause a temporary visual blur. Patients may be allergic to the vehicle and the ointment base with this as well as any other medication.

It is desirable that the patient be kept under supervision for several hours after the first instillation of the long-acting anticholinesterase drops, since a paradoxical rise in pressure may occur in certain susceptible individuals.

Any of the miotic drops can cause an allergic reaction involving the conjunctiva, globe, and eyelids as a conjunctival congestion; conjunctivitis; blepharitis; dermatitis; the limbus with a ciliary flush, the cornea as a keratitis; and the lacrimal passages by stenosis.

Side effects are generally more marked with the higher concentrations, and increased frequency of use of the medication. This is why it is important to begin with the lower concentrations and increase gradually according to the needs of the patient. Symptoms may include visual blur, induced myopia, slow dark-adaptation with poor vision in dim light, ciliary spasm, headache, browache, fibrinous iritis, vitreous detachment, and retinal detachment. In the very young patient few complaints are voiced, but symptoms are undoubtedly present. The milder symptoms are likely to disappear after several days of continued treatment. In young adults the discomfort from the ciliary spasm, brow, and headache are often intolerable. The induced myopia often necessitates a change in prescription or the use of clip-on lenses.

When a narrow angle is present it is wise to avoid the stronger miotics (Floropryl, Humersol, and Phospholine iodide). These drugs relax the zonules of the lens causing an increased shallowness of the anterior chamber, thus accentuating the narrow angle. The result may be a paradoxical rise in the intraocular pressure. In addition, while pupillary constriction pulls the iris root away from the trabecular meshwork and opens the angle (Fig. 1), the area of contact between iris and lens is increased, resulting in a physiologic pupil block in susceptible eyes. The increased resistance to aqueous flow between the posterior and anterior chambers, produced by the

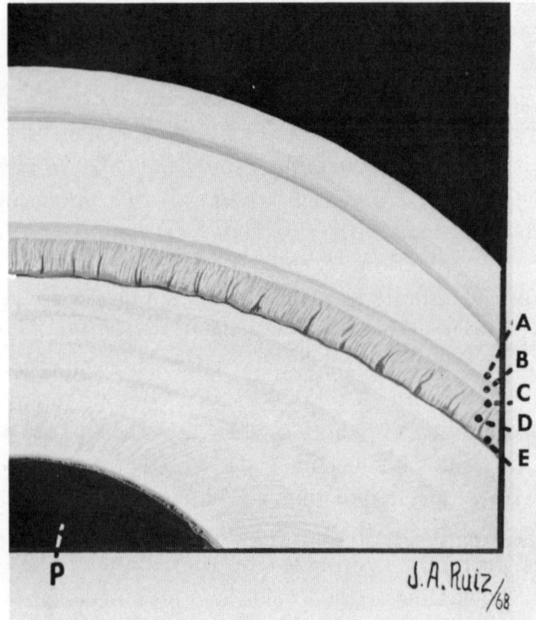

FIG. 1. The open filtration angle. (A) Schwalbe's line; (B) trabeculum; (C) scleral spur; (D) ciliary body; (E) angle recess; (P) pupil.

intense miosis, may lead to a forward displacement of the iris-lens diaphragm and angle closure. Vasodilation of the intraocular vessels results in vascular congestion about the filtration angle which aggravates the condition. Cases of hemorrhagic glaucoma noted in juvenile diabetics would be especially susceptible. These reactions have been observed even with the weaker miotics.

Depending on the frequency of administration of phospholine iodide, DFP, and the other long-acting anticholinesterase drugs, young children tend to produce nodular excrescences ("iris cysts") at the pupil margin owing to proliferation of the pigment epithelium. They may occasionally rupture or break free of the iris and float in the anterior chamber. The cysts may become large enough to occlude the pupil but almost invariably subside when the drug is discontinued. The addition of 10 percent phenylephrine hydrochloride (Neosynephrine) drops to the phospholine iodide solution seems to eliminate this difficulty.

An annoying but otherwise insignificant side effect may be the development of muscular twitching of the eyelids, resulting from locally increased skeletal muscle tonus.

The long-acting anticholinesterase drops, e.g., phospholine iodide, have been shown to produce cataracts in susceptible individuals. This complication has not been noted in infants but has been observed in young patients and is much more common in adults over 60 years of age.

Since the long-acting anticholinesterase drugs may be absorbed systemically through the skin, a thorough washing with voluminous amounts of water should be undertaken if the skin is thus contaminated.

The systemic absorption of anticholinesterase agents can significantly reduce the serum cholinesterase and pseudocholinesterase levels (see Chap. 7). The affected patient may show signs of weakness, diarrhea, nausea, vomiting, salivation, slow heart beat, and other evidence of parasympathetic nervous system stimulation. A treated child playing in an area sprayed with an insecticide containing anticholinesterase may be further depleted of his cholinesterase reserve. This becomes particularly dangerous if surgery is contemplated, since succinylcholine is commonly employed as a muscle relaxant during general anesthesia. This drug persists at the nerve endings. Normally, it is promptly hydrolyzed by the action of the cholinesterase. However, when the cholinesterase level is low, prolonged apnea can result. If, for any reason, the patient is receiving other anticholinesterase drugs systemically, the possibility of drug interaction should be considered.

Parasympathomimetic agents are contraindicated in marked vagotonia and pronounced vasomotor instability, bronchial asthma, spastic gastrointestinal disturbances, peptic ulcer, high degree of bradycardia, hypotension, and epilepsy.

An effective way to prevent systemic spread of any eye drop is to first position the eyeball in the horizontal plane by hyperextending the head or placing the body in the horizontal supine position. Secondly, press on the lacrimal puntum with the index finger for a minute or two, as the drop is instilled on the lateral aspect of the eyeball, before allowing the eyelid to close. This maneuver will prevent the drug from overflowing into the nasal and pharyngeal passages, which could induce systemic complications.

Atropine is the antidote for parasympathetic overstimulation. Should the drug be taken systemically by accident, or should systemic effects occur after topical administration, atropine sulfate in a dose of 0.4 to 0.6 mg or more should be given parenterally. A proportionately smaller amount should be given to young children. The atropine should be repeated as needed for 48 hrs. However, it should not be used if cyanosis is present, as ventricular fibrillation can be induced. Protopam iodide (2-pyridine aldoxime methiodide, or P_2AM) releases reactivated cholinesterase, and is available in 500 mg tablets; or 1,000 mg may be given intravenously at a slow rate. This dose may be repeated if muscle weakness persists after one hr. It is fortunate when these complications occur in the presence of the anesthetist and stress the importance of having the same one working on each case; one that would be acquainted with these problems. It is vital to remember to discontinue these long-acting anticholinesterase drugs long before surgery is planned.

The local ocular effects of the strong cholinesterase inhibitors on intraocular pressure, outflow facility, and pupil size may all be reversed with a subconjunctival injection of P_2AM. The drug is administered in a dose of 0.2 ml of a 4 percent solution.

Sympathomimetic Drugs

Sympathomimetic drugs lower the intraocular pressure by decreasing aqueous humor production and increasing the facility of outflow in glaucomatous eyes. The exact mechanism is still unclear. These solutions are intended solely for local corneal instillation and should never by used orally or by injection. When the glaucoma state is not severe, one of these eye drops, given once or twice a day, is often sufficient to control the intraocular pressure. If required, additional control can be achieved by adding a miotic followed in 2 to 3 min by the sympathomimetic. If necessary, the miotic may be used as often as 4 times a day, and the sympathomimetic drop up to 4 times to achieve optimum control of tension. Combinations of these two drops (miotic-sympathomimetic) are presently available commercially in one package.

Since sympathomimetic drugs dilate the pupil, even when used in conjunction with a miotic, they should not be used in eyes with narrow angles for fear of producing an acute glaucoma. However, this function makes them valuable drugs to be used in treating glaucoma, secondary to uveitis, or trauma where dilating the pupil is desirable.

There are 3 forms of the levo-epinephrine salts commercially available; all are about equally effective. They are L-epinephrine hydrochloride (Glaucon, 1 and 2 percent; Epifrin, 2 percent); L-epinephrine bitartrate, 2 percent (Epitrate, Lyophrin); and L-epinephrine borate, 0.5 and 1 percent (Eppy, Epinal). Because the hydrochloride and the bitartrate salts produce an acidic solution of about pH 3.5, a burning sensation is experienced after the drop is instilled. This may result in poor cooperation on the part of the young patient. L-epinephrine borate has a higher pH (about 7), and is therefore more comfortable to use. The drops are administered every 12 to 24 hrs. Up to a 30 percent reduction in aqueous humor production may result after the use of this medication.

The combination drugs utilize pilocarpine hydrochloride (1 to 6 percent) with L-epinephrine bitartrate (1 percent).

These drops may be better tolerated than the miotics because they produce less visual disturbances (except for the semidilated pupil; however, the burning, stinging sensation experienced by the patient may be severe enough to cause the drops to be discontinued. Often the discomfort becomes less noticeable with continued use of the medication. As sympathomimetic drugs they can produce systemic symptoms of sympathetic nervous system stimulation in the predisposed patient, e.g., pulse and blood pressure changes, palpitation, tachycardia, and extrasystoles. The most obvious sign is pupillary dilatation. Other side effects include headaches, faintness, trembling, paleness, and perspiration.

A reactive conjunctival hypermia may occur following the initial vasoconstriction. After prolonged use melanin-like adrenachrome deposits may be noted in the conjunctival glands and occasionally in the cornea. L-epinephrine causes an allergic conjunctivitis and blepharitis in over 30 percent of treated cases. All of these symptoms may be severe enough to cause the eye drops to be discontinued.

Sympathomimetic drugs can produce macular edema in aphakic eyes, which results in a central scotoma. Complete recovery is possible if the drug is discontinued promptly.

Carbonic Anhydrase Inhibitors

By supressing the rate of aqueous humor production by 40 to 60 percent, systemic carbonic anhydrase inhibitors, administered in a maximum dosage, reduce the intraocular pressure. However, even with massive dosages, some 50 percent persists. This reduction in aqueous production is additive to the 30 percent reduction which may be obtained with the sympathomimetic agents when the different agents are used together. The first of these carbonic anhydrase inhibitors to be tested was acetazolamide (Diamox). Several others, all of which are sulfonamides, have been introduced and at appropriate dosages appear equally effective to acetazolamide, but none have had the same extensive laboratory and clinical study in children.

Acetazolamide (Diamox), 250 mg pills: 500 mg sequels; 500 mg ampules (to be dissolved in 5 to 10 ml distilled water). In adults the pill is used two to 4 times daily by mouth, depending on the need and the side effects experienced. The pill may be halved to alter the dosage; long acting sequels, 500 mg are taken one to two times daily. The ampule is used in emergency situations by intravenous or intramuscular injection. For use in infants, acetazolamide is crushed into a powder and given in the formula or other food. Dosage in the very young infant is up to 15 mg/kg of body weight/day in divided portions. In older babies, 5 to 10 mg/kg of body weight every 4 to 6 hrs may be given. In children this dosage may be doubled.

Other carbonic anhydrase inhibitors used orally in adults include methazolamide (Neptazane), 50 to 100 mg, 3 to 4 times daily; dichlorphenamide (Daranide, Oratrol) 50 to 200 mg, 3 to 4 times daily; and ethoxzolamide (Cardrase, Ethamide), 50 to 250 mg, 3 to 6 times daily. There is little experience for the use of these latter drugs in children.

Dichlorphenamide has been found to cause birth anomalies in experimental animals. Acetazolamide is valuable in lowering the intraocular pressure in the self-limited secondary glaucomas such as trauma, glaucomatocyclitic crisis, and iritis. It may also be used preoperatively in infantile glaucoma, as described in Chapter 7. There is no place for the long-term use of this drug in young patients.

The inhibition of carbonic anhydrase, which is present throughout the body, may result in a variety of widespread systemic side effects including paresthesias seen as numbness and tingling of the fingers, toes, and tongue; dizziness; mental depression; generalized fatigue; sedation; ataxia; tremor; and occasional disorientation. Side effects in infants and young children are rare. Gastrointestinal symptoms of anorexia leading to weight loss, globus hystericus, distaste for carbonated beverages, nausea, and either diarrhea or constipation may occur. Genitourinary problems include frequency of urination, which diminishes after two or 3 weeks of use, urethral colic, and stone formation. Shortness of breath may appear if the patient has pulmonary or cardiac problems. As in the use of other sulfonamides, a sensitivity manifested as a skin eruption and pruritis may occur. The electrolyte balance of the patient must be under surveillance at all times during therapy. Dichlorphenamide effects an increase in chloride excretion that reduces the possibility of acidosis, which may occur with the other carbonic anhydrase inhibitors. Potassium depletion may be treated with Elizir Kaon or orange juice (see Chap. 7). Blood analysis should be performed at regular intervals during therapy, to detect the onset of agranulocytosis and thrombocytopenia in those rare, unfortunate instances when it occurs. There have been no reports of ocular damage or functional alterations attributed to the inhibition of carbonic anhydrase.

Osmotic Agents

The administration of osmotic agents causes a fluid loss from the eye and other tissues, leading to a reduction in the intraocular pressure in 20 to

45 min. The effect may last up to 10 hrs. This treatment is used in glaucoma secondary to trauma, and angle closure glaucoma. It may be used preoperatively when the tension of adolescent or aphakic glaucoma remains uncontrolled. However, its use is limited in inflamed eyes and neovascular glaucoma because the osmotic gradient is diminished. The commonly used osmotic agents include the following.

Glycerol (Glycerine)

The drug is administered in a dose of 0.75 to 1.5 ml/kg of body weight, orally in a 50 percent solution. The very sweet taste may be partially masked by the dilutent, which may be cracked ice with lemon or orange juice, a carbonated beverage, or instant coffee. It produces less diuresis than the intravenous agents, since it is largely metabolized by the body, whereas urea and mannitol must be excreted. If the patient is nauseated, one of the intravenous osmotic agents must be used.

Mannitol (20% Solution) or Lyophilized Urea (Urevert, Ureaphil)

Urea is prepared in a solid form which must be dissolved in 10 percent invert sugar to make a 30 percent solution.

This drug is administered intravenously in a dose of 0.5 to 1.5 g/kg of body weight, at approximately 60 drops per min. A rapid fall in pressure occurs in 20 to 30 min and lasts for 4 to 10 hrs. Tonometry should be performed at regular intervals during the infusion to determine when the

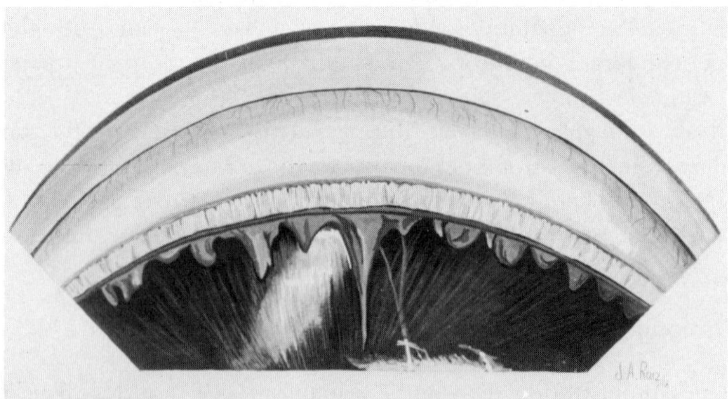

FIG. 2. Aniridia. Filtration angle illustrating rudimentary iris root.

glaucoma cycle has been broken. Urea must be prepared immediately before use, contrary to mannitol, and may cause tissue sloughing if the infusion leaks out of the vein. This does not occur with mannitol. Both appear to be equally effective. Patients may experience headaches, dehydration, nausea, vomiting, vertigo, and chills. The drugs result in a profuse diuresis, so that the preoperative patient should be asked to void or have an indwelling catheter inserted if general anesthesia is contemplated. Mannitol requires a larger volume to produce the same effect and penetrates into the ocular fluids less readily than urea, which makes it more effective in the presence of active inflammation.

SURGICAL MANAGEMENT

Goniotomy

The goniotomy procedure, as outlined in Chapter 12, can be used as a primary procedure in many forms of glaucoma in the young. Barkan advised goniotomy as the treatment for aniridia. He noted that residual embryonic tissue may pull the rudimentary root of the iris toward the line of Schwalbe, sealing off the filtration angle (Fig. 2). The purpose of the goniotomy

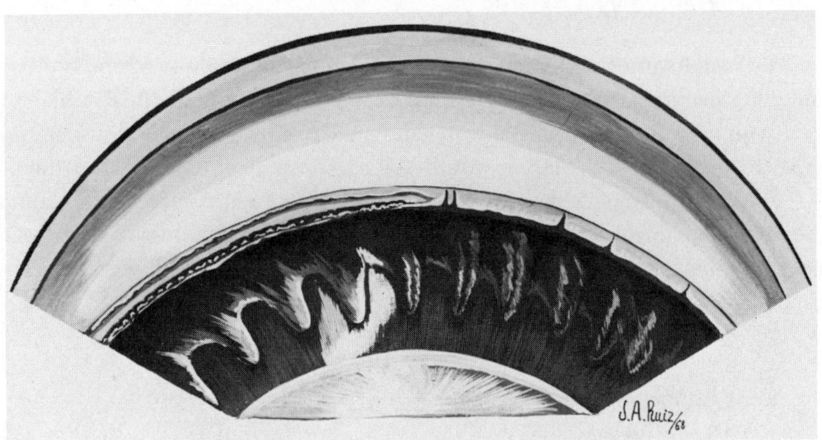

FIG. 3. Aniridia. Filtration angle after a goniotomy. (Modified from Barkan. **Arch. Ophthalmol.** 49:1, 1953.)

procedure would be to release the adhesions of the iris stump (Fig. 3). There is by no means general agreement that goniotomy is the treatment of choice in aniridia. However, the experienced goniotomist may observe an area of the filtration angle which seems amenable to this treatment and an attempt may be made.

The congenital glaucoma case associated with congenital syphilis, naevus flammeus (Sturge-Weber's syndrome) and neurofibromatosis, may display the same typical filtration angle features seen in spontaneous congenital glaucoma and respond in the same favorable way to goniotomy. When the angle exhibits markedly abnormal features, including large blood vessels, the goniotomy procedure should not be used.

Goniopuncture

It may be impossible to perform a goniotomy upon a case with well developed mesodermalis dysgenesis (Rieger's anomaly or Axenfeld's syndrome) because of the extensive adhesions of the stroma of the iris to Schwalbe's line. Sweeping the knife along such an angle would only result in a badly torn iris, hemorrhage, and a disorganized angle. Goniopuncture may be considered as the primary procedure. The accessible portions of the angle located between the adhesions are selected, and the goniopunctures performed in these areas.

Trabeculotomy ab Externo

Trabeculotomy ab externo has been performed on most of the types of glaucoma occurring in young patients. In experienced hands the results have been generally good. Any type of glaucoma resulting from an obstruction prior to the canal of Schlemm would seem to be amenable to this treatment.

Burian described a case of Marfan's syndrome with bilateral glaucoma. The filtration angle was crowded with large blood vessels in the thin tissue covering the angle. For this reason, a trabeculotomy ab externo was performed.

Lens Abnormalities

Ectopia Lentis

The mode of treatment for the dislocated lens continues to be controversial. In most cases vision may be maintained at a functional level

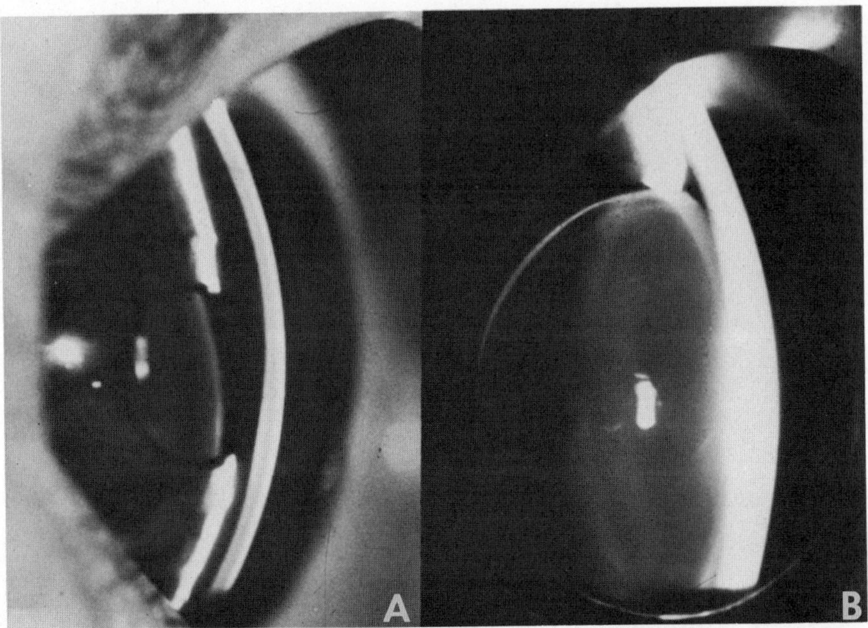

FIG. 4. Ectopia lentis. (A) The lens rests in its normal location posterior to the pupil; (B) the lens dislocated into the anterior chamber and trapped by the iris. (Courtesy of J. Barraquer.)

with a careful refraction. When the lens dislocates forward into the anterior chamber through the pupil, causing pupillary block, secondary glaucoma occurs. The pressure must first be normalized with osmotic agents, while the pupil is being constricted with miotics (Fig. 4). This will minimize vitreous loss. The lens is extracted through a limbal incision.

Cataract

A thorough discussion on the origin of cataracts in young patients is beyond the scope of this book. Similarly, a description of cataract surgery as a treatment in the nonglaucomatous eye is not included here. For this purpose the reader is referred to appropriate books on cataracts and cataract surgery. However, the presence of a cataract in a young patient either of congenital, metabolic, or traumatic origin must signal a warning to the attending ophthalmologist that secondary glaucoma is an ever-present possibility.

Once lens changes in children have taken place, they may remain stationary or maturation may occur as in adults. The cataract may progress

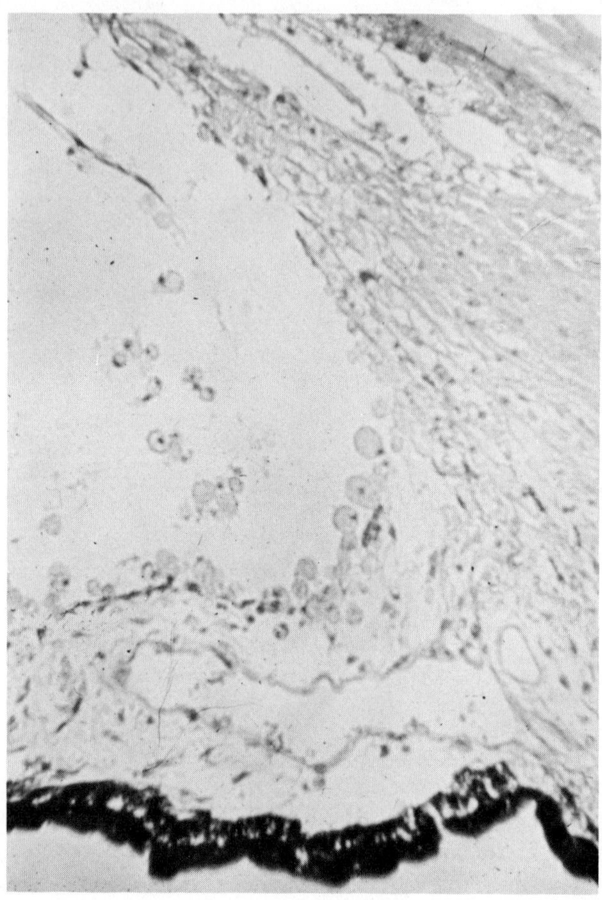

FIG. 5. Phacolytic glaucoma. Lens material is engulfed by macrophages which block the trabecular spaces.

to a stage that results in secondary glaucoma, by swelling which results in a forward displacement of the iris-lens diaphragm (intumescent cataract) and angle closure (phacomorphic glaucoma). The cataract may advance in maturity (hypermature cataract) and leak lens material through a damaged lens capsule which is engulfed by macrophages (Fig. 5). These are carried to the filtration angle, causing blockage (phacolytic glaucoma).

The pressure is controlled by intravenous urea or mannitol, the pupil is widely dilated with mydriatics, and the cataract extraction is performed. The aspiration-irrigation technique is the preferred treatment (Fig. 6). Kelman's phacoemulsification procedure is an alternative method.

Glaucoma as a Complication to Cataract Surgery

Glaucoma is known to occur as a complication following cataract surgery in young patients.

DISCISSION OPERATION, FAULTY TECHNIQUE. When an inadequate opening is made in the lens capsule during a discission operation, swelling of lens material within the capsule may occur. The iris is pushed forward against the filtration angle, producing angle closure glaucoma.

The intraocular pressure must first be controlled by osmotic agents; then through a widely dilated pupil a linear extraction or aspiration of lens material is performed.

BLOCKAGE OF THE FILTRATION ANGLE BY LENS MATERIAL. Secondary glaucoma can occur when an excessive amount of lens material remains in the anterior chamber following congenital cataract surgery. The lens cortex swells and may be swept toward the filtration angle by aqueous currents, causing a blockage. If the pressure remains elevated, the lens material must be removed by the aspiration technique after the pressure is brought under control with osmotic agents.

SEVERE POSTOPERATIVE REACTION. A stormy postoperative course following a linear extraction may result in the production of peripheral anterior synechiae, iris bombé, and secondary glaucoma. An iridectomy or transfixation of the iris must be performed after the pressure is controlled with osmotic agents to relieve the pupillary block. This complication is seen much less commonly following the aspiration-irrigation operation. Intensive use of mydriatics and local corticosteroid drops will shorten the course of the reaction and prevent the development of iris adhesions to surrounding structures.

While on this regime, it is important to assess the ocular pressure on frequent occasions, either directly with the tonometer (where possible) or via the judicial use of the fingers, since the steroid drops themselves can cause an elevated intraocular tension. The local steroids must therefore be terminated as soon as the anterior segment reaction has subsided. The mydriatics which cause no adverse effects should be maintained for several months after cataract surgery in children.

PUPILLARY BLOCK. Vitreous may block the pupil following cataract surgery. An inflammatory reaction may result in an adherence between the pupil border and the vitreous face, resulting in iris bombé and secondary glaucoma. The diagnosis may be missed, owing to the difficulty in using the tomometer and slit lamp in young children. A peripheral iridectomy or transfixation of the iris is performed after the pressure is

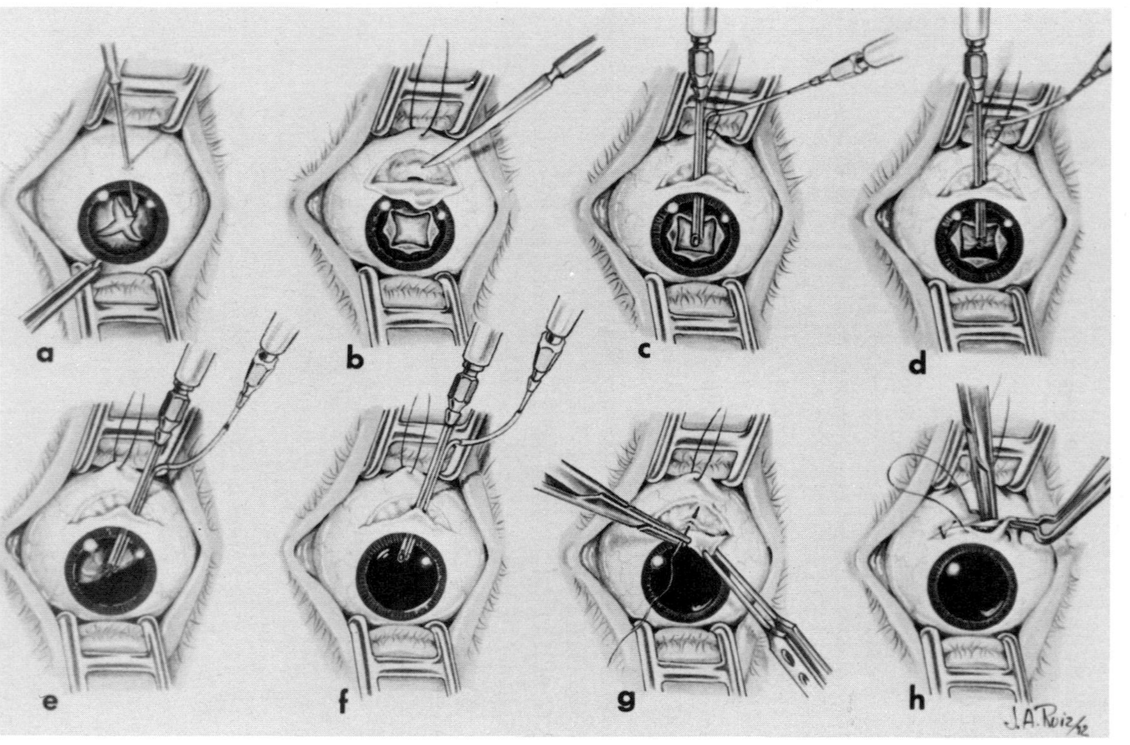

FIG. 6. A. Aspiration-irrigation technique for congenital cataract. (A) A cruciate incision is made in the anterior lens capsule with the knife needle. Care must be exercised to spare the posterior lens capsule. (B) Knife needle is withdrawn. A small, narrow, limbal-based conjunctival flap is made over the puncture site. The limbal opening is enlarged with the graefe knife, the width of which is sufficient to allow an 18-gauge needle to enter the anterior chamber.

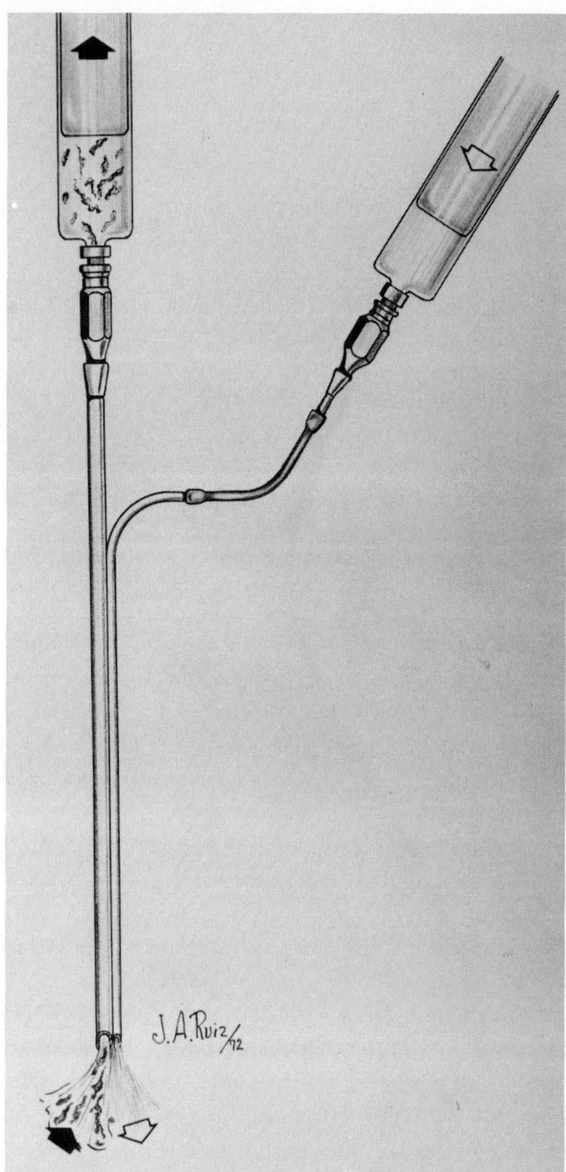

FIG. 6. (Cont.) A blunt, thin-wall 18 gauge needle attached to a 2-cc syringe, containing 0.25 cc of saline solution, enters the anterior chamber. This needle may be fitted with an accompanying 22-gauge needle, attached separately to another 2-cc syringe filled with saline (Fig. 6.**B.**). This auxiliary system is used to keep the anterior chamber filled, while the 18-gauge needle aspirates the broken down pieces of lens material and accompanying fluid. Otherwise there is considerable flattening of the cornea and anterior movement of the posterior capsule during aspiration. (D) Aspiration of lens material. (E) The needle may be directed to various positions to gather remaining lens material. (F) The anterior chamber is clear and the needle is withdrawn. It is not necessary to remove the last bit of lens material. (G) Suturing of limbal incision. (H) Suturing of conjunctival incision. (Modified from Scheie. **Am. J. Ophthalmol.** 50:1048, 1960.)

brought under control with osmotic agents.

The ophthalmologist should look for an unevenness in the depth of the anterior chamber which may develop into a loss of the chamber itself: an early sign of pupil block. A flat anterior chamber which remains unchecked predisposes to the development of peripheral anterior synechiae and a permanent glaucoma state. For this reason, the pupil must be fully dilated following cataract surgery in young patients, and be maintained at full dilation for at least 4 to 6 months, even though the eye appears completely quiet. If peripheral anterior synechiae form, the condition must be treated as a case of aphakic glaucoma. One of the strong, long-acting anticholinesterase drops, administered once or twice a day may give adequate control. The cyclodialysis operation is probably the best surgical option if medical management fails.

VITREOUS LOSS. Owing to the high rate of vitreous loss associated with intracapsular cataract extraction in children, this method must be considered unsuitable. The use of α-chymotrypsin has not improved the outlook for the intracapsular technique in young patients, and may itself cause a transient rise in intraocular pressure. This could be a serious complication in this age group, where any excessive pressure on the limbal wound should be avoided.

Whatever the technique used in children, the posterior capsule must remain intact. Rupture of this structure causes a break in the vitreous face and the entrance of vitreous into the anterior chamber. Once here, any excessive manipulation by the surgeon will result in vitreous loss. This complication may occur with the linear extraction, the irrigation-aspiration operation, and phacoemulsification. For this reason, it is important that the microscope be used, no matter what surgical option is chosen, to perform cataract surgery in young patients. It is only under high magnification that the posterior capsule can be observed and thus avoided.

Although many eyes sustain vitreous loss without further difficulties, a careful examination must be performed at regular intervals to detect the onset of detachment of the retina and aphakic glaucoma.

The detachment must be treated in the appropriate manner. Glaucoma is best treated with one of the strong, long-acting anticholinesterase agents administered once or twice a day. If medical management fails, the cyclodialysis operation should be performed.

Ocular Perforation with Lens Involvement

Perforation of the anterior segment may result from (1) a sharp instrument (e.g., scissors, ice pick); (2) a fast moving projectile (e.g., metal fragment resulting with hammer blow to metal object (metallic), exploding bullet casing (non-metallic)); (3) an accident with a bursting firecracker held near the face; or (4) a surgically induced injury (e.g., corneal transplant trephine striking lens, iris forceps entering anterior chamber during filtration operation and striking lens). The lens may be involved either directly from the injury or secondarily during surgical repair.

The eye should be carefully examined and the accident assessed with the slit lamp, avoiding completely any external pressure to the globe. If a retained radioopaque foreign body is suspected, the ophthalmologist should accompany the patient during the x-ray examinations to prevent nonexperienced x-ray technicians from pushing on the eyeball.

The patient should be anesthetized, prepared, and draped in the usual way. No pressure should be exerted on the eye at this time. If a retained foreign body is present it should be localized and removed in the prescribed manner. The anterior segment perforation should be repaired. The slit lamp examination will have revealed any lens damage. If perforation has occurred, the lens may have *matured* by the time surgery is undertaken. Secondary glaucoma may result from a forward displacement of the iris-lens diaphragm, which occurs with lens swelling, or a blockage of the filtration angle by macrophages that have engulfed leaking lens material. The rupture in the lens capsule may be large enough to allow lens material to escape, swell up, and be carried to the filtration angle. Therefore, if the lens is damaged it is best removed at the same time the perforation is repaired. The aspiration-irrigation technique should be performed in the normal fashion from the limbus at 12 o'clock. The lens should not be removed from the perforation site except when the accident takes place during a corneal transplant operation. If the lens appears clear at the time of surgery or if the surgeon chooses not to remove the damaged lens, the patient should be carefully followed, since maturation may take place at a later date and result in secondary glaucoma. If this occurs, the pressure should be brought under control with osmotic agents and the lens removed through a widely dilated pupil with the aspiration-irrigation technique.

Lens Induced Angle Closure Glaucoma

RETROLENTAL FIBROPLASIA. Elevation of the intraocular pressure is not an infrequent complication of retrolental fibroplasia. The mechanism by which glaucoma arises is likely a forward movement of the lens-iris diaphragm and angle closure, possibly resulting from a contracture of the retrolental membrane. The pressure may be controlled by aspiration of the lens.

PERSISTENT HYPERPLASTIC PRIMARY VITREOUS. Persistent

hyperplastic primary vitreous (PHPV) may be complicated by angle closure glaucoma. When indications are present for the treatment of PHPV, the lens must first be removed, preferably by the aspiration-irrigation technique, followed by removal or incision of the retrolental membrane. The mechanism for the occurrence of secondary angle closure glaucoma in PHPV is still unclear. It may be caused by swelling of the lens which results from a rupture of the posterior capsule (see Chap. 9), or because of a forward movement of the iris-lens diaphragm associated with a contracture of the retrolental membrane.

Iridectomy

Iridectomy is rarely indicated in the young patient. It is mainly useful in relieving pupillary block from iris bombé which can occur following iritis, cataract surgery, or trauma. The iridectomy operation is also the treatment of choice in plateau iris. In this condition, the iris leaf is inserted anteriorly on the ciliary body. The iris plane is flat, running directly toward Schwalbe's line, and then dips sharply backward to the ciliary body leaving a narrow entrance to the angle. When the pupil is dilated, the peripheral portion of the iris is crowded into the angle, causing angle closure glaucoma. The central portion of the anterior chamber is deeper than the typical case of angle closure; there is only a minimal bulge of the iris contrary to that seen in iris bombé, and pupillary block is minimal. After the peripheral iridectomy has been performed, miotic therapy is often necessary to prevent further acute attacks.

Cyclodialysis

Since Heine published his report on the cyclodialysis operation in 1905, the operation has been used for many different types of glaucoma. The technique is unique in its approach, since it provides the only means of producing a communication between the anterior chamber and the supra-choroidal space. This is accomplished by making a cleft between uveal tissue on one side, and the outer coat of the eyeball on the other. The cleft provides a substitute for normal aqueous outflow, so the aqueous humor may seep into the suprachoroidal space and be absorbed.

Cyclodialysis has a high failure rate in young patients because the suprachoroidal cleft has a tendency to seal over. Intraocular hemorrhage following surgery is also seen more frequently in children than in the adult. This would be another factor leading to failure, if the clot organizes in the area of the cleft. Other complications include injury to the lens, peeling of Descemet's membrane, iridodialysis, and perforation of the choroid with vitreous loss at the site of the scleral incision. There is a place for this operation in the young patient: in aphakic glaucoma following congenital cataract surgery.

Cyclodiathermy

The cyclodiathermy operation is a last resort in pediatric glaucoma surgery, except in cases of aniridia and hemorrhagic glaucoma where it may be the only suitable choice. The purpose of the technique is to reduce aqueous humor production by destroying a portion of the ciliary body or its blood supply.

The operation is performed as follows. A 1.0 mm insulated penetrating electrode is applied through the conjunctiva into the sclera, in the inferior or superior half of the globe in one or two rows. The different diathermy machines vary, but the equivalent of 50 mA of current is applied through the electrode for 3 sec, much as is done in retinal detachment surgery. The applications are evenly spaced in an arc 4 to 6 mm from the limbus, several mm apart. A second row may be made 8 mm from the limbus, giving a total of about 15 applications.

The applications may be directly to the sclera, after the conjunctiva is incised and cleared from the operative site. The rectus muscle must be isolated and drawn away from the field by a traction suture. An alternative route is to make a small perforation in the conjunctiva at 6 or 12 o'clock, and undermine the tissue. The electrode is then slid sideways under the conjunctiva and turned, so that the point engages the sclera. Vitreous may extrude from the puncture sites. The conjunctival wound is closed with interrupted virgin or 10-0 silk sutures. The procedure may be repeated, if necessary, in the opposite half of the globe at a later time.

Postoperative reaction is usually slight. Treatment consists of the instillation of 1 percent atropine, and chloramphenicol drops or ointment applied 3 times a day, for about 4 days. Corticosteroid drops or ointment may be added if warranted. Initially, the intraocular pressure may be high because of shrinkage of the sclera, later falling to normal levels.

Complications associated with cyclodiathermy include phthisis bulbi, anterior chamber hemorrhage, vitreous hemorrhage, iritis, uveitis, cataract formation, retinal detachment, bullous keratitis, sympathetic ophthalmia, and scleral ectasia. Iritis, peripheral anterior synechia, and corneal damage may result when the applications are made less than 2 mm from the limbus.

Cyclocryotherapy

Cyclocryotherapy has the advantage of causing only minimal tissue destruction; ectasia of the sclera is thus unlikely to occur. The operation is performed as follows. The cryoprobe is applied in an arc, about the circumference of the globe, 5 mm from the limbus. The cryoprobe is set at -70° C and applied for 30 to 45 sec. Approximately 8 applications are administered. Little has been reported about the usefulness of this technique in the glaucomas of young patients.

Glaucoma Due to Secondary Hyphema

Secondary hyphema, which occurs spontaneously on the second to the fifth day following the initial ocular injury, may result in a blockage of the trabecular filtration area and cause a severe uncontrolled secondary glaucoma. The pressure may force red blood cells into the substantia propria of the cornea ("blood staining") so that the final visual outcome is often disappointing, even after surgical evacuation of the blood clot.

Kwitko and Costenbader reported on the use of intravenous urea in glaucoma due to secondary hyphema. In all cases, the plan was to remove the blood clot by surgical intervention after the intraocular pressure was brought under control. Following the administration of intravenous urea, there was such a dramatic response that no further treatment was necessary, except in one case where a second infusion of urea was required. The elevated pressure was brought to within normal limits, as expected, but during the infusion, the blood escaped from the anterior chamber at a surprisingly rapid rate. Cole and Byron made similar observations in a later report. Kwitko and Costenbader speculated that the urea-induced artificial withdrawal of fluid from the eye caused a secondary over-production of intraocular fluid from the ciliary body epithelium. With this increased circulation of fluid, red blood cells would be irrigated from the anterior chamber in a more efficient manner. This clinical observation awaits laboratory verification.

Control of intraocular pressure in the secondary hyphemas is vital since, with a normal pressure, the complication of a blood-stained cornea is avoided.

The administration of intravenous urea in a healthy young patient even several times, causes little harm. In addition to parenteral therapy, which is used only when the pressure rises and remains elevated, the child should be placed on complete bed rest, both eyes should be patched, and the head of the bed raised about 30 ° to allow the blood to settle below the pupillary area. There is little agreement over the use of mydriatics and miotics, since movement of the iris may massage the torn blood vessel and aggravate the condition. The author prefers to avoid the use of these drugs. Oral enzymes (Orenzyme®), vitamin K, vitamin B_{12}, calcium gluconate, and conjugated estrogen (Premarin®) in appropriate dosages may have some beneficial effect.

If a large blood clot remains lodged in the anterior chamber without definite improvement, in spite of this treatment, surgical intervention is indicated. The anterior chamber is irrigated with saline through an ab externo incision made at the limbus. A fibrinolytic agent (Urokinase®, 5,000 units, made up in 2 ml of sterile distilled water) may be used to wash out the anterior chamber. Kelman and Brooks described the use of the phacoemulsification apparatus to fragment and aspirate the blood clot.

Enucleation

The state of therapy in glaucoma of the young patient is such that all cases are not saved. When the eye is distorted, blind, and painful, particularly after a retrobulbar alcohol injection has been made, enucleation may be the only suitable treatment available. It is important to remember, while performing the enucleation, that the scleral coat is abnormally thinned. It is not improbable, while isolating and incising the recti muscles at their insertions where the thinning may be exaggerated, that the sclera might be picked up and cut, causing a perforation of the globe. This complication might also occur when severing the optic nerve. Meticulous dissection and sufficient exposure is vital to insure the successful performance of this operation.

DISCUSSION

When using eye drop solutions, care should be exercised to not contaminate the dropper tip, by avoiding contact with the eye, eyelid, eyelashes, or any other object (Fig. 7A and B), and by replacing the cap of the bottle immediately after use.

The treatment of glaucoma in young patients should begin with the use of the weaker concentrations of the parasympathomimetic (cholinergic)

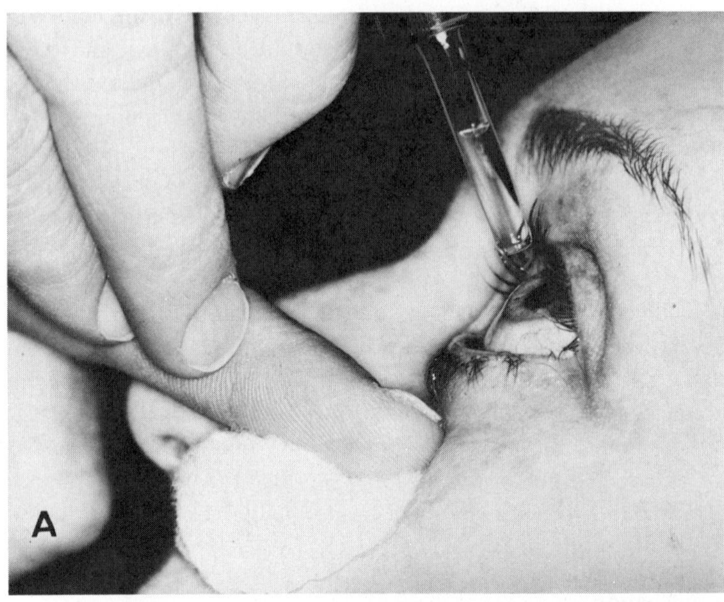

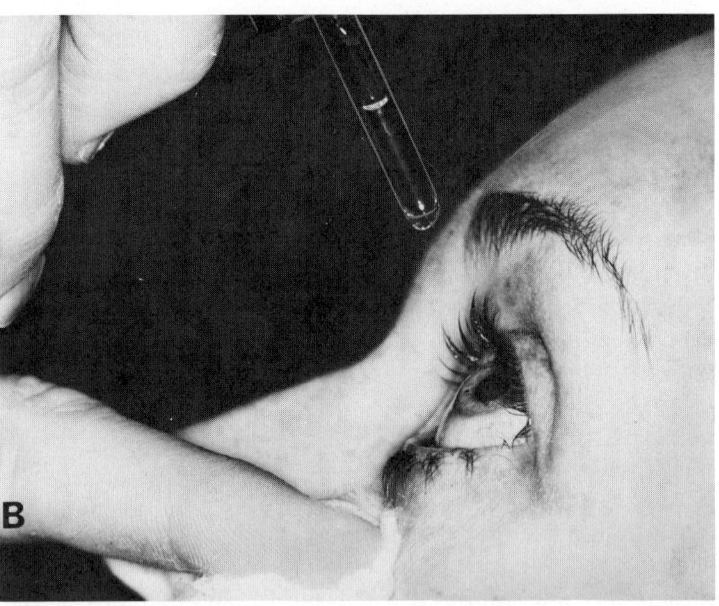

FIG. 7. Installation of eyedrops. (A) Improper method. The dropper tip touching the eyelashes; (B) Proper method. The dropper is held well back from the eye and the drop instilled. (Courtesy of H. A. Stein and B. J. Slatt.)

drops. The stronger medications are then used as needed, slowly titrating the drops, in concentration and frequency, to produce the optimal intraocular pressure. After prolonged use, a specific agent can begin to show diminished effectiveness in lowering the intraocular pressure. Another drug must then be substituted. Often the original drops may be restarted with original effectiveness after a period of several months. This is the case with pilocarpine and carbachol. The stable, strong, long-acting anticholinesterase agents produce good control in younger patients with perhaps only a single dose at bed time. The accommodative spasm is fairly constant and may be corrected with glasses. An occasional patient may not respond at all to a specific eye drop. The ophthalmologist must be aware of this possibility so that other forms of therapy may be explored.

A tension of under 22 mm Hg is satisfactory when there is no optic nerve cupping substantiated by a normal visual field. Once the optic nerve is damaged a much lower pressure is required, but, more important than visual acuity assessment, tonometry and tonography, it is essential to repeat the visual fields at frequent intervals to insure that the treatment is effective. A satisfactory pressure and 20/20 vision with progressive field loss cannot long be tolerated by the eyeball or the ophthalmologist. In this case management must be reassessed, and different agents in various combinations introduced.

If surgery becomes necessary because of failure of medical control, it is wise to discontinue the anticholinesterase agent one to two weeks beforehand. These drugs seem to be associated with a greater postoperative inflammatory response if continued up to the time of surgery. Their effect on the serum cholinesterase and pseudocholinesterase levels when a general anesthetic is employed is of even greater importance.

SUMMARY

While the delineation of the anatomic abnormalities of infantile glaucoma requires additional histologic study, the mechanism of action of the surgery used to correct these abnormalities is in equal need of such study. Goniotomy has been used for about 20 years and has proven to be an effective surgical procedure. However, the few follow-up studies of eyes which have had successful goniotomies as well as tonographic, gonioscopic, and histologic evaluation, have not yet determined the exact mechanism of action of goniotomy. This would also apply to the newer microsurgical techniques, trabeculotomy ab externo, and trabeculectomy.

While presently used surgical methods are successful in most eyes with infantile glaucoma, many eyes are not controlled and continue to show progressive damage. There is good reason to suggest that the failure of some surgical procedures may be as much related to the scarring and damage produced by the surgery as to the disease itself. Present surgical techniques are far too gross to perform accurately—a procedure may be so delicate that it requires the incision of a membrane one cell-layer thick. New methods of carefully controlled microsurgery, perhaps using a refined laser beam, microcryo impulses of energy, or some form of energy not presently known, are needed, with visualization of the angle structures, in high magnification and perhaps even with motor-driven stereotactic instruments which can be accurately positioned. It may be that only with such techniques, the surgical procedures can be accurately defined and their mechanisms of action more accurately studied.

In addition to the surgical technique itself, more information must be added to our knowledge of wound healing and the effects of enzymatic, chemical, or other mechanisms that retard or inhibit what otherwise appears to be a successful technical procedure. In addition to this information, we must search for a substance that renders tissue such as Tenon's capsule or the subconjunctival tissue more permeable or more absorbent. Chemicals which reduce fibroblastic proliferation would be very helpful. Our knowledge about the treatment of vitreous loss, a not unlikely problem in the treatment of congenital glaucoma, is still in its infancy. Seton operations have never found great favor and are largely experimental, but mechanisms may be found to create a new conduit when birth finds the eyeball without means of excreting the fluid it is producing.

References

Acers, T. E., and Coston, T. O. Persistent hyperplastic primary vitreous, early surgical management. Am. J. Ophthalmol., 64:734, 1967.

Anderson, T. R. Hydrophthalmia or Congenital Glaucoma. Cambridge Univ. Press, London, 1939.

Ascher, K. W. Some details on the technique of cyclodialysis. Am. J. Ophthalmol., 50:1207, 1960.

Barkan, O. Operation for congenital glaucoma. Am. J. Ophthalmol., 25:552, 1942.

——— Goniotomy for glaucoma associated with aniridia. Arch. Ophthalmol., 49:1, 1953.

——— Goniotomy for glaucoma associated with nevus flammeus. Am. J. Ophthalmol., 43:545, 1959.

Becker, B. Decrease in intraocular pressure in man by carbonic anhydrase inhibitor, Diamox. Preliminary report. Am. J. Ophthalmol., 37:13, 1954.

——— and Shaffer, R. N. Diagnosis and Therapy of the Glaucomas, 2nd ed. Mosby, St. Louis, 1965.

Berens, C., and King, J. H. An Atlas of Ophthalmic Surgery. Lippincott, Philadelphia, 1961.

Blake, E. M. The surgical treatment of glaucoma complicating congenital aniridia. Am. J. Ophthalmol., 36:907, 1953.

Burian, H. M. A case of Marfan's syndrome with bilateral glaucoma, with a description of a new type of operation for developmental glaucoma (trabeculotomy ab externo). Am. J. Ophthalmol., 50:1187, 1960.

Byron, H. M. Ocular trauma, importance, prevention, therapy. Eye, Ear, Nose, Throat Mon., 42:48, 1963.

Cole, J. G., and Byron, H. M. Evaluation of 100 eyes with traumatic hyphema. Intravenous urea. Arch. Ophthalmol., 71:35, 1964.

Collier, R., Arstikaitis, M., and Pashby, T. Glaucoma in children. Trans. Can. Ophthalmol., Soc., 21:92, 1959.

Cordes, F. H. Evaluation of the surgery of congenital cataracts. Arch. Ophthalmol., 46:133, 1951.

Costenbader, F. D., and Albert, D. G. Conservatism in the management of congenital cataract. Arch. Ophthalmol., 58:426, 1957.

Cotlier, E. Surgical results in rubella and nonrubella congenital cataracts. Am. J. Ophthalmol., 66:539, 1968.

Ellis, G. S., and Haik, G. M. Management of congenital cataracts in children. J. St. Louis Med. Soc., 111:56, 1959.

Francois, J. Angiomatose oculo-cutaneé de Lawford (Angiome facial et glaucoma tradif). Ophthalmologica, 122:215, 1951.

Francois, J. Persistent hyperplastic primary vitreous. Trans. Can. Ophthalmol. Soc., 23:141, 1960.

Fuchs, J. Die Zweiwegespritze e-in neuartiges Instrument zur Absaugung weicher Stare. Klin. Monatsbl. Augenheilkd., 121:592, 1952.

Galin, M. A., Aizawa, F., and McLean, J. Urea as an osmotic hypotensive agent in glaucoma. Arch. Ophthalmol., 62:347, 1959.

Gallenga, R. L'operazione della cataratta, nell'aniridia congenita. Ress. Ital. Ottalmol., 7:168, 1938.

Gass, J. D. M. Surgical excision of persistent hyperplastic primary vitreous. Arch. Ophthalmol., 83:163, 1970.

Girard, L. J. Aspiration-irrigation of congenital and traumatic cataracts. Arch. Ophthalmol., 77:387, 1967.

Heine, L. Die Cyklodialyse eine neue Glaukomoperation. Dtsch. Med. Wchnschr., 31:825, 1905.

Holmes, W. J. Congenital buphthalmos complicated by dislocation of lens and hemorrhage into vitreous with complete recovery of central vision. Arch. Ophthalmol., 20:757, 1938.

Jauernig,. Primarer und sekundarer hydrophthalmus. Klin. Monatsbl. Augenheilkd., 99:542, 1937.

Joy, H. M. Nevus flammues associated with glaucoma. Am. J. Ophthalmol., 33:1401, 1950.

Kelman, C. D. Phacoemulsification and aspiration, a new technique of cataract removal. Am. J. Ophthalmol., 64:23, 1967.

Phacoemulsification and aspiration. Am. J. Ophthalmol., 67:464, 1969.

and Brooks, D. L. Ultrasonic emulsification and aspiration of traumatic hyphema, a preliminary report. Am. J. Ophthalmol., 71:1289, 1971.

Kwitko, M. L. Glaucoma due to hypermature cataract, the use of urea in diagnosis. Can. Med. Assoc. J., 89:569, 1963.

Urea therapy in lens induced glaucoma. Eye, Ear, Nose, Throat Mon., 42:55, 1963.

Glaucoma due to hypermature cataract, the use of urea in diagnosis. Can. Med. Assoc. J., 89:569, 1963.

Adverse effects of intravenous urea. Eye, Ear, Nose, Throat Dig., 26:61, 1964.

Urea therapy in ophthalmology. Survey Ophthalmol., 9:371, 1964.

Postoperative open-angle glaucoma following topical application of steroids. Can. Med. Assoc. J., 94:966, 1966.

Secondary glaucoma in infancy and childhood. Can. J. Ophthalmol., 4:231, 1969.

and Costenbader, F. D. Glaucoma due to secondary hyphema, a report of two cases treated with intravenous urea. Am. J. Ophthalmol., 53:590, 1962.

and Costenbader, F. D. Urea therapy in glaucoma due to secondary hyphema. Can. Med. Assoc. J. 86:447, 1962.

Maumenee, E. A. External filtering operations for glaucoma. The mechanism of function and failure. Trans. Am. Ophthalmol. Soc., 58:319, 1960.

McCormick, A. G., and Pratt-Johnson, J. A. Angle closure glaucoma in infancy. Can. J. Ophthalmol., 6:38, 1971.

Meller, J. Hydrophthalmus als Folge Einer Entwicklungsanomalie der Iris. Arch. Ophthalmol., 92:34, 1917.

Rakusin, W. Urokinase in the management of traumatic hyphemas. Br. J. Ophthalmol., 55:826, 1971.

Traumatic hyphema. Am. J. Ophthalmol., 74:284, 1972.

Raskind, R. H. Persistent hyperplastic primary vitreous. Am. J. Ophthalmol., 62:1072, 1966.

Reese, A. B. Persistent hyperplastic primary vitreous. Am. J. Ophthalmol., 40:317, 1955.

Scheie, H. G. Aspiration of congenital or soft cataracts, a new technique. Am. J. Ophthalmol., 50:1048, 1960.

Shaffer, R. N., and Weiss, D. I. Congenital and Pediatric Glaucomas. Mosby, St. Louis, 1970.

Wilson, W. A. Congenital cataracts, a review of 72 cases including the use of enzymatic zonulysis in 15 patients. Arch. Ophthalmol., 67:143, 1962.

Wolfe, O., and Wolfe, R. M. Removal of soft cataract by suction. A new double-barreled aspiration needle. Arch. Ophthalmol., 26:127, 1941.

14

Clinical Cases

From 55 patients affected by congenital glaucoma, 86 eyes were available for study. The cases are analyzed according to the classification described in Chapter 5.

Each of the groups of eyes outlined in Tables 1-4 are analyzed according to *sex, age of onset, eye involved, initial signs and symptoms noted, surgical procedures performed, and final result obtained.* Under initial signs and symptoms, the cases are classified with regard to *photophobia, haziness of the cornea, tearing, enlargement of the eye, corneal diameter, and intraocular pressure.* Surgical procedures are divided into *goniotomy or goniotomy-type operations and other filtering procedures. In final result the visual acuity and intraocular pressure on the last postoperative examination* are outlined.

The intraocular pressure measurement was made with the Schiötz tonometer in most of the eyes at the level of deep surgical anesthesia. When a series of measurements were not identical, the average was taken. In the assessment of visual acuity, the Snellen chart was used whenever possible. In younger children the vision was assessed according to fixation ability with the involved eye. Central and maintained fixation suggested good visual acuity. An enlarged eye was the manner of appearance to the observer. The symptoms were either those reported by the parents or noted by the observer. A follow-up on all the patients was not always possible. Some patients were seen in consultation, operated upon and never seen again, many being from distant cities. Other patients simply eluded follow-up after surgery.

In the assessment of final result the two important measurements are the intraocular pressure and the visual acuity. However, this may not be the best way to determine a cure in congenital glaucoma. The intraocular pressure measurement, as noted in Chapter 7, is dependent on many other independent factors—such as the level of anesthesia, type of anesthetic used, degree of dehydration, and so on. Therefore a pressure in excess of 22 mm Hg does not constitute a failure in therapy. Visual acuity in these cases must be assessed in the light of several important factors. Damage to ocular structures may already be present before surgery is instituted. In addition these eyes suffer often from conditions which by themselves can affect visual acuity. Such conditions include strabismus, nystagmus, congenital cataracts, corneal opacities, anisometropia, and retinal dysplasia. The nystagmoid movement may be ameliorated following normalization of the intraocular pressure.

It is the *total* assessment of the case which determines a cure—that is, the arrest of progressive corneal enlargement, the disappearance of corneal

TABLE 1

NEWBORN GLAUCOMA–
Age: Birth to Five Days

				Initial Signs and Symptoms						Surgical Procedure*	Final Result	
Patient	Sex	Age of Onset	Eye Examined	Photophobia	Hazy Cornea	Tearing	Enlarged Eye	Corneal Diam.	Tension (mm Hg)		Vision†	Tension (mm Hg)
JK	M	birth	OD		X		X	13	50	G		
			OS		X		X	13	50	G		
CP	M	birth	OD		X		X	13	35	GP,G	GC	26
		1m.	OS		X		X	13	55	GP(2),CY		26
WR	M	birth	OD	X	X			13	40	G		
			OS	X	X			13	45	G		
CF	F	birth	OD					13	40	G	GMC	20
			OS					13	40	G	GMC	22
AL	F	birth	OD	X	X		X	14	40	G,GP(2),S,S	GMC	19
			OS	X	X		X	14	40	G,GP(2),S,S	M	19
LP	M	2 d	OD	X	X			13	50	G		E
			OS	X	X			13	50	G(3)		E
HC	M	3 d	OD		X			13	61	G,GP(2),G,I,I,CY(3)		E
			OS		X			13	47	G,GP,G,CY,I,C,C		E
LL	F	4 d	OD	X	X			12	40	G(3),S	MC	
			OS	X	X			12	40	G(3),I	MC	
RH	M	4 d	OD		X			13	53	GP,G(2),CY(2),S		E
			OS		X			12	35	G,CY(5),T		E

*G, goniotomy; GP, with goniopuncture; P, goniopuncture; I, iridenclesis; CY, cyclodiathermy; T, trephine; S, Scheie type procedure.

†In this and the following tables: GMC, good maintained and central fixation; LP, light perception; NLP, no light perception; N, tension below 22 mm Hg; E, elevated above 35 mm Hg; Cat. ext., cataract extraction.

See J. Pediatr. Ophthalmol., 4:9, 1967.

TABLE 2

INFANTILE GLAUCOMA–
Age: Five Days to Six Months

Patient	Sex	Age of Onset	Eye Examined	Initial Signs and Symptoms: Photophobia	Hazy Cornea	Tearing	Enlarged Eye	Corneal Diam.	Tension (mm Hg)	Surgical Procedure*	Final Result: Vision†	Tension (mm Hg)
JW	M	14 d	OD					13	17		GMC	
			OS	X	X	X	X	15	35	G(3),GP,I		
CH	F	1 m	OD	X	X	X		13	40	GP	GMC	20
			OS	X	X	X		13	40	GP	GMC	20
AMc		1 m	OD		X		X	13	33	CY		
			OS					10	29			
CEE	F	1 m	OD	X	X			13	33	GP(3)	GMC	25
			OS	X	X			13	44	G(2),GP,S	GMC	29
AS	M	2 m	OD				X	17	40	P,cat.ext.	GC	N
			OS				X	17	40	P,cat.ext.	GC	N
EC	M	3 m	OD					12	25		20/15	26
			OS		X		X	14	45	G	20/200	26
VO	M	3 m	OD		X		X	13	50	GP	20/200	23
			OS					10	35		20/20	26
RB		3 m	OD	X		X	X	11	40	G		27
			OS	X		X		11	40	G		20
RL		3 m	OD		X		X	14	33	G,GP	GMC	35
			OS		X		X	14	31	G(2),GP,I	GMC	12
JR	F	3 m	OD		X	X	X	13	41	G,GP	MC	
			OS		X	X	X	13	43	G,GP(2)	GMC	N
FC	F	3 m	OD		X			12	60	GP	GMC	17
			OS		X			12	50	GP	GMC	18
DW	F	4 m	OD	X				14	50	GP(3),G		28
			OS	X				14	50	GP(3)		
SK	F	4 m	OD		X		X	12	25	G	GMC	N
			OS				X	14	30	GP	GMC	N
TM	F	4 m	OD	X	X			13	45	G(2),S	20/20	35
			OS	X	X			13	45	G(2),S,I	NLP	37
DJ		4 m	OD		X		X	13	40	GP		24
			OS					12	25		GMC	20
DI	M	4 m	OD	X	X		X	14	44	G(2)	20/30	16
			OS					11	18			18
DF	M	4 m	OD		X			13	50	GP,S		N
			OS		X			13	50	S		N
MD	F	5 m	OD	X	X		X	13	28	T	10/200	
			OS					11	24		20/15	

TABLE 2 (Cont.)

				Initial Signs and Symptoms						Surgical Procedure*	Final Result	
Patient	Sex	Age of Onset	Eye Examined	Photophobia	Hazy Cornea	Tearing	Enlarged Eye	Corneal Diam.	Tension (mm Hg)		Vision†	Tension (mm Hg)
PR	M	5 m	OD	X	X			12	40	I		23
			OS	X	X			13	40	I,T		47
SB	F	5 m	OD		X		X	13	48	G(2),C,I	20/50	N
			OS					11	30		20/20	N
RP	M	5 m	OD					13	22		GMC	22
			OS		X		X	14	34	G	GMC	16
JC	M	5 m	OD	X		X	X	14	24	GP	GMC	18
			OS	X		X	X	14	35	GP	GC	18
PC	F	5 m	OD					12	42		20/30	33
			OS		X		X	13	52	G(2),I	NLP	soft
PT	M	5 m	OD		X			14	41	G(2)		
			OS		X			12	36	G(2)		
AW	M	5 m	OD					12	28			
			OS				X	13	40	GP		
AM	M	5 m	OD		X		X	14	37	GP	10/200	24
			OS					11	20		20/20	21

*See Footnote to Table 1.
†See Footnote to Table 1.
See J. Pediatr. Ophthalmol., 4:9, 1967.

haze, the gonioscopic appearance of the surgical site, the ophthalmoscopic appearance of the optic nerve head and associated blood vessels, the subsidence of tearing, photophobia, and blepharospasm, visual field examination and visual acuity measurement.

Every eye treated for congenital glaucoma is a potential candidate for amblyopia. As soon as normalization of the pressure and arrest of the condition have been obtained, antiamblyopia treatment should be instituted. This includes patching the good eye, treatment of the anisometropia, and correction of the muscle imbalance when present by appropriate medical and surgical means. This treatment will often restore vision to an eye that might otherwise be lost if the ophthalmologist is content to be satisfied with only the immediate results of surgery.

TABLE 3

INFANTILE GLAUCOMA–
Age: Six Months to Thirty-Six Months

				Initial Signs and Symptoms						Surgical Procedure*	Final Result	
Patient	Sex	Age of Onset	Eye Examined	Photophobia	Hazy Cornea	Tearing	Enlarged Eye	Corneal Diam.	Tension (mm Hg)		Vision†	Tension (mm Hg)
JL	F	6 m	OD				X	13	50	GP	20/30	20
			OS					10	30		20/20	23
TW	M	6 m	OD	X	X	X		12	30	G(2).		20
			OS	X	X	X		12	28	CY		15
ST	M	6 m	OD				X	13	40	GP		
			OS		X		X	13	74	G		
DP	M	6 m	OD	X	X	X	X	15	50	GP	20/50	18
			OS					11	20		20/30	24
MG	F	7 m	OD					10	18		20/20	18
			OS		X			12	30	G,C	20/20	18
NF	F	7 m	OD	X	X	X	X	13	80	G,GP	GMC	22
			OS	X	X	X	X	14	80	G,GP,G(2),I	GMC	36
DJ	M	8 m	OD				X	13	40	GP	NLP	
			OS					12	17		20/50	
TP	F	8 m	OD		X	X	X	13	45	GP		25
			OS					12	25			30
DS	F	8 m	OD		X	X		11	27			23
			OS		X	X		13	45	GP(2),enucleated		
DA	M	9 m	OD	X	X		X	14	40	GP	20/20	18
			OS				X	13	40	GP	20/20	11
SC	M	9 m	OD	X			X	14	30	GP	20/200	30
			OS	X			X	16	50	GP(2)	20/200	18
NFB		11 m	OD				X	13	20			
			OS	X	X	X	X	15	45	GP		10
KH	F	12 m	OD					10	25			
			OS				X	13	35	G(2)		
TS	M	18 m	OD		X		X	13	40	G,GP,G	MC	22
			OS		X		X	13	40	G(2),I	GMC	19
CH	F	30 m	OD		X			13	40	G	GMC	15
			OS		X		X	15	40	G,S	LP	60

*See Footnote to Table 1.
†See Footnote to Table 1.
See J. Pediatr. Ophthalmol., 4:9, 1967.

TABLE 4

JUVENILE GLAUCOMA–
Age: Thirty-Six Months and Over

				Initial Signs and Symptoms						Surgical Procedure*	Final Result	
Patient	Sex	Age of Onset	Eye Examined	Photophobia	Hazy Cornea	Tearing	Enlarged Eye	Corneal Diam.	Tension (mm Hg)		Vision†	Tension (mm Hg)
RB	F	3 yr	OD		X	X		14	45	G(2),GP	20/30	24
			OS					12	20		20/20	20
LB	M	4 yr	OD					13	E	I	20/200	N
			OS					11	N		20/30	N
VBR	F	4 yr	OD		X		X	13	55	I	LP	E
			OS					11	17		GMC	16
DD‡	M	5 yr	OD				X	14	44	I	NLP	Soft
			OS				X	14	40	I	20/80	18
WW	M	9 yr	OD				X	15	30	CY	20/40	35
			OS					13	21		20/20	22

*See Footnote to Table 1.
†See Footnote to Table 1.
‡The right eye was successfully treated with an iridencleisis procedure but became phthesical after being struck with a baseball.
See J. Pediatr. Ophthalmol., 4:9, 1967.

References

Chavez, E., and Galin, M. A. Surgery of congenital glaucoma. Exerpta Medica Found., Amsterdam. 2:1188, 1971.

Costenbader, F. D., and Kwitko, M. L. Congenital glaucoma. Clin. Proc. Child Hosp. (Wash.), 17:100, 1961.

Congenital glaucoma, an analysis of seventy seven consecutive eyes. J. Pediatr. Ophthalmol., 4:9, 1967.

Galin, M. A., Binkhorst, R. D., and Kwitko, M. L. Ocular dehydration. Am. J. Ophthalmol., 66:233, 1968.

Galin, M. A., and Restrepo, N. Influence of diphenylhydantoin on accommodative esotropia. Trans. Int. Strab. Assoc. C. V. Mosby, St. Louis, 1971, p. 201.

Kwitko, M. L. Congenital glaucoma, a clinical study. Can. J. Ophthalmol., 2:91, 1967.

Congenital anterior segment anomalies. Am. J. Ophthalmol., 64:477, 1967.

Congenital glaucoma and anterior chamber cleavage defects. Am. J. Ophthalmol. Otolaryngol. Instruction Course, Chicago, 1967.

Genetic aspects of the anterior chamber cleavage syndrome. Exerpta Medica No. 154. Exerpta Medica Found., Amsterdam, 1967, p. 80.

Anterior segment anomalies; a clinical pathologic report of conditions simulating congenital glaucoma. Can. J. Ophthalmol., 3:120, 1968.

Glaucoma in infants and children. Modern Med. Can., 23:1, 1968.

Glaucoma in infants and children. Am. Acad. Ophthalmol. Otolaryngol. Instruction Course, Chicago, 1968.

Anterior segment anomalies, a clinical embryological study. Trans. VIII Cong. Panam. Oftalmol., 2:273, 1968.

Secondary glaucoma in infancy and childhood. Can. J. Ophthalmol., 4:231, 1969.

Glaucoma in infants and children. Am. Acad. Ophthalmol. Otolaryngol. Instruction Course, Chicago, 1969.

Glaucoma in infants and children. Mod. Med. Australia, 3:11, 1969.

Anterior chamber cleavage syndrome, anterior segment malformations. Progress in Neuro-ophthalmol. and Neuro-genetics, Exerpta Medica Found., Amsterdam, 2:313, 1969 (ICS 176).

Glaucoma in children. Am. Acad. Ophthalmol. Otolaryngol. Instruction Course, Las Vegas, 1970.

Pathogenesis of symptoms in congenital glaucoma. XXI Cong. Ophthalmologicum Pt. II, Mexico, 1970. Exerpta Medica Found., Amsterdam, 1971, p. 1188.

The opaque cornea in childhood. Trans VI Panhellenic Cong. Ophthalmol. Diagnosis and Treatment of Corneal Disease. Corfu, 1972, p. 238.

and Kronenberg, B., and Galin, M. A. The effect of intravenous urea on ocular fluid dynamics. Anali Ottalmol. Clin. Oculist. (Parma), XCIV:1309, 1968.

and Worst, J. G. F., and Galin, M. A. Congenital glaucoma. Am. Acad. Ophthalmol. Otolaryngol. Exhibit, Chicago, 1969.

Worst, J. G. F., and Galin, M. A. Pediatric and adolescent glaucoma. XXI Cong. Ophthalmologicum. Exhibit, Mexico City, 1970.

INDEX

Page numbers in italics refer to figures and tables.